ADVANCE PRAISE FOR PLUM AND POSNER'S DIAGNOSIS AND TREATMENT OF STUPOR AND COMA

"Facing patients with impaired consciousness or coma is among the most urgent and difficult medical emergencies. The 1966 first edition of the 'Diagnosis of Stupor and Coma' by Plum and Posner illuminated medical science with an orderly approach in dealing with the comatose patient. In this fifth edition, Saper and colleagues provide a concise state of the art update of this topic necessary for patient care and is a must read for all health care providers who wish to acquire or hone their knowledge to care for these patients."

—David A. Hafler, MD, William S. and Lois Stiles Edgerly Professor of Neurology and Immunobiology, Chairman, Department of Neurology, Yale School of Medicine, Neurologist-in-Chief, Yale New Haven Hospital, CT

"*Plum and Posner's Diagnosis and Treatment of Stupor and Coma* has long provided the best description of both the pathophysiology and the diagnostic approach to disorders of consciousness. Remarkably, this edition was able to integrate the many new diagnostic and therapeutic tools that have become available while still maintaining the clarity and logic that made the book so useful. Every neurologist should read it!"

—John Kessler, MD, Davee Professor, Davee Department of Neurology, Northwestern University, Chicago, IL

"This new 5th Edition of the seminal Plum and Posner's 'Stupor and Coma' contributed by a brilliant, and partly renewed, band associating Posner, Saper, Schiff, and Claassen is not a 'USA dormant cop' (anagram of the title), but a worldwide must-read for all those interested by the neurology, physiology and anatomy of consciousness, and by its disorders. Keeping with the very insightful and hitherto unseen tone of the 1972 first edition, this new opus covers almost exhaustively the rich and fast-growing relevant literature, and it can be read at different levels of expertise ranging from fresh college students to emeritus professors, including active neurologists, intensivists, and medical practitioners."

—Prof. Lionel Naccache, Sorbonne University, Pitié-Salpêtrière Hospital, Paris, France

"As both the authoritative text on the subject, and compulsory reading for all neurologists, neurosurgeons, intensivists and ER physicians, the 5th edition of *Plum and Posner's Diagnosis and Treatment of Stupor and Coma* is as indelible a contribution as its four prior editions. Continuing in the tradition of the first edition's 1966 grounding in brain structure-function relationships as they apply to disorders of consciousness, this edition is a welcome update to 2007's 4th edition capturing important advances in knowledge in the field. It is a comprehensive, yet succinct, well referenced, scholarly summary of our present day understanding of the molecular basis of consciousness as much as it is a practical clinician's guide to evaluation, treatment, and prognosis. A triumph—indeed! A wonderful and necessary addition to the bookshelf of a wide audience whose interests include the brain's role in modulating normal and disturbed states of consciousness."

—David B. Rye, MD, PhD, Professor of Neurology, Emory University School of Medicine, Atlanta, GA

"This new edition provides a comprehensive update of a classic and essential text. It preserves the best elements of the original—the succinct formulation of the pathophysiology of coma, the approach to examining a comatose patient—but brings the book solidly into the 21st Century with inclusion of modern technologies and methods. The expanded discussion of the treatment of comatose patients is most welcome, delivering a wealth of information in a concise format. This remains a remarkable book: at once both comprehensive and accessible, equally suitable for extended study and as a quick bedside reference. It deserves a place in the library of every practicing neurologist."

—David G. Standaert, MD, PhD, John N. Whitaker Professor and Chair, Department of Neurology, The University of Alabama at Birmingham, AL

Contemporary Neurology Series

PLUM AND POSNER'S DIAGNOSIS AND TREATMENT OF STUPOR AND COMA

Fifth Edition

Jerome B. Posner
George C. Cotzias Chair of Neuro-oncology Emeritus
Evelyn Few American Cancer Society Clinical Research Professor Emeritus
Memorial-Sloan Kettering Cancer Center
Weill Cornell Medical College
New York, NY

Clifford B. Saper
James Jackson Putnam Professor of Neurology and Neuroscience
Chairman, Department of Neurology
Beth Israel Deaconess Medical Center
Harvard Medical School
Boston, MA

Nicholas D. Schiff
Jerold B. Katz Professor of Neurology and Neuroscience
Brain Mind Research Institute
Weill Cornell Medical College
New York, NY

Jan Claassen
Associate Professor of Neurology
Department of Neurology
New York Presbyterian Hospital
Columbia University School of Medicine
New York, NY

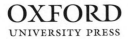
OXFORD
UNIVERSITY PRESS

OXFORD
UNIVERSITY PRESS

Oxford University Press is a department of the University of Oxford. It furthers
the University's objective of excellence in research, scholarship, and education
by publishing worldwide. Oxford is a registered trade mark of Oxford University
Press in the UK and certain other countries.

Published in the United States of America by Oxford University Press
198 Madison Avenue, New York, NY 10016, United States of America.

Library of Congress Cataloging-in-Publication Data
Names: Posner, Jerome B., 1932– editor. | Saper, C. B. (Clifford B.), editor. |
Schiff, Nicholas D., editor. | Claassen, Jan, editor.
Title: Plum and Posner's diagnosis and treatment of stupor and coma /
edited by Jerome B. Posner, Clifford B. Saper, Nicholas D. Schiff, and Jan Claassen.
Other titles: Diagnosis and treatment of stupor and coma |
Contemporary neurology series ; 94. 0069-9446
Description: Fifth edition. | Oxford ; New York : Oxford University Press, [2019] |
Series: Contemporary neurology series ; #94 |
Includes bibliographical references and index.
Identifiers: LCCN 2019006311 | ISBN 9780190208875 (hardback : alk. paper) |
ISBN 9780190208882 (updf) | ISBN 9780190208899 (epub) | ISBN 9780190208905 (on-line)
Subjects: | MESH: Coma—diagnosis | Stupor—diagnosis |
Brain Diseases—diagnosis | Brain Injuries—diagnosis
Classification: LCC RB150.C6 | NLM WB 182 | DDC 616.8/49—dc23
LC record available at https://lccn.loc.gov/2019006311

9 8 7 6 5 4 3 2 1

Printed by Sheridan Books, Inc., United States of America

Contents

Preface to the Fifth Edition

The first three editions of *The Diagnosis of Stupor and Coma* were prepared by Fred Plum and Jerry Posner, based on their experiences in diagnosis of patients with disorders of consciousness, first at King County Hospital in Seattle, and then at New York Hospital. During those three editions, medicine in general and neurology in particular underwent a revolution with the introduction of computerized tomography. Nevertheless, the principles of applying the clinical neurological exam to the comatose patient for the purpose of rapid diagnosis and treatment did not change.

The fourth edition of this book was published in 2007, and it incorporated the many advances made in the previous two decades, including the use of magnetic resonance imaging in the diagnosis of comatose patients. The need for the neurological examination to determine the best course for workup of the comatose patient, however, remained paramount. Drs. Clifford Saper and Nicholas Schiff, two former residents of Drs. Plum and Posner, were added to update the basic science of consciousness and the outcomes of patients with disorders of consciousness. Although Fred Plum could not participate in the final text of the fourth edition, we tried to the greatest extent possible to preserve his approach and his voice in the text. Out of respect for the original authors and to recognize their indelible contribution to the concept and structure of the text, Drs. Plum and Posner's names were formally added to the title of the book: *Plum and Posner's Diagnosis and Treatment of Stupor and Coma*.

With this fifth edition, both the book and the field have evolved further. Dr. Plum has passed on, and Dr. Posner participated in overseeing but not writing the revision. We have added Dr. Jan Claassen, Director of the Neurological Intensive Care Unit at Columbia University, as an additional author. His expertise has greatly expanded our section on the treatment of comatose patients so that we have again changed the title to reflect that refocusing of the book to *Plum and Posner's Diagnosis and Treatment of Stupor and Coma*. We once again had the honor to have a final chapter contributed by Dr. Joseph J. Fins on the ethical, legal and policy considerations of managing patients with disorders of consciousness. This chapter has been greatly updated and expanded from the portion of a chapter that he prepared for the fourth edition.

The primary text of Chapters 1–4 and 6 were prepared by Dr. Saper, that of Chapter 5 by Drs. Saper and Claassen, Chapters 7 and 8 by Dr. Claassen, Chapters 9 and 10 by Dr. Schiff, and Chapter 11 by Dr. Fins. However, all chapters were read and edited by Drs. Saper, Claassen, and Schiff who now bear the responsibility for the text and for any errors it may contain.

We owe a great debt of gratitude to Dr. Eva Feldman, who has taken over editing the Contemporary Neurology Series and who worked with the authors to keep us on time. However, it was the tireless work of Craig Panner and Emily Samulski at Oxford University Press who drew together the disparate schedules of the authors, herded us through the preparation of the chapters, and now provide the final oversight of the editing and production of the book.

Finally, we would like to thank our families for putting up with our extended reveries and writing time in order to finish this volume. A work like this always takes more time than anyone can expect, but it once again has been a labor of love. We have learned a great deal from preparing it, and we hope you will find it equally informative and thought-provoking as a companion to the management of patients with disorders of consciousness.

Jerome B. Posner, MD
Jan Claassen, MD, PhD
Clifford B. Saper, MD, PhD
Nicholas D. Schiff, MD
November 29, 2018

Chapter 1

Pathophysiology of Signs and Symptoms of Coma

ALTERED STATES OF CONSCIOUSNESS

And men should know that from nothing else but
from the brain come joys, delights, laughter and jests,
and sorrows, griefs, despondency and lamentations.
And by this, in an especial manner, we acquire
wisdom and knowledge, and see and hear and know
what are foul, and what are fair, what sweet and what
unsavory . . .

—The Hippocratic Writings

Impaired consciousness is among the most difficult and dramatic of clinical problems. The an-
cient Greeks knew that normal consciousness
depends on an intact brain and that impaired

consciousness signifies brain failure. The brain
tolerates only limited physical or metabolic injury, so that impaired consciousness is often a
sign of impending irreparable damage to the
brain. Stupor and coma imply advanced brain
failure just as, for example, uremia means renal
failure, and the longer such brain failure lasts,
the narrower the margin between recovery and
the development of permanent neurologic injury. The limited time for action and the mul-
tiplicity of potential causes of brain failure
challenge the physician and frighten both
the physician and the family; only the patient
escapes anxiety.

Many conditions cause coma. Table 1.1 lists
some of the common and often perplexing

1

Table 1.1 Cause of Stupor or Coma in 500 Patients Initially Diagnosed as "Coma of Unknown Etiology"[a]

	Subtotals
I. Supratentorial lesions	101
A. Rhinencephalic and subcortical destructive lesions	2
1. Thalamic infarcts	2
B. Supratentorial mass lesions	99
1. Hemorrhage	76
a. Intracerebral	44
(1) Hypertensive	36
(2) Vascular anomaly	5
(3) Other	3
b. Epidural	4
c. Subdural	26
d. Pituitary apoplexy	2
2. Infarction	9
a. Arterial occlusions	7
(1)Thrombotic	5
(2)Embolic	2
b. Venous occlusions	2
3. Tumors	7
a. Primary	2
b. Metastatic	5
4. Abscess	6
a. Intracerebral	5
b. Subdural	1
5. Closed head injury	1
II. Subtentorial lesions	65
A. Compressive lesions	12
1. Cerebellar hemorrhage	5
2. Posterior fossa subdural or extradural hemorrhage	1
3. Cerebellar infarct	2
4. Cerebellar tumor	3
5. Cerebellar abscess	1
6. Basilar aneurysm	0
B. Destructive or ischemic lesions	53
1. Pontine hemorrhage	11
2. Brainstem infarct	40
3. Basilar migraine	1
4. Brainstem demyelination	1
III. Diffuse and/or metabolic brain dysfunction	326
A. Diffuse intrinsic disorders of brain	38
1. "Encephalitis" or encephalomyelitis	14
2. Subarachnoid hemorrhage	13
3. Concussion, nonconvulsive seizures, and postictal states	9
4. Primary neuronal disorders	2
B. Extrinsic and metabolic disorders	288
1. Anoxia or ischemia	10
2. Hypoglycemia	16
3. Nutritional	1
4. Hepatic encephalopathy	17
5. Uremia and dialysis	8
6. Pulmonary disease	3
7. Endocrine disorders (including diabetes)	12
8. Remote effects of cancer	0
9. Drug intoxication	149

Table 1.1 **Cause of Stupor or Coma in 500 Patients Initially Diagnosed as "Coma of Unknown Etiology"ᵃ (cont.)**

	Subtotals
10. Ionic and acid-base disorders	12
11. Temperature regulation	9
12. Mixed or nonspecific metabolic coma	1
IV. Psychiatric "coma"	8
A. Conversion reactions	4
B. Depression	2
C. Catatonic stupor	2

ᵃRepresents only patients for whom a neurologist was consulted because the initial diagnosis was uncertain and in whom a final diagnosis was established. Thus, obvious diagnoses such as known poisonings, meningitis, and closed head injuries and cases of mixed metabolic encephalopathies in which a specific etiologic diagnosis was never established are underrepresented.

causes of unconsciousness that the physician may encounter in the emergency department or intensive care unit of a general hospital. The purpose of this monograph is to describe a systematic approach to the diagnosis of the patient with reduced consciousness, stupor, or coma based on anatomic and physiologic principles. Accordingly, this book divides the causes of unconsciousness into two major categories: structural and metabolic. This chapter provides background information on the pathophysiology of impaired consciousness, as well as on the signs and symptoms that accompany it. In Chapter 2, this information is used to define a brief but informative neurologic examination that is necessary to determine if the reduced consciousness has a structural cause (and therefore may require immediate imaging and perhaps surgical treatment) or a metabolic cause (in which case the diagnostic approach can be more lengthy and extensive). Chapters 3 and 4 discuss pathophysiology and specific causes of structural injury to the brain that result in defects of consciousness. Chapter 5 examines the broad range of metabolic causes of unconsciousness and the specific treatments they require. Chapter 6 explores psychiatric causes of unresponsiveness, which must be differentiated from organic causes of stupor and coma. Chapters 7 and 8 provide a systematic discussion of the treatment of both structural and nonstructural coma. Chapter 9 reviews the determination of brain death and the examination necessary for making that diagnosis. Chapter 10 explores the outcomes of coma of different causes, including the prognosis for useful recovery and the states of long-term

impairment of consciousness. Chapter 11 reviews some ethical problems encountered in treating unconscious individuals.

DEFINITIONS

Consciousness

Consciousness is the state of full awareness of the self and one's relationship to the environment. Clinically, the level of consciousness of a patient is defined operationally at the bedside by the responses of the patient to the examiner. It is clear from this definition that it is possible for a patient to be conscious yet not responsive to the examiner, for example, if the patient lacks sensory inputs, is paralyzed (see *locked-in syndrome*, page 6), or for psychologic reasons decides not to respond. Thus, the determination of the state of consciousness can be a technically challenging exercise. In the definitions that follow, we assume that the patient is not unresponsive due to sensory or motor impairment or psychiatric disease.

Consciousness has two major dimensions: content and arousal. The *content* of consciousness represents the sum of all functions mediated at a cerebral cortical level, including both cognitive and affective responses. These functions are subserved by unique networks of cortical neurons, and it is possible for a lesion that is strategically placed to disrupt one of the networks, causing a *fractional loss of consciousness*.[1] Such patients may have preserved awareness of most stimuli, but, having suffered the loss of a critical population of neurons (e.g., for recognizing language symbol content, differences between colors or faces, or the presence of the left side of space), the patient literally becomes unconscious of that class of stimuli. Patients with these deficits are often characterized as "confused" by inexperienced examiners because they do not respond as expected to behavioral stimuli. More experienced clinicians recognize the focal cognitive deficits and that the alteration of consciousness is confined to one class of stimuli. Occasionally, patients with right parietotemporal lesions may be sufficiently inattentive as to appear to be globally confused, but they are not sleepy and, in fact, are usually agitated.[2]

Thus, unless the damage to cortical networks is diffuse or very widespread, the level of consciousness is not reduced. For example, patients with advanced Alzheimer's disease may lose memory and other cognitive functions but remain awake and alert until the damage is so extensive and severe that response to stimuli is reduced as well (see *vegetative state,* page 7). Hence, a reduced *level of consciousness* is not due to focal impairments of cognitive function, but rather to a global reduction in the level of behavioral responsiveness. In addition to being caused by widespread cortical impairment, a reduced level of consciousness can result from injury to a specific set of brainstem and diencephalic pathways that regulate the overall *level* of cortical function and hence consciousness.

Of course, the content and level of consciousness interact. The arousal system receives extensive inputs from medial prefrontal cognitive areas, which can drive arousal even under adverse conditions if the behavioral situation demands it (e.g., a doctor who is taking care of a very sick patient in the emergency department late at night).[3,4] Conversely, a very sleepy patient may not be able to participate meaningfully in cognitive testing.

Sleep is a recurrent, physiologic form of reduced consciousness in which the responsiveness of brain systems responsible for cognitive function is globally reduced so that the brain does not respond readily to environmental stimuli. Pathologic alteration of the relationships between the brain systems that are responsible for wakefulness and sleep can impair consciousness. The systems subserving normal sleep and wakefulness are reviewed later in this chapter. A key difference between

sleep and coma is that sleep is intrinsically reversible: sufficient stimulation will return the individual to a normal waking state. In contrast, if patients with pathologic alterations of consciousness can be awakened at all, they rapidly fall back into a sleep-like state when stimulation ceases.

Patients who have a sleep-like appearance and remain behaviorally unresponsive to all external stimuli are unconscious clinically. However, continuous sleep-like coma as a result of brain injury rarely lasts more than 2–4 weeks. Like the emergence of spasticity from the initial flaccid state after spinal cord transection (spinal shock), the "forebrain shock" due to damage to the intrinsic arousal systems gives way to reorganization of that circuitry, and there is gradual emergence of wake–sleep cycles over a period of weeks after the injury. But, like spinal spasticity, which supplies tone but not complex functions, those wake–sleep cycles may be useless for performing daily tasks if there is extensive damage also to cognitive networks. Wakefulness in the absence of such content is called a *vegetative state* or *unresponsive wakefulness syndrome* (UWS). Recent studies using functional imaging have found that some UWS patients may retain contextually relevant cortical activation yet lack an external response (see Chapter 9). However, similar studies have not been done in acutely comatose patients.

Acutely Altered States of Consciousness

The terms used to describe altered states of consciousness break down into two groups: those that indicate depressed level of consciousness and those that describe a mixture of drowsiness with hyperexcitability. Within these categories, there are relatively mild states and those with more profound behavioral disruption (see Table 1.2).

Clouding of consciousness, for example, is a term applied to minimally reduced wakefulness or awareness, which may include hyperexcitability and irritability alternating with drowsiness. A key distinction must be made in such patients between those who are confused (i.e., do not respond appropriately to their environment) because of a focal deficit

Table 1.2 **Terms Used to Describe Disorders of Consciousness**

Acute	Subacute or chronic
Clouding	Dementia
Delirium	Hypersomnia
Obtundation	Abulia
Stupor	Akinetic mutism
Coma	Minimally conscious state
Locked-in (must be distinguished from coma)	Vegetative or unresponsive wake state
	Brain death

of cognitive function versus those who have more global impairment. The beclouded patient is usually incompletely oriented to time and sometimes to place. Such patients are inattentive and perform poorly on repeating numbers backward (the normal range is at least four or five) and remembering details or even the meaning of stories. Drowsiness is often prominent during the day, but agitation may predominate at night.

The pathophysiology of brain function in such patients has rarely been studied, but there is evidence that the clouding of consciousness is associated with reduced cerebral blood flow and oxygen consumption in a wide range of pathologies, from hepatic encephalopathy to Wernicke's encephalopathy.[5,6] The pathogenesis of clouding of consciousness and delirium is discussed in more detail in Chapter 5.

Delirium, from the Latin "to go out of the furrow," is a more floridly abnormal mental state characterized by misperception of sensory stimuli and, often, vivid hallucinations. Delirium is defined by the *Diagnostic and Statistical Manual of Mental Disorders,* 5th edition (DSM-5)[7] as follows: "A. Disturbance of attention (i.e., reduced ability to direct, focus, sustain, and shift attention) and awareness (reduced orientation to the environment). B. The disturbance develops over a short period of time (usually hours to a few days), representing an acute change from baseline attention and awareness, and tends to fluctuate in severity during the course of the day. C. An additional disturbance in cognition (e.g., deficit in memory, orientation, language, visuospatial ability, or perception). D. The condition is not better explained by a pre-existing, established, or evolving neurocognitive disorder. E. The condition is a direct physiological consequence of another medical condition."

Delirious patients are disoriented, first to time, next to place, and then to persons in their environment. Rarely are patients unaware of who they are, although sometimes married women will revert to their maiden name. Patients are often fearful or irritable and may overreact or misinterpret the normal activities of physicians and nurses. Delusions or hallucinations may place the patient completely out of contact with the environment and the examiner. Full-blown delirious states tend to come on rapidly and rarely last more than 4–7 days. However, fragments of misperceptions may persist for several weeks, especially among alcoholics and patients with cerebral involvement from collagen vascular diseases.

Delirium is often seen in hospitalized patients, particularly the elderly. The occurrence of delirium in an elderly patient is both a risk factor for developing dementia and often a turning point, one at which the decline in cognitive function accelerates.[8] In recent years, there has been a tendency to equate delirium with acute confusional states, and the most common way of assessing delirium has been the Confusion Assessment Method (CAM).[9,10] The CAM and other methods of assessing delirium rely predominantly on testing attention, which is largely a right parietal lobe function. However, neurologists also see many patients with right parietal lobe lesions who are inattentive and confused but not delirious. Delirium also includes an element of sensory misperception that suggests a more widespread degradation of cortical sensory processing. In fact, most delirious patients are suffering from a toxic-metabolic state, such as an anticholinergic or sedative drug, hepatic or renal failure, or a systemic infection (see Chapter 5). One of the few exceptions to this rule is the rare group of patients with focal lesions of the right parieto-occipitotemporal cortex.[2,11] Lesions in this area can produce a florid state of multimodal sensory hallucination that transcends the confusional states seen in patients with purely right parietal attentional disorders.

Obtundation, by contrast, denotes a relatively mild state of reduced arousal. From the Latin "to beat against or blunt," it literally means mental blunting or torpidity. In a medical setting, such patients have a mild to moderate reduction in alertness accompanied by a lesser interest in the environment. Obtunded patients have slower psychologic responses to stimulation. They may have an increased number of hours of sleep and may be drowsy between sleep bouts, but they still are responsive and can maintain a waking state.

Stupor, from the Latin "to be stunned," is a condition of deep sleep or similar behavioral unresponsiveness from which the subject can be aroused only with vigorous and continuous stimulation. Even when maximally aroused, the level of cognitive function may be impaired. Such patients can be differentiated from those with psychiatric impairment, such as catatonia or severe depression, because they can be aroused by vigorous stimulation to respond to simple stimuli.

Coma, from the Greek "deep sleep or trance," is a state of unresponsiveness in which the patient lies with eyes closed and cannot be aroused to respond appropriately to stimuli even with vigorous stimulation. The patient may grimace in response to painful stimuli and limbs may demonstrate stereotyped withdrawal responses, but the patient does not make localizing responses or discrete defensive movements. As coma deepens, the responsiveness of the patient, even to painful stimuli, may diminish or disappear. However, it is difficult to equate the lack of motor responses to the depth of the coma because the neural structures that regulate motor responses differ from those that regulate consciousness, and they may be differentially impaired by specific brain disorders.

The locked-in syndrome describes a state in which the patient is de-efferented, resulting in paralysis of all four limbs and the lower cranial nerves. This condition has been recognized at least as far back as the nineteenth century, but its distinctive name was applied in the first edition of this monograph (1966), reflecting the implications of this condition for the diagnosis of coma and for the specialized care such patients require. Although not unconscious, locked-in patients are unable to respond to most stimuli. A high level of clinical suspicion is required on the part of the examiner to distinguish a locked-in patient from one who is comatose. The most common cause is a lesion of the base and tegmentum of the midpons that interrupts descending cortical control of motor functions. Such patients usually retain control of vertical eye movements and eyelid opening, which can be used to verify their responsiveness. They may be taught to respond to the examiner by using eye blinks as a code. Rare patients with subacute motor neuropathy, such as Guillain-Barré syndrome, also may become completely de-efferented, but there is a history of progressive, subacute paralysis. In both instances, electroencephalographic (EEG) examination discloses a reactive posterior alpha rhythm[12] (see EEG section, page 87).

It is important to identify locked-in patients so that they may be treated appropriately by the medical and nursing staff. At the bedside, discussion should be *with* the patient, not, as with an unconscious individual, *about* the patient. Patients with lower pontine lesions that cause a locked-in state often are awake most of the time, with greatly diminished sleep on physiologic recordings.[13] They may suffer greatly if they are treated by hospital staff as if they are nonresponsive. For this reason, and because some patients even with extensive brain injury may retain some cognitive ability on functional MRI (fMRI) scanning (see Chapter 9), many clinicians treat all patients in an unresponsive state as if they could potentially be sentient but unable to respond.

As the preceding definitions imply, each of these conditions includes a fairly wide range of behavioral responsiveness, and there may be some overlap among them. Therefore, it is generally best to describe a patient by indicating what stimuli do or do not result in responses and the kinds of responses that are seen, rather than using less precise terms.

Subacute or Chronic Alterations of Consciousness

Dementia defines an enduring and often progressive decline in mental processes owing to an organic disorder not usually accompanied by a reduction in arousal. Conventionally, the term implies a diffuse or disseminated reduction in cognitive functions rather than the impairment of a single cognitive modality such as language. DSM-5 avoids the term "dementia," which it considered to be stigmatizing, and instead divides such individuals into minor and major neurocognitive disorders. Both involve chronic and usually progressive decline in cognitive function in one or more domains, with the difference being that the declines in minor neurocognitive disorder do not interfere with independent living and are typically within 1 or 2 standard deviations of normal (a range that neurologists and gerontologists usually call *minor cognitive impairment* or MCI), whereas the major neurocognitive disorder does interfere with independent living and typically includes deficits of 2 or more standard deviations below the norm. This definition is difficult to apply to individuals whose function begins several standard deviations above the norm, and who thus may have substantial decline without meeting the definition.

The term "dementia" as applied by neurologists refers to the effects of primary disorders of the cerebral hemispheres, such as degenerative conditions, traumatic injuries, and neoplasms. Occasionally, dementia can be at least partially reversible, such as when it accompanies thyroid or vitamin B_{12} deficiency or results from a reversible communicating hydrocephalus[14]; more often, however, the term applies to chronic conditions carrying limited hopes for improvement.

Patients with dementia are usually awake and alert but, as the dementia worsens, may become less responsive and eventually evolve into a vegetative state (see later discussion). Patients with dementia are at significantly increased risk of developing delirium when they become medically ill or develop comorbid brain disease.[15]

Hypersomnia refers to a state characterized by excessive but normal-appearing sleep from which the subject readily, even if briefly, awakens when stimulated. Many patients with either acute or chronic alterations of consciousness sleep excessively. However, when awakened, consciousness is clearly clouded. In the truly hypersomniac patient, sleep appears normal and cognitive functions are normal when patients are awakened. Hypersomnia due to a brain injury typically results from posterior

hypothalamic or midbrain dysfunction, as indicated later in this chapter.[16,17]

Abulia (from the Greek for "lack of will") is an apathetic state in which the patient responds slowly if at all to verbal stimuli and generally does not initiate conversation or activity. When sufficiently stimulated, however, cognitive functions may be normal. Unlike hypersomnia, the patient usually appears fully awake. Abulia is usually associated with bilateral frontal lobe disease and, when severe, may evolve into akinetic mutism.

Akinetic mutism describes a condition of silent, alert-appearing immobility that characterizes certain subacute or chronic states of altered consciousness in which sleep–wake cycles have returned, but externally obtainable evidence for mental activity remains almost entirely absent and spontaneous motor activity is lacking. Such patients generally have lesions including the hypothalamus and adjacent basal ganglia.

The term *minimally conscious state* (MCS) was developed by the Aspen Workgroup, a consortium of neurologists, neurosurgeons, neuropsychologists, and rehabilitation specialists.[18] MCS identifies a condition of severely impaired consciousness in which minimal but definite behavioral evidence of self or environmental awareness is demonstrated. Like the vegetative state, MCS often exists as a transitional state arising during recovery from coma or worsening of progressive neurologic disease. In some patients, however, it may be an essentially permanent condition. Preserved pockets of cognitive function seen on fMRI scans in some MCS patients have prompted the suggestion to rename MCS "cortically mediated state."[19] However, because virtually all states of consciousness are mediated by the cerebral cortex, we prefer the term MCS for this distinct group of patient. For a detailed discussion of the clinical criteria for the diagnosis of the MCS, see Chapter 9.

The *vegetative state* (VS; now often called the *unresponsive wakefulness syndrome*,[20] UWS) denotes the recovery of crude cycling of arousal states heralded by the appearance of "eyes-open" periods in an unresponsive patient. Very few surviving patients with severe forebrain damage remain in eyes-closed coma for more than 2–4 weeks. In most patients, vegetative behavior usually replaces coma by that time. Patients in the vegetative state, like comatose patients, show no evidence of awareness of self or their environment. Unlike brain death, in which the cerebral hemispheres and the brainstem both undergo overwhelming functional impairment, patients in vegetative states retain brainstem regulation of cardiopulmonary function and visceral autonomic regulation. Although the original term *persistent vegetative state* (PVS) was not associated with a specific timeframe, the use of PVS is now commonly reserved for patients remaining in a vegetative state for at least 30 days. The American Neurological Association advises that PVS be applied only to patients in the state for 1 month, although some patients recover from PVS even after that interval.[21] On the other hand, most patients who have recovered consciousness after months or years have been in a MCS, not PVS or UWS (see Chapter 9). Other terms in the older literature designating the vegetative state include *coma vigil* and the *apallic state*.

Brain death is defined as the irreversible loss of all functions of the entire brain.[22] Although vigorous supportive care may keep the body processes going for some time, particularly in an otherwise healthy young person, the complete loss of brain function (including loss of hypothalamic homeostatic control) eventually results in failure of the systemic circulation within a few days or, rarely, after several weeks. It is clear that the brain has been dead for some time prior to the cessation of the heartbeat in such cases because the brain is usually autolyzed (respirator brain) when examined postmortem.[23] Current criteria for demonstrating brain death have been criticized, however, because they depend primarily on the absence of purposive behavior as well as brainstem reflexes.[24,25] However, in cases of purely brainstem injury, damage to the ascending arousal system (see later discussion) will cause loss of wakefulness in the forebrain. As a result, the usual US criteria for brain death are not greatly different from those developed by physicians in the United Kingdom for *brainstem death*,[26] defined as "irreversible loss of the capacity for consciousness, combined with irreversible loss of the capacity to breathe." It should be apparent that these criteria may include patients with survival of appreciable forebrain tissue, and some of those patients have a prolonged survival or may even recover consciousness. This disparity has caused some critics to suggest that the declaration of brain death should depend on the absence of blood flow to the brain, rather than physical examination.[27] These concepts are discussed in greater detail in Chapters 9 and 10.

Acute alterations of consciousness are discussed in Chapters 2 through 5. Subacute and chronic alterations of consciousness are discussed in Chapter 9.

APPROACH TO THE DIAGNOSIS OF THE COMATOSE PATIENT

Determining the cause of an acutely depressed level of consciousness is a difficult clinical challenge. The clinician must determine rapidly whether the cause of the impairment is structural or metabolic and what treatments must be instituted to save the life of the patient. In this era of readily available computed tomographic (CT) and MRI scans, this may seem like a trivial distinction to make. However, a brief examination by a skillful clinician will reveal those patients for whom even a short delay in treatment would be life-threatening and immediate intervention will be life-saving. In addition, some structural causes of coma (e.g., acute brainstem or global ischemia) may be difficult to detect on CT scan, or findings on scanning may be misleading. The clinician must be able to differentiate structural and metabolic causes of coma on the initial exam, as these require quite different responses.

If the cause of coma is structural, it generally is due to a focal injury along the course of the neural pathways that generate and maintain a normal waking brain. *Therefore, the clinical diagnosis of structural coma depends on the recognition of the signs of injury to structures that accompany the arousal pathways through the brain.* Structural processes that impair the function of the arousal system fall into two categories: (1) supratentorial mass lesions, which may compress deep diencephalic structures and hence impair the function of both hemispheres, and (2) infratentorial mass or destructive lesions, which directly damage the arousal system at its source in the upper brainstem. The remainder of this chapter will systematically examine the major arousal systems in the brain and the physiology and pathophysiology of consciousness. Chapter 2 addresses examination of the patient with a disturbance of consciousness, particularly those components of the examination that assay the function of the arousal systems and the major sensory, motor, and autonomic systems that accompany them. Once the examination is completed, the examiner should be able to determine whether the source of the impairment of consciousness is caused by a focal structural lesion (Chapters 3 and 4) or a diffuse and therefore presumably metabolic process (Chapter 5) and should be able to choose the best course for further investigation and treatment (Chapters 7 and 8).

Although it is important to question family members or attendants who may have details of the history, including emergency medical personnel who bring the patient into the emergency department, the history for comatose patients is often scant or absent. The neurologic examination of a patient with impaired consciousness, fortunately, is brief because the patient cannot participate in detailed cognitive or sensory testing or provide voluntary motor responses. The key components of the examination, which can be completed by a skilled physician in just a few minutes, include (1) the level of consciousness of the patient, (2) the pattern of breathing, (3) the size and reactivity of the pupils, (4) the eye movements and oculovestibular responses, and (5) the skeletal motor responses. From this information, the examiner must be able to reconstruct the type of lesion and move swiftly to life-saving measures. Before reviewing the components of the coma examination in detail, however, it is necessary to understand the basic pathways in the brain that sustain wakeful, conscious behavior. Only from this perspective is it possible to understand how the components of the coma examination test pathways that are intertwined with those that maintain consciousness.

PHYSIOLOGY AND PATHOPHYSIOLOGY OF CONSCIOUSNESS AND COMA

The Ascending Arousal System

In the late nineteenth century, the great British neurologist John Hughlings-Jackson proposed that consciousness in humans was the sum total of the activity in their cerebral hemispheres.[28]

A corollary was that consciousness could only be eliminated by lesions that simultaneously damaged both cerebral hemispheres. However, several clinical observations challenged this view. As early as 1890, Mauthner reported that stupor in patients with Wernicke's encephalopathy was associated with lesions involving the gray matter surrounding the cerebral aqueduct and the caudal part of the third ventricle.[29] The nascent field of neurosurgery also began to contribute cases in which loss of consciousness was associated with lesions confined to the upper brainstem or caudal diencephalon. However, the most convincing body of evidence was assembled by Baron Constantin von Economo,[30] a Viennese neurologist who recorded his observations during an epidemic of a unique disorder, *encephalitis lethargica*, that occurred in the years surrounding World War I. Most victims of encephalitis lethargica were very sleepy, spending 20 or more hours per day asleep and awakening only briefly to eat. When awakened, they could interact in a relatively unimpaired fashion with the examiner, but soon fell asleep if not continuously stimulated. Many of these patients suffered from oculomotor abnormalities, and, when they died, they were found to have lesions involving the paramedian reticular formation of the midbrain at the junction with the diencephalon. Other patients during the same epidemic developed prolonged wakefulness, sleeping at most a few hours per day. Movement disorders were also common in this latter group. Von Economo identified the causative lesion in the gray matter surrounding the anterior part of the third ventricle in the hypothalamus and extending laterally into the basal ganglia at that level.

Von Economo suggested that there was specific brainstem circuitry that causes arousal or wakefulness of the forebrain and that the hypothalamus contains circuitry for inhibiting this system to induce sleep. However, it was difficult to test these deductions because naturally occurring lesions in patients (or experimental lesions in animals) that damaged the brainstem almost invariably destroyed important sensory and motor pathways that complicated the interpretation of the results. As long as the only tool for assessing activity of the cerebral hemispheres remained the clinical examination, this problem could not be resolved (see Box 1.1).

Box 1.1 Constantin von Economo and the Discovery of Intrinsic Wake and Sleep Systems in the Brain

Baron Constantin von Economo von San Serff was born in 1876, the son of Greek parents. He was brought up in Austrian Trieste, studied medicine in Vienna, and, in 1906, took a post in the Psychiatric Clinic under Professor Julius Wagner-Jauregg. In 1916, during World War I, he began seeing cases of a new and previously unrecorded type of encephalitis and published his first report of this illness in 1917. Although subsequent accounts have often confused this illness with the epidemic of influenza that swept through Europe and then the rest of the world during World War I, von Economo was quite clear that encephalitis lethargica was not associated with respiratory symptoms and that its appearance preceded the onset of the latter epidemic. Von Economo continued to write and lecture about this experience for the remainder of his life, until his premature death in 1931 from heart disease.

Based on his clinical observations, von Economo proposed a dual-center theory for regulation of sleep and wakefulness: a waking influence arising from the upper brainstem and passing through the gray matter surrounding the cerebral aqueduct and the posterior third ventricle, and a rostral hypothalamic sleep-promoting area. These observations became the basis for lesion studies done by Ranson in 1939,[31] by Nauta in 1946,[32] and by Swett and Hobson in 1968,[33] in which they showed that the posterior lateral hypothalamic lesions in monkeys, rats, and cats could reproduce the prolonged sleepiness that von Economo had observed. The rostral hypothalamic sleep-promoting area was confirmed experimentally by lesions causing insomnia in rats by Nauta in 1946[32] and in cats by McGinty and Sterman in the 1960s.[34]

Interestingly, von Economo also identified a third clinical syndrome, which appeared some months after the acute encephalitis in some patients who had posterior hypothalamic lesions, as they were beginning to recover. These individuals would develop episodes of sleep attacks during which they had an overwhelming need to sleep. He noted that they also had attacks of cataplexy in which they lost all muscle tone, often when excited emotionally. Von Economo noted accurately that these symptoms were similar to the rare condition previously identified by Westphal[35] and Gelinau[36] as narcolepsy. S. A. Kinnier Wilson described a cohort of similar patients in London in 1928.[37] He also noted that they had developed symptoms of narcolepsy after recovering from encephalitis lethargica with posterior hypothalamic lesions. This work was the first to identify symptomatic narcolepsy with lesions of the region including the orexin (or hypocretin) neurons in the posterior lateral hypothalamus. Wilson even described examining a patient in his office, with the young house officer McDonald Critchley, and that the patient indeed had atonic paralysis with loss of tendon reflexes and an extensor plantar response during the attack, indicating that cataplexy is related to rapid eye movement (REM) sleep atonia which directly hyperpolarizes α-motor neurons, not due to paralysis of the descending pyramidal motor system.

Von Economo's theory was highly influential during this period, and a great deal of what was subsequently learned about the organization of brain systems controlling sleep and wakefulness owes its origins to his careful clinicopathologic observations and his imaginative and far-reaching vision about brain organization.

Box 1.1 Constantin von Economo and the Discovery of Intrinsic Wake and Sleep Systems in the Brain (cont.)

(A) Sleep as a Problem of Localization*

Baron

Constantin von Economo

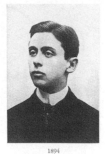

1894

* Read before the College of Physicians and Surgeons, Columbia University, December 3, 1929. Reprinted, by permission, from *The Journal of Nervous and Mental Disease*, Vol. 71, No. 3, March, 1930.

Figure B1.1A Baron Constantin von Economo and excerpts from the title page of his lecture on the localization of sleep- and wake-promoting systems in the brain.
From von Economo,[30] with permission.

(B)

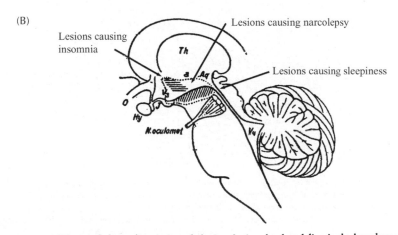

Schema of the median section of the interbrain; the dotted line is the boundary of the field, in which the center for sleep regulation is lying.

Figure B1.1B Von Economo's original drawing of the localization of the lesions in the brain that caused excessive sleepiness and insomnia.
Modified from von Economo,[30] with permission.

In 1929, Hans Berger, a German psychiatrist, reported a technologic innovation, the EEG, which he developed to assess the cortical function of his psychiatric patients with various types of functional impairment of responsiveness.[38]

He noted that the waveform pattern that he recorded from the scalps of his patients was generally sinusoidal and that the amplitude and frequency of the waves in the EEG correlated closely with the level of consciousness of the

(A)

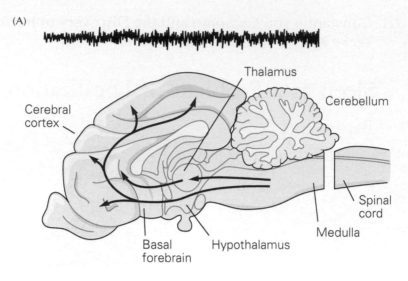

(B)

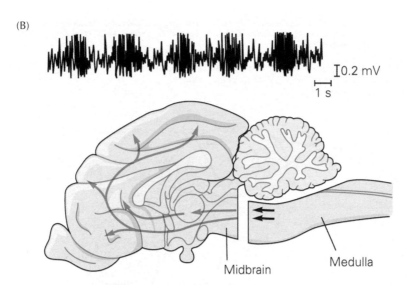

Figure 1.1 Electroencephalogram (EEG) from a cat in which Frederic Bremer transected the cervicomedullary junction (A), showing a normal, desynchronized waking activity. However, after a transection at the midcollicular level (B), the EEG consisted of higher voltage slow waves, more typical of sleep or coma.

From Richerson GB, Aston-Jones G, Saper C. The modulatory functions of the brain stem. Chapter 46 in: Kandel ER, Schwartz JH, Jessel TM., Siegelbaum SA, Hudspeth AJ. *Principles of Neural Science*. 5th ed. McGraw-Hill, New York, 2013, pp. 1038–1055. By permission of McGraw-Hill.

patient. This report was met with skepticism that the waveforms that were recorded were due to brain, as opposed to scalp muscles, and it was not until Sir Edgar Adrian confirmed in 1934 that similar waveforms could be recorded directly from the surface of the cerebral cortex in a cat[39] that this advance became widely recognized.

Shortly afterward, the Belgian neurophysiologist Frederic Bremer examined the EEG waveforms in cats with lesions of the brainstem.[40] He found that after a transection between the medulla and the spinal cord, a preparation that he called the *encéphale isolé*, or isolated brain, animals showed a desynchronized (low voltage, fast; i.e., waking) EEG pattern and appeared to be fully awake (see Figure 1.1). However, when he transected the neuraxis at the level between the superior and inferior colliculus, a preparation he called the *cerveau isolé*, or isolated cerebrum, the EEG showed a synchronized, or high-voltage, slow-wave pattern indicative of deep sleep and the animals were behaviorally unresponsive. Bremer concluded that the forebrain fell asleep due to the lack of somatosensory and auditory sensory inputs. He did not address why the animals failed to respond to visual inputs either with EEG desynchronization or by making vertical eye movements (as do patients who are locked-in).

This issue was addressed after World War II by Moruzzi and Magoun,[41] who placed more selective lesions in the lateral part of the midbrain tegmentum in cats, interrupting the ascending somatosensory and auditory lemniscal pathways but leaving the paramedian reticular core of the midbrain intact. Such animals were deaf and did not appear to appreciate somatosensory stimuli, but they were fully awake, as indicated both by EEG desynchronization and motor responses to visual stimuli. Conversely, when they placed lesions in the paramedian reticular formation of the midbrain, the animals still showed cortical-evoked responses to somatosensory or auditory stimuli, but the background EEG was synchronized (high-voltage, slow-wave) and the animals were behaviorally unresponsive. Later studies showed that electrical stimulation of the midbrain reticular core could excite forebrain desynchronization.[42] These observations emphasized the midbrain reticular core as relaying important arousing influences to the cerebral cortex, and this pathway was labeled the "ascending reticular activating system" because it was assumed that the pathway took its origin from neurons in the reticular formation, although this was not established in this early work.

Subsequent studies in which transecting lesions were placed sequentially at different levels of the brainstem in cats demonstrated that transections at the midpontine level or caudally down to the lower medulla resulted in animals that acutely spent most of their time in a wakeful state.[43] Thus, the lower brainstem was thought to play a synchronizing, or sleep-promoting, role.[44] Transections from the rostral pons forward produced EEG slowing and behavioral unresponsiveness. Periods of forebrain arousal returned after several days if the animals were kept alive. However, it is clear that the slab of tissue from the rostral pons through the caudal midbrain (the mesopontine tegmentum) contains neural structures that are critically important to forebrain arousal, at least in the acute setting.

At the time of Moruzzi and Magoun, little was known about the origins of ascending projections from the mesopontine tegmentum to the forebrain, and the arousal effect to midbrain reticular formation stimulation was attributed to activation of neurons in the reticular formation. However, more recent studies have shown that projections from the mesopontine tegmentum to the forebrain arise from several well-defined populations of neurons. The major source of mesopontine afferents that span the entire thalamus is a collection of cholinergic neurons that form two large clusters, the pedunculopontine and laterodorsal tegmental nuclei.[45] These neurons project through the paramedian midbrain reticular formation to the relay nuclei of the thalamus (which innervate specific cortical regions), as well as to the midline and intralaminar nuclei (which innervate the entire cortex more diffusely) and the reticular nucleus. As noted in Box 1.2, the reticular nucleus plays a critical role in regulating thalamocortical transmission by profoundly hyperpolarizing thalamic relay neurons via gamma-aminobutyric acid $(GABA)_B$ receptors.[46] Cholinergic inputs in turn hyperpolarize the reticular nucleus. Other neurons in the cholinergic pedunculopontine and laterodorsal tegmental nuclei send axons into the lateral hypothalamus and basal forebrain, where they contact populations of neurons with diffuse cortical projections (see later discussion). Neurons in the pedunculopontine and laterodorsal tegmental nuclei fire fastest during rapid eye movement (REM) sleep (see Box 1.3) and wakefulness,[47] two conditions that are characterized by a low-voltage, fast (desynchronized) EEG. They slow down during non-REM (NREM) sleep, when the EEG is dominated by high-voltage slow waves (Figure B1.3A).

In addition, at the mesopontine level, the brainstem contains at least three different monoamine groups whose axons project through the hypothalamus to the cerebral cortex.[48] The noradrenergic locus coeruleus projects through the paramedian midbrain reticular formation and the lateral hypothalamus, innervating the

Box 1.2 What Is the Origin of EEG Waves?

It has been known since the pioneering work of Mountcastle (in somatosensory cortex) and of Hubel and Wiesel (in visual cortex) in the 1960s that cortical neurons fire in patterns that represent various aspects of the incoming sensory stimuli. However, the waveforms in the electroencephalogram (EEG) are sinusoidal and their frequency is more closely related to the level of arousal. This disparity occurs because the EEG does not represent the action potentials generated by cortical neurons but rather the summation of excitatory postsynaptic potentials (EPSPs) on dendrites of cortical neurons. More recent studies have addressed what drives these sinusoidal EEG waves.

An isolated slab of cerebral cortex, not receiving any input from its usual subcortical or cortical afferents, produces a high-voltage, slow EEG (0.5–2.0 Hz), indicating that this EEG pattern represents an intrinsic oscillation within the cerebral cortex.[49] Intracellular recordings show that the neurons oscillate between up and down states, with the up states representing relatively depolarized membrane potential when the neurons are most likely to fire.

EEG waves in the mid-frequency range (3–10 Hz) have been thought to represent incoming activity from subcortical afferents. Because the thalamocortical projections are so extensive, it was assumed for many years that this input was mainly from the thalamus. This idea was reinforced by the finding that many thalamocortical relay neurons fire single actions potentials that transmit sensory or other information when their membrane potential is near to threshold. However, when the relay neuron has been hyperpolarized to a membrane potential far below its usual threshold for firing sodium action potentials, a low-threshold calcium channel is deinactivated. A small membrane depolarization at this point can open the calcium channel, bringing the cell's membrane potential to a plateau that is above the threshold for firing sodium action potentials. As a result, a series of sodium spikes is fired in a high-frequency burst until sufficient calcium has entered the cell to activate a calcium-activated potassium current. This potassium current then brings the cell back to a hyperpolarized state, terminating the burst.[46]

The bursting behavior of neurons in the thalamic relay nuclei, which are a major source of cortical inputs, is often thought to be a major source of cortical EEG. The synchrony is credited to the thalamic reticular nucleus, which is a thin sheet of GABAergic neurons that covers the thalamus like a shroud. Thalamic axons on their way to the cerebral cortex, and cortical projections to the thalamus, give off collaterals to the reticular nucleus as they pass through it. Neurons in the reticular nucleus provide GABAergic inputs to the thalamic relay nuclei, which hyperpolarize them and set them into bursting mode.

However, there is evidence that the synchrony of EEG rhythms across the cerebral cortex is due in large part to corticocortical connections and that even very large thalamic lesions fail to cause much change in the mid-range EEG oscillations.[50] These thalamic lesions mainly suppress spindles (8–13 Hz EEG waves that wax and wane, particularly during light sleep) and higher frequency EEG (which is due to cortico-cortical activity). On the other hand, there are also neurons in the basal forebrain that show bursting behavior, with the bursts time-locked to the mid-frequency waves in the EEG.[51,52] Some of the basal forebrain neurons that project to the cerebral cortex are cholinergic, and these largely contact and excite pyramidal cells. However, many of the basal forebrain neurons that project to the cerebral cortex contain GABA and the calcium-buffering protein parvalbumin. The latter cells tend to contact cortical GABAergic interneurons, thus disinhibiting the

Box 1.2 What Is the Origin of EEG Waves? (cont.)

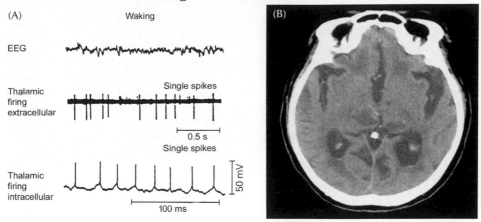

Figure B1.2 Thalamic relay neurons have transmission and burst modes of firing. (A) During transmission mode, which operates mainly during wakefulness, individual neurons in the thalamus fire single spikes in patterns that reflect their incoming afferent inputs. This correlates with a desynchronized electroencephalogram. (B) Computed tomography (CT) scan from Case Presentation below, 3.5 weeks after second thalamic hemorrhage. Note that the left thalamus is atrophic and the right is still swollen but largely infarcted.

Panel A: From Saper C. Brain stem modulation of sensation, movement, and consciousness. In: Kandel ER, Schwartz JH, Jessel TM. *Principles of Neural Science*. 4th ed. New York: McGraw-Hill; 2000:871–909. By permission of McGraw-Hill.

cerebral cortex.[53] One class of these GABAergic interneurons that also contain parvalbumin is involved in intracortical circuits that generate most of the high-frequency oscillations in the cortical EEG.[54] Large lesions of the basal forebrain cause loss of midrange and higher frequency EEG, suggesting that the basal forebrain keeps the cerebral cortex awake and that the thalamus provides the content of consciousness.

Thus, the waveforms of the cortical EEG appear to be due to complex interactions among the burst neurons in the thalamus, cortex, and basal forebrain, all of which receive substantial inputs from the ascending arousal system.[49]

Case Presentation

A 73-year-old woman with a history of hypertension and a left thalamic infarct causing a right hemiparesis complained of a headache; 5 minutes later her speech became slurred and then she lost consciousness. Emergency medical technicians found her to be minimally responsive, unable to speak, with unresponsive pupils and extensor posturing. She was transported to the emergency department where a computed tomography (CT) scan of the head disclosed a 1.7 × 2.7-cm right thalamic hemorrhage (see Fig. B1.2). Over the next 3 weeks, she developed spontaneous cycles of eye opening during the day, with eyes closed at night, but remained in a vegetative state, with no purposive responses to her environment. This did not change during the remainder of her 7-week hospital stay. Her EEG 7 weeks after the second thalamic hemorrhage showed a continuous 6–7 Hz theta rhythm during the day, with slowing into the 4 Hz range during the night. No spindles, slow waves, or higher frequency activity was noted.

Box 1.3 Wake–Sleep States

In the early days of EEG recording, it was widely assumed that sleep, like coma, represented a period of brain inactivity. Hence, it was not surprising when the EEG appearance of deep sleep was found to resemble the high-voltage, slow waves that appear during coma. However, in 1953, Aserinsky and Kleitman[55] reported the curious observation that, when they recorded the EEG as well as the electromyogram (EMG) and the electro-oculogram (EOG) overnight, their subjects would periodically enter a state of sleep in which their eyes would move and their EEG would appear to be similar to waking states, yet their eyes were closed and they were deeply unresponsive to external stimuli.

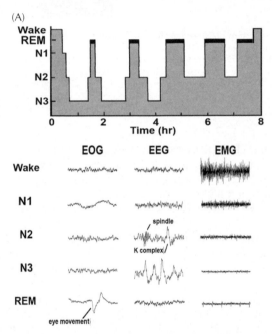

Figure B1.3A The main features of a polysomnogram showing the electroencephalogram (EEG), muscle tone (electromyogram [EMG]), and eye movements (electro-oculogram [EOG]), across the different stages of sleep and wakefulness. During wakefulness, the EEG is desynchronized, the EMG is active, and there are spontaneous eye movements. During progressively deeper stages of non-rapid eye movement (NREM) sleep (N1 through N3), the EEG becomes progressively slower, the EMG less active, and eye movements slow down or become slowly roving. The EEG demonstrates waxing and waning bouts of 12–14 Hz activity (sleep spindles) and occasional high-voltage slow waves (K complexes) in stage N2 and is dominated by high voltate slow waves in N3. During REM sleep, there is a rapid transition to a desynchronized EEG and irregular, rapid eye movements, but the EMG becomes nearly silent, consistent with atonia. As the night progresses, the subject typically will spend progressively less time in the deeper stages of NREM sleep and more time in REM sleep, so that most of the REM sleep for the night comes in the last few bouts. Spontaneous awakenings during the night typically occur from the lighter stages of NREM sleep. Active dreams occur predominantly during REM sleep, although many subjects report passive dreams and ideation during NREM sleep as well.

From Scammel TE, Saper CB. Sleep and wakefulness. In: Kandel ER, Jessel TM, Siegelbaum S, Hudspeth A, eds. *Principles of Neural Science*. 6th ed. New York: McGraw-Hill; 2019. By permission of McGraw-Hill.

Box 1.3 Wake–Sleep States (cont.)

This condition of rapid eye movement (REM) sleep has also been called *desynchronized sleep* (from the appearance of the EEG) as well as *paradoxical sleep*. More detailed study of the course of a night of sleep revealed that the REM and non-REM (NREM) periods tend to alternate in a rhythmic pattern throughout the night.[56,57]

During active wakefulness, the EEG gives the appearance of small, desynchronized waves and the EMG is active, indicating muscle activity associated with waking behavior. In quiet wakefulness, the EEG often begins to synchronize, with 8- to 12-Hz alpha waves predominating, particularly posteriorly over the hemisphere. Muscle tone may diminish as well. As sleep begins, the EEG rhythm drops to the 4- to 7-Hz theta range, muscle tone is further diminished, and slowly roving eye movements emerge (Stage I NREM). The appearance of sleep spindles (waxing and waning runs of alpha frequency waves) and large waves in the 1- to 3-Hz delta range, called K complexes, denotes the onset of Stage II NREM. The subject may then pass into the deeper stages of NREM (Stage III), sometimes called slow-wave sleep, in which delta waves become a progressively more prominent feature. During these periods, eye movements are few and muscle tone drops to very low levels. This usually takes about 45–60 minutes, and then the subject often will gradually emerge from the first bout of slow-wave sleep to Stage I again.

(B)

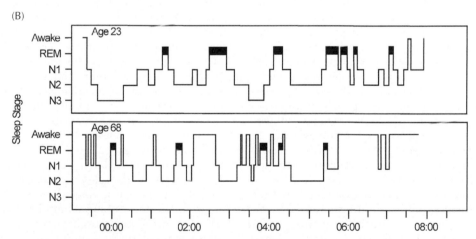

Figure B1.3B The stages of sleep through the night in a young adult and older person. There is usually regular progression from wakefulness through the stages of non-rapid eye movement (NREM) sleep into its deepest stages, then progression back to light NREM sleep before the first REM episode of the night. With successive cycles through the night, the amount of deeper NREM sleep becomes less, and the amount of REM becomes greater. This pattern, which is typical of young adults, changes dramatically across a lifetime. Infants spend much more time asleep, and much more time in the deeper stages of NREM sleep, than do adults. The amount of Stage III NREM sleep diminishes as children enter puberty, and it may not occur at all in some older adults. With aging, there is sleep fragmentation with more frequent awakenings and often early awakening with fewer hours of sleep.[58]

From Scammell TE, Saper CB, Czeisler CA. Sleep disorders. In: Jameson JL, Fauci AS, Kasper DL, Hauser SL, Longo D L, Loscalzo J, eds. *Harrison's Principles of Internal Medicine*. 20th ed. New York: McGraw-Hill; 2018. By permission of McGraw-Hill.

Box 1.3 Wake–Sleep States (cont.)

At this point, the first bout of REM sleep of the night often occurs. The subject abruptly transitions into a desynchronized, low-voltage EEG, with rapid and vigorous eye movements and virtually complete loss of muscle tone, except in the muscles of respiration. The first bout of REM sleep during the night typically lasts only 5–10 minutes, and then the subject will transition into Stage I NREM and again begin to descend gradually into deeper stages of NREM sleep.

entire cerebral cortex diffusely.[59] Projections from the serotoninergic neurons in the dorsal and median raphe nuclei take a similar course.[60] Mixed in with the serotoninergic neurons are a smaller number of dopaminergic cells, which are an extension of the ventral tegmental dopamine group along the midline of the midbrain, into the area under the cerebral aqueduct.[61,62] These dopaminergic neurons also project through the paramedian midbrain reticular formation. Some of them innervate the midline and intralaminar nuclei of the thalamus, and others pass through the lateral hypothalamus to the basal forebrain and prefrontal cortex. Evidence from single-unit recording studies in behaving animals indicates that neurons in these monoaminergic nuclei are most active during wakefulness, slow down during slow-wave sleep, and stop almost completely during REM sleep.[63–66] Driving these monoamine pathways optogenetically produces wakefulness.[62,67–70]

Application of monoaminergic neurotransmitters to cortical neurons produces complex responses.[46,71–73] In most cases, there is inhibition resulting in a decrease in background firing, although firing induced by the specific stimulus to which the neuron is best tuned may not be reduced to as great a degree as background firing. In an awake and aroused individual, this alteration in firing may result in an improvement in the signal-to-noise ratio, which may be critical in sharpening cortical information processing to avoid misperception of stimuli, such as occurs during a delirious state.

Although the cholinergic and monoaminergic neurons in the mesopontine tegmentum have traditionally been thought to play a major role in regulating wake–sleep states, lesions of these cell groups have relatively little effect on wake–sleep states or cortical EEG.[72] On the other hand, glutamatergic neurons in the laterodorsal and pedunculopontine tegmental and parabrachial nuclei also have intense inputs to the basal forebrain.[51,74] Cell-specific lesions of these neurons produce profound coma, suggesting that they may be a major source of the ascending arousal influence (Figure 1.2).

In addition, along the course of the ascending cholinergic and monoaminergic axons through the rostral midbrain reticular formation, there are many additional neurons that project to the thalamic midline and intralaminar nuclei.[75,76] Many of these neurons appear to be glutamatergic, and they may amplify the arousal signal that arises in the mesopontine tegmentum. On the other hand, they do not appear to be capable of maintaining a waking state on their own after acute mesopontine lesions.

As axons from brainstem ascending arousal neurons pass through the hypothalamus, they are augmented by neurons in several hypothalamic cell groups that also project to the basal forebrain and cerebral cortex. These include histaminergic neurons in the tuberomammillary nucleus as well as glutamatergic neurons in the supramammillary area and orexin neurons in the lateral hypothalamic area, all of which project diffusely to the cerebral cortex and innervate the intralaminar and midline thalamus.[77–82] There is considerable evidence that the histaminergic input plays a role in maintaining a wakeful state. Histamine H_1 blockers impair wakefulness in both animals and humans,[83] and transgenic mice lacking histidine decarboxylase show a deficit in wakefulness induced by a novel environment, whereas mice injected with an inhibitor of this

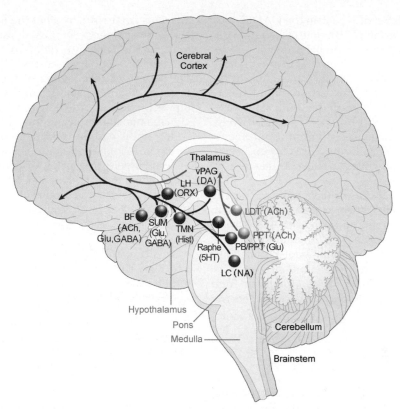

Figure 1.2 A summary diagram of the ascending arousal system. The cholinergic system, shown in yellow, provides the main input to the relay and reticular nuclei of the thalamus from the upper brainstem. This inhibits the reticular nucleus and activates the thalamic relay nuclei, allowing the thalamus to relay sensory information to the cerebral cortex. The cortex is activated simultaneously by a series of direct inputs, shown in red. These include glutamatergic (Glu) neurons in the parabrachial nucleus (PB) and pedunculopontine tegmental nucleus (PPT); monoaminergic inputs from the upper brainstem and posterior hypothalamus, such as noradrenaline (NA) from the locus coeruleus (LC), serotonin (5-HT) from the dorsal and median raphe nuclei, dopamine (DA) from the ventral periaqueductal gray matter (vPAG), and histamine (His) from the tuberomammillary nucleus (TMN); glutamatergic inputs from the supramammillary nucleus in the hypothalamus as well as peptidergic hypothalamic inputs from the orexin (ORX) neurons in the lateral hypothalamus (LH); and cholinergic (ACh), gamma-aminobutyric acid (GABA)-ergic and glutamatergic inputs from the basal forebrain (BF). Activation of the brainstem yellow pathway in the absence of the red pathways occurs during rapid eye movement (REM) sleep, resulting in the cortex entering a dreaming state. LDT, laterodorsal tegmental nucleus.
Modified from Saper CB, Scammell TE, Lu J. Hypothalamic regulation of sleep and circadian rhythms. *Nature* 437: 1257–1263, 2005. By permission of Nature Publishing Group.

key enzyme for histamine synthesis similarly show less wakefulness.[84] However, acute excitation or inhibition of the histamine neurons has relatively modest effects on either acute wakefulness or long-term wake–sleep.

By contrast, acute chemogenetic excitation of the supramammillary glutamatergic neurons causes a prolonged (6–8 hours) period of sleeplessness in mice, and inhibiting them causes somnolence.[78] The supramamillary neurons have a particularly intense input to the dentate gyrus and CA2 field of the hippocampus,[77,78,82] and some of these glutamatergic neurons also,

paradoxically, release GABA.[78,85] The reason for this colocalization is not known, but knocking out the GABA vesicular transporter from these cells causes mice to have seizures, so it may play a protective role to prevent overexcitation of target neurons.

Some of the lateral hypothalamic neurons that project to the basal forebrain and cerebral cortex contain orexin,[79] a peptide that is associated with arousal, and others contain melanin-concentrating hormone.[86,87] The orexin neurons also use glutamate as a neurotransmitter,[88] as do many of the melanin-concentrating hormone neurons; the latter also contain the GAD65, the enzyme for making GABA, but lack the GABA vesicular transporter, so probably do not release GABA from their terminals.[89] Many neurons in the lateral hypothalamic area, including those that contain orexin, fire fastest during wakefulness and slow down during both slow-wave and REM sleep (see Box 1.4).[90,91] Alternatively, the firing of melanin-concentrating hormone neurons increases during REM sleep,[92] and activating them causes a selective increase in REM sleep.[93–95]

In addition, the ascending monoaminergic and hypothalamic projections pass through the basal forebrain, and, along their pathway to the cerebral cortex, they encounter and are augmented further by additional populations of cholinergic and noncholinergic neurons in the magnocellular basal forebrain nuclei.[96–98] The large cholinergic neurons receive afferents from virtually all of the hypothalamic and monoaminergic brainstem ascending systems and accompany them to diffusely innervate the cerebral cortex.[99–101] However, the pattern of termination of the cholinergic neurons is more specific than the monoamine inputs to the cortex. Whereas axons from individual monoaminergic neurons typically ramify widely in the cerebral cortex, axons from basal forebrain cholinergic neurons each innervate pyramidal cells in a patch of cortex of only a few millimeters in diameter.[96,102] Recordings from basal forebrain neurons in rats across the wake–sleep cycle indicate that they have a wide range of activity patterns. Many are most active during wakefulness or during slow-wave sleep, and they fire in bursts that correlate with EEG wave patterns.[52] Interestingly, in behaving monkeys, firing of basal forebrain neurons correlates best with the reward phase

Box 1.4 Orexin and Narcolepsy

From the first use of the term by Gelineau in 1880,[38] narcolepsy has puzzled clinicians and scientists alike. Although Gelineau included within his definition a wide range of disorders with excessive daytime sleepiness, Gowers has been credited with limiting the term to cases with brief periods of sleep that interrupt a normal waking state. Kinnier Wilson firmly identified it with attacks of cataplexy, during which "the patient's knees give way and he may sink to the ground, without any loss of consciousness."[39] Wilson pointed out that narcolepsy had been considered a very rare condition of which he had seen only a few cases during the first 20 years of his practice but that, in the mid-1920s, there was a sudden increase in the number of cases, so that he had seen six within a year in 1927; Spiller reported seeing three within a year in 1926. Wilson opined that the epidemic of new cases of narcolepsy in those years was due to the worldwide epidemics of influenza and encephalitis from about 1918 to 1925. During the H1N1 influenza epidemic in China in 2009, there was also a spike in narcolepsy cases,[103] and a sudden rash of narcolepsy cases followed attempts to immunize the Swedish and Finnish population with a vaccine (Pandemrix) that contained an AS03 adjuvant.[104] These observations have suggested that narcolepsy is typically an autoimmune condition due to autoantibodies that attack the brain. Consistent with that hypothesis, the incidence of narcolepsy is seasonal, with increases following the winter influenza season each year, and is highest during the second and third decades of life, leading to a background prevalence of one per 2,000 population.[105]

About half of patients with narcolepsy report sleep paralysis, a curious state of inability to move during the transition from sleep to wakefulness or from wakefulness to sleep.[105] However, up to 20% of normal individuals may also experience this condition occasionally, especially during periods of sleep deprivation. More characteristic of narcolepsy, but occurring in only about 20% of cases, are episodes

Box 1.4 Orexin and Narcolepsy (cont.)

of hypnagogic hallucinations during which the patient experiences a vivid, cartoon-like hallucination, with movement and action against a background of wakefulness. The patient can distinguish that the hallucination is not real. Electroencephalogram (EEG) and electromyelogram (EMG) recordings during sleep and wakefulness show that narcoleptic patients fall asleep more frequently during the day, but they also awaken more frequently at night, so that they get about the same amount of sleep as normal individuals. However, they often enter into rapid eye movement (REM) sleep very soon after sleep onset (short-onset REM periods [SOREMPs]), and, during cataplexy attacks, they show muscle atonia consistent with intrusion of a REM-like state into consciousness. On a multiple sleep latency test (MSLT), where the patient lies down in a quiet room five times during the course of the day at 2-hour intervals, narcoleptics typically fall asleep much faster than normal individuals (often in less than 5 minutes on repeated occasions) and show SOREMPs, which normal individuals rarely, if ever, experience.

There is a clear genetic predisposition to narcolepsy, as individuals with a first-degree relative with the disorder are 40 times more likely to develop it themselves.[105] However, there are clearly environmental factors involved, consistent with an autoimmune pathogenesis: among monozygotic twins, if one twin develops narcolepsy, the other will develop it only about 25% of the time. The relationship of narcolepsy to the immune system is further underscored by the finding that the HLA allele DQB1*0602 is present in 88–98% of individuals with narcolepsy with cataplexy, but only in about 12% of white Americans and 38% of African Americans in the general population.

Scientists worked fruitlessly for decades to unravel the pathophysiology of this mysterious illness until, in 1999, two dramatic and simultaneous findings suddenly brought the problem into focus. The previous year, two groups of

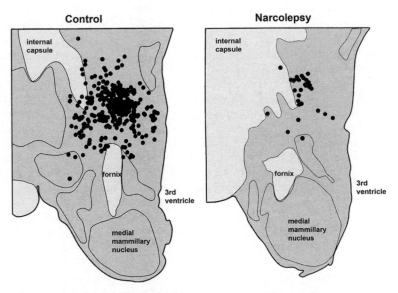

Figure B1.4 Narcolepsy is caused by loss of the orexin neurons in the posterior and lateral hypothalamus of the human brain. The panels plot the location of orexin neurons (*black dots*) in the posterior hypothalamus in a healthy control subject on the left and in a patient with narcolepsy on the right. There is typically about a 90% loss of orexin neurons in patients who have narcolepsy with cataplexy.
From Scammel TE, Saper CB. Sleep and wakefulness. In: Kandel ER, Jessel TM, Siegelbaum S, Hudspeth A. *Principles of Neural Science*. 6th ed. New York: McGraw-Hill; 2019. By permission of McGraw-Hill.

Box 1.4 Orexin and Narcolepsy (cont.)

scientists, Masashi Yanagisawa and colleagues at the University of Texas Southwestern Medical School, and Greg Sutcliffe and coworkers at the Scripps Institute, had simultaneously identified a new pair of peptide neurotransmitters made from the same precursor by neurons in the lateral hypothalamus, which Yanagisawa called "orexins" (based on the presumption of a role in feeding)[106] and Sutcliffe called "hypocretins" (because this hypothalamic peptide has a sequence similar to secretin).[107] Yanagisawa further showed that the type 1 orexin receptor had 10-fold specificity for orexin A, whereas the type 2 receptor was activated equally well by both orexins.[108] The orexin neurons in the lateral hypothalamus were found to have wide-ranging projections from the cerebral cortex to the spinal cord, much like the monoaminergic neurons in the brainstem.[79,109]

When Yanagisawa's group prepared mice in which the orexin gene had been deleted, they initially found that the animals had normal sleep behavior during the day.[109] However, when the mice were observed under infrared video monitoring during the night, they showed intermittent attacks of behavioral arrest during which they would suddenly fall over onto their side, twitch a bit, lie still for a minute or two, then just as suddenly get up and resume their normal behaviors. EEG and EMG recordings demonstrated that these attacks have the appearance of cataplexy (sudden loss of muscle tone, EEG showing either an awake pattern or large amounts of theta activity typical of rodents during REM sleep). The animals also had short-onset REM periods when asleep, another hallmark of narcolepsy.

At the same time, Emmanuel Mignot had been working at Stanford for nearly a decade to determine the cause of genetically inherited canine narcolepsy. He finally determined that the dogs had a genetic defect in the type 2 orexin receptor.[110] The nearly simultaneous publication of the two results firmly established that narcolepsy could be produced in animals by impairment of orexin signaling.

The presence of orexin receptors on many of the hypothalamic and brainstem cell groups that are known to regulate REM sleep[111] suggests that one or more of these targets may be critical for regulating the transitions to REM sleep that are disrupted in patients with narcolepsy.

Over the following year, it became clear that most humans with narcolepsy do not have a genetic defect either of the orexin gene or of its receptors, although a few cases with onset during infancy and particularly severe narcolepsy were found to be due to this cause.[91] Instead, postmortem studies showed that narcoleptics with cataplexy lose about 90% of their orexin neurons and that the spinal fluid levels of orexin often are very low.[91-93] However, the nearby melanin-concentrating hormone neurons were not affected. This specificity suggested either an autoimmune or neurodegenerative cause of the orexin cell loss. Recent data demonstrating increased numbers of new cases of narcolepsy after the H1N1 influenza epidemic in China and the vaccination of children in Scandinavia against H1N1 virus strongly suggest that most cases of sporadic narcolepsy are autoimmune in origin.[103,104]

of complex behaviors, suggesting that these neurons may be involved in some highly specific aspect of arousal, such as focusing attention on rewarding tasks, rather than in the general level of cortical activity.[112] Optical calcium imaging of basal forebrain neurons in mice found that cholinergic neurons were especially active during motor activity but that all three classes of basal forebrain neuron were activated during behavioral punishment, again suggesting a role in motivated behavior as opposed to baseline wakefulness.[113]

Many GABAergic basal forebrain neurons also display a wake-active firing pattern.[52] They are believed to innervate cortical GABAergic interneurons, particularly of the parvalbumin or somatostatin-containing type.[54] This would disinhibit the cortex, and recent findings from opto- or chemogenetic studies have found that driving the basal forebrain GABA neurons produces wakefulness as well as high-frequency (gamma) oscillations in the EEG, indicative of cortical processing activity.[114–117] Neurons of both the GABAergic and cholinergic type in the basal forebrain may play an important role in maintaining a normal waking state.[115] The basal forebrain also contains some glutamatergic neurons that innervate the cerebral cortex. They also appear to be arousing, although perhaps less potent than the GABAergic and cholinergic neurons.[115,116]

Surprisingly, large cell-specific bilateral basal forebrain lesions (i.e., not damaging fibers of passage) have been shown in experimental animals to cause a deeply comatose state.[51] This observation implies that the bulk of the influence of the ascending arousal system is mediated by its input to the basal forebrain neurons and, consequently, their input to the cerebral cortex. Neither lesions of just the cholinergic nor just the noncholinergic neurons in the basal forebrain was able to cause coma, consistent with observations that both types of neurons have potent arousing effects.[115,116] Such bilateral basal forebrain lesions would be rare in humans, as the area lies just above the circle of Willis where it is supplied by small feeding vessels directly off the anterior cerebral arteries on each side. However, Fisher indicated that he did observe coma in patients with bilateral

anterior cerebral artery occlusions,[118] which may be explained by bilateral acute damage to the basal forebrain.

Thus, the ascending arousal system consists of multiple ascending pathways originating in the mesopontine tegmentum but augmented by additional inputs at virtually every level through which it passes on its way to the basal forebrain, thalamus, and cerebral cortex. These different pathways may fire independently under a variety of different conditions, modulating the functional capacities of cortical neurons during a wide range of behavioral states.

Behavioral State Switching

An important feature of the ascending arousal system is its interconnectivity: the cell groups that contribute to the system also maintain substantial connections with other components of the system. Another important property of the system is that nearly all of these components receive inputs from the ventrolateral preoptic nucleus.[48,119–121] Ventrolateral preoptic neurons contain the inhibitory transmitters GABA and galanin; they fire fastest during sleep.[120,122,123] Lesions of the ventrolateral preoptic nucleus cause a state of profound insomnia in animals,[124,125] and loss of ventrolateral preoptic neurons with aging in humans is associated with sleep fragmentation and loss of consolidated periods of sleep.[59] Conversely, opto- or chemogenetic driving of the ventrolateral preoptic neurons causes sleep.[126,127] Additional sleep-active GABAergic neurons in the median preoptic nucleus also are thought to contribute to sleep promotion,[128] and chemogenetic driving of median preoptic glutamatergic neurons produces NREM sleep.[129] Lesions involving this region presumably accounted for the insomnia described by von Economo in patients with encephalitis involving the rostral third ventricular region[30] (see Box 1.1).

The ventrolateral preoptic neurons also receive extensive inhibitory inputs from many components of the ascending arousal system.[130–132] This mutual inhibition between the ventrolateral preoptic nucleus and the ascending arousal system has interesting implications for the mechanisms of the natural switching from wakefulness to sleep over the course of the day and from slow-wave to REM sleep over the course of the night (Figure 1.3). Electrical engineers call a circuit in which the two sides inhibit each other a "flip-flop" switch.[48,121] Each side of a flip-flop circuit is self-reinforcing (i.e., when the neurons are firing, they inhibit neurons that would otherwise turn them off, and hence they are disinhibited by their own activity). As a result, firing by each side of the circuit tends to be self-perpetuating, and the circuit tends to spend nearly all of its time with either one side or the other in ascendancy and very little time in transition. These sharp boundaries between wakefulness and sleep are a key feature of normal physiology, as it would be maladaptive for animals to walk around half-asleep or to spend long portions of their normal sleep cycle half-awake (Figure 1.4).

During REM sleep, the brain enters a very different state from the high-voltage slow waves that characterize NREM sleep. As indicated in Box 1.3, during REM sleep, the forebrain shows low-voltage, fast EEG activity similar to wakefulness, and the ascending cholinergic system is even more active than during a wakeful state. However, the ascending

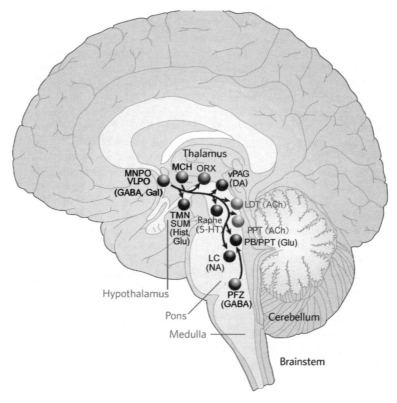

Figure 1.3 The ventrolateral preoptic nucleus (VLPO) and median preoptic nucleus (MnPO), shown in purple, inhibit the components of the ascending arousal system during sleep. Both VLPO and MnPO neurons contain gamma-aminobutyric acid (GABA) and VLPO neurons also contain inhibitory peptide, galanin (Gal). Together, they send axons to most of the cell groups that compose the ascending arousal system. This unique relationship allows the VLPO and MnPO neurons effectively to turn off the arousal systems during sleep. Loss of VLPO neurons results in profound insomnia. Other GABAergic neurons in the parafacial zone (PFZ) primarily inhibit the parabrachial nucleus (PB) and also produce sleep. Neurons in the lateral hypothalamus that contain melanin-concentrating hormone (MCH) primarily promote REM sleep. 5-HT, serotonin; ACh, acetylcholine; DA, dopamine; Glu, glutamate; His, histamine; LC, locus coeruleus; LDT, laterodorsal tegmental nuclei; NA, noradrenaline; ORX, orexin; PeF; PPT, pedunculopontine; TMN, tuberomammillary nucleus; vPAG, ventral periaqueductal gray matter.
Modified from Saper CB, Scammell TE, Lu J. Hypothalamic regulation of sleep and circadian rhythms. *Nature* 437:1257–1263, 2005. By permission of Nature Publishing Group.

monoaminergic systems cease firing virtually completely during REM sleep,[63–66] so that the increased thalamocortical transmission seen during REM sleep falls on a cerebral cortex that lacks the priming to maintain a wakeful state. As a result, REM sleep is sometimes called *paradoxical sleep* because the cortex gives an EEG appearance of wakefulness, and yet the individual is profoundly unresponsive to external stimuli.

A second flip-flop switch in the pons for switching from NREM to REM sleep (and back again) has been identified in the rostral pons. Many GABAergic neurons in the extended part of the ventrolateral preoptic

nucleus are specifically active during REM sleep, suggesting that they inhibit a population of REM-off neurons.[133,134] In addition, the orexin neurons in the lateral hypothalamus are excitatory, but their firing inhibits REM sleep, suggesting that they may activate REM-off neurons because patients or animals with narcolepsy who lack orexin neurons transition into REM sleep exceptionally quickly.[113] By searching for the intersection of these two pathways, a population of neurons was defined in the rostral pons, including the ventrolateral periaqueductal gray matter and the lateral pontine tegmentum at the level where they are adjacent to the dorsal raphe nucleus.[133] These sites

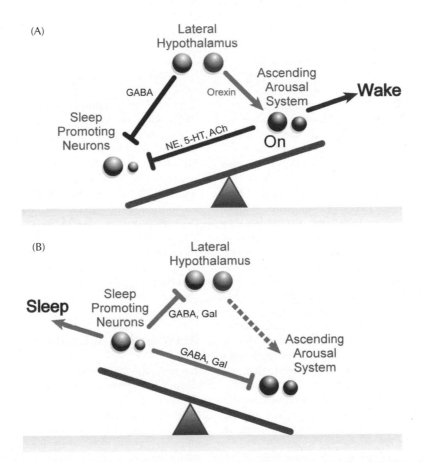

Figure 1.4 A diagram of the flip-flop relationship between the ventrolateral preoptic nucleus (VLPO), which promotes sleep, and several monoaminergic cell groups that contribute to the arousal system, including the locus coeruleus (LC), the tuberomammillary nucleus (TMN), and raphe nuclei. During wakefulness (A), the orexin neurons (ORX) are active, stimulating the monoamine nuclei, which both cause arousal and inhibit the VLPO to prevent sleep. During sleep (B), the VLPO and extended VLPO (eVLPO) inhibit the monoamine groups and the orexin neurons, thus preventing arousal. This mutually inhibitory relationship ensures that transitions between wake and sleep are rapid and complete.

From Saper CB, Scammell TE, Lu J. Hypothalamic regulation of sleep and circadian rhythms. *Nature* 437:1257–1263, 2005. By permission of Nature Publishing Group.

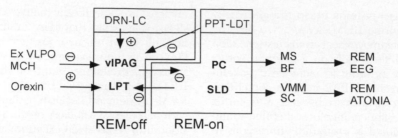

Figure 1.5 The control elements for rapid eye movement (REM) sleep also form a flip-flop switch. Gamma-aminobutyric acid (GABA)-ergic REM-off neurons in the ventrolateral periaqueductal gray matter (vlPAG) and the lateral pontine tegmentum (LPT) inhibit the REM-on neurons in the sublaterodorsal (SLD) and the precoeruleus (PC) areas, whereas GABA-ergic SLD neurons inhibit the vlPAG and the LPT. This mutual inhibition forms a second flip-flop switch that regulates transitions into and out of REM sleep, which also are generally rapid and complete. Other modulatory systems, such as the extended ventrolateral preoptic nucleus (Ex VLPO) and the melanin-concentrating hormone (MCH) and orexin neurons in the hypothalamus, regulate REM sleep by their inputs to this switch. Similarly, the monoaminergic dorsal raphe nucleus (DRN) and locus coeruleus (LC) inhibit REM sleep by activating the REM-off neurons, and cholinergic neurons in the pedunculopontine (PPT) and laterodorsal tegmental nuclei (LDT) activate REM sleep by inhibiting neurons in the REM-off region. Neurons in the SLD cause motor atonia during REM sleep by excitatory inputs to inhibitory interneurons in the ventromedial medulla (VMM) and the spinal cord (SC), which inhibit alpha motor neurons. Neurons in the PC contact the medial septum (MS) and basal forebrain (BF), which drive the electroencephalogram (EEG) phenomena associated with REM sleep.
Modified from Lu, Sherman, Devor, et al.,[133] by permission.

contain many GABAergic neurons, and lesions of this region increase REM sleep, confirming a REM-off influence.[111,112] GABAergic neurons in the REM-off area innervate an adjacent region including the sublaterodorsal nucleus and pre-coeruleus region that contain REM-active neurons. This REM-on region contains two types of neurons. GABAergic neurons, mainly in the sublaterodorsal nucleus, project back to the REM-off area.[133] This produces a flip-flop switch relationship accounting for the tendency for transitions into and out of REM sleep to be relatively abrupt. A second population of neurons is glutamatergic. Glutamatergic REM-on neurons in the sublaterodorsal nucleus project to the brainstem and spinal cord, where they are thought to be responsible for the motor manifestations of REM sleep, including atonia and perhaps the rapid eye movements that are the hallmarks of the state.[133] Glutamatergic REM-on neurons in the pre-coeruleus region target the basal forebrain, where they appear to be critical for maintaining EEG phenomena associated with REM sleep (Figure 1.5).

Cholinergic and monoaminergic influences may have a modulatory effect on REM sleep by playing upon this flip-flop switch mechanism. Although lesions of the cholinergic or monoaminergic systems do not have a major effect on REM sleep, the response to over-activity may be quite dramatic. For example,

injections of cholinomimetic agents into the region containing the REM switch can trigger prolonged bouts of a REM-like state in animals.[135] Whether this is due to activating REM-on neurons or inhibiting REM-off neurons (or both) is not known. On the other hand, patients who take antidepressants that are either serotonin or norepinephrine reuptake inhibitors (or both) have very little REM sleep. This effect may be due to the excess monoamines activating the REM-off neurons or inhibiting the REM-on neurons (or both) and thereby locking the individual out of REM sleep.[136,137]

Relationship of Coma to Sleep

Because the brain enters a state of quiescence during sleep on a daily basis, it is natural to wonder whether coma may not be a pathologic entrance into the sleep state. In fact, both impaired states of consciousness and NREM sleep are characterized by EEG patterns that include increased amounts of high-voltage slow waves. Both conditions are due, ultimately, to lack of activity by the ascending arousal system. However, in sleep, the lack of activity is due to an intrinsically regulated inhibition of the arousal system, whereas in coma the impairment of the arousal system is due either to damage to the arousal system or to diffuse dysfunction of its diencephalic or forebrain targets.

Because sleep is a regulated state, it has several characteristics that distinguish it from coma. A key feature of sleep is that the subject can be aroused from it to wakefulness. Patients who are obtunded may be aroused briefly, but they require continuous stimulation to maintain a wakeful state, and comatose patients may not be arousable at all. In addition, sleeping subjects undergo a variety of postural adjustments, including yawning, stretching, and turning, which are not seen in patients with pathologic impairment of level of consciousness.

The most important difference, however, is the lack of cycling between NREM and REM sleep in patients in coma. Sleeping subjects undergo a characteristic pattern of waxing and waning depth of NREM sleep during the night, punctuated by bouts of REM sleep, usually beginning when the NREM sleep reaches its lightest phase (see Box 1.3). The monotonic high-voltage slow waves in the EEG of the comatose patient indicate that although coma may share with NREM sleep the property of a low level of activity in the ascending arousal systems, it is a fundamentally different and pathologic state.

The Cerebral Hemispheres and Conscious Behavior

The cerebral cortex acts like a massively parallel processor that breaks down the components of sensory experience into a wide array of abstractions that are analyzed independently and in parallel during normal conscious experience.[1] This organizational scheme predicts many of the properties of consciousness, and it sheds light on how these many parallel streams of cortical activity are reassimilated into a single conscious state.

The cerebral neocortex of mammals, from rodents to humans, consists of a sheet of neurons divided into six layers. Inputs from the thalamic relay nuclei arrive mainly in layer IV, which consists of small granule cells. Inputs from other cortical areas arrive into layers II, III, and V. Layers II and III consist of small- to medium-sized pyramidal cells, arrayed with their apical dendrites pointing toward the cortical surface. Layer V contains much larger

pyramidal cells, also in the same orientation. The apical dendrites of the pyramidal cells in layers II, III, and V receive afferents from thalamic and cortical axons that course through layer I parallel to the cortical surface. Layer VI comprises a varied collection of neurons of different shapes and sizes (the polymorph layer). Layer III provides most projections to other cortical areas, whereas layer V provides long-range projections to the brainstem and spinal cord. The deep part of layer V projects to the striatum. Layer VI provides the reciprocal output from the cortex back to the thalamus (Figure 1.6).[138-140]

It has been known since the 1960s that the neurons in successive layers along a line drawn through the cerebral cortex perpendicular to the pial surface all tend to be concerned with similar sensory or motor processes.[141,142] These neurons form columns, of about 0.3–0.5 mm in width, in which the nerve cells share incoming signals in a vertically integrated manner. Recordings of neurons in each successive layer of a column of visual cortex, for example, all respond to bars of light in a particular orientation in a particular part of the visual field. Columns of neurons send information to one another and to higher order association areas via projection cells in layer III and, to a lesser extent, layer V.[143] In this way, columns of neurons are able to extract progressively more complex and abstract information from an incoming sensory stimulus. For example, neurons in a primary visual cortical area may be primarily concerned with simple lines, edges, and corners, but, by integrating their inputs, a neuron in a higher order visual association area may respond only to a complex shape, such as a hand or a brush.

The organization of the cortical column does not vary much from mammals with the most simple cortex, such as rodents, to primates with much larger and more complex cortical development. The depth or width of a column, for example, is only about two times larger in a primate brain compared to a rat brain. What has changed most across evolution has been the number of columns. The sheet of cortical columns in a human brain occupies approximately 2,500 cm^2, compared to 1 cm^2 in a mouse, a 2,500-fold difference that provides the massively parallel processing power needed to perform a sonata on the piano, solve a differential equation, or send a rocket to another planet.

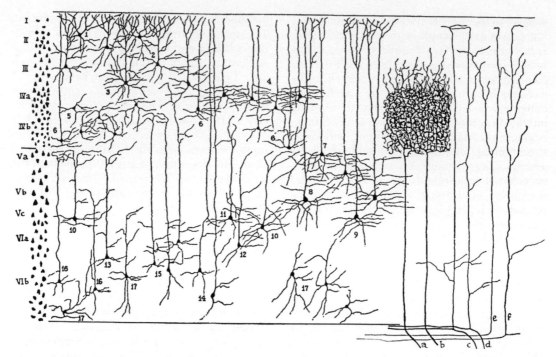

Figure 1.6 A summary drawing of the laminar organization of the neurons and inputs to the cerebral cortex. The neuronal layers of the cerebral cortex are shown at the left, as seen in a Nissl stain, and in the middle of the drawing as seen in Golgi stains. Layer I has few if any neurons. Layers II and III are composed of small pyramidal cells, and layer V of larger pyramidal cells. Layer IV contains very small granular cells, and layer VI, the polymorph layer, cells of multiple types. Axons from the thalamic relay nuclei (a, b) provide intense ramifications mainly in layer IV. Inputs from the "nonspecific system," which includes the ascending arousal system, ramify more diffusely, predominantly in layers II, III, and V (c, d). Axons from other cortical areas ramify mainly in layers II, III, and V (e, f).

From Lorente de No R. Cerebral cortex: architecture, intracortical connections, motor projections. In Fulton JF. *Physiology of the Nervous System*. Oxford University Press, New York, 1938, pp. 291–340. By permission of Oxford University Press.

An important principle of cortical organization is that neurons in different areas of the cerebral cortex specialize in certain types of operations. In a young human brain, before school age, it is possible for cortical functions to reorganize themselves to an astonishing degree if one area of cortex is damaged. However, the organization of cortical information processing goes through a series of critical stages during development, in which the maturing cortex gives up a degree of plasticity but demonstrates improved efficiency of processing.[144,145] In adults, the ability to perform a specific cognitive process may be irretrievably assigned to a region of cortex, and, when that area is damaged, the individual not only loses the ability to perform that operation, but also loses the very concept that information of that type exists. Hence, the individual with a large right parietal infarct not only loses the ability to appreciate stimuli from the left side of space,

but also loses the concept that there is a left side of space.[146] We have witnessed a patient with a large right parietal lobe tumor who ate only the food on the right side of her plate; when done, she would get up and turn around to the right until the remaining food appeared on her right side because she was entirely unable to conceive that the plate or space itself had a left side. Similarly, a patient with aphasia due to damage to Wernicke's area in the dominant temporal lobe not only cannot appreciate the language symbol content of speech, but also can no longer comprehend that language symbols are an operative component of speech. Such a patient continues to speak meaningless babble and is frustrated that others no longer understand his speech because the very concept that language symbols are embedded in speech eludes him.

This concept of fractional loss of consciousness is critical because it explains confusional states caused by focal cortical lesions.[1] It is also a common observation by clinicians that, if the cerebral cortex is damaged acutely and bilaterally in multiple locations by a multifocal disorder, it can cause an impairment of consciousness that, at its most severe, can verge on coma. However, this is never seen with purely unilateral cortical damage. The best example of this is the Wada test, a procedure in which the localization of language function can be assessed prior to surgery by an injection of a short-acting barbiturate into the carotid artery to anesthetize one hemisphere at a time. When the left hemisphere is acutely anesthetized, the patient gives the appearance of confusion and is typically placid but difficult to test due to the absence of language skills. When the patient recovers, he or she typically is amnestic for the event because much of memory is encoded verbally. Following a right hemisphere injection, the patient also typically appears to be confused and is unable to orient to his or her surroundings, but can answer simple questions and perform simple commands. The experience also may not be remembered clearly, perhaps because of the sudden inability to encode visuospatial memory.

However, the patient does not appear to be unconscious when either hemisphere is acutely anesthetized. An important principle is that *impairment of consciousness with a lesion that apparently affects only a single hemisphere implies that the injury is more widespread* (e.g., a unilateral space-occupying lesion may compress the diencephalon or midbrain, or an acute infarct of one hemisphere may be accompanied by more widespread ischemia). However, loss of consciousness is not a feature of unilateral carotid disease unless both hemispheres are supplied by a single carotid artery or the patient has had a subsequent seizure.

The concept of the cerebral cortex as a massively parallel processor introduces the question of how all of these parallel streams of information are eventually integrated into a single consciousness, a conundrum that has been called the *binding problem*.[147,148] Embedded in this question, however, is a supposition: that it is necessary to reassemble all aspects of our experience into a single whole so that they can be monitored by an internal being, like a small person or *homunculus* watching a television screen. Although most people believe that they

experience consciousness in this way, there is no a priori reason why such a self-experience cannot be the neurophysiologic outcome of the massively parallel processing (i.e., the illusion of reassembly, without the brain actually requiring that to occur in physical space). For example, people experience the visual world as an unbroken scene. However, each of us has a pair of holes in the visual fields where the optic nerves penetrate the retina. This blind spot can be demonstrated by passing a small, brightly colored object along the visual horizon until it crosses the macula, at which point it disappears. However, the visual field is "seen" by the conscious self as a single unbroken expanse, and this hole is papered over with whatever visual material borders it. If the brain can produce this type of conscious impression in the absence of reality, there is no reason to think that it requires a physiologic reassembly of other stimuli for presentation to a central homunculus. Rather, consciousness may be conceived as a property of the integrated activity of the two cerebral hemispheres and not in need of a separate physical manifestation.

Despite this view of consciousness as an "emergent" property of hemispheric information processing, the hemispheres do require a mechanism for arriving at a singularity of thought and action. If each of the independent information streams in the cortical parallel processor could separately command motor responses, human movement would be a hopeless confusion of jumbled activities. A good example is seen in patients in whom the corpus callosum has been transected to prevent spread of epileptic seizures.[149] In such "split-brain" patients, the left hand may button a shirt and the right hand follow along right behind it unbuttoning. If independent action of the two hemispheres can be so disconcerting, one could only imagine the effect of each stream of cortical processing commanding its own plan of action.

The brain requires a funnel to narrow down the choices from all of the possible modes of action to the single plan of motor behavior that will be pursued. The physical substrate of this process is the basal ganglia. All cortical regions provide input to the striatum (caudate, putamen, nucleus accumbens, and olfactory tubercle). The output from the striatum is predominantly to the globus pallidus, which it inhibits by using the neurotransmitter

GABA.[150,151] The pallidal output pathways, in turn, also are GABAergic and constitutively inhibit the motor thalamus, so that when the striatal inhibitory input to the pallidum is activated, movement is disinhibited. By constricting all motor responses that are not specifically activated by this system, the basal ganglia ensure a smooth and steady unitary stream of action. Basal ganglia disorders that permit too much striatal disinhibition of movement (hyperkinetic movement disorders) result in the emergence of disconnected movements that are outside this unitary stream (e.g., tics, chorea, athetosis).

Similarly, the brain is capable of following only one line of thought at a time. The conscious self is prohibited even from seeing two equally likely versions of an optical illusion simultaneously (e.g., the classic case of the ugly woman vs. the beautiful woman illusion; Figure 1.7). Rather, the self is aware of the two alternative visual interpretations alternately. Hence, if it is necessary to pursue two different tasks at the same time, they are pursued alternately rather than simultaneously until they become so automatic that they can

be performed with little conscious thought. The striatal control of thought processes is implemented by the outflow from the ventral striatum to the ventral pallidum, which in turn inhibits the mediodorsal thalamic nucleus, the relay nucleus for the prefrontal cortex.[151,152] By selectively disinhibiting prefrontal thought processes, the striatum ensures that a single line of thought and a unitary view of self will be expressed from the multipath network of the cerebral cortex.

An interesting philosophic question is raised by the hyperkinetic movement disorders, in which the tics, chorea, and athetosis are thought to represent "involuntary movements." But the use of the term "involuntary" again presupposes a homunculus that is in control and making "voluntary" decisions. Instead, the interrelationship of involuntary movements, which the self feels "compelled" to make, with "self-willed" movements is complex. Patients with movement disorders often can inhibit the unwanted movements for a while but feel uncomfortable doing so, and they often report pleasurable release when they can carry out the action. Again, the

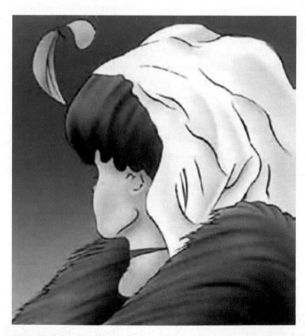

Figure 1.7 A classic optical illusion, illustrating the inability of the brain to view the same scene simultaneously in two different ways. The image of the ugly, older woman or the pretty younger woman may be seen alternately, but not at the same time, as the same visual elements are used in two different percepts.
From Hill WE, "My Wife and My Mother-in-Law," 1915, for *Puck* magazine. Used by permission. All rights reserved.

conscious state is best considered as an emergent property of brain function, rather than directing it.

Similarly, hyperkinetic movement disorders may be associated with disinhibition of larger scale behaviors and even thought processes. In this view, thought disorders can be conceived as chorea (derailing) and dystonia (fixed delusions) of thought. Inappropriate release of prefrontal cortex inhibition may even permit the striatum to drive mental imagery, producing hallucinations. Under such conditions, we have a tendency to believe that somehow the conscious self is a homunculus that is being tricked by hallucinatory sensory experiences or is unable to command thought processes. In fact, it may be more accurate to view the sensory experience and the behavior as manifestations of an altered consciousness due to malfunction of the brain's machinery for maintaining a unitary flow of thought and action.

Neurologists tend to take the mechanistic perspective that all that we observe is due to action of the nervous system behaving according to fundamental principles. Hence, the evaluation of the comatose patient becomes an exercise in applying those principles to the evaluation of a human with brain failure.

Structural Lesions that Cause Altered Consciousness in Humans

To produce stupor or coma in humans, a disorder must damage or depress the function of either extensive areas of both cerebral hemispheres or the ascending arousal system, including the paramedian region of the upper brainstem or the diencephalon on both sides of the brain. Figure 1.8 illustrates examples of such lesions that may cause coma. Conversely, unilateral hemispheric lesions, or lesions of the brainstem at the level of the midpons or below, do not cause coma. Figure 1.9 illustrates several such cases that may cause profound sensory and motor deficits but do not impair consciousness.

BILATERAL HEMISPHERIC DAMAGE

Bilateral and extensive damage to the cerebral cortex occurs most often in the context of hypoxic-ischemic insult. The initial response

to loss of cerebral blood flow (CBF) or insufficient oxygenation of the blood includes loss of consciousness. Even if blood flow or oxygenation is restored after 5 or more minutes, there may be widespread cortical injury and neuronal loss even in the absence of frank infarction.[153,154] The typical appearance pathologically is that neurons in layers III and V (which receive the most glutamatergic input from other cortical areas) and in the CA1 region of the hippocampus (which receives extensive glutamatergic input from both the CA3 fields and the entorhinal cortex) demonstrate eosinophilia in the first few days after the injury. Later, the neurons undergo pyknosis and apoptotic cell death (Figure 1.10). The net result is pseudolaminar necrosis, in which the cerebral cortex and the CA1 region both are depopulated of pyramidal cells.

Alternatively, in some patients with less extreme cortical hypoxia, there may be a lucid interval in which the patient appears to recover, followed by a subsequent deterioration. Such a case is described in Historical Vignette Patient 1.1. (Throughout this book we will use historical vignettes to describe cases that occurred before the modern era of neurologic diagnosis and treatment in which the natural history of a disorder unfolded in a way in which it would seldom do today. Fortunately, most such cases included pathologic assessment, which is also all too infrequent in modern cases.)

Historical Vignette Patient 1.1

A 59-year-old man was found unconscious in a room filled with natural gas. A companion already had died, apparently the result of an attempted double suicide. On admission, the man was unresponsive. His blood pressure was 120/80 mm Hg, pulse 120, and respirations 18 and regular. His rectal temperature was 102°F. His stretch reflexes were hypoactive, and plantar responses were absent. Coarse rhonchi were heard throughout both lung fields.

He was treated with nasal oxygen and began to awaken in 30 hours. On the second hospital day he was alert and oriented. On the fourth day he was afebrile, his chest was clear, and he ambulated. The neurologic examination was normal, and an evaluation by a psychiatrist revealed a clear sensorium with "no evidence of organic brain damage." He was

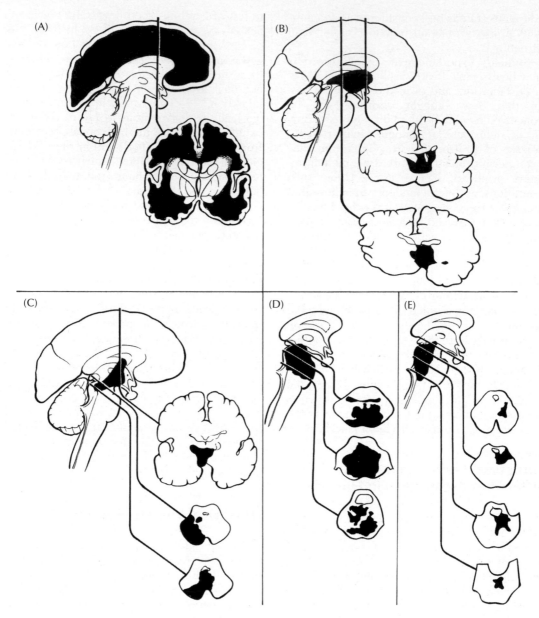

Figure 1.8 Brain lesions that cause coma. (A) Diffuse hemispheric damage, for example, due to hypoxic-ischemic encephalopathy (see Patient Vignette 1.1). (B) Diencephalic injury, as in a patient with a tumor destroying the hypothalamus. (C) Damage to the paramedian portion of the upper midbrain and caudal diencephalon, as in a patient with a tip of the basilar embolus. (D) High pontine and lower midbrain paramedian tegmental injury (e.g., in a case of basilar artery occlusion). (E) Pontine hemorrhage, because it produces compression of the surrounding brainstem, can cause dysfunction that extends beyond the area of the tissue loss. This case shows the residual area of injury at autopsy 7 months after a pontine hemorrhage. The patient was comatose during the first 2 months.

discharged to the care of relatives 9 days after the anoxic event.

At home he remained well for 2 days but then became quiet, speaking only when spoken to. The following day he merely shuffled about

and responded in monosyllables. The next day (13 days after the anoxia) he became incontinent and unable to walk, swallow, or chew. He neither spoke to nor recognized his family. He was admitted to a private psychiatric hospital

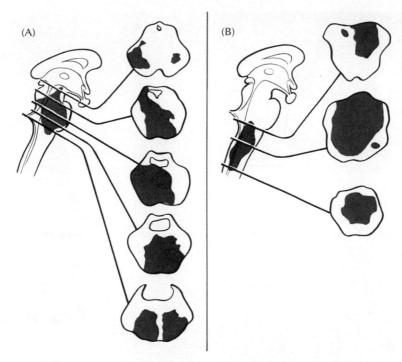

Figure 1.9 Lesions of the brainstem may be very large without causing coma if they do not involve the ascending arousal system bilaterally. (A) Even an extensive infarction at the mesopontine level that does not include the dorsolateral pons on one side and leaves intact the paramedian midbrain can result in preservation of consciousness. (B) Lesions at a low pontine and medullary level, even if they involve a hemorrhage, do not impair consciousness. (Patient Vignette 1.2, p. 33)

with the diagnosis of depression. Deterioration continued, and 28 days after the initial anoxia he was readmitted to the hospital. His blood pressure was 170/100 mm Hg, pulse 100, respirations 24, and temperature 101°F. There were coarse rales at both lung bases. He perspired profusely and constantly. He did not respond to pain, but would open his eyes momentarily to loud sounds. His extremities were flexed and rigid, his deep tendon reflexes were hyperactive, and his plantar responses extensor. Laboratory studies, including examination of the spinal fluid, were normal. He died 3 days later.

An autopsy examination showed diffuse bronchopneumonia. The brain was grossly normal. There was no cerebral swelling. Coronal sections appeared normal with no evidence of pallidal necrosis. Histologically, neurons in the motor cortex, hippocampus, cerebellum, and occipital lobes appeared generally well preserved, although a few sections showed minimal cytodegenerative changes and reduction of neurons. There was

occasional perivascular lymphocytic infiltration. Pathologic changes were not present in blood vessels, nor was there any interstitial edema. The striking alteration was diffuse demyelination involving all lobes of the cerebral hemispheres and sparing only the arcuate fibers (the immediately subcortical portion of the cerebral white matter). Axons were also reduced in number but were better preserved than was the myelin. Oligodendroglia were preserved in demyelinated areas. Reactive astrocytes were considerably increased. The brainstem and cerebellum were histologically intact. The condition of delayed postanoxic cerebral demyelination observed in this patient is discussed at greater length in Chapter 5.

Another major class of patients with bilateral hemispheric damage causing coma is those who suffer brain trauma.[155] These cases usually do not present a diagnostic dilemma as there is usually history or external evidence

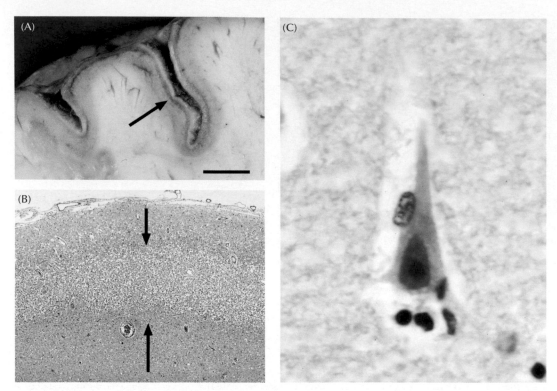

Figure 1.10 Hypoxia typically causes more severe damage to large pyramidal cells in the cerebral cortex and hippocampus compared to surrounding structures. (A) shows a low magnification view of the cerebral cortex illustrating pseudolaminar necrosis (arrow), which parallels the pial surface. At higher magnification (B), the area of necrosis involves layers II to V of the cerebral cortex, which contains the large pyramidal cells (region between the two arrows). (C) At high magnification, surviving neurons are pyknotic and eosinophilic, indicating hypoxic injury. Scale in A = 8 mm, B = 0.6 mm, and C = 15 micrometers. Photographs courtesy of Dr. Jeffrey Joseph.

of trauma to suggest the cause of the impaired consciousness. On the other hand, bilateral subdural hematomas can compress both hemispheres and the diencephalon, but the trauma that caused them may have been so mild it is not recalled. The compression is generally worsened by edema of the underlying brain, and the clinical state of the patient can fluctuate, making it very difficult to diagnose (see Chapter 4).

DIENCEPHALIC INJURY

The relay nuclei of the thalamus provide the largest ascending source of input to the cerebral cortex. As a result, it is no exaggeration to say that virtually any deficit due to injury of a discrete cortical area can be mimicked by injury to its thalamic relay

nucleus.[156] Hence, thalamic lesions that are sufficiently extensive can produce the same result as bilateral cortical injury. The most common cause of such lesions is the "tip of the basilar" syndrome, in which vascular occlusion of the perforating arteries that arise from the basilar apex or the first segment of the posterior cerebral arteries can produce bilateral thalamic infarction.[157] In the syndrome of the artery of Percheron, there can be a single vessel emerging from the tip of the basilar that supplies the medial thalamus on both sides.[158] However, careful examination of the MRI scans of such patients (or of their brains postmortem) usually shows some damage as well to the paramedian midbrain reticular formation and often to the posterior hypothalamus. Other causes of primarily thalamic damage include thalamic hemorrhage, local infiltrating tumors, and rare cases of diencephalic inflammatory lesions (e.g., Behçet's syndrome).[159,160] However, there are no convincing cases of isolated thalamic lesions that caused a comatose state. Rather, such patients, as in Box 1-2, appear to be in a persistent vegetative state, with preserved arousal and sleep cycles, but without content.

Another example of severe thalamic injury causing coma was reported by Kinney and colleagues in the brain of Karen Anne Quinlan, a famous medicolegal case of a woman who remained in a PVS (Chapter 9) for many years after a hypoxic brain injury.[161] Examination of her brain at the time of death disclosed unexpectedly widespread thalamic neuronal loss. There was also extensive damage to other brain areas, including the cerebral cortex, so that the thalamic damage alone may not have caused the clinical loss of consciousness. However, thalamic injury is frequently found in patients with brain injuries who eventually enter a PVS (Chapter 9).[155]

Ischemic lesions of the hypothalamus are rare because the hypothalamus is literally encircled by the main vessels of the circle of Willis and is fed by local penetrating vessels from all the major arteries.[146] However, the location of the hypothalamus above the pituitary gland results in localized hypothalamic damage in cases of pituitary tumors.[162] The hypothalamus also may harbor primary lymphomas of brain, gliomas, or sarcoid granulomas. Patients with hypothalamic lesions often appear to be hypersomnolent rather than comatose. They may yawn, stretch, or sigh, features that are usually lacking in patients with coma due to brainstem lesions.

UPPER BRAINSTEM INJURY

Evidence from clinicopathologic analyses firmly establishes that the midbrain and pontine area critical to consciousness in humans includes the paramedian tegmental zone immediately ventral to the periaqueductal gray matter, from the caudal diencephalon through the rostral pons.[163,164] Numerous cases are on record of small lesions involving this territory bilaterally in which there was profound loss of consciousness (see Figure 1.11). On the other hand, we have not seen loss of consciousness with lesions confined to the medulla or the caudal pons. This

principle is illustrated by Historical Vignette Patients 1.2 and 1.3.

Historical Vignette Patient 1.2

A 62-year-old woman was referred for evaluation. Twenty-five years earlier she had developed weakness and severely impaired position and vibration sense of the right arm and leg. Two years before we saw her, she developed paralysis of the right vocal cord and wasting of the right side of the tongue, followed by insidiously progressing disability with an unsteady gait and more weakness of the right limbs. Four days before coming to the hospital, she became much weaker on the right side, and 2 days later she lost the ability to swallow.

When she entered the hospital she was alert and in full possession of her faculties. She had no difficulty breathing and her blood pressure was 162/110 mm Hg. She had upbeat nystagmus on upward gaze and decreased appreciation of pinprick on the left side of the face. The right sides of the pharynx, palate, and tongue were paralyzed. The right arm and leg were weak and atrophic, consistent with disuse. Stretch reflexes below the neck were bilaterally brisk, and the right plantar response was extensor. Position and vibratory sensations were reduced on the right side of the body, and the appreciation of pinprick was reduced on the left.

The next day she was still alert and responsive, but she developed difficulty in coughing and speaking, and finally she ceased breathing. An endotracheal tube was placed and mechanical ventilation was begun. Later, on that third hospital day, she was still bright and alert and quickly and accurately answered questions by nodding or shaking her head. The opening pressure of cerebrospinal fluid (CSF) at lumbar puncture was 180 mm of water (normal <160), and the xanthochromic fluid contained 8,500 red blood cells/mm^3 (normal <5) and 14 white blood cells/mm^3 (normal <5).

She lived for 23 more days. During that time she developed complete somatic motor paralysis below the face. Several hypotensive crises were treated promptly with infusions of pressor agents, but no pressor drugs were needed during the last 2 weeks of life. Intermittently during those final days, she had brief periods of unresponsiveness, but

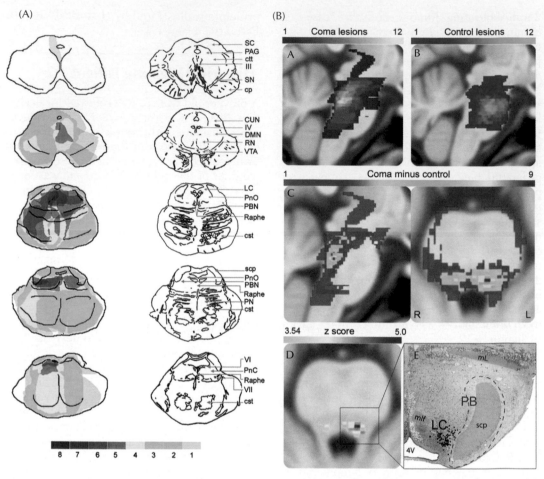

Figure 1.11 Brainstem lesions that cause coma. (A) shows a series of drawings illustrating levels through the brain-stem at which lesions caused impairment of consciousness. For each case, the extent of the injury at each level was plotted, and the colors indicate the number of cases that involved injury to that area. (B) shows a subtractive analysis, comparing the brainstem lesions in 13 patients with coma (subpanel A) to those in 12 patients without coma (subpanel B). Subpanels C subtract the control lesions from the coma lesions, and subpanel D shows the site that most intensely correlates with loss of consciousness. This region (red and yellow pixels) is just ventral to the locus coeruleus (LC) and includes the medial parabrachial nucleus (PB) on the left side of the brain (subpanel E). mL, medial lemniscus; mlf, medial longitudinal fasciculus; scp, superior cerebellar peduncle.

Panel A from Parvizi and Damasio[163] with permission. Panel B. subpanels A–E from Fischer et al.,[164] with permission.

then awakened and signaled quickly and appropriately to questions demanding a yes or no answer and opened or closed her eyes and moved them laterally when commanded to do so. There was no other voluntary movement. Four days before she died, she developed ocular bobbing when commanded to look laterally, but although she consistently responded to commands by moving her eyes, it was difficult to know whether or not her responses were appropriate. During the ensuing 3 days, evidence of wakefulness decreased. She died of

gastrointestinal hemorrhage 26 days after entering the hospital.

The brain at autopsy contained a moderate amount of dark, old blood overlying the right lateral medulla adjacent to the fourth ventricle. A raspberry-appearing arteriovenous malformation, 1.4 cm in greatest diameter, protruded from the right lateral medulla, beginning with its lower border 2.5 cm caudal to the obex. On section, the vascular malformation was seen to originate in the central medulla and to extend rostrally to approximately

2 mm above the obex. From this point, a large hemorrhage extended forward to destroy the central medulla all the way to the pontine junction (Figure 1.9B). Microscopic study demonstrated that, at its most cranial end, the hemorrhage destroyed the caudal part of the right vestibular nuclei and most of the adjacent lower pontine tegmentum on the right. Caudal to this, the hemorrhage widened and destroyed the entire dorsal center of the medulla from approximately the plane of the nucleus of the glossopharyngeal nerve down to just below the plane of the nucleus ambiguus. From this latter point caudally, the hemorrhage was more restricted to the reticular formation of the medulla. The margins of this lesion contained an organizing clot with phagocytosis and reticulum formation indicating a process at least 2 weeks old. The center of the hemorrhage contained a degenerating clot estimated to be at least 72 hours old; at several places along the lateral margin of the lesion were small fresh hemorrhages estimated to have occurred within a few hours of death. It was considered unlikely that the lesion had changed substantially in size or extent of destruction in the few days before death.

Historical Vignette Patient 1.3

A 65-year-old woman was admitted to the neurology service for "coma" after an anesthetic procedure. She had rheumatoid arthritis with subluxation of C1 on C2, and compression of the C2 root causing occipital neuralgia. An anesthesiologist attempted to inject the root with ethanol to eliminate the pain. Almost immediately after the injection, the patient became flaccid and experienced a respiratory arrest. On arrival in the neurology intensive care unit she was hypotensive and apneic. Mechanical ventilation was instituted and blood pressure was supported with pressors.

On examination she had spontaneous eye movements in the vertical direction only and her eyelids fluttered open and closed. There was complete flaccid paralysis of the hypoglossal, vagal, and accessory nerves, as well as all spinal motor function. Twitches of facial and jaw movement persisted. There was no

response to pinprick over the face or body. CT scan showed hypodensity of the medulla and lower pons.

The patient responded to commands to open and close her eyes and learned to communicate in this way. She lived another 12 weeks in this setting, without regaining function, and rarely was observed to sleep. No postmortem examination was permitted. However, the injection of ethanol had apparently entered the C2 root sleeve and fixed the lower brainstem up through the facial and abducens nuclei without clouding the state of consciousness of the patient.

Comment

Both of these cases demonstrate the preservation of consciousness in patients with a locked-in state due to destruction of motor pathways below the critical level of the rostral pons. Chapter 2 will explore the ways in which the neurologic examination of a comatose patient can be used to differentiate these different causes of loss of consciousness.

REFERENCES

1. Saper CB, Plum F. Disorders of consciousness. In: Frederiks JAM, ed. *Handbook of Clinical Neurology, Vol 45: Clinical Neuropsychology.* Amsterdam: Elsevier; 1985:107–128.
2. Mesulam MM, Waxman SG, Geschwind N, Sabin TD. Acute confusional states with right middle cerebral artery infarctions. *J Neurol Neurosurg Psychiatry* 1976;39:84–89.
3. Gompf HS, Mathai C, Fuller PM, et al. Locus ceruleus and anterior cingulate cortex sustain wakefulness in a novel environment. *J Neurosci* 2010;30:14543–14551.
4. Aston-Jones G, Cohen JD. Adaptive gain and the role of the locus coeruleus-norepinephrine system in optimal performance. *J Comp Neurol* 2005;493:99–110.
5. Posner JB, Plum F. The toxic effects of carbon dioxide and acetazolamide in hepatic encephalopathy. *J Clin Invest* 1960;39:1246–1258.
6. Shimojyo S, Scheinberg P, Reinmuth O. Cerebral blood flow and metabolism in the Wernicke-Korsakoff syndrome. *J Clin Invest* 1967;46:849–854.
7. American Psychiatric Association. *Diagnostic and Statistical Manual of Mental Disorders.* 5th edition. Washington, DC: American Psychiatric Association; 2013.
8. Fong TG, Jones RN, Shi P, et al. Delirium accelerates cognitive decline in Alzheimer disease. *Neurology* 2009;72:1570–1575.

9. Inouye SK, van Dyck CH, Alessi CA, Balkin S, Siegal AP, Horwitz RI. Clarifying confusion: the confusion assessment method. A new method for detection of delirium. *Ann Intern Med* 1990;113:941–948.
10. Marcantonio ER. Delirium in hospitalized older adults. *N Engl J Med* 2018;378:96–97.
11. Guan X-M, Peroutka SJ. Basic mechanisms of action of drugs used in treatment of essential tremor. *Clin Neuropharmacol* 1990;13:210–223.
12. Markand ON. Eectroencephalogram in "locked-in" syndrome. *Electroencephalogr Clin Neurophysiol* 1976;40:529–534.
13. Markand ON, Dyken ML. Sleep abnormalities in patients with brain stem lesions. *Neurology* 1976;26:769–776.
14. Saper CB. Is there even such a thing as "idiopathic normal pressure hydrocephalus"? *Ann Neurol* 2017;82:514–515.
15. Davis DH, Muniz-Terrera G, Keage HA, et al. Association of delirium with cognitive decline in late life: a neuropathologic study of 3 population-based cohort studies. *JAMA Psychiatry* 2017;74:244–251.
16. Saini P, Rye DB. Hypersomnia: evaluation, treatment, and social and economic aspects. *Sleep Med Clin* 2017;12:47–60.
17. Leu-Semenescu S, Quera-Salva MA, Dauvilliers Y. French consensus. Idiopathic hypersomnia: investigations and follow-up. *Rev Neurol (Paris)* 2017;173:32–37.
18. Giacino JT. The vegetative and minimally conscious states: consensus-based criteria for establishing diagnosis and prognosis. *NeuroRehabilitation* 2004;19:293–298.
19. Naccache L. Minimally conscious state or cortically mediated state? *Brain* 2018;141:949–960.
20. Laureys S, Celesia GG, Cohadon F, et al. Unresponsive wakefulness syndrome: a new name for the vegetative state or apallic syndrome. *BMC Med* 2010;8:68.
21. American Neurological Association. Persistent vegetative state: report of the American Neurological Association Committee on Ethical Affairs. ANA Committee on Ethical Affairs. *Ann Neurol* 1993;33:386–390.
22. Wijdicks EFM. How Harvard defined irreversible coma. *Neuro Crit Care* 2018;29:136–141.
23. Towbin A. The respirator brain death syndrome. *Human Pathol* 1973;4:583–594.
24. Wijdicks EF, Varelas PN, Gronseth GS, Greer DM. Evidence-based guideline update: determining brain death in adults: report of the Quality Standards Subcommittee of the American Academy of Neurology. *Neurology* 2010;74:1911–1918.
25. Practice parameters for determining brain death in adults (summary statement). The Quality Standards Subcommittee of the American Academy of Neurology. *Neurology* 1995;45:1012–1014.
26. Criteria for the diagnosis of brain stem death. Review by a working group convened by the Royal College of Physicians and endorsed by the Conference of Medical Royal Colleges and their Faculties in the United Kingdom. *J R Coll Phys London* 1995;29:381–382.
27. McDonald D, Stewart-Perrin B, Shankar JJS. The role of neuroimaging in the determination of brain death. *J Neuroimaging* 2018;28:374–379.
28. Jackson JH. *Selected Writings of John Hughlings Jackson*. London: Hode and Stoughton; 1931.
29. Mauthner L. Sur pathologie und physiologie des schlafes nebst bermerkungen ueher die "nona." *Wien Klin Wochenschr* 1890;40:961–1185.
30. Von Economo C. Sleep as a problem of localization. *J Nerv Ment Dis* 1930;71:249–259.
31. Ranson SW. Somnolence caused by hypothalamic lesions in monkeys. *Arch Neurol Psychiatr* 1939;41:1–23.
32. Nauta WJH. Hypothalamic regulation of sleep in rats. An experimental study. *J Neurophysiol* 1946;9:285–314.
33. Swett CP, Hobson JA. The effects of posterior hypothalamic lesions on behavioral and electrographic manifestations of sleep and waking in cat. *Arch Ital Biol* 1968;106:270–282.
34. McGinty DJ, Sterman MB. Sleep suppression after basal forebrain lesions in the cat. *Science* 1968;160:1253–1255.
35. Westphal C. Eigenthümlichemit einschläfen verbundene anfälle. *Arch Psychiat* 1877;7:631–635.
36. Gelineau JB. De la narcolepsie. *Gaz Hop (Paris)* 1880;53:626f.
37. Wilson SAK. *The Narcolepsies. Modern Problems in Neurology*. London: Edward Arnold & Co.; 1928:76–119.
38. Berger H. Ueber das electroenkephalogramm des menschen. *Arch Psychiatr Nervenkr* 1929;87:527–570.
39. Adrian ED, Matthews BH. The interpretation of potential waves in the cortex. *J Physiol* 1934;81:440–471.
40. Bremer F. Cerveau "isole" et physiologie du somneil. *C R Soc Biol* 1935;118:1235–1241.
41. Moruzzi G, Magoun HW. Brain stem reticular formation and activation of the EEG. *Electroencephalogr Clin Neuro* 1949;1:455–473.
42. Starzl TE, Taylor CW, Magoun HW. Ascending conduction in reticular activating system, with special reference to the diencephalon. *J Neurophysiol* 1951;14:461–477.
43. Zernicki B, Gandolfo G, Glin L, Gottesmann C. Cerveau isole and pretrigeminal rat preparations. *Physiol Bohemoslov* 1985;34 Suppl:183–185.:183–185.
44. Magni F, Moruzzi G, Rossi GF, Zanchetti A. EEG arousal following inactivation of the lower brainstem by selective injection of barbiturate into the vertebral circulation. *Arch Ital Biol* 1959;97:33–46.
45. Hallanger AE, Levey AI, Lee HJ, Rye DB, Wainer BH. The origins of cholinergic and other subcortical afferents to the thalamus in the rat. *J Comp Neurol* 1987;262:105–124.
46. McCormick DA, Bal T. Sleep and arousal: thalamocortical mechanisms. *Annu Rev Neurosci* 1997;20:185–215.
47. Boucetta S, Cisse Y, Mainville L, Morales M, Jones BE. Discharge profiles across the sleep-waking cycle of identified cholinergic, GABAergic, and glutamatergic neurons in the pontomesencephalic tegmentum of the rat. *J Neurosci* 2014;34:4708–4727.
48. Saper CB, Fuller PM, Pedersen NP, Lu J, Scammell TE. Sleep state switching. *Neuron* 2010;68:1023–1042.
49. Steriade M. Synchronized activities of coupled oscillators in the cerebral cortex and thalamus at different levels of vigilance. *Cereb Cortex* 1997;7:583–604.
50. Fuller PM, Sherman D, Pedersen NP, Saper CB, Lu J. Reassessment of the structural basis of the ascending arousal system. *J Comp Neurol* 2011;519:933–956.

51. Hassani OK, Lee MG, Henny P, Jones BE. Discharge profiles of identified GABAergic in comparison to cholinergic and putative glutamatergic basal forebrain neurons across the sleep-wake cycle. *J Neurosci* 2009;29:11828–11840.

52. Hangya B, Borhegyi Z, Szilagyi N, Freund TF, Varga V. GABAergic neurons of the medial septum lead the hippocampal network during theta activity. *J Neurosci* 2009;29:8094–8102.

53. Freund TF, Meskenaite V. Gamma-aminobutyric acid-containing basal forebrain neurons innervate inhibitory interneurons in the neocortex. *Proc Natl Acad Sci U S A* 1992;89:738–742.

54. Hu H, Gan J, Jonas P. Interneurons. Fast-spiking, parvalbumin(+) GABAergic interneurons: from cellular design to microcircuit function. *Science* 2014; 345:1255263.

55. Aserinsky E, Kleitman N. Regularly occurring periods of eye motility, and concomitant phenomena, during sleep. *Science* 1953;118:273–274.

56. Kales A, Vela-Bueno A, Kales JD. Sleep disorders: sleep apnea and narcolepsy. *Ann Intern Med* 1987; 106:434–443.

57. Vgontzas AN, Kales A. Sleep and its disorders. *Annu Rev Med* 1999;50:387–400.

58. Lim AS, Ellison BA, Wang JL, et al. Sleep is related to neuron numbers in the ventrolateral preoptic/intermediate nucleus in older adults with and without Alzheimer's disease. *Brain* 2014;137:2847–2861.

59. Loughlin SE, Foote SL, Fallon JH. Locus coeruleus projections to cortex: topography, morphology and collateralization. *Brain Res Bull* 1982;9:287–294.

60. Bobillier P, Seguin S, Petitjean F, Salvert D, Touret M, Jouvet M. The raphe nuclei of the cat brain stem: a topographical atlas of their efferent projections as revealed by autoradiography. *Brain Res* 1976;113:449–486.

61. Lu J, Jhou TC, Saper CB. Identification of wake-active dopaminergic neurons in the ventral periaqueductal gray matter. *J Neurosci* 2006;26:193–202.

62. Cho JR, Treweek JB, Robinson JE, et al. Dorsal raphe dopamine neurons modulate arousal and promote wakefulness by salient stimuli. *Neuron* 2017;94:1205–1219.

63. Foote SL, Bloom FE, Aston-Jones G. Nucleus locus ceruleus: new evidence of anatomical and physiological specificity. *Physiol Rev* 1983;63:844–914.

64. Steininger TL, Alam MN, Gong H, Szymusiak R, McGinty D. Sleep-waking discharge of neurons in the posterior lateral hypothalamus of the albino rat. *Brain Res* 1999;840:138–147.

65. Jacobs BL. Single unit activity of locus coeruleus neurons in behaving animals. *Prog Neurobiol* 1986;27:183–194.

66. Trulson ME, Jacobs BL, Morrison AR. Raphe unit activity during REM sleep in normal cats and in pontine lesioned cats displaying REM sleep without atonia. *Brain Res* 1981;226:75–91.

67. Eban-Rothschild A, Rothschild G, Giardino WJ, Jones JR, de LL. VTA dopaminergic neurons regulate ethologically relevant sleep-wake behaviors. *Nat Neurosci* 2016;19:1356–1366.

68. Carter ME, Yizhar O, Chikahisa S, et al. Tuning arousal with optogenetic modulation of locus coeruleus neurons. *Nat Neurosci* 2010;13:1526–1533.

69. Fujita A, Bonnavion P, Wilson MH, et al. Hypothalamic tuberomammillary nucleus neurons: electrophysiological diversity and essential role in arousal stability. *J Neurosci* 2017;37:9574–9592.

70. Ito H, Yanase M, Yamashita A, et al. Analysis of sleep disorders under pain using an optogenetic tool: possible involvement of the activation of dorsal raphe nucleus-serotonergic neurons. *Molecular brain* 2013;6:59.

71. Sato H, Fox K, Daw NW. Effect of electrical stimulation of locus coeruleus on the activity of neurons in the cat visual cortex. *J Neurophysiol* 1989;62:946–958.

72. Bassant MH, Ennouri K, Lamour Y. Effects of iontophoretically applied monoamines on somatosensory cortical neurons of unanesthetized rats. *Neuroscience* 1990;39:431–439.

73. Salgado H, Garcia-Oscos F, Martinolich L, et al. Pre- and postsynaptic effects of norepinephrine on gamma-aminobutyric acid-mediated synaptic transmission in layer 2/3 of the rat auditory cortex. *Synapse* 2012;66:20–28.

74. Anaclet C, Ferrari L, Arrigoni E, et al. The GABAergic parafacial zone is a medullary slow wave sleep-promoting center. *Nat Neurosci* 2014;17:1217–1224.

75. Hallanger AE, Levey AI, Lee HJ, Rye DB, Wainer BH. The origins of cholinergic and other subcortical afferents to the thalamus in the rat. *J Comp Neurol* 1987;262:105–124.

76. Edwards SB, de Olmos JS. Autoradiographic studies of the projections of the midbrain reticular formation: ascending projections of nucleus cuneiformis. *J Comp Neurol* 165:417–431.

77. Saper CB. Organization of cerebral cortical afferent systems in the rat. II. Hypothalamocortical projections. *J Comp Neurol* 1985;237:21.

78. Pedersen NP, Ferrari L, Venner A, et al. Supramammillary glutamate neurons are a key node of the arousal system. *Nat Commun* 2017;8:1405.

79. Peyron C, Tighe DK, van den Pol AN, et al. Neurons containing hypocretin (orexin) project to multiple neuronal systems. *J Neurosci* 1998;18:9996–10015.

80. Panula P, Airaksinen MS, Pirvola U, Kotilainen E. A histamine-containing neuronal system in human brain. *Neuroscience* 1990;34:127–132.

81. Köhler C, Swanson LW, Haglund L, Wu JY. The cytoarchitecture, histochemistry and projections of the tuberomammillary nucleus in the rat. *Neuroscience* 1985;16:85–110.

82. Haglund L, Swanson LW, Kohler C. The projection of the supramammillary nucleus to the hippocampal formation: an immunohistochemical and anterograde transport study with the lectin PHA-L in the rat. *J Comp Neurol* 1984;229:171–185.

83. Welch MJ, Meltzer EO, Simons FE. H1-antihistamines and the central nervous system. *Clin Allergy Immunol* 2002;17:337–388.:337–388.

84. Parmentier R, Ohtsu H, Djebbara-Hannas Z, Valatx JL, Watanabe T, Lin JS. Anatomical, physiological, and pharmacological characteristics of histidine decarboxylase knock-out mice: evidence for the role of brain histamine in behavioral and sleep-wake control. *J Neurosci* 2002;22:7695–7711.

85. Boulland JL, Jenstad M, Boekel AJ, et al. Vesicular glutamate and GABA transporters sort to distinct sets of vesicles in a population of presynaptic terminals. *Cereb Cortex* 2009;19:241–248.

86. Bittencourt JC, Frigo L, Rissman RA, Casatti CA, Nahon JL, Bauer JA. The distribution of melanin-concentrating hormone in the monkey brain (*Cebus apella*). *Brain Res* 1998;804:140–143.
87. Bittencourt JC, Presse F, Arias C, et al. The melanin-concentrating hormone system of the rat brain: an immunization and hybridization histochemical characterization. *J Comp Neurol* 1992;319:218–245.
88. Torrealba F, Yanagisawa M, Saper CB. Colocalization of orexin a and glutamate immunoreactivity in axon terminals in the tuberomammillary nucleus in rats. *Neuroscience* 2003;119:1033–1044.
89. Chee MJ, Arrigoni E, Maratos-Flier E. Melanin-concentrating hormone neurons release glutamate for feedforward inhibition of the lateral septum. *J Neurosci* 2015;35:3644–3651.
90. Lee MG, Hassani OK, Jones BE. Discharge of identified orexin/hypocretin neurons across the sleep-waking cycle. *J Neurosci* 2005;25:6716–6720.
91. Mileykovskiy BY, Kiyashchenko LI, Siegel JM. Behavioral correlates of activity in identified hypocretin/orexin neurons. *Neuron* 2005;46:787–798.
92. Verret L, Goutagny R, Fort P, et al. A role of melanin-concentrating hormone producing neurons in the central regulation of paradoxical sleep. *BMC Neurosci* 2003;4:19.
93. Vetrivelan R, Kong D, Ferrari LL, et al. Melanin-concentrating hormone neurons specifically promote rapid eye movement sleep in mice. *Neuroscience* 2016;336:102–113.
94. Jego S, Glasgow SD, Herrera CG, et al. Optogenetic identification of a rapid eye movement sleep modulatory circuit in the hypothalamus. *Nat Neurosci* 2013;16:1637–1643.
95. Tsunematsu T, Ueno T, Tabuchi S, et al. Optogenetic manipulation of activity and temporally controlled cell-specific ablation reveal a role for MCH neurons in sleep/wake regulation. *J Neurosci* 2014;34:6896–6909.
96. Saper CB. Organization of cerebral cortical afferent systems in the rat. I. Magnocellular basal nucleus. *J Comp Neurol* 1984;222:313–342.
97. Rye DB, Wainer BH, Mesulam MM, Mufson EJ, Saper CB. Cortical projections from the basal forebrain: a study of cholinergic and non-cholinergic components employing combined retrograde tracing and immunohistochemical localization of choline acetyltranferase. *Neuroscience* 1984;13:627–643.
98. Henny P, Jones BE. Projections from basal forebrain to prefrontal cortex comprise cholinergic, GABAergic and glutamatergic inputs to pyramidal cells or interneurons. *Eur J Neurosci* 2008;27:654–670.
99. Zaborszky L, Brownstein MJ, Palkovits M. Ascending projections to the hypothalamus and limbic nuclei from the dorsolateral pontine tegmentum: a biochemical and electron microscopic study. *Acta Morphol Acad Sci Hung* 1977;25:175–188.
100. Zaborszky L, Cullinan WE, Luine VN. Catecholaminergic-cholinergic interaction in the basal forebrain. *Prog Brain Res* 1993;98:31–49.:31–49.
101. Khateb A, Fort P, Pegna A, Jones BE, Muhlethaler M. Cholinergic nucleus basalis neurons are excited by histamine in vitro. *Neuroscience* 1995;69:495–506.
102. Price JL, Stern R. Individual cells in the nucleus basalis-diagnoal band complex have restricted axonal

projections to the cerebral cortex in the rat. *Brain Res* 1983;269:352–356.
103. Han F, Lin L, Warby SC, et al. Narcolepsy onset is seasonal and increased following the 2009 H1N1 pandemic in China. *Ann Neurol* 2011;70:410–417.
104. Partinen M, Kornum BR, Plazzi G, Jennum P, Julkunen I, Vaarala O. Narcolepsy as an autoimmune disease: the role of H1N1 infection and vaccination. *Lancet Neurol* 2014;13:600–613.
105. Scammell TE. The neurobiology, diagnosis, and treatment of narcolepsy. *Ann Neurol* 2003;53:154–166.
106. Sakurai T, Amemiya A, Ishii M, et al. Orexins and orexin receptors: a family of hypothalamic neuropeptides and G protein-coupled receptors that regulate feeding behavior. *Cell* 1998;92:573–585.
107. de Lecea L, Kilduff TS, Peyron C, et al. The hypocretins: hypothalamus-specific peptides with neuroexcitatory activity. *Proc Natl Acad Sci U S A* 1998;95:322–327.
108. Willie JT, Chemelli RM, Sinton CM, Yanagisawa M. To eat or to sleep? Orexin in the regulation of feeding and wakefulness. *Annu Rev Neurosci* 2001;24:429–458.:429–458.
109. Chemelli RM, Willie JT, Sinton CM, et al. Narcolepsy in orexin knockout mice: molecular genetics of sleep regulation. *Cell* 1999;98:437–451.
110. Lin L, Faraco J, Li R, et al. The sleep disorder canine narcolepsy is caused by a mutation in the hypocretin (orexin) receptor 2 gene. *Cell* 1999;98:365–376.
111. Marcus JN, Aschkenasi CJ, Lee CE, et al. Differential expression of orexin receptors 1 and 2 in the rat brain. *J Comp Neurol* 2001;435:6–25.
112. Richardson RT, DeLong MR. Context-dependent responses of primate nucleus basalis neurons in a go/no-go task. *J Neurosci* 1990;10:2528–2540.
113. Harrison TC, Pinto L, Brock JR, Dan Y. Calcium imaging of basal forebrain activity during innate and learned behaviors. *Front Neural Circuits* 2016;10:36.
114. Kim T, Thankachan S, McKenna JT, et al. Cortically projecting basal forebrain parvalbumin neurons regulate cortical gamma band oscillations. *Proc Natl Acad Sci U S A* 2015;112:3535–3540.
115. Anaclet C, Pedersen NP, Ferrari LL, et al. Basal forebrain control of wakefulness and cortical rhythms. *Nat Commun* 2015;6:8744. doi:10.1038/ncomms9744.:8744.
116. Xu M, Chung S, Zhang S, et al. Basal forebrain circuit for sleep-wake control. *Nat Neurosci* 2015;18:1641–1647.
117. Sohal VS, Zhang F, Yizhar O, Deisseroth K. Parvalbumin neurons and gamma rhythms enhance cortical circuit performance. *Nature* 2009;459:698–702.
118. Fisher CM. The neurological examination of the comatose patient. *Acta Neurol Scand* 1969;45:Suppl 36:1–56.
119. Sherin JE, Shiromani PJ, McCarley RW, Saper CB. Activation of ventrolateral preoptic neurons during sleep. *Science* 1996;271:216–219.
120. Sherin JE, Elmquist JK, Torrealba F, Saper CB. Innervation of histaminergic tuberomammillary neurons by GABAergic and galaninergic neurons in the ventrolateral preoptic nucleus of the rat. *J Neurosci* 1998;18:4705–4721.
121. Saper CB, Chou TC, Scammell TE. The sleep switch: hypothalamic control of sleep and wakefulness. *Trends Neurosci* 2001;24:726–731.

122. Szymusiak R, Alam N, Steininger TL, McGinty D. Sleep-waking discharge patterns of ventrolateral preoptic/anterior hypothalamic neurons in rats. *Brain Res* 1998;803:178–188.

123. Gaus SE, Strecker RE, Tate BA, Parker RA, Saper CB. Ventrolateral preoptic nucleus contains sleep-active, galaninergic neurons in multiple mammalian species. *Neuroscience* 2002;115:285–294.

124. Sallanon M, Denoyer M, Kitahama K, Aubert C, Gay N, Jouvet M. Long-lasting insomnia induced by preoptic neuron lesions and its transient reversal by muscimol injection into the posterior hypothalamus in the cat. *Neuroscience* 1989;32:669–683.

125. Lu J, Greco MA, Shiromani P, Saper CB. Effect of lesions of the ventrolateral preoptic nucleus on NREM and REM sleep. *J Neurosci* 2000;20:3830–3842.

126. Chung S, Weber F, Zhong P, et al. Identification of preoptic sleep neurons using retrograde labelling and gene profiling. *Nature* 2017;545:477–481.

127. Kroeger DA, Absi G, Gagliardi C, et al. Galanin neurons in the ventrolateral preoptic area promote sleep and heat loss in mice. *Nat Commun* 2018;9:4129.

128. Gong H, McGinty D, Guzman-Marin R, Chew KT, Stewart D, Szymusiak R. Activation of c-fos in GABAergic neurones in the preoptic area during sleep and in response to sleep deprivation. *J Physiol* 2004;556:935–946.

129. Harding EC, Yu X, Miao A, et al. A neuronal hub binding sleep initiation and body cooling in response to warm external stimuli. *Curr Bio* 2018;28:2263–2273.

130. Gallopin T, Fort P, Eggermann E, et al. Identification of sleep-promoting neurons in vitro. *Nature* 2000;404:992–995.

131. Nelson LE, Lu J, Guo T, Saper CB, Franks NP, Maze M. The alpha2-adrenoceptor agonist dexmedetomidine converges on an endogenous sleep-promoting pathway to exert its sedative effects. *Anesthesiology* 2003;98:428–436.

132. Yu X, Franks NP, Wisden W. Sleep and sedative states induced by targeting the histamine and noradrenergic systems. *Front Neural Circuits* 2018;12:4.

133. Lu J, Sherman D, Devor M, Saper CB. A putative flip-flop switch for control of REM sleep. *Nature* 2006;441:589–594.

134. Sapin E, Lapray D, Berod A, et al. Localization of the brainstem GABAergic neurons controlling paradoxical (REM) sleep. *PLoS One* 2009;4:e4272.

135. Lydic R, Douglas CL, Baghdoyan HA. Microinjection of neostigmine into the pontine reticular formation of C57BL/6J mouse enhances rapid eye movement sleep and depresses breathing. *Sleep* 2002;25:835–841.

136. McCarthy A, Wafford K, Shanks E, Ligocki M, Edgar DM, Dijk DJ. REM sleep homeostasis in the absence of REM sleep: effects of antidepressants. *Neuropharmacology* 2016;108:415–425.

137. Arrigoni E, Chen MC, Fuller PM. The anatomical, cellular and synaptic basis of motor atonia during rapid eye movement sleep. *J Physiol* 2016;594:5391–5414.

138. Lorente de No R. Cerebral cortex: architecture, intracortical connections, motor projections. In: Fulton JF, ed. *Physiology of the Nervous System*. New York: Oxford University Press; 1938:291–340.

139. Usrey WM, Sherman SM. Corticofugal circuits: communication lines from the cortex to the rest of the brain. *J Comp Neurol* 2018;547:640–650.

140. Palomero-Gallagher N, Zilles K. Cortical layers: cyto-, myelo-, receptor- and synaptic architecture in human cortical areas. *Neuroimage* 2017 Aug 12. pii: S1053-8119(17)30682-1.

141. Hubel DH, Wiesel TN. Shape and arrangement of columns in cat's striate cortex. *J Physiol* 1963;165:559–568.:559–568.

142. McCasland JS, Woolsey TA. High-resolution 2-deoxyglucose mapping of functional cortical columns in mouse barrel cortex. *J Comp Neurol* 1988;278:555–569.

143. Gilbert CD, Wiesel TN. Columnar specificity of intrinsic horizontal and corticocortical connections in cat visual cortex. *J Neurosci* 1989;9:2432–2442.

144. Hubel DH, Wiesel TN. The period of susceptibility to the physiological effects of unilateral eye closure in kittens. *J Physiol* 1970;206:419–436.

145. Frank MG, Issa NP, Stryker MP. Sleep enhances plasticity in the developing visual cortex. *Neuron* 2001;30:275–287.

146. Saper CB. Hypothalamus. In: Mai JK, Paxinos G, eds. *The Human Nervous System*. 3rd ed. Amsterdam: Elsevier; 2012:548–583.

147. Hardcastle VG. Consciousness and the neurobiology of perceptual binding. *Semin Neurol* 1997;17:163–170.

148. Revonsuo A. Binding and the phenomenal unity of consciousness. *Conscious Cogn* 1999;8:173–185.

149. Nishikawa T, Okuda J, Mizuta I, et al. Conflict of intentions due to callosal disconnection. *J Neurol Neurosurg Psychiatry* 2001;71:462–471.

150. Alexander GE, DeLong MR, Strick PL. Parallel organization of functionally segregated circuits linking basal ganglia and cortex. *Annu Rev Neurosci* 1986;9:357–381.:357–381.

151. Alexander GE, Crutcher MD, DeLong MR. Basal ganglia-thalamocortical circuits: parallel substrates for motor, oculomotor, "prefrontal" and "limbic" functions. *Prog Brain Res* 1990;85:119–146.

152. Chica AB, Bayle DJ, Botta F, Bartolomeo P, Paz-Alonso PM. Interactions between phasic alerting and consciousness in the fronto-striatal network. *Scientific reports* 2016;6:31868.

153. van der Knaap MS, Smit LS, Nauta JJ, Lafeber HN, Valk J. Cortical laminar abnormalities: occurrence and clinical significance. *Neuropediatrics* 1993;24:143–148.

154. Wytrzes LM, Chatrian GE, Shaw CM, Wirch AL. Acute failure of forebrain with sparing of brain-stem function. Electroencephalographic, multimodality evoked potential, and pathologic findings. *Arch Neurol* 1989;46:93–97.

155. Adams JH, Graham DI, Jennett B. The neuropathology of the vegetative state after an acute brain insult. *Brain* 2000;123:1327–1338.

156. Schmahmann JD. Vascular syndromes of the thalamus. *Stroke* 2003;34:2264–2278.

157. Caplan LR. "Top of the basilar" syndrome. *Neurology* 1980;30:72–79.

158. Caruso P, Manganotti P, Moretti R. Complex neurological symptoms in bilateral thalamic stroke due
to Percheron artery occlusion. *Vascular health and
risk management* 2017;13:11–14.
159. Wechsler B, Dellisola B, Vidailhet M, et al. MRI
in 31 patients with Behcet's disease and neurological involvement: prospective study with clinical correlation. *J Neurol Neurosurg Psychiatry*
1993;56:793–798.
160. Park-Matsumoto YC, Ogawa K, Tazawa T, Ishiai S,
Tei H, Yuasa T. Mutism developing after bilateral
thalamo-capsular lesions by neuro-Behcet disease.
Acta Neurol Scand 1995;91:297–301.

161. Kinney HC, Korein J, Panigrahy A, Dikkes P,
Goode R. Neuropathological findings in the brain
of Karen Ann Quinlan. The role of the thalamus
in the persistent vegetative state. *N Engl J Med*
1994;330:1469–1475.
162. Reeves AG, Plum F. Hyperphagia, rage, and dementia accompanying a ventromedial hypothalamic
neoplasm. *Arch Neurol* 1969;20:616–624.
163. Parvizi J, Damasio AR. Neuroanatomical correlates
of brainstem coma. *Brain* 2003;126:1524–1536.
164. Fischer DB, Boes AD, Demertzi A, et al. A human
brain network derived from coma-causing brainstem
lesions. *Neurology* 2016;87:2427–2434.

Chapter 2

Examination of the Comatose Patient

OVERVIEW

Coma, indeed any alteration of consciousness, is a medical emergency. The physician encountering such a patient must begin examination and treatment simultaneously. The examination must be thorough, but brief. The examination begins by informally assessing the patient's level of consciousness. First, the physician addresses the patient verbally. If the patient does not respond to the physician's voice, the physician may speak more loudly or shake the patient. When this fails to produce a response, the physician begins a more formal coma evaluation.

The examiner must systematically assess the arousal pathways. To determine if there is a structural lesion involving those pathways, it is necessary also to examine the function of brainstem sensory and motor pathways that are adjacent to the arousal system. In particular, because the oculomotor circuitry enfolds and surrounds most of the arousal system, this part of the examination is particularly informative. Fortunately, the examination of the comatose patient can usually be accomplished very quickly because the patient has such a limited range of responses. However, the examiner must become conversant with the meaning of the signs elicited in that examination so that decisions that may save the patient's life can then be made quickly and accurately.

The evaluation of the patient with a reduced level of consciousness, like that of any patient, requires a history (to the extent possible), physical examination, and laboratory evaluation. These are considered, in turn, in this chapter. However, *as soon as it is determined that a patient has a depressed level of consciousness, the next step is to ensure that the patient's brain is receiving adequate blood and oxygen*. The emergency treatment of the comatose patient is detailed in Chapters 7 and 8. The physiology and pathophysiology of the cerebral circulation and of respiration are considered in the upcoming paragraphs.

HISTORY

Although the history is the most important part of the evaluation for most neurological disorders (Table 2.1), patients with disorders

Table 2.1 Examination of the Comatose Patient

History (from relatives, friends, or attendants)
Onset of coma (abrupt, gradual)
Recent complaints (e.g., headache, depression, focal weakness, vertigo)
Recent injury
Previous medical illnesses (e.g., diabetes, renal failure, heart disease)
Previous psychiatric history
Access to drugs (sedatives, psychotropic drugs)
General physical examination
Vital signs: Respiration, blood pressure, heart rate
Evidence of trauma
Evidence of acute or chronic systemic illness
Evidence of drug ingestion (needle marks, alcohol on breath)
Nuchal rigidity (assuming that cervical trauma has been excluded)
Neurologic examination
Verbal responses
Eye opening
Optic fundi
Pupillary reactions
Spontaneous eye movements
Oculocephalic responses (assuming cervical trauma has been excluded)
Oculovestibular responses
Corneal responses
Respiratory pattern
Motor responses
Deep tendon reflexes
Skeletal muscle tone

of consciousness by definition are not able to give a history. Thus, this information must be obtained if possible from relatives, friends, or the individuals, usually the emergency medical personnel who brought the patient to the hospital.

The onset of coma is often important. In a previously healthy, young patient, the sudden onset of coma may be due to drug poisoning, subarachnoid hemorrhage, or head trauma; in the elderly, sudden coma is more likely caused by cerebral hemorrhage or infarction. Most patients with lesions compressing the brain either have a clear history of trauma (e.g., epidural hematoma; see Chapter 4) or a more gradual rather than abrupt impairment of consciousness. Gradual onset is also true of most patients with metabolic disorders (see Chapter 5).

The examiner should inquire about previous medical symptoms or illnesses or any recent trauma. A history of headache of recent onset points to a compressive lesion, whereas the history of depression or psychiatric disease may suggest drug intoxication. Patients with known diabetes, renal failure, heart disease, or other chronic medical illness are more likely to be suffering from metabolic disorders or perhaps brainstem infarction. A history of premonitory signs, including focal weakness, such as dragging of the leg or complaints of unilateral sensory symptoms or diplopia, suggests a cerebral or brainstem mass lesion.

GENERAL PHYSICAL EXAMINATION

The general physical examination is an important source of clues as to the cause of unconsciousness. After stabilizing the patient (Chapter 7), one should search for signs of head trauma. Bilateral symmetric black eyes suggest basal skull fracture, as does blood behind the tympanic membrane or under the skin overlying the mastoid bone (Battle's sign). Examine the neck with care; if there is a possibility of trauma, the neck should be immobilized until cervical spine instability has been excluded by imaging. Resistance to neck flexion in the presence of easy lateral movement suggests meningeal inflammation, such as meningitis or subarachnoid hemorrhage. Flexion of the legs upon flexing the neck (Brudzinski's sign) confirms meningismus. Examination of the skin is also useful. Needle marks suggest drug ingestion. Petechiae may suggest meningitis or intravascular coagulation. Pressure sores or bullae indicate that the patient has been unconscious and lying in a single position for an extended period of time, and these signs are especially frequent in patients with barbiturate overdosage.[1]

LEVEL OF CONSCIOUSNESS

After conducting the brief history and examination as just outlined and stabilizing the patients' vital functions, the examiner should conduct a formal coma evaluation. In assessing the level of consciousness of the patient, it is necessary to determine the intensity of stimulation necessary to arouse a response and the quality of the response that is achieved. When the patient does not respond to voice or vigorous shaking, the examiner next provides a source of pain to arouse the patient. Several methods for providing a sufficiently painful stimulus to arouse the patient without causing tissue damage are illustrated in Figure 2.1. It is best to begin with a modest, lateralized stimulus, such as compression of the nail beds, the supraorbital ridge, or the temporomandibular joint. These give information about the lateralization of motor response (see later discussion) but must be repeated on each side in case there is a focal lesion of the pain pathways on one side of the brain or spinal cord. If there is no response to the stimulus, a more vigorous midline stimulus may be given by the sternal rub. By vigorously pressing the examiner's knuckles into the patient's sternum and rubbing up and down the chest, it is possible to create a sufficiently painful stimulus to arouse any subject who is not deeply comatose.

The response of the patient is noted and graded. The types of motor responses seen are

(A)   (B)   (C)   (D)

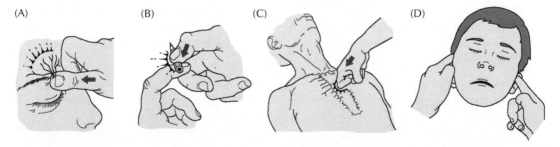

Figure 2.1 Methods for attempting to elicit responses from unconscious patients. Noxious stimuli can be delivered with minimal trauma to the supraorbital ridge (A), the nail beds or the fingers or toes (B), the sternum (C) or the temporomandibular joints (D).

considered in the section on *motor responses* (page 76). However, the level of response is important to the initial consideration of the depth of impairment of consciousness. In descending order of arousability, a sleepy patient who responds to being addressed verbally or light shaking, or one who responds verbally to more intense mechanical stimulation, is said to be lethargic or obtunded. A patient whose best response to deep pain is to attempt to push the examiner's arm away is considered to be stuporous, with localizing responses. Patients who make only nonspecific motor responses (wincing, restlessness, withdrawal reflexes) without a directed attempt to defend against the stimulus are considered to have a nonlocalizing response and are comatose. Patients who fail to respond at all are in the deepest stage of coma.

This rough grading system, from verbal responsiveness, to localizing responses, to nonlocalizing responses, to no response, is all that is needed for an initial assessment of the depth of unresponsiveness that can be used to follow the progress of the patient. If the initial evaluation of the level of consciousness demonstrates impairment, it is essential to progress through the next steps of the coma examination as rapidly as possible to safeguard the patient's life. More elaborate coma scales are described in Box 2.1, but many of these depend on the results of later stages in the examination, and it is never justified to delay attending to the basics of airway, breathing, and circulation while performing a more elaborate scoring evaluation.

Box 2.1 Coma Scales

A number of different scales have been devised for scoring patients with coma. While each patient is different, and a clinician faced with a single patient must rely on a careful and complete history and exam, scales are useful for comparing groups of patients and can be useful in estimating the prognosis for recovery. We discuss several simple scales that are often used at the bedside here; the more complex Coma Recovery Scale-Revised (CRS-R) is typically used in a research setting (see Chapter 9).

The prognosis, of course, depends both on the cause of the coma as well as the status of the examination. For example, the widely known Glasgow Coma Scale (GCS) was devised by Teasdale and Jennett to categorize patients with head trauma and predict outcome.[2,3] The GCS is widely used and still is probably the best for most trauma patients. GCS scores can also be compared against large databases to evaluate prognosis for specific etiologies of coma (see Chapter 9). Unfortunately, when used by emergency room physicians, interrater agreement is only moderate.[4]

Two simple scales, ACDU (alert, confused, drowsy, unresponsive) and AVPU (alert, response to voice, response to pain, unresponsive) correspond well to the GCS and are easier to use.[5] The ACDU scale appears better at identifying early deterioration in level of consciousness.

A recently validated coma scale, the FOUR (full outline of unresponsiveness) score, provides more neurologic detail than the GCS.[6] However, no scale is adequate for all patients; hence, the best policy in recording the results of the coma examination is simply to describe the findings.

Glasgow Coma Scale

Eye Response

   4 = eyes open spontaneously
   3 = eye opening to verbal command
   2 = eye opening to pain
   1 = no eye opening

Box 2.1 Coma Scales (cont.)

Motor Response

    6 = obeys commands
    5 = localizing pain
    4 = withdrawal from pain
    3 = flexion response to pain
    2 = extension response to pain
    1 = no motor response

Verbal Response

    5 = oriented
    4 = confused
    3 = inappropriate words
    2 = incomprehensible sounds
    1 = no verbal response

A GCS score of 13 or higher indicates mild brain injury, 9–12 moderate brain injury, and 8 or less severe brain injury.

AVPU	ACDU
Is the patient	Is the patient
Alert and oriented?	Alert and oriented?
Responding to voice?	Confused?
Responding to pain?	Drowsy?
Unresponsive?	Unresponsive?

FOUR (Full Outline of Unresponsiveness) Score

Eye Response

    4 = eyelids open or opened, tracking, or blinking to command
    3 = eyelids open but not tracking
    2 = eyelids closed but open to loud voice
    1 = eyelids closed but open to pain
    0 = eyelids remain closed with pain

Motor Response

    4 = thumbs-up, fist, or peace sign
    3 = localizing to pain
    2 = flexion response to pain
    1 = extension response to pain
    0 = no response to pain or generalized myoclonus status

(continued)

Box 2.1 Coma Scales (cont.)

Brainstem Reflexes

4 = pupil and corneal reflexes present
3 = one pupil wide and fixed
2 = pupil or corneal reflexes absent
1 = pupil and corneal reflexes absent
0 = absent pupil, corneal, and cough reflex

Respiration

4 = not intubated, regular breathing pattern
3 = not intubated, Cheyne-Stokes breathing pattern
2 = not intubated, irregular breathing
1 = breathes above ventilator rate
0 = breathes at ventilator rate or apnea

ABC: AIRWAY, BREATHING, CIRCULATION

It is critical to ensure that the patient's airway is maintained, that he or she is breathing adequately, and that there is sufficient arterial perfusion pressure. The first goal must be to correct any of these conditions if they are found inadequate (see Chapter 7). In addition, blood pressure, heart rate, and respiration may provide valuable clues to the cause of coma.

Circulation

It is critical first to ensure that the brain is receiving adequate blood flow. Cerebral perfusion pressure is the systemic blood pressure minus the intracranial pressure (ICP). The physician can measure blood pressure but, in the initial examination, can only estimate ICP. Over a wide range of blood pressures, cerebral perfusion remains stable because the brain autoregulates its blood flow by mechanisms described in the following paragraphs and illustrated in Figure 2.2. If the blood pressure falls too low or becomes too high, autoregulation fails and cerebral perfusion follows perfusion pressure passively; that is, cerebral perfusion pressure falls as the blood pressure falls and rises as the blood pressure rises. In this

situation, both too low (ischemia) and too high (hypertensive encephalopathy; see Chapter 5) a blood pressure can damage the brain. To ensure adequate brain perfusion, the physician should attempt to maintain the blood pressure at a level normal for the individual patient. For example, a patient with chronic hypertension autoregulates at a higher level than a normotensive patient. Lowering the blood pressure to a "normal level" may deprive the brain of an adequate blood supply (see Figure 2.2). Conversely, the cerebral blood flow (CBF) in children and pregnant women, who normally run low blood pressures, is autoregulated at lower blood pressures, and these patients may develop excessive perfusion if the blood pressure is raised into a "high normal" range (e.g., preeclampsia).

The perfusion pressure of the brain may be influenced by the position of the head. In a normal individual, as the head is raised, the systemic arterial pressure is maintained by blood pressure reflexes. At the same time, the arterial perfusion pressure to the head is reduced by the distance the head is raised above the heart, but the ICP is also reduced because of the improved venous and cerebrospinal fluid (CSF) drainage. The net effect is that there is very little change in brain perfusion pressure or CBF. On the other hand, in a patient with stenosis of a carotid or vertebral artery, the

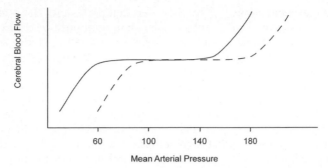

Figure 2.2 Cerebral autoregulation in hypertension. Schematic representation of autoregulation of cerebral blood flow (CBF) in normotensive (solid line) and hypertensive (dashed line) subjects. In both groups, within a range of about 100 mm Hg, increases or decreases in mean arterial pressure are associated with maintenance of CBF due to appropriate changes in arteriolar resistance. Changes in pressure outside this range are eventually associated with loss of autoregulation, leading to a reduction (with hypotension) or an elevation (with marked hypertension) in CBF. Note that hypertensive encephalopathy (increased blood flow with pressures exceeding the autoregulatory range) may occur with a mean arterial pressure below 200 mm Hg in the normotensive individual, but may require a much higher mean arterial pressure in patients who have sustained hypertension. Conversely, acutely lowering blood pressure of a hypertensive patient to the "normal range" of a mean arterial pressure of 80 mm Hg (equivalent to 120/60) may produce a clinically significant fall in CBF, particularly if there is a preexisting cerebrovascular stenosis.

perfusion pressure for that vessel may be much lower than systemic arterial pressure. If the head of the bed is raised, perfusion pressure may fall below the threshold for autoregulation, and blood flow may be diminished below the level needed to support neurologic function. Such patients may show improvement in neurologic function when the head of the bed is flat. Conversely, in cases of head trauma where there is increased ICP, it may be important to raise the head of the bed 15–30 degrees to improve venous drainage to maximize cerebral perfusion pressure.[7] Similarly, it is necessary to remove tight neckwear and ensure that a cervical spine collar is not applied too tightly to a victim of head injury to avoid diminishing venous outflow from the brain.

In a patient with impaired consciousness, the blood pressure can give important clues to the level of the nervous system that has been damaged. *Damage to the descending sympathetic pathways that support blood pressure may result in a fall to levels seen after spinal transection (mean arterial pressure about 60–70 mm Hg).* Blood pressure is supported by a descending sympathoexcitatory pathway from the rostral ventrolateral medulla to the spinal cord, and so damage along the course of this pathway can result in spinal levels of blood pressure. The hypothalamus in turn provides a descending sympathoexcitatory input to the medulla and the spinal cord.[8,9] As

a consequence, bilateral diencephalic lesions result in a fall in sympathetic tone, including meiotic pupils (see later discussion), decreased sweating responses, and a generally low level of arterial pressure.[10]

However, persistent hypotension below these levels in a comatose patient is almost never caused by an acute neurologic injury. A common mistake in evaluation of a comatose patient with a mean arterial pressure below 60 mm Hg is the assumption that a neurologic event may have caused the hypotension. This is almost never the case. A mean arterial pressure at or above 60 mm Hg is generally sufficient in a supine patient to support cerebral and systemic function. On the other hand, acute hypotension due to cardiogenic or vasomotor shock is a common cause of loss of consciousness and a threat to the patient's life. Thus, the initial evaluation of a comatose patient with low blood pressure should focus on identifying the cause of and correcting the hypotension.

On the other hand, *lesions that result in stimulation of the sympathoexcitatory system may cause an increase in blood pressure.* For example, pain is a major ascending sympathoexcitatory stimulus, which acts via direct collaterals from the ascending spinothalamic tract into the rostral ventrolateral medulla. The elevation of blood pressure in response to a painful stimulus applied to the body (pinch of skin, sternal rub) is evidence of intact medullospinal connections.[11,12] In a patient who is still semi-wakeful after subarachnoid hemorrhage, blood pressure may be elevated as a response to headache pain. Each of these conditions is associated with a rise in heart rate as well. The ciliospinal reflex is typically exaggerated in a patient in pentobarbital coma (e.g., used to treat status epilepticus), and even routine nursing maneuvers (e.g., tracheal suction) can cause bilateral pupillary dilatation that can persist for up to 6 minutes.[13]

Direct pressure to the floor of the medulla can activate the Cushing reflex, an increase in blood pressure and a decrease in heart rate.[14] In children, the Cushing reflex may be seen when there is a generalized increased ICP, even above the tentorium. However, the more rigid compartmentalization of intracranial contents in adults usually prevents this phenomenon unless there is an expansile mass in the posterior fossa.

Activation of descending sympathoexcitatory pathways from the forebrain may also elevate blood pressure. Irritative lesions of the hypothalamus, such as occur with subarachnoid hemorrhage, may result in an excess hypothalamic input to the sympathetic and parasympathetic control systems.[15] This condition can trigger virtually any type of cardiac arrhythmia, from sinus pause to supraventricular tachycardia to ventricular fibrillation.[16] However, the most common electrocardiographic (EKG) finding in subarachnoid hemorrhage is a pattern of ST segment elevation, QT prolongation, and T wave inversion. This pattern, which is believed to be due to high levels of circulating catecholamines acting on the heart, may be associated with *tako-tsubo cardiomyopathy*, with ballooning of the apical segment of the heart. Such patients may have enzyme evidence of myocardial infarction and at autopsy can demonstrate contraction band necrosis of the myocardium.[17]

Sympathoexcitation is also seen in patients who are delirious. The infralimbic and insular cortex and the central nucleus of the amygdala provide important inputs to sympathoexcitatory areas of the hypothalamus and the medulla.[9] Activation of these areas due to misperception of stimuli in the environment causing emotional responses such as fear or anger may result in hypertension, tachycardia, and enlarged pupils.

Stokes-Adams attacks are periods of brief loss of consciousness due to lack of adequate cerebral perfusion. These almost always occur in an upright position. In recumbent positions, when the head is at the same height as the heart, it takes a much steeper fall in blood pressure (below 60–70 mm Hg mean pressure) to cause loss of consciousness. The fall in blood pressure during a Stokes-Adams attack may be due to a cardiac arrhythmia[18] and thus requires careful cardiologic evaluation, but it also can reflect a failure of the baroreceptor reflex arc to stabilize blood pressure in the upright position (in which case it can be reproduced by testing orthostatic blood pressure and heart rate responses in the office). Alternatively, hyperactivity of the baroreceptor reflex nerves may occasionally cause hypotension (e.g., in patients with carotid sinus hypersensitivity or glossopharyngeal neuralgia, where brief bursts of activity in baroreceptor nerves trigger a rapid fall in heart rate and blood pressure).[19,20]

PATHOPHYSIOLOGY

The brain ordinarily tightly controls the circulation to provide an adequate level of cerebral perfusion. It does this in two ways. First, across a wide range of arterial blood pressures, it autoregulates its own blood flow.[21–23] The mechanism for this remarkable stability of blood flow is not entirely understood, although it appears to be due to intrinsic innervation of the cerebral blood vessels and may also be regulated by local metabolism.[21,24] In general, local increases in CBF correspond to increases in local metabolic rate, allowing the use of blood flow (in positron emission tomography [PET] imaging or arterial spin labeling magnetic resonance imaging [MRI]) or local blood oxygen level (in functional MRI) to approximate neuronal activity. However, there are also neuronal networks that regulate cerebral perfusion distinct from metabolic need. The two systems normally act in concert to ensure sufficient blood supply to allow normal cerebral function over a wide range of blood pressures but are dysregulated following some brain injuries.

Second, the brain acts through the autonomic nervous system to acutely adjust systemic arterial pressure in order to maintain a pressure head that is within the range that allows cerebral autoregulation. Blood pressure is the product of the cardiac output times the total vascular peripheral resistance. Cardiac output in turn is the product of heart rate and stroke volume. Both heart rate and stroke volume are increased by beta-1 adrenergic stimulation from sympathetic nerves (or adrenal catechols), which play a key role in regulating cardiac output. Heart rate is slowed by muscarinic cholinergic action of the vagus nerve, and hence, increased vagal tone decreases cardiac output. Peripheral resistance is regulated mainly by the level of alpha-1 adrenergic tone in small arterioles, the most important resistance vessels. Therefore, the blood pressure is regulated by the balance of sympathetic tone, which increases both cardiac output and vasoconstrictor tone, versus parasympathetic tone, which slows heart rate and therefore decreases cardiac output. The cardiac vagal tone is maintained by the nucleus ambiguus in the medulla, which contains most of the cardiac parasympathetic preganglionic neurons.[25] Sympathetic vascular and cardiac sympathetic tone is set by neurons in the rostral ventrolateral medulla that provide a tonic activating input to the sympathetic preganglionic neurons in the thoracic spinal cord.[26]

When in a lying position, the brain is at the same level as the heart, but as one rises, the brain elevates to a position 20–30 cm above the heart. This drop in cerebral perfusion pressure (arterial pressure minus ICP) is equivalent to 15–23 mm Hg, and it may be sufficient to cause a drop in cerebral perfusion pressure that would make it difficult to maintain CBF necessary to allow conscious brain function.

To defend against such a precipitous fall in perfusion pressure, the brain maintains reflex mechanisms to compensate for the hydrodynamic consequences of gravity. The level of arterial pressure is sensed at two sites, the aortic arch (by the aortic depressor nerve, a branch of the vagus nerve) and the carotid bifurcation (by the carotid sinus nerve, a branch of the glossopharyngeal nerve). These two nerves terminate in the brain in the nucleus of the solitary tract, which is the main relay for all visceral sensory information in the brain.[9]

The nucleus of the solitary tract then provides an excitatory input to the caudal ventrolateral medulla.[27] The caudal ventrolateral medulla in turn provides an ascending inhibitory input to the tonic vasomotor neurons in the rostral ventrolateral medulla.[28] In addition, the nucleus of the solitary tract provides both direct and relayed excitatory inputs to the cardiac decelerator neurons in the nucleus ambiguus.[27] Thus,

a rise in blood pressure results in a reflex fall in heart rate and vasomotor tone, re-establishing a normal arterial pressure. Conversely, a fall in blood pressure causes a reflex tachycardia and vasoconstriction, re-establishing the necessary arterial perfusion pressure. As a result, on assuming an upright posture, there is normally a small increase in both heart rate and blood pressure.

On occasion, loss of consciousness may result from failure of this baroreceptor reflex arc. In such patients, measurement of standing and supine blood pressure and heart rate discloses a fall in blood pressure on assuming an upright posture that is clinically associated with symptoms of insufficient CBF. Rigid criteria for diagnosing orthostatic hypotension (e.g., a fall in blood pressure of 10 or 15 mm Hg) are not useful as systemic arterial pressure is usually measured in the arm but the symptoms are produced by decreased blood flow to the brain. A pressure head that is adequate to perfuse the arm (which is at the same elevation as the heart) will be reduced by 15–23 mm Hg at the brain in an upright posture, and if perfusion pressure to the brain falls even a few mm Hg below the level needed to maintain autoregulation, the drop in cerebral perfusion may be precipitous.

The most common nonneurologic causes of orthostatic hypotension, including low intravascular volume (often a consequence of diuretic administration or inadequate fluid intake), cardiac pump failure, and medications that impair arterial constriction (e.g., alpha blockers or direct vasodilators), do not impair the tachycardic response. Most neurologic cases of orthostatic hypotension, including peripheral autonomic neuropathy or central or peripheral autonomic degeneration (e.g., in Parkinson's disease or multiple systems atrophy), impair both the heart rate and the blood pressure responses. Put in other words, the hallmark of baroreceptor reflex failure is absence of the elevation of heart rate when arterial pressure falls in response to an orthostatic challenge.[29]

Respiration

The brain cannot long survive without an adequate supply of oxygen. Within seconds of being deprived of oxygen, brain function begins to fail, and within minutes neurons begin to die. The physician must ensure that respiration is supplying adequate oxygenation. To do this requires examination of both respiratory exchange and respiratory pattern. Listening to the chest will ensure that there is adequate movement of air. A normal patient at rest will regularly breathe at about 14 breaths per minute and the exchange of air can be heard at both lung bases. The physician should estimate from the rate and depth of respiration whether the patient is hypo- or hyperventilating or whether respiration is normal. The patient's color is a gross indicator of oxygenation: cyanosis indicates deficient oxygenation, although a cherry red color may also indicate deficient oxygenation because of carbon monoxide (CO) intoxication. A better estimate of oxygenation can be achieved by placing an oximeter on the finger; many intensive care units and some emergency departments also measure expired carbon dioxide (CO_2), which correlates well with partial pressure of CO_2 (PCO_2) as long as the relationship between ventilation and pulmonary perfusion remains stable.

This section considers the neuroanatomic basis of respiratory abnormalities that accompany coma (Table 2.2, Figure 2.3). Chapter 5 discusses respiratory responses to metabolic

Table 2.2 Neuropathologic Correlates of Breathing Abnormalities

Forebrain damage
  Epileptic respiratory inhibition
  Apraxia for deep breathing or breath holding
  "Pseudobulbar" laughing or crying
  Posthyperventilation apnea
  Cheyne-Stokes respiration
Hypothalamic-midbrain damage
  Central reflex hyperpnea (neurogenic pulmonary edema)
Basis pontis damage
  Pseudobulbar paralysis of voluntary control
Lower pontine tegmentum damage or dysfunction
  Apneustic breathing
  Cluster breathing
  Short-cycle anoxic-hypercapnic periodic respiration
  Ataxic breathing (Biot)
Medullary dysfunction
  Ataxic breathing
  Slow regular breathing
  Loss of automatic breathing with preserved voluntary control (Ondine's curse)
  Gasping
Apnea

disturbances. Because neurogenic and metabolic influences on breathing interact extensively, respiratory changes must be interpreted cautiously if there is evidence of pulmonary disease.

The pattern of respiration can give important clues concerning the level of brain damage. Once assured that there is adequate exchange of oxygen, the physician should watch the patient spontaneously breathe. Irregularities of the respiratory pattern that provide clues to the level of brain damage are described in the following paragraphs.

PATHOPHYSIOLOGY

Breathing is a sensorimotor act that integrates nervous influences arising from nearly every level of the brain and upper spinal cord. In humans, respiration subserves two major functions: one of metabolism and the other behavioral. Metabolically, respiratory control is directed principally at maintaining tissue oxygenation and normal acid–base balance. It is regulated mainly by reflex neural mechanisms located in the posterior-dorsal region of the pons and in the medulla. Behavioral control of breathing allows it to be integrated with swallowing and with verbal and emotional communication, as well as with other behaviors.

Respiratory rhythm is an intrinsic property of the brainstem that is generated by a network of neurons that lie in the ventrolateral medulla, including the pre-Bötzinger complex (see Figure 2.3).[30,31] This rhythm is regulated in the intact brain by a number of influences that enter via the vagus and glossopharyngeal nerves. The carotid sinus branch of the glossopharyngeal nerve brings afferents that carry information about blood oxygen and carbon dioxide content, whereas the vagus nerve conveys pulmonary stretch afferents. These terminate in the nucleus of the solitary tract.[9] Chemoreceptor afferents can increase respiratory rate and depth, whereas pulmonary stretch receptors tend to inhibit lung inflation (the Herring-Breuer reflex). These influences are relayed to reticular areas in the ventrolateral medulla that regulate the onset of inspiration and expiration.[31] In addition, the glutamatergic retrotrapezoid nucleus and the serotoninergic neurons in the ventral medulla also serve as CO_2 chemoreceptors and directly influence the nearby circuitry that generates the respiratory rhythm.[32,33]

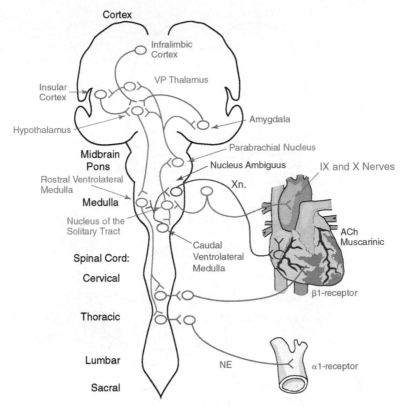

Figure 2.3 A diagram summarizing the cardiovascular control pathways in the brain. Visceral afferent information (gray) arrives from nerves IX and X into the nucleus of the solitary tract. This information is then distributed to the parabrachial nucleus, which relays it to the forebrain, and to the ventrolateral medulla, which controls cardiovascular reflexes. Inputs to the nucleus ambiguous modulate vagal control of heart rate (red); inputs to the caudal (purple) and rostral (orange) ventrolateral medulla regulate sympathetic outflow to both the heart and the blood vessels (dark green). Forebrain areas that influence the cardiovascular system (brown) include the insular cortex (a visceral sensory area), the infralimbic cortex (a visceral motor area), and the amygdala, which produces autonomic emotional responses. All of these act on the hypothalamic sympathetic activating neurons (orange) in the paraventricular and lateral hypothalamic areas to provide behavioral and emotional influence over the blood pressure and heart rate. ACh, acetylcholine; NE, norepinephrine; VP, ventroposterior.

The medullary circuitry that controls respiration is under the control of pontine cell groups that integrate breathing with ongoing orofacial stimuli and behaviors (Figure 2.4).[34] Neurons in the parabrachial nucleus primarily increase the rate and depth of respiration, presumably in relation to emotional responses or in anticipation of metabolic demand during various behaviors. On the other hand, neurons located more ventrally in the intertrigeminal zone, between the principal sensory and motor trigeminal nuclei, produce apneas, which are necessary during swallowing and in response to noxious chemical irritation of the airway (e.g., smoke or water in the nasal passages).[35]

Superimposed on these metabolic demands and basic reflexes, the forebrain can command a wide range of respiratory responses. Respiration can be altered by emotional response, and it increases in anticipation of metabolic demand during voluntary exercise (i.e., as a consequence of central command rather than metabolic reflex).[36] The pathways that control vocalization in humans originate in the frontal opercular cortex, which provides premotor and motor integration of orofacial motor actions.[37] However, there is also a prefrontal contribution to the maintenance of respiratory rhythm, even in the absence of metabolic demand (the basis for posthyperventilation apnea, described later).

These considerations make the recognition of respiratory changes useful in the diagnosis of coma (Figure 2.5).

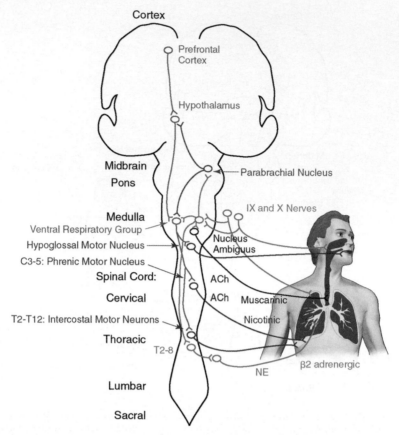

Figure 2.4 A diagram summarizing the respiratory control pathways in the brain. Afferents from the lung (pulmonary stretch), upper airway (cough reflexes), and carotid body arrive via cranial nerves IX and X in the nucleus of the solitary tract (gray), also called the dorsal respiratory group. These control airway and respiratory reflexes, analogous to the cardiovascular system, by inputs to the ventrolateral medulla. These include outputs to the airways via the vagus nerve (red) and outputs from the ventral respiratory group (orange) to the spinal cord, controlling sympathetic airway responses (green) and respiratory motor (phrenic motor nucleus, blue) and accessory motor (hypoglossal and intercostal, blue) outputs. The ventral respiratory group is responsible for generating respiratory rhythm. However, it is assisted in this process by the parabrachial nucleus (or pontine respiratory group, purple), which receives ascending respiratory afferents and integrates them with other brainstem reflexes (e.g., swallowing). The prefrontal cortex (brown) provides behavioral regulation of breathing, producing a continual breathing rhythm even in the absence of metabolic need. This influences the hypothalamus (orange), which may vary respiratory pattern in coordination with behavior or emotion. ACh, acetylcholine; NE, norepinephrine.

POSTHYPERVENTILATION APNEA

If the arterial CO_2 tension is lowered by a brief period of hyperventilation, a healthy awake subject will nevertheless continue to breathe with a normal rhythm, at least initially[38] and albeit at reduced volume, until the PCO_2 returns to its original level. By contrast, subjects with diffuse metabolic impairment of the forebrain or bilateral structural damage to the frontal lobes commonly demonstrate posthyperventilation apnea.[39] Their respirations stop after deep breathing has

lowered the CO_2 content of the blood below its usual resting level. Rhythmic breathing returns when endogenous CO_2 production raises the arterial level back to normal.

The demonstration of posthyperventilation apnea requires that the patient voluntarily take several deep breaths, so it is useful in the differential diagnosis of lethargic or confused patients but not in cases of stupor or coma. One instructs the subject to take five deep breaths. No other instructions are given. It is useful for the examiner to place a hand on the patient's chest to make it easier later to detect when breathing has

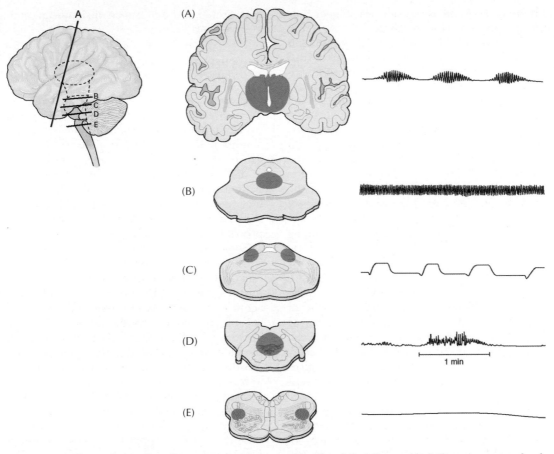

Figure 2.5 Different abnormal respiratory patterns are associated with pathologic lesions (shaded areas) at various levels of the brain. Tracings by chest-abdomen pneumography, inspiration reads up. (A) Cheyne-Stokes respiration is seen with metabolic encephalopathies and with lesions that impair forebrain or diencephalic function. (B) Central neurogenic hyperventilation is most commonly seen in metabolic encephalopathies, but may rarely be seen in cases of high brainstem tumors. (C) Apneusis, consisting of inspiratory pauses, may be seen in patients with bilateral pontine lesions. (D) Cluster breathing and ataxic breathing are seen with lesions at the pontomedullary junction. (E) Apnea occurs when lesions encroach on the ventral respiratory group in the ventrolateral medulla bilaterally.

From Saper C. Brain stem modulation of sensation, movement, and consciousness. Chapter 45 in: Kandel ER, Schwartz JH, Jessel TM. *Principles of Neural Science*. 4th ed. McGraw-Hill, New York, 2000, pp. 871–909. By permission of McGraw-Hill.

restarted and to count the breaths. If the lungs function well, the maneuver usually lowers the arterial CO_2 by 8–14 torr. At the end of the deep breathing, wakeful patients without brain damage show little or no apnea (less than 10 seconds). However, in patients with forebrain impairment, the period of apnea may last from 12–30 seconds. The neural substrate that produces a continuous breathing pattern even in the absence of metabolic need is believed to include the same frontal pathways that regulate behavioral alterations of breathing patterns, as the continuous breathing pattern disappears with sleep, bilateral frontal

lobe damage, or diffuse metabolic impairment of the hemispheres.[39,40]

CHEYNE-STOKES RESPIRATION

Cheyne-Stokes respiration is a pattern of periodic breathing with phases of hyperpnea alternating regularly with apnea.[41] The depth of respiration waxes from breath to breath in a smooth crescendo during onset of the hyperpneic phase and then, once a peak is reached, wanes in an equally smooth decrescendo until a period of apnea, usually from 10–20 seconds, is reached.

The hyperpneic phase usually lasts longer than the apneic phase (Figure 2.5).

This rhythmic alternation in Cheyne-Stokes respiration results from the interplay of normal brainstem respiratory reflexes. When the medullary chemosensory circuits sense adequate oxygen and CO_2 tension, they reduce the rate and depth of respiration, causing a gradual rise in arterial CO_2 tension. There is normally a short delay of a few seconds, representing the transit time for fresh blood from the lungs to reach the left heart and then the chemoreceptors in the carotid artery and the brain. By the time the brain begins increasing the rate and depth of respiration, the alveolar CO_2 has reached even higher levels, and so there is a gradual ramping up of respiration as the brain sees a rising level of CO_2, despite its additional efforts. By the time the brain begins to see a fall in CO_2 tension, the levels in the alveoli may be quite low. When blood containing this low level of CO_2 reaches the brain, respiration slows or may even cease, thus setting off another cycle. Hence, the periodic cycling is due to the delay (*hysteresis*) in the feedback loop between alveolar ventilation and brain chemoreceptor sensory responses.

The Cheyne-Stokes respiratory cycle is not usually seen in normal individuals because the circulatory delay between a change in alveolar blood gases and CO_2 tension in the brain is only a few seconds. Even as circulatory delay rises with cardiovascular or pulmonary disease, during waking, the descending pathways that prevent posthyperventilation apnea also ensure the persistence of respiration even during periods of low metabolic need, thus damping the oscillations that produce Cheyne-Stokes respiration. However, during sleep or with bilateral forebrain impairment, due either to a diffuse metabolic process such as uremia, hepatic failure, or bilateral damage such as cerebral infarcts or a forebrain mass lesion with diencephalic displacement, periodic breathing may emerge. In patients with heart failure, the transit time for blood from the lungs to reach the carotid and cerebral chemoreceptors can become so prolonged as to produce a Cheyne-Stokes pattern of respiration even in the absence of forebrain impairment. Thus, Cheyne-Stokes respiration is mainly useful as a sign of intact brainstem respiratory reflexes in patients with forebrain impairment, but it cannot be interpreted in the presence of significant congestive heart failure.

HYPERVENTILATION IN COMATOSE PATIENTS

Sustained hyperventilation is often seen in patients with impaired consciousness but is usually a result of either hepatic coma or sepsis, conditions in which circulating chemical stimuli cause hyperpnea, or a metabolic acidosis, such as diabetic ketoacidosis (see Chapter 5). Other patients have meningitis caused either by infection or subarachnoid hemorrhage, which stimulates chemoreceptors in the brainstem, probably by altering CSF pH.[42]

Some patients hyperventilate when intrinsic brainstem injury or subarachnoid hemorrhage or seizures cause neurogenic pulmonary edema.[42] Hyperventilation following acute brain injury is frequent and associated with brain tissue hypoxia leading to worse outcomes.[43] The ventilatory response is driven by pulmonary mechanosensory and chemosensory receptors. The pulmonary congestion lowers both the arterial CO_2 and the oxygen tension. Stimulation of pulmonary stretch receptors is apparently sufficient to cause reflex hyperpnea as oxygen therapy sufficient to raise the arterial oxygen level does not always correct the overbreathing.

Another small group of patients has been identified who have hyperventilation associated with brainstem gliomas or lymphomas.[44,45] These patients have spinal fluid that is acellular, but generally acidotic compared to arterial pH. In others, the lumbar CSF may have a normal pH, but it is believed that the tumor causes local lactic acidosis, which may trigger brain chemoreceptors to cause hyperventilation (Figure 2.5).

It is theoretically possible for an irritative lesion in the region of the parabrachial nucleus or other respiratory centers to produce hyperpnea. The diagnosis of such true "central neurogenic hyperventilation" requires that, with the subject breathing room air, the blood gases show elevated arterial oxygen tension, decreased CO_2 tension, and an elevated pH. The CSF likewise must show an elevated pH and be acellular. The respiratory changes must persist during sleep to eliminate psychogenic hyperventilation, and one must exclude the presence of stimulating drugs, such as salicylates, or disorders that stimulate respiration, such as hepatic failure or underlying systemic infection. Cases fulfilling all of these criteria have rarely been reported,[46,47] and none that we are aware of has come to postmortem examination of the brain.

APNEUSTIC BREATHING

Apneusis is a respiratory pause at full inspiration. Fully developed apneustic breathing, with each cycle including an inspiratory pause, is rare in humans but of considerable localizing value. Experiments in animals indicate that apneusis develops with injury to the pontine respiratory nuclei described earlier, and experience with rare human cases would support this view (see Figure 2.5).[48]

Clinically, end-inspiratory pauses of 2–3 seconds usually alternate with end-expiratory pauses, and both are most frequently encountered in the setting of pontine infarction due to basilar artery occlusion. However, apneustic breathing may rarely be observed in metabolic encephalopathies, including hypoglycemia, anoxia, or meningitis. It is sometimes observed in cases of transtentorial herniation as the brainstem dysfunction advances. At least one patient with apneusis due to a brainstem infarct responded to buspirone, a serotonin 1A receptor agonist.[48]

ATAXIC BREATHING

Irregular, gasping respiration implies damage to the respiratory rhythm generator at the pre-Bötzinger level of the upper medulla.[31] This cell group can be specifically eliminated in experimental animals by the use of a toxin that binds to neurons in the ventrolateral medulla that express NK-1 receptors.[49] The resulting irregular, gasping breathing is eerily similar to humans with bilateral rostral medullary lesions, and it indicates that sufficient neurons survive in the medullary reticular formation to drive primitive ventilatory efforts despite the loss of the neurons that cause smooth to-and-fro respiration.[50] More complete bilateral lesions of the ventrolateral medullary reticular formation cause apnea, which is not compatible with life unless the patient is artificially ventilated (Figure 2.5).

A variety of intermediate types of breathing patterns are also seen with high medullary lesions. Some patients may breathe in irregular clusters or ratchet-like breaths separated by pauses.[51] In other cases, particularly during intoxication with opiates or sedative drugs, the breathing may slow and decline in depth gradually until it fades into complete arrest.

There is a tendency in modern hospitals to intubate and ventilate patients with structural coma to protect the airway and permit treatment of respiratory failure. If the patient fights intubation or ventilation, paralytic drugs are often administered. This compromises the ability of the neurologist to assess brainstem reflexes and, in some cases, may delay diagnosis and compromise care. Thus, it is important, whenever possible, to delay intubation until after the brief coma examination described here has been completed.

SLEEP APNEA AND ONDINE'S CURSE

Obstructive sleep apnea is a common disorder in which the cross-section of the upper airway is anatomically narrow.[52] During sleep, there is gradual loss of tone in the muscles that keep the upper airway open, including the genioglossus muscle that pulls the tongue forward. This results in critical narrowing of the airway, and the increased rate of movement of air tends to further reduce airway pressure resulting in sudden closure. Patients who are liable to this disorder include obese individuals, where adipose deposits in neck tissue reduces airway diameter; men, because the increased ratio of the length of the airway to its diameter predisposes to collapse; and middle-aged or older patients, because muscle tone is more reduced during sleep with age. However, cases may occur in thin, young adults, or even in children. Sleep apnea typically occurs in cycles lasting a few minutes each when the patient falls asleep, airway tone fails and an obstructive apnea occurs, blood oxygen levels fall, CO_2 rises, and the patient is aroused sufficiently to resume breathing. This cycle may be repeated many times over the course of a night. The fragmentation of sleep and intermittent hypoxia result in chronic daytime sleepiness and impairment of cognitive function, particularly vigilance.

Excessive drowsiness during the day and loud snoring at night may be the only clues. Lethargy or drowsiness due to neurologic injury may induce apneic cycles in a patient with obstructive sleep apnea. However, as the level of consciousness becomes more impaired, it may be difficult to achieve the periodic arousals necessary to resume breathing, resulting in intermittent severe hypoxia.

Other patients with pauses in ventilation have central sleep apnea. Most such patients have congestive heart failure, and the pauses are thought to be analogous to the periodic breathing that is seen in patients who develop Cheyne-Stokes respiration when they fall asleep.

Failure of automatic breathing during sleep is a rare condition, sometimes called Ondine's curse, named after the mythologic wood nymph whose mortal lover pledged his love to her "with every waking breath." When she found him sleeping with another woman, she cursed him to lose automatic breathing whenever he went to sleep. In adults, failure of automatic breathing during sleep is seen after lesions of the ventrolateral medullary chemosensory areas or bilateral damage to the descending pathways that control automatic respiration in the lateral columns of the spinal cord (e.g., as a complication of cordotomy to relieve cancer pain).[53,54] A variety of interventions have been successful, ranging from a rocking bed, which provides continuous somatic sensory and vestibular stimulation, to negative pressure ventilation, or even diaphragmatic pacing.[55]

In children, central hypoventilation is most frequently seen as a congenital condition in infants associated with a mutation in the *Phox2B* gene, a transcription factor that is necessary for the normal production of chemosensory neurons of the retrotrapezoid nucleus.[56] *Phox2B* is also necessary for normal development of the neural crest, and patients with mutations may also have Hirschsprung's disease, neuroblastoma, or pheochromocytoma.[57]

YAWNING, HICCUPPING, VOMITING

The neuronal pattern generators responsible for coordinating respiratory-related behaviors also are located in the ventrolateral medulla, in close proximity to the nucleus ambiguus.

Yawning is a motor pattern that involves deep inspiration associated with wide opening of the jaw and generalized muscle stretching.[58] It apparently is caused by a medullary pattern generator, as it is seen in anencephalic children who lack a forebrain and even in patients who are locked-in due to extensive pontine level injury. Yawning may improve the compliance of the lungs and chest wall, but its function is not understood. It may be seen in lethargic patients, but yawning is also seen in complex partial seizures emanating from the medial temporal lobe and is not of great localizing value.

Hiccups occur in patients with abdominal or subphrenic pathology (e.g., pancreatic cancer) that impinges on the vagus nerve.[59,60] Dexamethasone may induce hiccups; the mechanism is unknown.[61] Hiccups occasionally occur with lesions in the medullary tegmentum, including neoplasms, infarction, hematomas, vascular malformations, infections, or syringobulbia.[62–64] Because stuporous patients with intracranial mass lesions are often treated with corticosteroids to reduce brain edema, it may be difficult to determine whether pressure on the floor of the fourth ventricle from the mass lesion or the treatment with corticosteroids is causing the hiccups.[65]

Pathologic hiccupping is peculiarly more common in men; in a study of 220 patients at the Mayo Clinic with pathologic hiccupping, all but 39 were men.[66]

The hiccup reflex consists of a spasmodic burst of inspiratory activity, followed 35 milliseconds later by abrupt glottic closure, so that the ventilatory effect is negligible. On the other hand, if the airway is kept open artificially (e.g., by tracheostomy), the inrush of air can be sufficient to hyperventilate the patient. As an example, one patient in our experience with a low brainstem infarct and tracheostomy maintained his total ventilation for several days by hiccups alone.

Pathologic hiccups are difficult to treat.[67] A number of drugs and physical approaches have been tried, most of which do not work well. Agents used to treat hiccups include phenothiazines, calcium channel blockers, baclofen, and anticonvulsants, including gabapentin and pregabalin.[59,68] In steroid-induced hiccups, decreasing the dose usually reduces the hiccups.

Vomiting is a reflex response involving coordinated somatomotor (posture, abdominal muscle contraction), gastrointestinal (reversal of peristalsis), and respiratory (retching, breath holding) components that are coordinated by neurons in the ventrolateral medullary tegmentum near the compact portion of the nucleus ambiguus. The vomiting reflex may be triggered by vagal afferents or by chemosensory neurons in the area postrema, a small group of nerve cells that sits atop the nucleus of the solitary tract in the floor of the fourth ventricle, just at the level of the obex.[60,69] Because the area postrema lacks a blood–brain barrier, neurons in the area postrema may initiate vomiting in response to emetic molecules in the bloodstream, such as dopamine or glucagon-like peptide 1 (GLP-1).[70,71] The area postrema contains both dopaminergic and serotonergic neurons, which produce emesis by means of contacting dopamine (D_2) and serotonin ($5HT_3$) receptors, respectively.[72] In addition, there are neurokinin-1 receptors located in the nucleus of the solitary tract and ventrolateral medulla. Hence, drugs that block dopamine D_2 receptors (e.g., chlorpromazine, metoclopramide), serotonin $5HT_3$ receptors (ondansetron), or NK-1 receptors (aprepitant) are effective antiemetics.[73]

In patients with impaired consciousness, vomiting is frequently due to lesions involving the lateral pons or medulla. It occasionally occurs in patients with irritative lesions limited to the region of the nucleus of the solitary tract.[72] Such vomiting is typically preceded by intense nausea. More commonly, however, vomiting is due to a sudden increase in ICP, such as occurs in subarachnoid hemorrhage. The pressure wave may stimulate the emetic response directly by pressure on the floor of the fourth ventricle, resulting in sudden, "projectile" vomiting, without warning. This type of vomiting is particularly common in children with posterior fossa tumors. It is also seen in adults with brain tumors who hypoventilate during sleep, resulting in cerebral vasodilation. The small increase in intravascular blood volume in a patient whose ICP is already elevated may cause a sharp increase in ICP (see Chapter 3), resulting in onset of an intense headache that may awaken the patient, followed shortly thereafter by sudden projectile vomiting. Children with posterior fossa tumors may simply vomit without headache.

Vomiting is also commonly seen in patients with brain tumors during chemotherapy or even radiation therapy. Tissue injury, particularly in the gut, may release emetic hormones, such as GLP-1, which act at the area postrema to induce vomiting.[70,74]

The integrity of lower medullary pathways should be tested with the gag reflex. The ability of the sensory input from the IX and X nerves to cause reflex palatal elevation via the IX and X nerve motor pathways can be tested by stroking the posterior pharyngeal wall with a cotton swab. Bilateral palatal elevation is normal. Unilateral lack of elevation of the soft palate suggests medullary damage on that side. However, some normal people have bilateral absence of the gag reflex, and it is often suppressed by the presence of an endotracheal tube or by a depressed level of consciousness, so the significance of bilateral lack of a gag reflex cannot be determined.

PUPILLARY RESPONSES

The pupillary light reflex is one of the most basic and easily tested nervous system responses. It is controlled by a complex balance of sympathetic (pupillodilator) and parasympathetic (pupilloconstrictor) pathways (see Figure 2.6). The anatomy of these pathways is closely intertwined with the components of the ascending arousal system. In addition, the pupillary pathways are among the most resistant to metabolic insult. *Hence, abnormalities of pupillary responses are of great localizing value in diagnosing the cause of stupor and coma, and the pupillary light reflex is the single most important physical sign in differentiating metabolic from structural coma.*

Examine the Pupils and Their Responses

If possible, inquire if the patient has suffered eye disease or uses eyedrops. Observe the pupils in ambient light; if room lights are bright and pupils are small, dimming the light may make it easier to see the pupillary responses. They should be equal in size and about the same size as those of normal individuals in the same light (8–18% of normal individuals have anisocoria greater than 0.4 mm). Unequal pupils can result from sympathetic paralysis making the pupil smaller or parasympathetic paralysis making the pupil larger. If one suspects sympathetic paralysis (see *Horner's syndrome*, pages 62–63), dim the lights in the room, allowing the normal pupil to dilate and thus bringing out the pupillary inequality. Unless there is specific damage to the pupillary

(A)   (B)

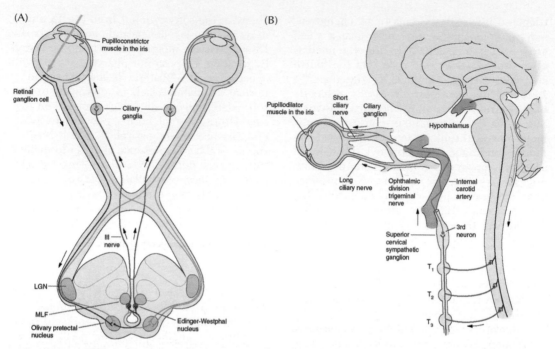

Figure 2.6 Two summary drawings indicating the (A) parasympathetic pupilloconstrictor pathways and (B) sympathetic pupillodilator pathways. LGN, lateral geniculate nucleus; MLF, medial longitudinal fasciculus.
From Saper C. Brain stem modulation of sensation, movement, and consciousness. Chapter 45 in: Kandel ER, Schwartz JH, Jessel TM. *Principles of Neural Science*. 4th ed. McGraw-Hill, New York, 2000, pp. 871–909. By permission of McGraw-Hill.)

system, pupils of stuporous or comatose patients are usually smaller than normal pupils in awake subjects. Pupillary responses must be examined with a bright light. The eyelids can be held open while the light from a bright flashlight illuminates each pupil. Shining the light into one pupil should cause both pupils to react briskly and equally. Because the pupils are often small in stuporous or comatose patients and the light reflex may be through a small range, one may want to view the pupil through the bright light of an ophthalmoscope using a plus 20 lens or through the lens of an otoscope. Most pupillary responses are brisk, but a tonic pupil may react slowly, so the light should illuminate the eye for at least 10 seconds. Moving the light from one eye to the other may result in constriction of both pupils when the light is shined into the first eye but, paradoxically, pupillary dilation when the light is shined in the other eye. This aberrant pupillary response results from damage to the retina or optic nerve on the side on which the pupil dilates (relative afferent pupillary defect [RAPD]), although it may rarely result from injury to the contralateral optic tract.[75]

One of the most ominous signs in neurology is a unilateral dilated and unreactive pupil. In a comatose patient, this usually indicates oculomotor nerve compromise either by a posterior communicating artery aneurysm or by temporal lobe herniation. However, the same finding can be mimicked by unilateral instillation of atropine-like eye drops. Occasionally this happens by accident, as when a patient who is using a scopolamine patch to avert motion sickness inadvertently gets some scopolamine onto a finger when handling the patch and then rubs the eye; it is also seen in cases of factitious presentation. At still other times, unilateral pupillary dilation may occur in the setting of ciliary ganglion dysfunction from head or facial trauma. In most of these cases there is a fracture in the posterior floor of the orbit that interrupts the fibers of the inferior division of the oculomotor nerve.[76] Injury to the third nerve can be distinguished from atropinic blockade at the bedside by instilling a dilute solution of pilocarpine into the eye (see *Pharmacology*, below). The denervated pupil will respond briskly, whereas one that is blocked by atropine will not.[77]

Once both the ipsilateral and consensual pupillary light reflexes have been noted, the next step is to induce a ciliospinal reflex.[11] This can be done by pinching the skin of the neck or the face. The pupils should dilate 1–2 mm bilaterally. This reflex is an example of a spinobulbospinal response (i.e., the pain stimulus arises from the trigeminal or spinal dorsal horn, must ascend to brainstem autonomic control areas, and then descend again to the C8–T2 sympathetic preganglionic neurons). A normal ciliospinal response ensures integrity of these circuits from the lower brainstem to the spinal cord, thus usually placing the lesion in the rostral pons or higher.

Pathophysiology of Pupillary Responses: Peripheral Anatomy of the Pupillomotor System

The pupil is a hole in the iris; thus, change in pupillary diameter occurs when the iris contracts or expands. The pupillodilator muscle is a set of radially oriented muscle fibers running from the edge of the pupil to the limbus (outer edge) of the iris. When these muscles contract, they open the pupil in much the way a drawstring pulls up a curtain. The pupillodilator muscles are innervated by sympathetic ganglion cells in the superior cervical ganglion. These axons pass along the internal carotid artery, joining the ophthalmic division of the trigeminal nerve in the cavernous sinus and accompanying it through the superior orbital fissure into the orbit. Sympathetic input to the lid retractor muscle takes a similar course, but sympathetic fibers from the superior cervical ganglion that control facial sweating travel along the external carotid artery.[10] Hence, lesions of the ascending cervical sympathetic chain up to the superior cervical ganglion typically give rise to Horner's syndrome (ptosis, miosis, and facial anhydrosis). However, lesions along the course of the internal carotid artery may give only the first two components of this syndrome (Raeder's paratrigeminal syndrome).[10] The sympathetic preganglionic neurons for pupillary control are found in the intermediolateral column of the first three thoracic segments. Lesions of those roots, or of the ascending sympathetic trunk between T1 and the superior cervical ganglion (e.g., an apical sulcus lung

tumor causing Pancoast syndrome), may also cause a Horner's syndrome with, depending on the exact site of the lesion, anhydrosis of the ipsilateral face or the face and arm.

The pupilloconstrictor muscle consists of circumferentially oriented muscle fibers that narrow the pupil when they contract, in the same manner as the drawstring of a purse. The parasympathetic neurons that supply the pupilloconstrictor muscle are located in the ciliary ganglion and in episcleral ganglion cells within the orbit. The preganglionic neurons for pupilloconstriction are located in the oculomotor complex in the brainstem (Edinger-Westphal nucleus), and they arrive in the orbit via the oculomotor or third cranial nerve. The pupilloconstrictor fibers travel in the dorsomedial quadrant of the third nerve, where they are vulnerable to compression by a number of causes (Chapter 3), often before there is clear impairment of the third-nerve extraocular muscles. As a result, unilateral loss of pupilloconstrictor tone is of great diagnostic importance in patients with stupor or coma caused by supratentorial mass lesions.

Pharmacology of the Peripheral Pupillomotor System

Because the state of the pupils is of such importance in the diagnosis of patients with coma, it is sometimes necessary to explore the origin of aberrant responses. Knowledge of the pharmacology of the pupillomotor system is essential to properly interpret the findings.[78] The sympathetic preganglionic neurons in the thoracic spinal cord are cholinergic, and they act on a nicotinic type II receptor on the sympathetic ganglion cells. The sympathetic terminals onto the pupillodilator muscle in the iris are noradrenergic, and they dilate the pupil via a beta-1 adrenergic receptor.

In the presence of a unilateral small pupil, it is possible to determine whether the cause is failure of the sympathetic ganglion cells or of the preganglionic inputs to those cells.[10,78] In the latter case, the ganglion cells are intact, but not active. The pupil can then be dilated by instilling a few drops of 1% hydroxyamphetamine into the eye, which releases norepinephrine from surviving sympathetic terminals. Because the postsynaptic receptors have become hypersensitive due to the paucity of neurotransmitter being released, there is brisk pupillodilation after instilling the eye drops. Conversely, if the pupil is small due to loss of postganglionic neurons or receptor blockade, hydroxyamphetamine will have little if any effect. Postganglionic failure can be differentiated from receptor blockade (e.g., instillation of eyedrops containing a beta blocker such as are used to treat glaucoma) by administration of 0.1% adrenaline drops, which have direct beta agonist effects. Denervated receptors are hypersensitive and there is brisk pupillary dilation, but a pupil that is small due to a beta blocker does not respond.

The pupilloconstrictor neurons in the oculomotor complex use acetylcholine as a neurotransmitter, and they act on the ciliary and episcleral ganglion cells via a nicotinic II receptor. The parasympathetic ganglion cells, by contrast, activate the pupilloconstrictor muscle via muscarinic cholinergic receptors. In the presence of a dilated pupil due to an injury to the third nerve or the postganglionic neurons, the hypersensitive receptors will constrict the pupil rapidly in response to a dilute solution of the muscarinic agonist pilocarpine (0.125%). However, if the enlarged pupil is due to atropine, even much stronger solutions of pilocarpine (up to 1.0%) will be unable to constrict the pupil.

CENTRAL PATHWAYS CONTROLLING PUPILLARY RESPONSES

It is important to understand the central pathways that regulate pupillary light responses because dysfunction in these pathways causes the abnormal pupillary signs seen in patients with coma due to brainstem injury.

Preganglionic *sympathetic* neurons in the C8–T2 levels of the spinal cord, which regulate pupillodilation, receive inputs from several levels of the brain. The main input driving sympathetic pupillary tone derives from the ipsilateral hypothalamus. Neurons in the paraventricular nucleus and in the lateral hypothalamus innervate the upper thoracic sympathetic preganglionic neurons.[8] The orexin/hypocretin neurons in the lateral hypothalamus provide a particularly intense input to this area.[79] This input may be important because the activity of the orexin neurons is greatest during active wakefulness, when pupillodilation is

maximal.[80] The descending hypothalamic input runs through the lateral part of the pontine and medullary brainstem tegmentum, where it is vulnerable to damage.[8] Electrical stimulation of the descending sympathoexcitatory tract in cats demonstrates that it runs in a superficial position along the surface of the ventrolateral medulla, just dorsolateral to the inferior olivary nucleus.[81] Experience in patients with lateral medullary infarction supports a similar localization in humans.[10] Such patients may have a *central Horner's syndrome,* which includes not only miosis and ptosis, but also loss of sweating on the entire ipsilateral side of the body. Thus, the sympathoexcitatory pathway remains ipsilateral from the hypothalamus all the way to the spinal cord.

Other brainstem pathways also contribute to pupillodilation. Inputs to the C8–T2 sympathetic preganglionic column arise from a number of brainstem sites, including the Kölliker-Fuse nucleus, A5 noradrenergic neurons, C1 adrenergic neurons, medullary raphe serotoninergic neurons, and other populations in the rostral ventrolateral medulla that have not been chemically characterized in detail.[9] Ascending pain afferents from the spinal cord terminate both in these sites as well as in the periaqueductal gray matter. Brainstem sympathoexcitatory neurons can cause pupillodilation in response to painful stimuli (the *ciliospinal reflex*).[11] They also provide ascending inhibitory inputs to the pupilloconstrictor neurons in the midbrain. As a result, pinpoint pupils are seen in patients with lesions of the pontine tegmentum (often pontine hemorrhage), which destroy both the ascending inhibitory inputs to the pupilloconstrictor system as well as the descending excitatory inputs to the pupillodilator system.

Preganglionic *parasympathetic* neurons are located in the Edinger-Westphal nucleus in primates.[82] This complex cell group also contains peptidergic neurons that mainly provide descending projections to the spinal cord.[83] The main input to the Edinger-Westphal neurons of clinical interest is the afferent limb of the pupillary light reflex. The retinal ganglion cells that contribute to this pathway belong to a special class of irradiance detectors, most of which contain the photopigment melanopsin.[84] The same population of retinal ganglion cells that drives the pupillary light reflex also provides inputs to the suprachiasmatic nucleus in the circadian system, and, in many cases, individual ganglion cells send axonal branches to both systems.[85] Although these ganglion cells are activated by the traditional pathways from rods and cones, they also are directly light sensitive, and, as a consequence, pupillary light reflexes are preserved in animals and humans with retinal degeneration who lack rods and cones (i.e., are functionally blind).[86] This is in contrast to acute onset of blindness, in which preservation of the pupillary light reflex implies damage to the visual system beyond the optic tracts, usually at the level of the visual cortex.

The brightness-responsive retinal ganglion cells innervate the olivary pretectal nucleus.[85] Neurons in the olivary pretectal nucleus then send their axons through the posterior commissure to the Edinger-Westphal nucleus of both sides.[87] The Edinger-Westphal nucleus in humans, as in other species, lies very close to the midline, just dorsal to the main body of the oculomotor nucleus. As a result, lesions that involve the posterior commissure disrupt the light reflex pathway from both eyes, resulting in fixed, slightly large (5–6 mm) pupils.

Electrical stimulation of cortical sites can cause either pupillary constriction or dilation, which can either be ipsilateral, contralateral, or bilateral.[88] Sites that may produce pupillary responses are found in both the lateral and medial frontal lobes, the occipital lobe, and the temporal lobe. Unilateral pupillodilation has also been reported in patients during epileptic seizures. However, the pupillary response can be either ipsilateral or contralateral to the presumed origin of the seizures. Because so little is known about descending inputs to the pupillomotor system from the cortex and their physiologic role, it is not possible at this point to use pupillary responses during seizure activity to determine the lateralization, let alone localization, of the seizure onset. However, brief, reversible changes in pupillary size may be due to seizure activity rather than structural brainstem injury. We have also seen rapidly and spontaneously reversible and asymmetric changes in pupillary diameter in patients with oculomotor dysfunction due to tuberculous meningitis and with severe cases of Guillain-Barré syndrome that cause autonomic denervation. These probably represent hypersensitivity of a partially deafferented target during rapid fluctuations of autonomic tone.

Localizing Value of Abnormal Pupillary Responses in Patients in Coma

Characteristic pupillary responses are seen with lesions at specific sites in the neuraxis (Figure 2.7).

Diencephalic injuries typically result in small, reactive pupils. Bilateral, small, reactive pupils are typically seen when there is bilateral diencephalic injury or compression, but they also are seen in almost all types of metabolic encephalopathy, and therefore this finding is also of limited value in identifying structural causes of coma.

A unilateral, small, reactive pupil accompanied by ipsilateral ptosis is often of great diagnostic value. Because the sympathetic fibers causing facial sweating accompany the external carotid artery, while those causing ptosis and meiosis follow the internal carotid artery, the combination of the two (a full *peripheral Horner's syndrome*) implies a lesion between the T1 and T2 spinal cord and the carotid bifurcation. Meiosis and ptosis with no associated loss of sweating in the face or the body (after the patient is placed under a heating lamp that causes sweating of the contralateral face) indicates a lesion along the course of the internal carotid artery or in the cavernous sinus, superior orbital fissure, or the orbit itself (*Raeder's paratrigeminal syndrome*, although in some cases the Horner's syndrome is merely incomplete). If the loss of sweating involves the entire side of the body (*central Horner's syndrome*), it indicates a lesion involving the pathway between the hypothalamus and the spinal cord on the ipsilateral side. Although hypothalamic unilateral injury can produce this finding, lesions of the lateral brainstem tegmentum are a more common cause.

Midbrain injuries may cause a wide range of pupillary abnormalities, depending on the nature of the insult. Bilateral midbrain tegmental infarction, involving the oculomotor nerves or nuclei bilaterally, results in fixed pupils that are either large (if the descending sympathetic tracts are preserved) or midposition (if they are not). However, pupils that are fixed due to midbrain injury may dilate with the ciliospinal reflex. This response distinguishes midbrain pupils from

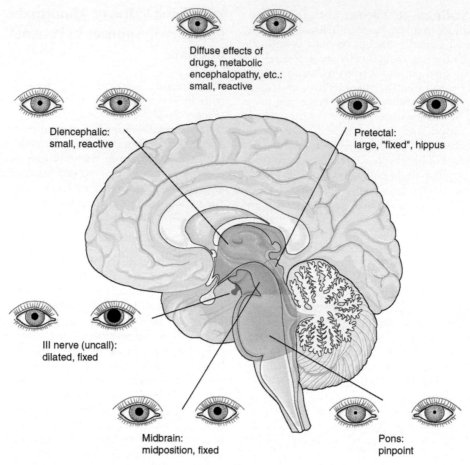

Diffuse effects of drugs, metabolic encephalopathy, etc.: small, reactive

Diencephalic: small, reactive

Pretectal: large, "fixed", hippus

III nerve (uncall): dilated, fixed

Midbrain: midposition, fixed

Pons: pinpoint

Figure 2.7 Summary of changes in pupils in patients with lesions at different levels of the brain that cause coma. From Saper C. Brain stem modulation of sensation, movement, and consciousness. Chapter 45 in: Kandel ER, Schwartz JH, Jessel TM. *Principles of Neural Science*. 4th ed. McGraw-Hill, New York, 2000, pp. 871–909. By permission of McGraw-Hill.

cases of brain death. It is often thought that pupils become fixed and dilated in death, but this is only true if there is a terminal release of adrenal catecholamines. The dilated pupils found immediately after death resolve over a few hours to the midposition, as are seen in patients who are brain dead or who have midbrain infarction.

More distal injury, after the *oculomotor nerve* leaves the brainstem, is typically unilateral. The oculomotor nerve's course makes it susceptible to damage by either the uncus of the temporal lobe as it herniates through the tentorial opening (see page 104) or an aneurysm of the posterior communicating artery. Either of these lesions may compress the oculomotor nerve from the dorsal direction. Because the pupilloconstrictor

fibers lie superficially on the dorsomedial surface of the nerve at this level,[89] the first sign of impending disaster may be a unilateral enlarged and poorly reactive pupil. These conditions are discussed in detail in Chapter 3.

Pontine tegmental injury typically results in pinpoint pupils. The pupils can often be seen under magnification to respond to bright light. However, the simultaneous injury to both the descending and ascending pupillodilator pathways causes near maximal pupillary constriction.[81] The most common cause is pontine hemorrhage.

Lesions involving the lateral *medullary* tegmentum, such as Wallenberg's lateral medullary infarction, may cause an ipsilateral central Horner's syndrome.[10]

Metabolic and Pharmacologic Causes of Abnormal Pupillary Response

Although the foregoing discussion illustrates the importance of the pupillary light response in diagnosing structural causes of coma, it is critical to be able to distinguish structural causes from metabolic and pharmacologic causes of pupillary abnormalities. Nearly any metabolic encephalopathy that causes a sleepy state may result in small, reactive pupils that are difficult to differentiate from pupillary responses caused by diencephalic injuries. However, the pupillary light reflex is one of the most resistant brain responses during metabolic encephalopathy. Hence, preservation of pupillary light responses in a comatose patient vouches for the structural integrity of the upper midbrain and thus suggests a metabolic cause for the coma.

During or following seizures, one or both pupils may transiently (usually for 15–20 minutes, and rarely as long as an hour) be large or react poorly to light. During hypoxia or global ischemia of the brain, such as during a cardiac arrest, the pupils typically become large and fixed due to a combination of systemic catecholamine release at the onset of the ischemia or hypoxia and lack of response by the metabolically depleted brain. If resuscitation is successful, the pupils usually return to a small, reactive state. Pupils that remain enlarged and nonreactive for more than a few minutes after otherwise successful resuscitation are indicative of profound brain ischemia and a poor prognostic sign (see discussion of outcomes from hypoxic/ischemic coma in Chapter 9).

Although most drugs that impair consciousness cause small, reactive pupils, a few produce quite different responses that may help to identify the cause of the coma. Opiates, for example, typically produce pinpoint pupils that resemble those seen in pontine hemorrhage. However, administration of an opioid antagonist such as naloxone results in rapid reversal of both the pupillary abnormality and the impairment of consciousness (naloxone must be given carefully to an opioid-intoxicated patient because, if the patient is opioid dependent, the drug may precipitate acute withdrawal). Chapter 7 discusses the use of naloxone. Muscarinic cholinergic antagonist drugs that cross the blood–brain barrier, such as scopolamine, may cause a confused, delirious state in combination with large, poorly reactive pupils. Lack of response to pilocarpine eye drops (see above) demonstrates the muscarinic blockade.[78] Overdose with glutethimide, a sedative-hypnotic drug that was popular in the 1960s, was notorious for causing large and poorly reactive pupils. Fortunately, it is not used anymore.

Visual assessments of pupillary reactivity with the naked eye have poor test–re-test and interrater reliability.[90] Automated quantification of the extent and speed of pupillary reactivity at the bedside is now possible using infrared pupillometry, and this method is increasingly being introduced in critical care settings. Automated and quantified pupillary reactivity correlates with uncal herniation,[91] carries prognostic significance in cardiac arrest, and predicts the development of delirium.[92,93] At this point it is unclear if patient care will be improved by the availability of these more accurate automated pupillary reactivity assessments.

OCULOMOTOR RESPONSES

The brainstem nuclei and pathways that control eye movements lie in close association with the ascending arousal system. Hence, it is unusual for a patient with a structural cause of coma to have entirely normal eye movements, and the type of oculomotor abnormality often identifies the site of the lesion that causes coma. A key clinical tenet of the coma examination is that, with rare exception (e.g., a comatose patient with a congenital strabismus), *asymmetric oculomotor function typically identifies a patient with a structural rather than metabolic cause of coma*.

Functional Anatomy of the Peripheral Oculomotor System

Eye movements are due to the complex and simultaneous contractions of six extraocular muscles controlling each globe. In addition, the muscles of the iris (see earlier description), the lens accommodation system, and the eyelid receive input from some of the same central cell groups and cranial nerves. Each of these can be used to identify the cause of an ocular motor disturbance and may shed light on the origin of coma (Figure 2.8).[94]

Lateral movement of the globes is caused by the lateral rectus muscle, which in turn is under the control of the abducens or sixth cranial nerve. The superior oblique muscle and trochlear or fourth cranial nerve have more complex actions. Because the trochlear muscle loops through a pulley, or trochleus, it attaches behind the equator of the globe and pulls it forward rather than back. When the eye turns medially, the action of this muscle is to pull the eye down and in. When the eye is turned laterally, however, the action of the muscle is to intort the eye (rotate it on its axis with the top of the iris moving medially).

All of the other extraocular muscles receive their innervation through the oculomotor or third cranial nerve. These include the medial rectus, whose action is to turn the eye inward; the superior rectus, which pulls the eye up and out; and the inferior rectus and oblique, which turn the eye down and out and up and in, respectively. It should be clear from this that, whereas impairment of mediolateral movements of the eyes mainly indicates imbalance of the medial and lateral rectus muscles, disturbances of upward or downward movement are far more complex to work out because they result from dysfunction of the complex set of balanced contractions of the other four muscles. This situation is reflected in the central control of these movements, as will be reviewed later.

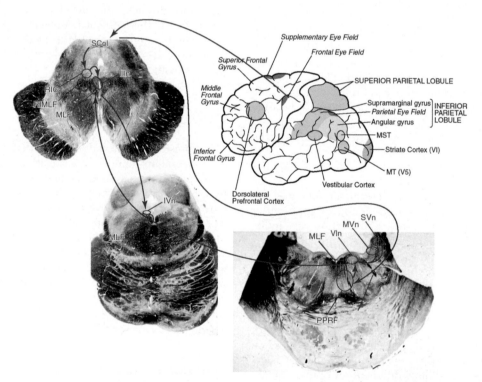

Figure 2.8 A summary diagram showing the major pathways responsible for eye movements. The frontal eye fields (A) provide input to the superior colliculus (SCol) to program saccadic eye movements. The superior colliculus then projects to a premotor area for horizontal saccades (the paramedian pontine reticular formation [PPRF]), which in turn contacts neurons in the abducens nucleus that abduct the ipsilateral eye. Abducens neurons (VIn) also send axons through the opposite medial longitudinal fasciculus (MLF) to the opposite oculomotor nucleus (IIIn) to activate medial rectus motor neurons and adduct the opposite eye. Vertical saccades are controlled by inputs from the superior colliculus to the rostral interstitial nucleus of the MLF (RIMLF) and rostral interstitial nucleus of Cajal (RIC), which act as a premotor area to instruct the neurons in the oculomotor and trochlear (IVn) nuclei to perform a vertical saccade. Vestibular and gaze-holding inputs come to the same ocular motor nuclei from the medial (MVN) and superior (SVN) vestibular nucleus. Note the intimate relationship of these cell groups and pathways with the ascending arousal system, whose axons run just ventral to the MLF.

The oculomotor nerve exits the brainstem through the medial part of the cerebral peduncle, then travels anteriorly between the superior cerebellar and posterior cerebral arteries. It passes through the tentorial opening and runs adjacent to the posterior communicating artery, where it is subject to injury by posterior communicating artery aneurysms. The nerve then runs through the cavernous sinus and superior orbital fissure to the orbit, where it divides into superior and inferior branches. The superior branch innervates the superior rectus muscle and the levator palpebrae superioris, which raises the eyelid, and the inferior branch supplies the medial and inferior rectus and inferior oblique muscles as well as the ciliary ganglion. The abducens nerve exits from the base of the pons, near the midline. This slender nerve, which is often avulsed when the brain is removed at autopsy, runs along the clivus, through the tentorial opening, and into the cavernous sinus and superior orbital fissure, on its way to the lateral rectus muscle. The trochlear nerve is a crossed nerve (i.e., it consists of axons whose cell bodies are on the other side of the brainstem), and it is the only cranial nerve that exits from the dorsal side of the brainstem. The axons emerge from the anterior medullary velum just behind the inferior colliculi, then wrap around the brainstem, pass through the tentorial opening, enter the cavernous sinus, and travel through the superior orbital fissure to innervate the superior oblique muscle.

Unilateral or even bilateral abducens palsy is commonly seen as a false localizing sign in patients with increased ICP. Although the long intracranial course of the nerve is often cited as the cause of its predisposition to injury, the trochlear nerve (which is rarely injured by diffusely increased intracranial pressure) is actually longer,[95] and the sharp bend of the abducens nerve as it enters the cavernous sinus may play a more decisive role. From a clinical point of view, however, it is important to remember that isolated unilateral or bilateral abducens palsy does not necessarily indicate a site of brain or nerve injury. The emergence of the trochlear nerve from the dorsal midbrain just behind the inferior colliculus makes it prone to injury by the tentorial edge (which runs along the adjacent superior surface of the cerebellum) in cases of severe head trauma. Thus, trochlear nerve palsy after head trauma does not necessarily represent a focal brainstem injury (although the dorsal brainstem at this level may be damaged by the same process).

The course of all three ocular motor nerves through the cavernous sinus and superior orbital fissure means that they are often damaged in combination by lesions at these sites. Thus, a lesion of all three of these nerves unilaterally indicates injury in the cavernous sinus or superior orbital fissure rather than the brainstem. Head trauma causing a blowout fracture of the orbit may trap the eye muscles, resulting in abnormalities of ocular motility unrelated to any underlying brain injury. The entrapment of the eye muscles is determined by forced duction (i.e., resistance to physically moving the globe) as described later in the examination.

Functional Anatomy of the Central Oculomotor System

The oculomotor nuclei receive and integrate a large number of inputs that control their activity and coordinate eye muscle movement to produce normal, conjugate gaze. These afferents arise from cortical, tectal, and tegmental oculomotor systems, as well as directly from the vestibular system and vestibulocerebellum. In principle, these classes of afferents are not greatly different from the types of inputs that control alpha-motor neurons concerned with striated muscles, except the oculomotor muscles do not contain muscle spindles and hence there is no somatosensory feedback.

The oculomotor nuclei are surrounded by areas of the brainstem tegmentum containing premotor cell groups that coordinate eye movements.[94,96,97] The premotor area for regulating lateral saccades consists of the paramedian pontine reticular formation (PPRF), which is just ventral to the abducens nucleus. The PPRF contains several different classes of neurons with bursting and pausing activities related temporally to horizontal saccades.[97–99] Their main effect is to allow conjugate lateral saccades to the ipsilateral side of space, and when neurons in this area are inactivated by injection of local anesthetic, ipsilateral saccades are slowed or eliminated. In addition, neurons in the dorsal pontine nuclei relay smooth pursuit signals to the flocculus, and the medial vestibular nucleus and flocculus are both important for holding eccentric gaze.[97] Inputs from these systems converge on the abducens nucleus, which contains two classes of neurons: those that directly innervate the lateral rectus muscle (motor neurons) and those that project through the medial longitudinal fasciculus (MLF) to the opposite medial rectus motor neurons in the oculomotor nucleus (premotor neurons). Axons from these premotor neurons cross the midline at the level of the abducens nucleus and ascend on the contralateral side of the brainstem to allow conjugate lateral gaze. Thus, pontine tegmental lesions typically result in the inability to move the eyes to the ipsilateral side of space (lateral gaze palsy). Similarly, the premotor area for vertical saccades and gaze holding, respectively, are found in the rostral interstitial nucleus of the MLF and rostral interstitial nucleus of Cajal, which surround the oculomotor nucleus laterally. A premotor area for vergence eye movements is found at the rostral tip of this region, near the midbrain–diencephalic junction. Unilateral lesions of the rostral interstitial nuclei typically reduce vertical saccades as well as causing torsional nystagmus.[100,101] Compression of the midbrain from the tectal surface and posterior commissure (e.g., by a pineal tumor) causes loss of vertical eye movements, usually beginning with upgaze (along with loss of pupillary light response).

The PPRF and rostral interstitial nuclei are under the control of descending inputs from the superior colliculus. Each superior colliculus contains a map of the visual world on the contralateral side of space, and electrical stimulation of a specific point in this visual map will command a saccade to the corresponding point in space. In nonmammalian vertebrates, such as frogs, this area is called the *optic tectum* and is the principal site for directing eye movement; in mammals, it can direct rapid, reflex eye movements but comes largely under the control of the cortical system for directing saccades.

The cortical descending inputs to the ocular motor system are complex.[102] The frontal eye fields (area 8) direct saccadic eye movements to explore behaviorally relevant features of the contralateral side of space.[103,104] However, it would be incorrect to think of this area as a motor cortex. Unlike neurons in the primary motor cortex, which fire in relation to movements of the limbs in particular directions

at particular joints, recordings from area 8 neurons in awake, behaving monkeys indicate that they do not fire during most random saccadic eye movements. However, they are engaged during tasks that require a saccade to a particular part of space only when the saccadic eye movement is part of a behavioral sequence that is rewarded. In this respect, neurons in area 8 are more similar to those in areas of the prefrontal cortex that are involved in planning movements toward the opposite side of space. Area 8 projects widely to both the superior colliculus as well as the premotor areas for vertical and lateral eye movements, and to the ocular motor nuclei themselves.[103,105] Descending axons from area 8 mainly run through the internal medullary lamina of the thalamus to enter the region of the rostral interstitial nucleus of the MLF. They then cross the midline to descend along with the MLF to the contralateral PPRF and abducens nucleus.

In the posterior part of the hemisphere, in the ventrolateral cortex near the occipitoparietal junction, is an area of visual cortex, sometimes called area V5 or area MT, that is important in judging movement of objects in contralateral space.[106] Cortex in this region plays a critical role in following movements originating in contralateral space, including movements toward the ipsilateral space. Thus, following an object that travels from the left to the right engages the right parietal cortex (area 7) to fix attention on the object, the right area 8 to produce a saccade to pick it up, the right occipital cortex to follow the object to the right, and, ultimately, the left occipital cortex as well to see the object as it enters the right side of space. Thus, following moving stripes to the right, as in testing optokinetic nystagmus, engages a number of important cortical as well as brainstem pathways necessary to produce eye movements. Although the test is fairly sensitive for picking up oculomotor problems at a cortical and brainstem level, the interpretation of failure of optokinetic nystagmus is a complex process.

In addition to these motor inputs, the ocular motor neurons also receive sensory inputs to guide them. Although there are no spindles in the ocular motor muscles to provide somatic sensory feedback, the ocular motor nuclei depend on two different types of sensory feedback. First, visual feedback allows the rapid correction of errors in gaze. Second, the ocular motor nuclei receive direct and relayed inputs from the vestibular system.[102] Because the eyes must respond to changes in head position very quickly to stabilize the visual image on the retina, the direct vestibular input, which identifies angular or linear acceleration of the head, is integrated to provide a signal for rapid correction of eye position. The abducens nucleus is located at the same pontine level as the vestibular complex, and it receives inputs from the medial and superior vestibular nuclei. Additional axons from these nuclei cross the midline and ascend in the contralateral MLF to reach the trochlear and oculomotor nuclei. These inputs from the vestibular system allow both horizontal and vertical eye movements (vestibulo-ocular reflexes) in response to vestibular stimulation.

Another sensory input necessary for the brain to calculate its position in space is head position and movement. Ascending somatosensory afferents, particularly from the neck muscles and vertebral joint receptors, arise from the C2–C4 levels of the spinal cord. They ascend through the MLF to reach the vestibular nuclei and cerebellum, where they are integrated with vestibular sensory inputs.

The vestibulocerebellum, including the flocculus, paraflocculus, uvula, and nodulus, receives extensive vestibular input as well as somatosensory and visual afferents.[97,102] The output from the flocculus ensures the accuracy of saccadic eye movements and contributes to pursuit eye movements and the ability to hold an eccentric position of gaze. The vestibulocerebellum is also critical in learning new relationships between eye movements and visual displacement (e.g., when wearing prism or magnification glasses). Lesions of the vestibulocerebellum cause ocular dysmetria (inability to perform accurate saccades), ocular flutter (rapid to-and-fro eye movements), and opsoclonus (chaotic eye movements).[107] It may be difficult to distinguish less severe cases of vestibulocerebellar function from vestibular dysfunction.

Because the MLF conveys so many classes of input from the pontine level to the midbrain, lesions of the MLF have profound effects on eye movements. After a unilateral MLF lesion, the eye ipsilateral to the lesion cannot follow the contralateral eye in conjugate lateral gaze to the other side of space (an *internuclear ophthalmoplegia*, a condition that occurs quite

commonly in multiple sclerosis and brainstem lacunar infarcts). The abducting eye shows horizontal gaze-evoked nystagmus (slow phase toward the midline, rapid jerks laterally), while the adducting eye stops in the midline (if the lesion is complete) or fails to fully adduct (if it is partial). Bilateral injury to the MLF caudal to the oculomotor complex not only causes a bilateral internuclear ophthalmoplegia, but also prevents vertical vestibulo-ocular responses or pursuit. Vertical saccades, however, are implemented by the superior colliculus inputs to the rostral interstitial nucleus of Cajal and are intact. Similarly, vergence eye movements are intact after caudal lesions of the MLF, which allows the paresis of adduction to be distinguished from a medial rectus palsy. More rostral MLF lesions, however, may also damage the closely associated preoculomotor areas for vertical or vergence eye movements.

The Ocular Motor Examination

The examination of the ocular motor system in awake, alert subjects involves testing both voluntary and reflex eye movements. In patients with stupor or coma, testing of reflex eyelid and ocular movements must suffice.[100]

EYELIDS AND CORNEAL RESPONSES

Begin by noting the position of the eyes and eyelids at rest and observing for spontaneous eye movements. The eyelids at rest in coma, as in sleep, are maintained in a closed position by tonic contraction of the orbicularis oculi muscles. (Patients with long-term impairment of consciousness who enter a persistent vegetative state have alternating cycles of eyes opening and closing; see Chapter 9.) Next, gently raise and then release the eyelids, noting their tone. The eyelids of a comatose patient close smoothly and gradually, a movement that cannot be duplicated by an awake individual simulating unconsciousness. Absence of tone or failure to close either eyelid can indicate facial motor weakness. Blepharospasm, or strong resistance to eyelid opening and then rapid closure, is usually voluntary, suggesting that the patient is not truly comatose. However, lethargic patients with either metabolic or structural lesions may resist eye opening, as do some patients with a nondominant parietal lobe infarct. In awake patients, ptosis may result from either brainstem or hemispheric injury. In patients with unilateral forebrain infarcts, the ptosis is often ipsilateral to hemiparesis.[108] In cases of brainstem injury, the ptosis may be part of a Horner's syndrome (i.e., accompanied by pupilloconstriction) due to injury to the lateral tegmentum, or it may be due to an injury to the oculomotor complex or nerve, in which case it is typically accompanied by pupillodilation. Tonically retracted eyelids (Collier's sign) may be found in patients with dorsal midbrain or, occasionally, pontine damage.

Spontaneous blinking usually is lost in coma as a function of the depressed level of consciousness and concomitant eye closure. However, in persistent vegetative state, it may return during cycles of eye opening (Chapter 9). Blinking in response to a loud sound or a bright light implies that the afferent sensory pathways are intact to the brainstem but does not necessarily mean that they are active at a forebrain level. Even patients with complete destruction of the visual cortex may recover reflex blink responses to light,[109] but not to threat.[110] A unilateral impairment of the speed or depth of the eyelid excursion during blinking occurs in patients with ipsilateral facial paresis.

The corneal reflex can be performed by approaching the eye from the side with a wisp of cotton that is then gently applied to the sclera and pulled across it to touch the corneal surface. Eliciting the corneal reflex in coma may require more vigorous stimulation than in an awake subject, but it is important not to touch the cornea with any material that might scratch its delicate surface. Corneal trauma can be completely avoided by testing the corneal reflex with sterile saline. Two to three drops of sterile saline are dropped on the cornea from a height of 4–6 inches.[6] Reflex closure of both eyelids and elevation of both eyes (Bell's phenomenon) indicates that the reflex pathways, from the trigeminal nerve and spinal trigeminal nucleus through the lateral brainstem tegmentum to the oculomotor and facial nuclei, remain intact. However, some patients who wear contact lenses may have permanent suppression of the corneal reflex. In other patients with an acute lesion of the descending corticofacial pathways, the blink reflex may be suppressed, but Bell's phenomenon should still occur. Some of these patients may have a jaw movement (thrusting of the jaw to the opposite side) as a synkinesis with spontaneous eye blinking; when this occurs during corneal stimulation, it is called a *corneomandibular reflex*.[111] This sign is not very useful in localization as it can occur with lesions from the cerebral hemispheres down to the pons. On the other hand, loss of Bell's phenomenon in the presence of an intact corneal blink response suggests a structural lesion at the midbrain level.[112]

EXAMINATION OF OCULAR MOTILITY

Hold the eyelids gently in an open position to observe eye position and movements in a comatose patient. A small flashlight or bright ophthalmoscope held about 50 cm from the face and shined toward the eyes of the patient should reflect off the same point in the cornea of each eye if the gaze is conjugate. Most patients with impaired consciousness demonstrate a slight exophoria. If it is possible to obtain a history, ask about eye movements, as a congenital strabismus may be misinterpreted as dysconjugate eye movements due to a brainstem lesion. Observe for a few moments for spontaneous eye movements. Slowly roving eye movements are typical of metabolic encephalopathy, and, if conjugate, they imply an intact ocular motor system.

The vestibulo-ocular responses are then tested by rotating the patient's head (*oculocephalic reflexes*).[100] In patients who may have suffered trauma, it is important first to rule out the possibility of a fracture or dislocation of the cervical spine; until this is done, it may be necessary to skip ahead to caloric testing (see later discussion). The head is rotated first in a lateral direction to either side while holding the eyelids open. This can be done by grasping the head on either side with both hands and using the thumbs to hold the eyelids open. The head movements should be brisk, and when the head position is held at each extreme for a few seconds, the eyes should gradually come back to midposition. Moving the head back to the opposite side then produces a maximal stimulus. The eye movements should be smooth and conjugate. The head is then rotated in a vertical plane (as in head nodding) and the eyes are observed for vertical conjugate movement. During downward head movement, the eyelids may also open (the doll's head phenomenon).[113]

The normal response generated by the vestibular input to the ocular motor system is for the eyes to rotate counter to the direction of the examiner's movement (i.e., turning the head to the right should cause the eyes to deviate to the left). In an awake patient, the voluntary control of gaze overcomes this reflex response. However, in patients with impaired consciousness, the oculocephalic reflex should predominate. This response is often colloquially called the *doll's eye response*, [113] and normal responses in both horizontal and vertical directions imply intact brainstem pathways from the vestibular nuclei through the lower pontine tegmentum and thence the upper pontine and midbrain paramedian tegmentum (i.e., along the course of the MLF; see later discussion). There may also be a small contribution from proprioceptive afferents from the neck,[114] which also travel through the medial longitudinal fasciculus. Because these pathways overlap extensively with the ascending arousal system (see Figure 2.8), it is quite unusual for patients with structural causes of coma to have a normal oculocephalic examination. In contrast, patients with metabolic encephalopathy, particularly due to hepatic failure, may have exaggerated or very brisk oculocephalic responses.

However, other patients with particularly deep metabolic coma may have sluggish eye movements or none at all during oculocephalic testing. In such cases, more intense vestibular stimulation may be obtained by testing *caloric vestibulo-ocular responses*. With appropriate equipment, vestibulo-ocular monitoring can be done using galvanic stimulation and video-oculography.[115] However, at the bedside, caloric stimuli and visual inspection are generally used (see Figure 2.9). The ear canal is first examined, and, if necessary, cerumen is removed to allow clear visualization that the tympanic membrane is intact. The head of the bed is then raised to about 30 degrees to bring the horizontal semicircular canal into a vertical position so that the response is maximal. If the patient is merely sleepy, the canal may be irrigated with cool water (15–20°C); this usually induces a brisk response and may occasionally cause nausea and vomiting. Fortunately, in practice, it is rarely necessary to use caloric stimulation in such patients. If the patient is deeply comatose, a maximal stimulus is obtained by using ice water. A large (50 mL)

syringe is used, attached to a plastic IV catheter (without a needle), which is gently advanced until it is near the tympanic membrane. An emesis basin can be placed below the ear, seated on an absorbent pad, to catch the effluent. The ice water is infused at a rate of about 10 mL/min for 5 minutes, or until a response is obtained. After a response is obtained, it is necessary to wait at least 5 minutes for the response to dissipate before testing the opposite ear. To test vertical eye movements, both external auditory canals are irrigated simultaneously with cold water (causing the eyes to deviate downward) or warm water (causing upward deviation).

The cold water induces a downward convection current, away from the ampulla, in the endolymph within the horizontal semicircular canal. The effect of the current upon the hair cells in the ampulla is to reduce tonic discharge of the vestibular neurons. Because the vestibular neurons associated with the horizontal canal fire fastest when the head is turning toward that side (and thus push the eyes to the opposite side), the result of cold water stimulation is to produce a stimulus as if the head were turning to the opposite side, thus activating the ipsilateral lateral rectus and contralateral medial rectus muscles to drive the eyes toward the side of cold water stimulation. Convection currents of the anterior canal (which activates the ipsilateral superior rectus and the contralateral inferior oblique muscles) and the posterior canal (which activates the ipsilateral superior oblique and contralateral inferior rectus muscles) by caloric stimulation cancel each other out.

When caloric stimulation is done in an awake patient who is trying to maintain fixation (e.g., in the vestibular testing laboratory), cool stimulation (about 30°C) causes a slow drift toward the side of stimulation, with a compensatory rapid saccade back to the midline (the direction of nystagmus is the direction of the fast component). Warm stimulation (about 44°C) induces the opposite response. The traditional mnemonic for remembering these movements is "COWS" (cold opposite, warm same), which refers to the direction of nystagmus in an awake patient. This mnemonic can be confusing for inexperienced examiners as the responses seen in a comatose patient with an intact brainstem are the opposite: cold water induces only tonic deviation (there is no little or no corrective nystagmus), so the eyes

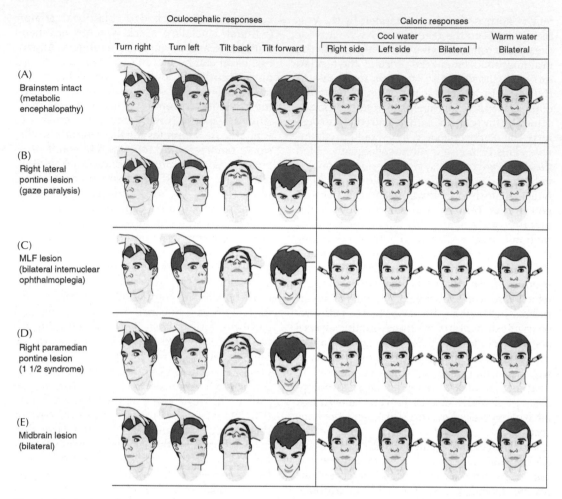

Figure 2.9 Ocular reflexes in unconscious patients. The left-hand side shows the responses to oculocephalic maneuvers (which should only be done after the possibility of cervical spine injury has been eliminated). The right-hand side shows responses to caloric stimulation with cold or warm water (see text for explanation). Normal brainstem reflexes in a patient with metabolic encephalopathy are illustrated in row (A). The patient shown in row (B) has a lesion of the right side of the pons (see Figure 2.8), causing a paralysis of gaze to that side with either eye. Row (C) shows the result of a lesion involving the medial longitudinal fasciculus (MLF) bilaterally (bilateral internuclear ophthalmoplegia). Only abducens responses with each eye persist. The patient in row (D) has a lesion involving both MLFs and the right abducens nucleus (one and a half syndrome). Only left eye abduction is retained. Row (E) illustrates a patient with a midbrain infarction eliminating both the oculomotor and trochlear responses, leaving only bilateral abduction responses. Note that the extraocular responses are identical to (C), in which there is a bilateral lesion of the MLF. However, pupillary light responses would be preserved after the MLF lesion.

From Saper C. Brain stem modulation of sensation, movement, and consciousness. Chapter 45 in: Kandel ER, Schwartz JH, Jessel TM. *Principles of Neural Science*. 4th ed. McGraw-Hill, New York, 2000, pp. 871–909. By permission of McGraw-Hill.

deviate toward the ear that is irrigated. The presence of typical vestibular nystagmus in a patient who is unresponsive suggests a psychogenic cause of unresponsiveness (i.e., the patient is actually awake). However, the absence of a response to caloric stimulation does not always imply brainstem dysfunction. Bilateral transient vestibular failure occurs with phenytoin or tricyclic antidepressant toxicity. Patients with chronic damage to the vestibular system (e.g., from aminoglycoside toxicity, Ménière's disease, vestibular schwannoma, or labyrinthine artery stroke) may also lack caloric vestibular responses, but oculocephalic responses may persist, with the neck muscles supplying the afferent information.[114]

On the other hand, because the oculomotor pathways are spatially so close to those involved in producing wakefulness, it is rare for a patient to have acute damage to the oculomotor control system without a change in consciousness.

Patient Vignette 2.1

A 56-year-old man with a 20-year history of poorly controlled hypertension came to the emergency department with a complaint of sudden onset of severe dizziness. On examination, he was fully awake and conversant. Pupils were 2.5 mm and constricted to 2.0 mm with light in either eye. The patient could not follow a moving light to either side or up or down. Hearing was intact, as were facial, oropharyngeal, and tongue motor and sensory responses. Motor and sensory examination was also normal, tendon reflexes were symmetric, and toes were downgoing.

The patient was sent for a computed tomography (CT) scan, which showed a hemorrhage into the periventricular gray matter in the floor of the fourth ventricle at a pontine level, which tracked rostrally into the midbrain. During the CT scan the patient lapsed into coma. At that point, the pupils were pinpoint and the patient was unresponsive with flaccid limbs. He subsequently died, but autopsy was not permitted.

Comment

The sudden onset of bilateral impairment of eye movements on the background of clear consciousness is rare and raised the possibility of a brainstem injury even without unconsciousness. Although the CT scan demonstrated a focal hemorrhage selectively destroying the abducens nuclei and medial longitudinal fasciculi, the proximity of these structures to the ascending arousal system was demonstrated by the loss of consciousness over the next few minutes.

Finally, if there has been head trauma, one or more eye muscles may become trapped by a blowout fracture of the orbit. It is important to distinguish this cause of abnormal eye movements from damage to neural structures, either peripherally or centrally. This is generally done by an ophthalmologist who applies topical anesthetics to the globe and uses a fine, toothed forceps to tug on the sclera to attempt to move the globe (*forced duction*). Inability to move the globe through a full range of movements may indicate a trapped muscle and requires evaluation for orbital fracture.

Interpretation of Abnormal Ocular Movements

A wide range of abnormal eye movements may be seen both at rest and during vestibular stimulation. Each presents clues about the nature of the insult that is causing the impairment of consciousness.

RESTING AND SPONTANEOUS EYE MOVEMENTS

A great deal of information may be gained by carefully noting the position of the eyes and any movements that occur without stimulation. Table 2.3 lists some of the spontaneous eye movements that may be observed in unconscious patients. Detailed descriptions are given in the following paragraphs. Most individuals have a mild degree of exophoria when drowsy and not maintaining active fixation. However, other individuals have varying types of strabismus, which may worsen as they become less responsive and no longer attempt to maintain conjugate gaze. Hence, it is very difficult to determine the meaning of dysconjugate gaze in a stuporous or comatose patient if nothing is known about the presence of baseline strabismus.

On the other hand, certain types of dysconjugate eye movements raise suspicion of brainstem injury that may require further examination for confirmation. For example, injury to the oculomotor nucleus or nerve produces exodeviation of the involved eye. Unilateral abducens injury causes the involved eye to deviate inward. In skew deviation,[116] in which one eye is deviated upward and the

Table 2.3 **Spontaneous Eye Movements Occurring in Unconscious Patients**

Term	Description	Significance
Ocular bobbing	Rapid, conjugate, downward movement; slow return to primary position	Pontine strokes; other structural, metabolic, or toxic disorders
Ocular dipping or inverse ocular bobbing	Slow downward movement; rapid return to primary position	Unreliable for localization; follows hypoxic-ischemic insult or metabolic disorder
Reverse ocular bobbing	Rapid upward movement; slow return to primary position	Unreliable for localization; may occur with metabolic disorders
Reverse ocular dipping or converse bobbing	Slow upward movement; rapid return to primary position	Unreliable for localization; seen with pontine infarction and with AIDS
Ping-pong gaze	Horizontal conjugate deviation of the eyes, alternating every few seconds	Bilateral cerebral hemispheric dysfunction; toxic ingestion
Periodic alternating gaze deviation	Horizontal conjugate deviation of the eyes, alternating every 2 minutes	Hepatic encephalopathy; cerebellar lesions and PRES
Vertical "myoclonus"	Vertical pendular oscillations (2–3 Hz)	Pontine strokes
Monocular movements	Small, intermittent, rapid monocular horizontal, vertical, or torsional movements	Pontine or midbrain destructive lesions, perhaps with coexistent seizures

Modified from Leigh and Zee,[94] with permission.

other downward, there typically is an injury to the brainstem (see later discussion).

CONJUGATE HORIZONTAL DEVIATION OF THE EYES

This is typically seen with destructive or irritative lesions, as compressive or metabolic disorders generally do not affect the supranuclear ocular motor pathways asymmetrically. A destructive lesion involving the frontal eye fields causes the eyes to deviate toward the side of the lesion (away from the side of the associated hemiparesis). This typically lasts for a few days after the onset of the lesion. An irritative lesion may cause deviation of the eyes away from the side of the lesion. These eye movements represent seizure activity, and often there is some evidence of quick, nystagmoid jerks toward the side of eye deviation indicative of continuing seizure activity. If seizure activity abates, there may be a Todd's paralysis of gaze for several hours, causing lateral gaze deviation toward the side of the affected cortex (i.e., opposite to the direction caused by the seizures). Hemorrhage into the thalamus may also produce "wrong-way eyes," which deviate away from the side of the lesion.[117,118]

This may be due to interruption of descending corticobulbar pathways for gaze control, which pass through the thalamic internal medullary lamina rather than the internal capsule. Damage to the lateral pons, on the other hand, may cause loss of eye movements toward that side (gaze palsy, Figure 2.9). The lateral gaze deviation in such patients cannot be overcome by vestibular stimulation, whereas vigorous oculocephalic or caloric stimulation usually overcomes lateral gaze deviation due to a cortical gaze paresis.

CONJUGATE VERTICAL DEVIATION OF THE EYES

Pressure on the tectal plate, as occurs with a pineal mass or sometimes with a thalamic hemorrhage, may cause conjugate downward deviation of the eyes.[119,120] Oculogyric crises may cause conjugate upward deviation. The classical cause of oculogyric crises was postencephalitic parkinsonism.[121] Few of these patients still survive, but a similar condition is frequently seen with dystonic crises in patients exposed to neuroleptics[122] and occasionally in patients with acute bilateral injury of the basal ganglia.[123]

NONCONJUGATE EYE DEVIATION

Whereas nonconjugate eye position may be due to an old baseline strabismus, failure of one eye to follow its mate during spontaneous or evoked eye movements is typically highly informative. Absence of abduction of a single eye suggests injury to the abducens nerve either within the brainstem or along its course to the orbit. However, either increased ICP or decreased pressure, as occurs with cerebral spinal fluid leaks, can cause either a unilateral or bilateral abducens palsy,[124] so the presence of an isolated abducens palsy may be misleading. Isolated loss of adduction of the eye contralateral to the head movement implies an injury to the medial longitudinal fasciculus (i.e., near the midline tegmentum) on that side between the abducens and oculomotor nuclei (Figure 2.9). Bilateral lesions of the medial longitudinal fasciculus impair adduction of both eyes as well as vertical oculocephalic and vestibuloocular eye movements, a condition that is distinguished from bilateral oculomotor nucleus or nerve injury in the comatose patient by preservation of the pupillary light responses. (Voluntary vergence and vertical eye movements remain intact, but require wakeful cooperation.)

Combined loss of adduction and vertical movements in one eye indicates an oculomotor nerve impairment. Typically, there is also severe ptosis on that side (so that if the patient is awake, he or she may not be aware of diplopia). In rare cases with a lesion of the oculomotor *nucleus*, the weakness of the superior rectus will be on the side *opposite* the other third-nerve muscles (as these fibers are crossed), and ptosis will be bilateral (but not very severe). Occasionally, oculomotor palsy may spare the pupillary fibers. This occurs most often when the paresis is due to ischemia of the oculomotor nerve (the smaller pupilloconstrictor fibers are more resistant to ischemia), such as in diabetic occlusion of the vasa nervorum.[125] Such patients are also typically awake and alert, whereas third-nerve paresis due to brainstem injury or compression of the oculomotor nerve by uncal herniation results in impairment of consciousness and early pupillodilation.

Trochlear nerve impairment causes a hyperopia of the involved eye, often with some exodeviation. If awake, the patient typically attempts to compensate by tilting the head toward the opposite shoulder. Because the trochlear nerve fibers cross to the opposite side before they exit the brainstem, a trochlear palsy in a comatose patient suggests damage either to the trochlear nerve on the same side as it exits the dorsolateral pons (e.g., in patients with severe head trauma) or to the trochlear nucleus on the opposite side of the brainstem.[126]

SKEW DEVIATION

Skew deviation refers to vertical dysconjugate gaze, with one eye displaced downward and the other upward, as if the head were tilted toward the side of the upper eye. In some cases, the eye that is elevated may alternate from side to side depending on whether the patient is looking to the left or the right.[127,128] Skew deviation is due either to a lesion in the lateral rostral medulla or lower pons, vestibular system, or vestibulo-cerebellum on the side of the inferior eye, or in the MLF on the side of the superior eye.[116,129]

ROVING EYE MOVEMENTS

These are slow, random deviations of eye position that are similar to the eye movements seen in normal individuals during light sleep. As in sleeping individuals who typically have some degree of exophoria, the eye positions may not be quite conjugate, but the ocular excursions should be conjugate. Most roving eye movements are predominantly horizontal, although some vertical movements may also occur. Most patients with roving eye movements have a metabolic encephalopathy, and oculocephalic and caloric vestibulo-ocular responses are typically preserved or even hyperactive. The roving eye movements may disappear as the coma deepens, although they may persist in quite severe hepatic coma. Roving eye movements cannot be duplicated by patients who are awake, and hence their presence indicates that unresponsiveness is not psychogenic. A variant of roving eye movements is periodic alternating or "ping-pong" gaze,[130] in which repetitive, rhythmic, and conjugate horizontal eye movements occur in a comatose or stuporous patient. The eyes move conjugately to the extremes of gaze and then rotate back again. The episodic movements of the eyes may continue uninterrupted for several hours to days. Periodic alternating eye movements

have been reported in patients with a variety
of structural injuries to the brainstem or even
bilateral cerebral infarcts that leave the oculomotor system largely intact but are most
common during metabolic encephalopathies.

RAPID EYE MOVEMENTS: NYSTAGMUS

Nystagmus refers to repetitive rapid (saccadic)
eye movements, generally alternating with a
slow drift in the opposite direction. Spontaneous
nystagmus is uncommon in coma because the
quick, saccadic phase is generally a corrective
movement generated by the voluntary saccade
system when the visual image drifts from the
point of intended fixation. However, continuous
seizure activity with versive eye movements
may give the appearance of nystagmus. In addition, several unusual forms of nystagmoid eye
movement do occur in comatose patients.

Retractory nystagmus consists of irregular jerks of both globes back into the orbit,
sometimes occurring spontaneously but other
times on attempted upgaze. Electromyography
during retractory nystagmus shows that the
retractions consist of simultaneous contractions
of all six extraocular muscles.[131] Retractory nystagmus is typically seen with dorsal midbrain
compression or destructive lesions[119] and is
thought to be due to impairment of descending
inputs that relax the opposing eye muscles
when a movement is made, so that all six muscles contract when attempts are made to activate any one of them.

Convergence nystagmus often accompanies
retractory nystagmus and also is typically seen
in patients with dorsal midbrain lesions.[132] The
eyes diverge slowly, and this is followed by a
quick convergent jerk.

Nystagmoid jerks of a single eye may occur
in a lateral, vertical, or rotational direction in
patients with pontine injury.

SLOWER EYE MOVEMENTS: OCULAR BOBBING AND DIPPING AND SEE-SAW NYSTAGMUS

C. Miller Fisher first described movements in
which the eyes make a brisk, conjugate downward movement, then "bob" back up more
slowly to primary position.[133] The patients
were comatose and the movements were not
affected by caloric vestibular stimulation. The
initially described patients had caudal pontine

injuries or compression, although later reports
described similar eye movements in patients
with obstructive hydrocephalus, uncal herniation, or even metabolic encephalopathy.
A variety of related eye movements have been
described including inverse bobbing (rapid elevation of the eyes, with bobbing downward
back to primary position) and both dipping
(downward slow movements with rapid and
smooth return to primary position) and inverse dipping (slow upward movements with
rapid return to primary position).[134,135] The
implications of these unusual eye movements
are similar to those of ocular bobbing: a lower
brainstem injury or compression of normal
vestibulo-ocular inputs.

See-saw nystagmus describes a rapid, pendular, disjunctive movement of the eyes in
which one eye rises and intorts while the
other descends and extorts, as with a head
tilt.[136,137] This is followed by reversal of the
movements. Although it is most commonly
seen during visual fixation in an awake patient
who has severe visual field defects or impairment of visual acuity, in a comatose patient
it appears to be due in most cases to lesions
near the rostral end of the periaqueductal
gray matter, perhaps involving the rostral
interstitial nucleus of Cajal.[138] In comatose
patients, see-saw nystagmus is sometimes
accompanied by ocular bobbing and, in such
a setting, may indicate severe, diffuse brainstem damage.[139]

MOTOR RESPONSES

The motor examination in a stuporous or comatose patient is, of necessity, quite different
from the patient who is awake and cooperative.
Rather than testing power in specific muscles,
it is focused on assessing the overall responsiveness of the patient (as measured by motor
response), the motor tone, and reflexes, and
identifying abnormal motor patterns, such as
hemiplegia or abnormal posturing.

Motor Tone

Assessment of *motor tone* is of greatest value
in patients who are drowsy but responsive to
voice. It may be assessed by gently grasping the

patient's hand as if you were shaking hands and lifting the arm while intermittently turning the wrist back and forth. Tone can also be assessed in the neck by gently grasping the head with two hands and moving it back and forth or up and down, and in the lower extremities by grasping each leg at the knee and gently lifting it from the bed or shaking it from side to side. Normal muscle tone provides mild resistance that is constant or nearly so throughout the movement arc and of similar intensity regardless of the initial position of the body part. Spastic rigidity, on the other hand, increases with more rapid movements and generally has a clasp-knife quality or a spastic catch, so that the movement is slowed to a near stop by the resistance, at which point the resistance collapses and the movement proceeds again. Parkinsonian rigidity remains equally intense despite the movement of the examiner (lead-pipe rigidity), but is usually diminished when the patient is asleep or there is impairment of consciousness. In contrast, during diffuse metabolic encephalopathies, many otherwise normal patients develop paratonic rigidity, also called *gegenhalten*. Paratonic rigidity is characterized by irregular resistance to passive movement that increases in intensity as the speed of the movement increases, as if the patient were willfully resisting the examiner. If the patient is drowsy but responsive to voice, urging him or her to "relax" may result in increased tone. Paratonia is often seen in patients with dementia and is normally found in infants between the second and eighth weeks of life, suggesting that it represents a state of loss of forebrain inhibition of motor tone as the level of consciousness becomes depressed. As patients become more deeply stuporous from a metabolic cause, tectospinal, reticulospinal, and vestibulospinal motor pathways that generate muscle tone may become less active, and motor tone may become minimal. Injury to these brainstem motor pathways may also cause a loss of motor tone, so the examiner is mainly searching for asymmetry of tone that may signal a focal lesion.

Motor Reflexes

Muscle stretch reflexes (sometimes erroneously referred to as "deep tendon reflexes" because they are typically elicited by tapping a

reflex hammer against a tendon) may be brisk or hyperactive in patients who are drowsy or confused and have increased motor tone. As the level of consciousness becomes further depressed, however, the muscle stretch reflexes tend to diminish in activity, until, in patients who are deeply comatose, they may be unobtainable.

Cutaneous reflexes, such as the abdominal or cremasteric reflex, typically become depressed as the level of consciousness wanes. On the other hand, in patients who are drowsy or confused, some abnormal cutaneous reflexes may be released. These may include extensor plantar responses. If the extensor plantar response is bilateral, this may signify nothing more than a depressed level of consciousness, but if it is asymmetric or unilateral, this implies injury to the descending corticospinal tract. However, in a patient with a preexisting neurological injury, the earlier deficits may become more apparent as the patient becomes more drowsy. It is important to distinguish this from a new deficit, which may signal the location of a structural lesion impairing the level of consciousness.

Prefrontal cutaneous reflexes, sometimes called "frontal release reflexes" or primitive reflexes,[140] may also emerge in drowsy or delirious patients with diffuse forebrain impairment. Rooting, glabellar, snout, palmomental, and other reflexes are often seen in such patients. However, these responses become increasingly common with advancing age in patients without cognitive impairment, so they are of limited value in elderly individuals.[141] On the other hand, the grasp reflex is generally seen only in patients who have some degree of bilateral prefrontal impairment.[142] It is elicited by gently stroking the palm of the patient with the examiner's fingers. The patient may grasp the examiner's fingers, as if grasping a branch of a tree. The pull reflex is a variant in which the examiner curls his or her fingers under the patient's as the patient attempts to grasp. The grasp is often so strong that it is possible to pull the patient from the bed. Many elderly patients with normal cognitive function will have a mild tendency to grasp the first time the reflex is attempted, but a request not to grasp the examiner quickly abolishes the response. Patients who are unable to inhibit the reflex invariably have prefrontal pathology. The grasp reflex may be asymmetric if the prefrontal injury is greater on one side, but probably requires some impairment of both hemispheres as small, unilateral lesions rarely cause grasping.[142] Grasping disappears when the lesion involves the motor cortex and causes hemiparesis. It is of greatest value in a sleepy patient who can cooperate with the exam; it disappears as the patient becomes more drowsy. Like paratonia, prefrontal reflexes are normally present in young infants but disappear as the forebrain matures.[140]

Nicolson and colleagues found that the presence in either the pre- or postoperative period of a single primitive reflex did not predispose surgical patients to developing delirium, but the presence of two or more such reflexes was predictive of delirium.[143]

Motor Responses

After assessing muscle tone, the examiner next tests the patient for best motor response to sensory stimulation (Figure 2.10). If the patient does not respond to voice or gentle shaking, arousability and motor responses are tested by painful stimuli. The maneuvers used to provide adequate stimuli without inducing actual tissue damage are shown in Figure 2.1. Responses are graded as appropriate, inappropriate, or no response. An appropriate response is one that attempts to escape the stimulus, such as pushing the stimulus away or attempting to avoid the stimulus. The motor response may be accompanied by a facial grimace or generalized increase in movement. It is necessary to distinguish an attempt to avoid the stimulus, which indicates intact sensory and motor connections within the spinal cord and brainstem, from a stereotyped withdrawal response, such as a triple flexion withdrawal of the lower extremity or flexion at the fingers, wrist, and elbow. The stereotyped withdrawal response is not responsive to the nature of the stimulus (e.g., if the pain is supplied over the dorsum of the toe, the foot will withdraw into, rather than away from, the stimulus) and thus is not appropriate to the stimulus that is applied. These spinal-level withdrawal patterns may occur in patients with severe brain injuries or even brain death.

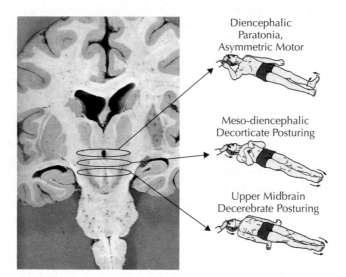

Figure 2.10 Motor responses to noxious stimulation in comatose patients with acute injury at different levels of the nervous system. Patients with deep hemispheric lesions that compress the diencephalon often have a contralateral hemiparesis (note lack of motor response with left arm, externally rotated left foot, and left extensor plantar response), but can generally make purposeful movements with the ipsilateral side. Lesions involving the junction of the diencephalon and the mid-brain may show decorticate posturing, including flexion of the upper extremities and extension of the lower extremities. As the lesion progresses into the midbrain, there is generally a shift to decerebrate posturing (C), in which there is extensor posturing of both upper and lower extremities.

Left hand panel modified from Wiliams P.L., Warwick R. *Functional Neuroanatomy of Man*. W.B. Saunders, Philadelphia, 1975, p. 975. By permission of Elsevier.

Right hand panel modified from Saper C. Brain stem modulation of sensation, movement, and consciousness. Chapter 45 in: Kandel ER, Schwartz JH, Jessel TM. *Principles of Neural Science*. 4th ed. McGraw-Hill, New York, 2000, pp. 871–909. By permission of McGraw-Hill.

It is also important to assess asymmetries of response. Failure to withdraw on one side may indicate either a sensory or a motor impairment, but if there is evidence of facial grimacing, an increase in blood pressure or pupillary dilation, or movement of the contralateral side, the defect is motor. Failure to withdraw on both sides, accompanied by facial grimacing, may indicate bilateral motor impairment below the level of the pons.

Posturing responses include several stereotyped postures of the trunk and extremities. Most appear only in response to noxious stimuli or are greatly exaggerated by such stimuli. Seemingly spontaneous posturing most often represents the response to endogenous stimuli, ranging from meningeal irritation to an occult bodily injury to a distended bladder. The nature of the posturing ranges from flexor spasms to extensor spasms to rigidity, and may vary according to the site and severity of the brain injury and the site at which the noxious stimulation is applied. In addition, the two sides of the body may show different patterns of response, reflecting the distribution of injury to the brain.

The terms *decerebrate rigidity* and *decorticate rigidity* were first applied to patterns of motor activity observed in experimental animals with various transections of the neuraxis between the diencephalon and midbrain[144,145] and later applied to similar patterns of motor abnormality seen in humans with brain injuries. This custom is unfortunate for two reasons. First, these terms imply more than we really know about the site of the underlying neurologic impairment. Even in experimental animals, these patterns of motor response may be produced by brain lesions of several different kinds and locations, and the patterns of motor response in an individual to any one of these lesions may vary across time. In humans, both types of responses can be produced by supratentorial lesions, although they imply at least incipient brainstem injury. There is a tendency for lesions that cause decorticate rigidity to be more rostral and less severe than those causing decerebrate rigidity. However, there is generally much greater agreement among observers if they simply describe the movements that are seen rather than attempt to fit them to complex patterns.

Flexor posturing of the upper extremities and extension of the lower extremities

corresponds to the pattern of movement also called *decorticate posturing*. The fully developed response consists of a relatively slow (as opposed to quick withdrawal) flexion of the arm, wrist, and fingers with adduction in the upper extremity and extension, internal rotation, and vigorous plantar flexion of the lower extremity. However, decorticate posturing is often fragmentary or asymmetric, and it may consist of as little as flexion posturing of one arm. Such fragmentary patterns have the same localizing significance as the fully developed postural change, but often reflect either a less irritating or smaller central lesion (or central lesions causing paralysis of the other limbs).

The decorticate pattern is generally produced by extensive lesions involving dysfunction of the forebrain down to the level of the rostral midbrain. Such patients typically have normal ocular motility. A similar pattern of motor response may be seen in patients with a variety of metabolic disorders or intoxications.[146] However, the presence of decorticate posturing in cases of brain injury is ominous. For example, in the series of Jennett and Teasdale, after head trauma, only 37% of comatose patients with decorticate (flexor) posturing recovered.[2] Chen and colleagues reported a similar experience if comatose patients showed flexor responses to pain on day 1 or 3 after cardiac arrest or severe hypotension.[147]

Even more ominous is the presence of *extensor posturing of both the upper and lower extremities*, often called *decerebrate posturing*. The arms are held in adduction and extension with the wrists fully pronated. Some patients assume an opisthotonic posture, with teeth clenched and arching of the spine. Tonic neck reflexes (rotation of the head causes hyperextension of the arm on the side toward which the nose is turned and flexion of the other arm; extension of the head may cause extension of the arms and relaxation of the legs, while flexion of the head leads to the opposite response) can usually be elicited. As with decorticate posturing, fragments of decerebrate posturing are sometimes seen. These tend to indicate a lesser degree of injury but in the same anatomic distribution as the full pattern. However, asymmetric posturing usually suggests an asymmetric structural lesion causing the coma.

Although decerebrate posturing usually is seen with noxious stimulation, in some patients it may occur spontaneously, often associated with waves of shivering and hyperpnea. Decerebrate posturing in experimental animals usually results from a transecting lesion at the level of the upper midbrain[145] and is believed to be due to the release of vestibulospinal, tectospinal, and reticulospinal postural reflexes from forebrain control. The level of brainstem dysfunction that produces this response in humans may be similar, as in most cases decerebrate posturing is associated with disturbances of ocular motility. However, electrophysiologic, radiologic, or even postmortem examination sometimes reveals pathology that is largely confined to the forebrain and diencephalon. Thus, decerebrate rigidity is a clinical finding that probably represents dysfunction, although not necessarily destruction extending into the upper brainstem. Nevertheless, it represents a more severe finding than decorticate posturing; for example, in the Jennett and Teasdale series, only 10% of comatose patients with head injury who demonstrated extensor (decerebrate) posturing recovered, and in the Chen et al. series of post–cardiac arrest patients, none with extensor posturing recovered.[2,147] Most patients with decerebrate rigidity have either massive and bilateral forebrain lesions causing rostrocaudal deterioration of the brainstem as diencephalic dysfunction evolves into midbrain dysfunction (see Chapter 3) or a posterior fossa lesion that compresses or damages the midbrain and rostral pons. However, the same pattern may occasionally be seen in patients with diffuse but fully reversible metabolic disorders, such as hepatic coma, hypoglycemia, or sedative drug ingestion.[146,148,149]

Extensor posturing of the arms with flaccid or weak flexor responses in the legs is typically seen in patients with injury to the lower brainstem, at roughly the level of the vestibular nuclei. This pattern was described in the 1972 edition of this monograph and has since been repeatedly confirmed. The physiologic basis of this motor pattern is not understood, but it may represent the transition from the extensor posturing seen with lower midbrain and high pontine injuries to the spinal shock (flaccidity) or even flexor responses seen from stimulating the isolated spinal cord.

FALSE LOCALIZING SIGNS IN PATIENTS WITH METABOLIC COMA

The main purpose of the foregoing review of the examination of a comatose patient is to distinguish patients with structural lesions of the brain from those with metabolic lesions. Most patients with structural lesions require urgent imaging. Patients with metabolic lesions often require an extensive laboratory evaluation to define the cause. When focal neurologic findings are observed, it becomes imperative to determine whether there is a destructive or compressive process that may become life-threatening or irreversibly damage the brain within a matter of minutes. On the other hand, even when there is no focal or lateralizing finding to suggest a structural lesion, it is important to know which signs point to specific metabolic causes, such as hypoglycemia or sepsis, that must be sought urgently. Therefore, the physician should become familiar with the few focal neurologic findings that are seen in patients with diffuse metabolic causes of coma and understand their implications for the diagnosis of the metabolic problem.

Respiratory Responses

Respiratory patterns seen in patients without structural brain lesions include the Cheyne-Stokes pattern of breathing, which is seen in many cognitively normal people with cardiac or respiratory disorders, particularly during sleep.[48–50] Sleep apnea must also be distinguished from pathologic breathing patterns. Patients with severe sleep apnea may stop breathing for 10–30 seconds or so every minute or two. Their color may become dusky during the oxygen desaturation that accompanies each period of apnea.

Kussmaul breathing, in which there are deep but slow rhythmic breaths, is seen in patients with coma due to an acidotic condition (e.g., diabetic ketoacidosis or intoxication with ethylene glycol). The low blood pH drives the deep respiratory efforts that reduce the PCO_2 in the blood, thus producing a compensatory respiratory alkalosis. It is common to see hyperventilation (rapid deep breathing) in patients with impairment of consciousness due to sepsis, hepatic encephalopathy, or cardiac dysfunction (see Chapter 5).[150–153]

Pupillary Responses

A key problem with interpreting pupillary responses is that either metabolic coma or diencephalic-level dysfunction from a structural lesion may cause bilaterally small and symmetric, reactive pupils. Thus, a patient with small pupils and little in the way of focal neurologic impairment may still have a diencephalic lesion or symmetric forebrain compression (e.g., by bilateral subdural hematomas). As a result, it is generally necessary to do an imaging study (see later discussion) within the first few hours in most comatose patients even if the cause is believed to be metabolic.

Very small pupils may be indicative of pontine-level dysfunction, often indicating an acute destructive lesion such as a hemorrhage. However, similar pinpoint but reactive pupils may be seen in opiate intoxication. Hence, in patients who present with pinpoint pupils and coma, it is necessary to administer an opiate antagonist such as naloxone to reverse potential opiate overdose. (Because an opioid antagonist can elicit severe withdrawal symptoms in a physically dependent patient, the drug should be diluted and delivered slowly, stopping as soon as one notes the pupils are enlarging and the patient is beginning to arouse. See Chapter 7 for details.)

Unreactive pupils usually indicate structural disease of the nervous system, but pupils may become unreactive briefly after a seizure. When a patient is seen who may have had an unobserved seizure within the past 30 minutes or so, it is necessary to re-examine the patient 15–30 minutes later to make sure that the lack of pupillary responses persists. Signs of major motor seizure, such as tongue biting or incontinence, or a transient metabolic acidosis are helpful in alerting the examiner to the possibility of a recent seizure. In addition, because the seizure usually results in the release of adrenalin, the pupils typically are large after a seizure.

Very deep coma due to sedative intoxication may suppress all brainstem responses, including pupillary light reactions, and simulate brain death (see Chapter 6). For this reason, it is critical to do urinary and blood toxin and drug screening on any patient who is so deeply comatose as to lack pupillary responses.

Ocular Motor Responses

Typical oculocephalic responses, as seen in a comatose patient with an intact brainstem, are not seen in awake subjects, whose voluntary eye movements supersede the brainstem vestibular responses. In fact, brainstem oculocephalic responses (as if the eyes were fixed on a point in the distance) are nearly impossible for an awake patient to simulate voluntarily and therefore are a useful differential point in identifying psychogenic unresponsiveness. On the other hand, oculocephalic responses may become particularly brisk in patients with hepatic coma.

Certain drugs may eliminate oculocephalic and even caloric vestibulo-ocular responses. Acute administration of phenytoin or fosphenytoin quite often has this effect, which may persist for 6–12 hours.[154] Occasionally, patients who have ingested an overdose of various tricyclic antidepressants may also have an absence of vestibulo-ocular responses.[155] Patients in very deep metabolic coma, particularly with sedative drugs, may also eventually lose vestibulo-ocular responses.

Ophthalmoplegia is also seen in combination with areflexia and ataxia in the Miller Fisher variant of Guillain-Barré syndrome. While such patients usually do not have impairment of consciousness, the Miller Fisher syndrome occasionally occurs in patients who also have autoimmune brainstem encephalitis (Bickerstaff's encephalitis), with impairment of consciousness and GQ1b autoantibodies.[156] In such cases, the relationship of the loss of eye movements to the impairment of consciousness may be confusing, and the prognosis may be much better than would be indicated by the lack of these brainstem reflexes, particularly if the patient receives early plasmapheresis or intravenous immune globulin. If breathing is also affected by the Guillain-Barré syndrome, the picture may even simulate brain death.[157] This condition must be considered among the reversible causes of coma that require exclusion before brain death is declared (see Chapter 8).

Isolated unilateral or bilateral abducens palsy may be seen in some patients with increased ICP, even due to nonfocal causes such as pseudotumor cerebri.[158] It may also occur with low CSF pressure, with a spontaneous leak, or after lumbar puncture.[159] In rare cases, the trochlear nerve may also be involved.[160]

Motor Responses

Patients with metabolic coma may have paratonia and/or extensor plantar responses. However, spastic rigidity should not be present. Rarely, patients with metabolic causes of coma, particularly hypoglycemia,[161] will present with asymmetric motor responses or even hemiplegia (see Chapter 5). Diffusion-weighted MRI may show a region of restricted diffusion over the internal capsule, but these are often reversible after administering glucose.[162] It has been suggested that the focal findings may be due to an underlying structural deficit brought out by the hypoglycemia, but the distribution of focal findings in patients with hypoglycemia may vary from one episode to the next. Furthermore, focal signs caused by hypoglycemia are more common in children than adults, again suggesting the absence of an underlying structural lesion. In contrast, focal deficits observed with hypertensive encephalopathy are usually due to brain edema consistent with the neurologic deficits. Cortical blindness is the most common of these deficits; edema of the occipital white matter is seen on MRI, the so-called *posterior reversible leukoencephalopathy syndrome* (PRES).[163] A number of severe metabolic causes of coma, especially hepatic coma, may also cause either decerebrate or decorticate posturing. In general, although it is important to be alert to the possibility of false localizing signs in patients with metabolic causes of coma,[146,148,149] it is still usually necessary to proceed as if the coma has a structural cause until proven otherwise.

MAJOR LABORATORY DIAGNOSTIC AIDS

The neurologic examination, as described earlier, is the cornerstone for the diagnosis of stupor and coma. It can be done at the bedside within a matter of a few minutes, and it provides critical diagnostic clues to determine the tempo of the further evaluation. If focal findings are seen, it may be necessary to institute treatment even before the remainder of the diagnostic testing can be completed. The same may be true for some types of metabolic coma, such as meningitis or hypoglycemia. On the other hand, if the evidence from a nonfocal examination points toward a diffuse metabolic encephalopathy, the examiner usually has time to employ additional diagnostic tools.

Blood and Urine Testing

Because of the propensity for some metabolic comas to cause focal neurologic signs, it is important to perform basic blood and urine testing on virtually every patient who presents with coma. It is important to draw blood for glucose and electrolytes, and to do toxin and drug screening almost immediately. The blood should not be drawn in a limb with a running intravenous line as this may alter the levels of glucose or electrolytes. Blood gases should be drawn if there is any suspicion of respiratory insufficiency or acid–base abnormality. Urine can then be collected for urinalysis and screening for toxic substances or drugs (which may no longer be detectable in the bloodstream). In a woman of reproductive age, pregnancy testing should also be done as this may affect the evaluation (e.g., MRI scan may be preferable to computed tomography [CT], if there is a choice). A bedside measurement of blood glucose is sufficiently accurate to rule out hypoglycemia and obviate the need for giving glucose. However, if glucose is given, 100 mg of parenteral thiamine should be given as well to prevent precipitating Wernicke encephalopathy (see Chapter 5).

Computed Tomography Imaging and Angiography

CT scanning is now ubiquitous, and it should be applied to any patient who does not have an immediately obvious source of coma (e.g., a hypoglycemic patient who arouses with injection of IV glucose). However, it is still necessary to complete the examination first, as a patient who is in incipient uncal herniation or whose fourth ventricle is compressed by a mass lesion may die even during the few minutes it takes to get a scan and may need to be treated emergently first. Similarly, for comatose patients in whom meningitis is suspected, it is now standard practice to give IV antibiotics before taking the patient for a CT scan to rule out a mass lesion prior to doing a lumbar puncture (but see later discussion on lumbar puncture and on meningitis in Chapters 4 and 5).

Emergency CT scans done for diagnostic purposes in patients with a depressed level of consciousness may appear to be simple to interpret. This is certainly the case for large, acute hemorrhages or extensive infarcts. However, subacute infarction may become isodense with brain during the second week, and hemorrhage may be isodense during the third week after onset. Acute infarcts may be difficult to identify, and bilateral edema may be quite difficult to distinguish from "hyper-normal brain" (i.e., small ventricles and general decrease in prominence of the sulci, which may be seen in young normal brains, particularly if the scan is not of good quality).

In such cases, it may be useful either to obtain a CT scan with contrast, or to have an MRI scan done (see later discussion). Current-generation CT scanners are fast enough so that it is rarely necessary to sedate a patient to eliminate motion artifact. However, many MRI examinations still take significantly longer, and they may be compromised if the patient moves. Such patients may be sedated with a short-acting benzodiazepine, which can be reversed if necessary with flumazenil. However, conscious sedation should only be done under the continuous supervision of a physician who is capable of intubating the patient if respirations are depressed or compromised.

CT angiography (CTA) involves reconstruction of images of the intracranial circulation from images acquired during an intravenous bolus injection of contrast dye. Perfusion CT may also identify areas of decreased perfusion, even in cases where the plain CT does not yet show an infarct (see Figure 2.11). CTA is highly accurate for demonstrating occlusions or stenoses of intracranial vessels, but it does not give the resolution of conventional direct imaging angiography. The images can be acquired quickly and the method is applicable to patients (see later discussion) who may not be eligible for magnetic resonance angiography (MRA). The use of large amounts of contrast dye can also be a drawback if the patient's history of dye reaction and renal function is not available.

Magnetic Resonance Imaging and Angiography

MRI scans take substantially longer than CT scans, and they are often less available and more cumbersome for emergency scanning, especially in patients who require ventilation during the scan. Hence, they are less often used for primary scanning of patients with coma. However, in many cases, it is necessary to obtain an MRI scan if a significant question remains about the origin of the coma after the CT imaging. Diffusion-weighted imaging may demonstrate an infarct that otherwise cannot be documented acutely. Additional sequences that measure the apparent diffusion coefficient of water in the brain (ADC mapping) and perfusion scanning can be used in cases where the standard diffusion imaging is confounded by background T2 bright lesions. This in turn may lead to a life-saving intervention (e.g., intra-arterial tissue plasminogen activator [tPA] in the case of basilar artery occlusion). MRA may also demonstrate arterial occlusion noninvasively, and MR venography may identify a dural sinus thrombosis. While T1 and T2 MRI sequences are not as sensitive as CT scanning for identifying acute blood, the combination of fluid-attenuated inversion recovery (FLAIR) and gradient echo T2° sequences is at least as sensitive in acute subarachnoid hemorrhage and may be more sensitive if the bleeding is subacute.[164]

On the other hand, MR scanning has significant limitations for its use in many comatose patients. Because MRI scanners use a high magnetic field, they are not compatible with certain types of implants in patients, including cardiac pacemakers and deep brain stimulators. Patients who require mechanical ventilation must either be ventilated by hand during the scan or placed on a specialized MR-compatible ventilator. In addition, most sequences take substantially longer than CT scans, so that clear images require that the patient not move.

MRA can reveal most stenoses or occlusions of cerebral blood vessels. However, the MRA is very flow dependent and tends to exaggerate the degree of stenosis in areas of slow flow.

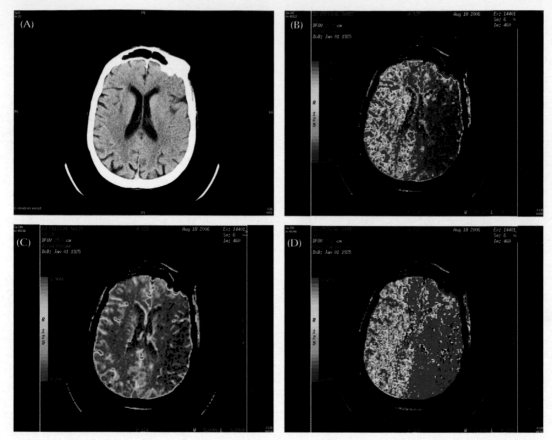

Figure 2.11 A series of computed tomography (CT) scans through the brain of a patient with a left internal carotid occlusion. Note that in the noncontrast CT scan in panel (A), there is loss of the gray-white differentiation and effacement of the sulci over the middle cerebral artery distribution on the left. Panel (B) shows the perfusion blood flow map, indicating that there is very low flow within the left middle cerebral artery distribution, but that there is also impairment of blood flow in both anterior cerebral arteries, consistent with loss of the contribution from the left internal carotid artery. Although the blood volume (C) is relatively normal in these areas, mean transit time (D) is also abnormal, indicating that tissue in the anterior cerebral distributions is at risk of infarction.

Magnetic Resonance Spectroscopy

Magnetic resonance spectroscopy (MRS) is becoming increasingly important in the diagnosis and prognosis of patients with a variety of illnesses that cause delirium, stupor, or coma (Figure 5.7).[165,166] The technique identifies neurochemicals in regions of both normal and abnormal brain. Although special techniques allow the identification of as many as 80 brain metabolites, most clinical centers using standard MRI machines perform proton (^{1}H) MRS that can identify about 13 brain metabolites (see Figure 5.8).

Myoinositol (mI) is a sugar-like molecule present in astrocytes. It helps to regulate cell volume.

Its presence serves as a marker of astrocytes. The metabolite is elevated in a number of disorders including hyperosmolar states, progressive multifocal leukoencephalopathy, renal failure, and diabetes. Levels are decreased in hyponatremia, chronic hepatic encephalopathy, tumor, and stroke.

Creatine (Cr) is actually the sum of creatine and phosphocreatine, a reliable marker of energy metabolism in both neurons and astrocytes. The total creatine peak remains constant, allowing other peaks to be calculated as ratios to the height of the creatine peak.

N-Acetylaspartate (NAA) is an amino acid derivative synthesized in neurons and transported down axons. It marks the presence of viable neurons, axons, and dendrites. Its levels may be increased in hyperosmolar states and are decreased in almost any disease that causes destruction of neurons or their processes.

The choline (Cho) peak represents several membrane components, primarily phosphocholine and glycerophosphocholine. Choline is found in higher concentration in glial cells and is thus higher in white matter than in gray matter. It is increased in tumors (particularly relative to NAA), strokes, and hyperosmolar states. It is decreased in liver disease and hyponatremia.

Glutamate/glutamine (Glx) represents a mixture of amino acids and amines involved in excitatory and inhibitory transmission as well as products of the Krebs cycle and mitochondrial redox systems. The peak is elevated in hypoxic encephalopathy and in hyperosmolar states; it is diminished in hyponatremia.

Lactate (Lac), not visible in normal brain, is a product of anaerobic glycolysis and is thus increased in hypoxic/ischemic encephalopathy, diabetic acidosis, stroke, and recovery from cardiac arrest. It is also increased in highly aggressive tumors.

A lipid peak is not present in normal brain but is identified in areas of brain necrosis, particularly in rapidly growing tumors. Cerebral fat embolism (see Chapter 5) can also cause a lipid peak.[167]

The clinical use of some of these spectra in stuporous or comatose patients is discussed in Chapter 5.

Neurosonography

Transcranial Doppler sonography identifies flow of blood in arteries, particularly the middle cerebral artery. The absence of flow in the brain has been used to confirm brain death, particularly in patients who have received sedative drugs that may alter some of the clinical findings (see Chapter 8).[168] The technique is also useful for following patients with strokes, head injuries, and hypoxic/ischemic encephalopathy. The injection of gas-filled microbubbles enhances the sonographic echo and provides better delineation of blood flow, occlusions, pseudo-occlusions, stenosis, and collateral circulation.[169]

Doppler studies of the extracranial carotid circulation are frequently done as a routine part of stroke evaluation at many centers. However, this is rarely helpful for patients in coma. If the coma is due to a reversible stenosis or occlusion of a single vessel, it almost always will be in the vertebrobasilar, not the carotid, circulation. If the patient is going to receive a CT or MRI scan, the CTA or MRA of the cervical vessels, which examines both the carotid and the vertebrobasilar circulation, is generally more revealing.

Lumbar Puncture

Although often overlooked in the technologic era, examination of the CSF still plays a central role in neurologic diagnosis, particularly in patients with a depressed level of consciousness. Once an imaging study has been performed, it is necessary to proceed with lumbar puncture as soon as possible for patients with no clear diagnosis. Rare patients in whom subarachnoid hemorrhage was not detected on imaging may demonstrate blood in the CSF. Similarly, occasional patients with bacterial meningitis or viral encephalitis may present with a depressed level of consciousness (sometimes after a missed seizure) and may not yet have sufficient meningismus to make the diagnosis of meningitis clear from examination. Meningismus may be particularly difficult to determine in patients who have underlying rigidity of the cervical spine (evidenced by resistance to lateral as well as flexion movements of the neck). Nevertheless, it is imperative to identify infection as early as possible to allow the administration of antibiotics or antiviral agents.

Patient Vignette 2.2

A 73-year-old woman who was taking 10 mg/day of prednisone for her ulcerative colitis had a 2-day history of presumed gastroenteritis, with fever, nausea, and vomiting. She awoke on the third day and found it difficult to walk to the bathroom. By the afternoon she had difficulty swallowing, her voice was hoarse, and her left limbs were clumsy. She was brought to the hospital by ambulance, and examination in the emergency department disclosed a lethargic patient who could be easily wakened.

Pupils were equal and constricted from 3 to 2 mm with light, but the left eye was lower than the right, she complained of skewed diplopia, and there was difficulty maintaining gaze to the left. There was left-sided facial numbness and lower motor neuron facial weakness. Hearing was intact, but her voice was hoarse. The tongue deviated to the right, there was distal weakness in her arms, and the left limbs were clumsy on fine motor tasks and showed dysmetria.

Magnetic resonance imaging (MRI) scan showed a left pontomedullary lesion surrounded by edema, which was bright on diffusion-weighted imaging, and she was diagnosed as having a brainstem infarct. However, despite normal MR angiography (MRA) of the vertebrobasilar system, her deficits progressed over the next day. A senior neuroradiologist noticed some enhancement at the periphery of the lesion on review of the MRI scan and suggested an abscess. Lumbar puncture disclosed 47 white blood cells/mm^3 and elevated protein, and she recovered after being treated for *Listeria monocytogenes*. An MRI scan much later in her course, disclosing a multiloculated abscess, is shown in Figure 4.12.

Comment

This case demonstrates the importance of examining the spinal fluid even when a presumptive diagnosis of vascular disease is entertained. This is particularly true in patients with fever, elevated white blood cell count, or stiff neck, where infectious disease is a consideration. However, every patient with an undetermined cause of coma requires lumbar puncture as part of the routine evaluation.

The timing of lumbar puncture with respect to CT scanning is discussed in Chapters 4 and 5. However, in some circumstances, scanning may not be not immediately available. In these cases, it is common to give antibiotics immediately and then do imaging and lumbar puncture up to a few hours later. However, once the antibiotics have penetrated the CSF, the ability to grow a bacterial pathogen and identify its susceptibilities may be permanently compromised. Hence, deferring

lumbar puncture in such cases until after the scanning procedure may do the patient harm. For this reason, when the evidence for meningitis is compelling and scanning would introduce a substantial delay that could compromise the microbiology, clinical judgment may dictate performing the lumbar puncture without benefit of prior imaging. Fortunately, that is rarely necessary in this era of ubiquitous CT scanners, but, as discussed in Chapters 4 and 5, the danger of this procedure is greatly overestimated. If the examination is nonfocal, and there is no evidence of papilledema on funduscopy, it is extremely rare to precipitate brain herniation by lumbar puncture. The benefit of establishing the exact microbial diagnosis far outweighs the risk of herniation.

A critical but often overlooked component of the lumbar puncture is to measure and record the opening pressure. Elevated pressure may be a key sign that leads to diagnosis of venous sinus thrombosis, cerebral edema, or other serious conditions that can cause coma. In addition to the routine cell count, protein, and glucose, CSF should be obtained for full cultures, including tuberculosis and fungal agents; serology and polymerase chain reaction (PCR) for specific agents such as syphilis, Lyme disease, and herpes encephalitis; and cytology, as cancer or leukemia sometimes may present with meningeal and subarachnoid infiltration. It is a good practice to set aside several milliliters of refrigerated CSF in case additional studies become necessary. This entire group of tests typically requires about 20 mL of CSF, an amount that the choroid plexus in the brain restores within about an hour.

One common problem is that the lumbar tap may be traumatic, yielding bloody CSF. This may make it difficult to determine the underlying numbers of both red and white blood cells in the CSF. If the cells come from the blood, the proportion of the red and white cells should remain the same as in the blood (usually 500–1,000 red cells per one white cell). If the tap is bloody, many clinicians send fluid from both tubes 1 and 4 for cell count. A falling count indicates that the tap was traumatic, but it does not tell you what the CSF was like prior to the tap. Nor does lack of a falling cell count indicate that the blood was there before the tap (the tip of the needle may be partially within or adjacent to a bleeding vein). An alternative approach is to examine the CSF for xanthochromia. However, CSF may be stained yellow due to high protein or bilirubin. Examination of the red blood cells under the microscope immediately after the tap may be helpful. Fresh red cells have the typical doughnut-shaped morphology, whereas crenelated cells indicate that they have been in the extravascular space for some time. Similarly, if the CSF sample is spun in a centrifuge until there are no red blood cells in the supernatant, the fluid can be tested for blood products with a urine dipstick. A positive test indicates breakdown of red blood cells, which typically takes at least 6 hours to occur after a subarachnoid hemorrhage, and demonstrates that the blood was there before the tap.

Electroencephalography and Evoked Potentials

Electroencephalography (EEG) is useful as an objective electrophysiologic assay of cortical function in patients who do not respond to normal sensory stimuli. A typical waking EEG is dominated anteriorly by low-voltage beta activity (faster than 13 Hz). During periods of quiet wakefulness, the EEG may slow into the alpha range (8–13 Hz) and the wave activity may be more rhythmic and symmetric. As the patient becomes more drowsy, higher voltage theta rhythms (4–7 Hz) become dominant; delta activity (1–3 Hz) predominates in patients who are deeply asleep or comatose. The EEG provides a rough but fairly accurate estimate of the degree to which a patient who is unresponsive may be simply uncooperative.

On the other hand, occasional patients with coma due to brainstem injury show an alpha EEG pattern. The alpha activity in such patients is usually more regular and less variable than in an awake patient, and it is not inhibited by opening the eyes.[170] It may be possible to drive the EEG by photic stimulation in alpha coma. Certain types of metabolic encephalopathy may also have characteristic EEG changes. For example, triphasic waves are often seen in patients with hepatic encephalopathy, but also can be seen in other metabolic disorders that cause coma.[171]

The EEG is most helpful in diagnosing impairment of consciousness due to nonconvulsive status epilepticus.[169] Such patients may lack the usual behavioral signs of complex partial seizures, such as lip smacking or blinking, and may present as merely confused, drowsy, or even stuporous or comatose. Some patients may demonstrate twitching movements of the eyelids or extremities, but others give no external sign of epileptic activity. In one series, 8% of comatose patients were found to be suffering from nonconvulsive status epilepticus.[173] When the EEG shows continuous epileptic activity, the diagnosis is easy and anticonvulsants are required. However, nonconvulsive status epilepticus may occur in patients without characteristic EEG changes, probably because the seizure activity is mainly in areas such as the medial temporal lobes that are not sampled by the surface electrodes. Accordingly, if one suspects that the patient's loss of consciousness is a result of nonconvulsive status epilepticus, it is probably wise to administer a short-acting benzodiazepine and observe the patient's response. If the patient improves, antiepileptic drugs should be administered. Unfortunately, some patients with a clinical and electroencephalographic diagnosis of nonconvulsive status epilepticus do not respond to anticonvulsant drugs because the underlying process causing the seizure activity is too severe to be suppressed by routine doses of drugs. Such patients are sometimes treated by large intravenous doses of gamma-aminobutyric acid agonist drugs, such as barbiturates or propofol, which at sufficiently high dosage can suppress all brain activity. However, unless the underlying brain process can be reversed, the prognosis of patients with nonconvulsive status epilepticus who do not awaken after anticonvulsant treatment is poor (see also "Seizures" in Chapter 5).[174]

Evoked potentials may also be used to test the integrity of brainstem and forebrain pathways in comatose patients. Although they do not provide reliable information on the location of a lesion in the brainstem, both auditory- and somatosensory-evoked potentials, and cortical event-related potentials, can provide information on the prognosis of patients in coma.[175] This use will be discussed in greater detail in Chapter 8.

REFERENCES

1. Chacon AH, Farooq U, Choudhary S, et al. Coma blisters in two postoperative patients. *Am J Dermatopathol* 2013;35:381–384.

2. Jennett B, Teasdale G, Braakman R, Minderhoud J, Knill-Jones R. Predicting outcome in individual patients after severe head injury. *Lancet* 1976;1:1031–1034.

3. Teasdale G, Jennett B. Assessment of coma and impaired consciousness. A practical scale. *Lancet* 1974;2:81–84.

4. Gill MR, Reiley DG, Green SM. Interrater reliability of Glasgow Coma Scale scores in the emergency department. *Annals of emergency medicine* 2004;43:215–223.

5. McNarry AF, Goldhill DR. Simple bedside assessment of level of consciousness: comparison of two simple assessment scales with the Glasgow Coma scale. *Anaesthesia* 2004;59:34–37.

6. Wijdicks EF, Bamlet WR, Maramattom BV, Manno EM, McClelland RL. Validation of a new coma scale: the FOUR score. *Ann Neurol* 2005;58:585–593.

7. Ropper AH, O'Rourke D, Kennedy SK. Head position, intracranial pressure, and compliance. *Neurology* 1982;32:1288–1291.

8. Saper CB, Loewy AD, Swanson LW, Cowan WM. Direct hypothalamo-autonomic connections. *Brain Res* 1976;117:305–312.

9. Saper CB, Stornetta RL. Central autonomic system. In: Paxinos G, ed. *The Rat Nervous System*. 4th ed. Amsterdam: Elsevier; 2015:627–671.

10. Martin TJ. Horner syndrome: A clinical review. *ACS Chem Neurosci* 2018;9:177–186.

11. Reeves AG, Posner JB. The ciliospinal response in man. *Neurology* 1969;19:1145–1152.

12. Vassend O, Knardahl S. Cardiovascular responsiveness to brief cognitive challenges and pain sensitivity in women. *Eur J Pain* 2004;8:315–324.

13. Andrefsky JC, Frank JI, Chyatte D. The ciliospinal reflex in pentobarbital coma. *J Neurosurg* 1999;90:644–646.

14. Aronovich D, Scumpia A, Edwards D. Cushing's reflex in a rare case of adult medulloblastoma. *World J Emerg Med* 2014;5:148–150.

15. Kawahara E, Ikeda S, Miyahara Y, Kohno S. Role of autonomic nervous dysfunction in electrocardio-graphic abnormalities and cardiac injury in patients with acute subarachnoid hemorrhage. *Circ J* 2003;67:753–756.

16. Lorsheyd A, Simmers TA, Robles De Medina EO. The relationship between electrocardiographic abnormalities and location of the intracranial aneurysm in subarachnoid hemorrhage. *Pacing Clin Electrophysiol* 2003;26:1722–1728.

17. Wybraniec MT, Mizia-Stec K, Krzych L. Neurocardiogenic injury in subarachnoid hemorrhage: A wide spectrum of catecholamine-mediated brain-heart interactions. *Cardiology journal* 2014;21:220–228.

18. Harbison J, Newton JL, Seifer C, Kenny RA. Stokes Adams attacks and cardiovascular syncope. *Lancet* 2002;359:158–160.

19. Cole CR, Zuckerman J, Levine BD. Carotid sinus "irritability" rather than hypersensitivity: a new name for an old syndrome? *Clin Auton Res* 2001;11:109–113.

20. Ferrante L, Artico M, Nardacci B, Fraioli B, Cosentino F, Fortuna A. Glossopharyngeal neuralgia with cardiac syncope. *Neurosurgery* 1995;36:58–63.

21. Wahl M, Schilling L. Regulation of cerebral blood flow—a brief review. *Acta Neurochir Suppl (Wien)* 1993;59:3–10.

22. Schondorf R, Benoit J, Stein R. Cerebral autoregulation in orthostatic intolerance. *Ann N Y Acad Sci* 2001;940:514–526.

23. Paulson OB, Strandgaard S, Edvinsson L. Cerebral autoregulation. *Cerebrovasc Brain Metab Rev* 1990;2:161–192.

24. Sato A, Sato Y, Uchida S. Regulation of cerebral cortical blood flow by the basal forebrain cholinergic fibers and aging. *Auton Neurosci* 2002;96:13–19.

25. Bieger D, Hopkins DA. Viscerotopic representation of the upper alimentary tract in the medulla oblongata in the rat: the nucleus ambiguus. *J Comp Neurol* 1987;262:546–562.

26. Ross CA, Ruggiero DA, Park DH, et al. Tonic vasomotor control by the rostral ventrolateral medulla: effect of electrical or chemical stimulation of the area containing Cl adrenaline neurons on arterial pressure, heart rate, and plasma catecholamines & vasopressin. *J Neurosci* 1984;4:474–496.

27. Ross CA, Ruggiero DA, Reis DJ. Projections from the nucleus tractus solitarii to the rostral ventrolateral medulla. *J Comp Neurol* 1985;242:511–534.

28. Blessing WW, Reis DJ. Inhibitory cardiovascular function of neurons in the caudal ventrolateral medulla of the rabbit: relationship to the area containing A1 noradrenergic cells. *Brain Res* 1982;253:161–171.

29. Norcliffe-Kaufmann L, Kaufmann H, Palma JA, et al. Orthostatic heart rate changes in patients with autonomic failure caused by neurodegenerative synucleinopathies. *Ann Neurol* 2018;83:522–531.

30. Smith JC, Ellenberger HH, Ballanyi K, Richter DW, Feldman JL. Pre-Bötzinger complex: a brainstem region that may generate respiratory rhythm in mammals. *Science* 1991;254:726–729.

31. Feldman JL, Del Negro CA, Gray PA. Understanding the rhythm of breathing: so near, yet so far. *Annu Rev Physiol* 2013;75:423–452.

32. Ray RS, Corcoran AE, Brust RD, et al. Impaired respiratory and body temperature control upon acute serotonergic neuron inhibition. *Science* 2011;333:637–642.

33. Guyenet PG, Stornetta RL, Bayliss DA. Central respiratory chemoreception. *J Comp Neurol* 2010;518:3883–3906.

34. Chamberlin NL, Saper CB. Topographic organization of respiratory responses to glutamate microstimulation of the parabrachial nucleus in the rat. *J Neurosci* 1994;14:6500–6510.

35. Chamberlin NL, Saper CB. A brainstem network mediating apneic reflexes in the rat. *J Neurosci* 1998;18:6048–6056.

36. Tobin MJ, Perez W, Guenther SM, D'Alonzo G, Dantzker DR. Breathing pattern and metabolic behavior during anticipation of exercise. *J Appl Physiol (Bethesda, Md. 1985)* 1986;60:1306–1312.

37. Dichter BK, Breshears JD, Leonard MK, Chang EF. The control of vocal pitch in human laryngeal motor cortex. *Cell* 2018;174:21–31.e9.

38. Meah MS, Gardner WN. Post-hyperventilation apnoea in conscious humans. *J Physiol* 1994;477(Pt 3):527–538.

39. Jennett S, Ashbridge K, North JB. Post-hyperventilation apnoea in patients with brain damage. *J Neurol Neurosurg Psychiatry* 1974;37:288–296.

40. Plum F, Brown HW, Snoep E. Neurologic significance of posthyperventilation apnea. *JAMA* 1962;181:1050–1055.
41. Cherniack NS, Longobardo G, Evangelista CJ. Causes of Cheyne-Stokes respiration. *Neurocrit Care* 2005;3:271–279.
42. Vespa PM, Bleck TP. Neurogenic pulmonary edema and other mechanisms of impaired oxygenation after aneurysmal subarachnoid hemorrhage. *Neurocrit Care* 2004;1:157–170.
43. Carrera E, Schmidt JM, Fernandez L, et al. Spontaneous hyperventilation and brain tissue hypoxia in patients with severe brain injury. *J Neurol Neurosurg Psychiatry* 2010;81:793–797.
44. Ledet D, Delos Santos NM, Khan R, Gajjar A, Broniscer A. Central neurogenic hyperventilation and renal tubular acidosis in children with pontine gliomas. *Neurology* 2014;82:1099–1100.
45. Gaviani P, Gonzalez RG, Zhu JJ, Batchelor TT, Henson JW. Central neurogenic hyperventilation and lactate production in brainstem glioma. *Neurology* 2005;64:166–167.
46. Rodriguez M, Baele PL, Marsh HM, Okazaki H. Central neurogenic hyperventilation in an awake patient with brainstem astrocytoma. *Ann Neurol* 1982;11:625–628.
47. Tarulli AW, Lim C, Bui JD, Saper CB, Alexander MP. Central neurogenic hyperventilation: a case report and discussion of pathophysiology. *Arch Neurol* 2005;62:1632–1634.
48. El-Khatib MF, Kiwan RA, Jamaleddine GW. Buspirone treatment for apneustic breathing in brain stem infarct. *Respir Care* 2003;48:956–958.
49. Gray PA, Janczewski WA, Mellen N, McCrimmon DR, Feldman JL. Normal breathing requires preBötzinger complex neurokinin-1 receptor-expressing neurons. *Nat Neurosci* 2001;4:927–930.
50. Bassetti C, Aldrich MS, Quint D. Sleep-disordered breathing in patients with acute supra- and infratentorial strokes. A prospective study of 39 patients. *Stroke* 1997;28:1765–1772.
51. Fisher CM. The neurological examination of the comatose patient. *Acta Neurol Scand* 1969;45(Suppl 36):1–56.
52. Osman AM, Carter SG, Carberry JC, Eckert DJ. Obstructive sleep apnea: current perspectives. *Nat Sci Sleep* 2018;10:21–34.
53. Tranmer BI, Tucker WS, Bilbao JM. Sleep apnea following percutaneous cervical cordotomy. *Can J Neurol Sci* 1987;14:262–267.
54. Vingerhoets F, Bogousslavsky J. Respiratory dysfunction in stroke. *Clin Chest Med* 1994;15:729–737.
55. Stankiewicz JA, Pazevic JP. Acquired Ondine's curse. *Otolaryngol Head Neck Surg* 1989;101:611–613.
56. Zaidi S, Gandhi J, Vatsia S, Smith NL, Khan SA. Congenital central hypoventilation syndrome: an overview of etiopathogenesis, associated pathologies, clinical presentation, and management. *Auton Neurosci* 2018;210:1–9.
57. Fernandez RM, Mathieu Y, Luzon-Toro B, et al. Contributions of PHOX2B in the pathogenesis of Hirschsprung disease. *PloS One* 2013;8:e54043.
58. Krestel H, Bassetti CL, Walusinski O. Yawning—its anatomy, chemistry, role, and pathological considerations. *Prog Neurobiol* 2018;161:61–78.
59. Steger M, Schneemann M, Fox M. Systemic review: the pathogenesis and pharmacological treatment of hiccups. *Aliment Pharmacol Ther* 2015;42:1037–1050.
60. Becker DE. Nausea, vomiting, and hiccups: a review of mechanisms and treatment. *Anesth Prog* 2010;57:150–156; quiz 7.
61. Jain R, Kumar B. Immediate and delayed complications of dexamethasone cyclophosphamide pulse (DCP) therapy. *J Dermatol* 2003;30:713–718.
62. Lee KH, Moon KS, Jung MY, Jung S. Intractable hiccup as the presenting symptom of cavernous hemangioma in the medulla oblongata: a case report and literature review. *J Korean Neurosurg Soc* 2014;55:379–382.
63. Park MH, Kim BJ, Koh SB, Park MK, Park KW, Lee DH. Lesional location of lateral medullary infarction presenting hiccups (singultus). *J Neurol Neurosurg Psychiatry* 2005;76:95–98.
64. Amirjamshidi A, Abbassioun K, Parsa K. Hiccup and neurosurgeons: a report of 4 rare dorsal medullary compressive pathologies and review of the literature. *Surg Neurol* 2007;67:395–402.
65. LeWitt PA, Barton NW, Posner JB. Hiccup with dexamethasone therapy. *Ann Neurol* 1982;12:405–406.
66. Souadjian JV, Cain JC. Intractable hiccup. Etiologic factors in 220 cases. *Postgrad Med* 1968;43:72–77.
67. Rouse S, Wodziak M. Intractable hiccups. *Curr Neurol Neurosci Rep* 2018;18:51.
68. Friauf E, Herbert H. Topographic organization of facial motoneurons to individual pinna muscles in rat (Rattus rattus) and bat (Rousettus aegyptiacus). *J Comp Neurol* 1985;240:161–170.
69. Yates BJ, Catanzaro MF, Miller DJ, McCall AA. Integration of vestibular and emetic gastrointestinal signals that produce nausea and vomiting: potential contributions to motion sickness. *Exp Brain Res* 2014;232:2455–2469.
70. Yamamoto H, Kishi T, Lee CE, et al. Glucagon-like peptide-1-responsive catecholamine neurons in the area postrema link peripheral glucagon-like peptide-1 with central autonomic control sites. *J Neurosci* 2003;23:2939–2946.
71. Al-Rasheid N, Gray R, Sufi P, et al. Chronic elevation of systemic glucagon-like peptide-1 following surgical weight loss: association with nausea and vomiting and effects on adipokines. *Obesity surgery* 2015;25:386–391.
72. Hornby PJ. Central neurocircuitry associated with emesis. *Am J Med* 2001;111(Suppl 8A):106S–112S.
73. Olver IN. Update on anti-emetics for chemotherapy-induced emesis. *Intern Med J* 2005;35:478–481.
74. Lu Z, Yeung CK, Lin G, Yew DTW, Andrews PLR, Rudd JA. Centrally located GLP-1 receptors modulate gastric slow waves and cardiovascular function in ferrets consistent with the induction of nausea. *Neuropeptides* 2017;65:28–36.
75. Chen CJ, Scheufele M, Sheth M, Torabi A, Hogan N, Frohman EM. Isolated relative afferent pupillary defect secondary to contralateral midbrain compression. *Arch Neurol* 2004;61:1451–1453.
76. Hornblass A. Pupillary dilatation in fractures of the floor of the orbit. *Ophthal Surg* 1979;10:44–46.
77. Antonio-Santos AA, Santo RN, Eggenberger ER. Pharmacological testing of anisocoria. *Exp Opin Pharmacother* 2005;6:2007–2013.

78. McLeod JG, Tuck RR. Disorders of the autonomic nervous system: Part 2. Investigation and treatment. Ann Neurol 1987;21:519–529.
79. Llewellyn-Smith IJ, Martin CL, Marcus JN, Yanagisawa M, Minson JB, Scammell TE. Orexin-immunoreactive inputs to rat sympathetic preganglionic neurons. Neurosci Lett 2003;351:115–119.
80. Lee MG, Hassani OK, Jones BE. Discharge of identified orexin/hypocretin neurons across the sleep-waking cycle. J Neurosci 2005;25:6716–6720.
81. Loewy AD, Araujo JC, Kerr FW. Pupillodilator pathways in the brain stem of the cat: anatomical and electrophysiological identification of a central autonomic pathway. Brain Res 1973;60:65–91.
82. Burde RM, Loewy AD. Central origin of oculomotor parasympathetic neurons in the monkey. Brain Res 1980;198:434–439.
83. Burde RM. Disparate visceral neuronal pools subserve spinal cord and ciliary ganglion in the monkey: a double labeling approach. Brain Res 1988;440:177–180.
84. Gooley JJ, Lu J, Chou TC, Scammell TE, Saper CB. Melanopsin in cells of origin of the retinohypothalamic tract. Nat Neurosci 2001;4:1165.
85. Gooley JJ, Lu J, Fischer D, Saper CB. A broad role for melanopsin in nonvisual photoreception. J Neurosci 2003;23:7093–7106.
86. Park JC, Moura AL, Raza AS, Rhee DW, Kardon RH, Hood DC. Toward a clinical protocol for assessing rod, cone, and melanopsin contributions to the human pupil response. Invest Ophthalmol Vis Sci 2011;52:6624–6635.
87. Buttner-Ennever JA, Cohen B, Horn AK, Reisine H. Pretectal projections to the oculomotor complex of the monkey and their role in eye movements. J Comp Neurol 1996;366:348–359.
88. Jampel RS. Convergence, divergence, pupillary reactions and accommodation of the eyes from faradic stimulation of the macaque brain. J Comp Neurol 1960;115:371–399.
89. Kerr FW, Hollowell OW. Location of pupillomotor and accommodation fibres in the oculomotor nerve: experimental observations on paralytic mydriasis. J Neurol Neurosurg Psychiatry 1964;27:473–481.
90. Olson DM, Stutzman S, Saju C, Wilson M, Zhao W, Aiyagari V. Interrater reliability of pupillary assessments. Neurocrit Care 2016;24:251–257.
91. Manley GT, Larson MD. Infrared pupillometry during uncal herniation. J Neurosurg Anesthesiol 2002;14:223–228.
92. Solari D, Rossetti AO, Carteron L, et al. Early prediction of coma recovery after cardiac arrest with blinded pupillometry. Ann Neurol 2017;81:804–810.
93. Yang E, Kreuzer M, Hesse S, Davari P, Lee SC, Garcia PS. Infrared pupillometry helps to detect and predict delirium in the post-anesthesia care unit. J Clin Monit Comput 2018;32:359–368.
94. Leigh RJ, Zee DS. The neurology of eye movements. 4th ed. New York: Oxford University Press; 2006.
95. Hanson RA, Ghosh S, Gonzalez-Gomez I, Levy ML, Gilles FH. Abducens length and vulnerability? Neurology 2004;62:33–36.
96. Strupp M, Kremmyda O, Adamczyk C, et al. Central ocular motor disorders, including gaze palsy and nystagmus. J Neurol 2014;261(Suppl 2):S542–S558.
97. Kheradmand A, Colpak AI, Zee DS. Eye movements in vestibular disorders. Handb Clin Neurol 2016;137:103–117.
98. Sparks DL, Mays LE. Signal transformations required for the generation of saccadic eye movements. Annu Rev Neurosci 1990;13:309–336.
99. Shinoda Y, Sugiuchi Y, Izawa Y, Takahashi M. Neural circuits for triggering saccades in the brainstem. Prog Brain Res 2008;171:79–85.
100. Buettner UW, Zee DS. Vestibular testing in comatose patients. Arch Neurol 1989;46:561–563.
101. Helmchen C, Rambold H, Kempermann U, Buttner-Ennever JA, Buttner U. Localizing value of torsional nystagmus in small midbrain lesions. Neurology 2002;59:1956–1964.
102. Goldberg ME, Walker MF, Hudspeth AJ. The vestibular system. In: Kandel ER, Schwartz JH, Jessell TM, Siegelbaum SA, Hudspeth AJ, eds. Principles of Neural Science. 5th ed. New York: McGraw Hill; 2013:917–934.
103. Vernet M, Quentin R, Chanes L, Mitsumasu A, Valero-Cabre A. Frontal eye field, where art thou? Anatomy, function, and non-invasive manipulation of frontal regions involved in eye movements and associated cognitive operations. Frontiers in Integr Neurosci 2014;8:66.
104. Goldberg ME, Bruce CJ. Primate frontal eye fields. III. Maintenance of a spatially accurate saccade signal. J Neurophysiol 1990;64:489–508.
105. Leichnetz GR. An anterogradely-labeled prefrontal cortico-oculomotor pathway in the monkey demonstrated with HRP gel and TMB neurohistochemistry. Brain Res 1980;198:440–445.
106. Born RT, Bradley DC. Structure and function of visual area MT. Annu Rev Neurosci 2005;28:157–189.
107. Cogan DG, Chu FC, Reingold DB. Ocular signs of cerebellar disease. Arch Ophthalmol 1982;100:755–760.
108. Caplan LR. Ptosis. J Neurol Neurosurg Psychiatry 1974;37:1–7.
109. Hackley SA, Johnson LN. Distinct early and late subcomponents of the photic blink reflex: response characteristics in patients with retrogeniculate lesions. Psychophysiology 1996;33:239–251.
110. Liu GT, Ronthal M. Reflex blink to visual threat. J Clin Neuroophthalmol 1992;12:47–56.
111. Pullicino PM, Jacobs L, McCall WD Jr, Garvey M, Ostrow PT, Miller LL. Spontaneous palpebromandibular synkinesia: a localizing clinical sign. Ann Neurol 1994;35:222–228.
112. Ogasawara K. Neural pathways mediating the corneal blink reflex and Bell's phenomenon in the cat. Neurosci Res 1985;2:309–320.
113. Roberts TA, Jenkyn LR, Reeves AG. On the notion of doll's eyes. Arch Neurol 1984;41:1242–1243.
114. Schubert MC, Das V, Tusa RJ, Herdman SJ. Cervico-ocular reflex in normal subjects and patients with unilateral vestibular hypofunction. Otol Neurotol 2004;25:65–71.
115. Schlosser HG, Unterberg A, Clarke A. Using video-oculography for galvanic evoked vestibulo-ocular monitoring in comatose patients. J Neurosci Methods 2005;145:127–131.
116. Brandt TH, Dieterich M. Different types of skew deviation. J Neurol Neurosurg Psychiatry 1991;54:549–550.
117. Fisher CM. Some neuro-ophthalmological observations. J Neurol Neurosurg Psychiatry 1967;30:383–392.

118. Chung CS, Caplan LR, Han WC, Pessin MS, Lee KH, Kim JM. Thalamic haemorrhage. *Brain* 1996;119:1873–1886.
119. Baloh RW, Furman JM, Yee RD. Dorsal midbrain syndrome: clinical and oculographic findings. *Neurology* 1985;35:54–60.
120. Choi KD, Jung DS, Kim JS. Specificity of "peering at the tip of the nose" for a diagnosis of thalamic hemorrhage. *Arch Neurol* 2004;61:417–422.
121. Litvan I, Jankovic J, Goetz CG, et al. Accuracy of the clinical diagnosis of postencephalitic parkinsonism: a clinicopathologic study. *Eur J Neurol* 1998;5:451–457.
122. Frucht SJ. Treatment of movement disorder emergencies. *Neurotherapeutics* 2014;11:208–212.
123. Kim JS, Kim HK, Im JH, Lee MC. Oculogyric crisis and abnormal magnetic resonance imaging signals in bilateral lentiform nuclei. *Mov Disord* 1996;11:756–758.
124. Peeraully T, Rosenberg ML. Spontaneous intracranial hypotension without intracranial hypotension. *J Neuroophthalmol* 2011;31:248–251. doi: 10.1097/WNO.0b013e3181fcc04a.
125. Lajmi H, Hmaied W, Ben Jalel W, et al. Oculomotor palsy in diabetics. *Journal francais d'ophtalmologie* 2018;41:45–49.
126. Kwee IL, Matsuzawa H, Nakada K, Fujii Y, Nakada T. Inferior colliculus syndrome: Clinical magnetic resonance microscopy anatomic analysis on a 7 T system. *Sage Open Med Case Rep* 2017;5:2050313x17745209.
127. Zee DS. Brain stem and cerebellar deficits in eye movement control. *Trans Ophthalmol Soc U K* 1986;105:599–605.
128. Keane JR. Alternating skew deviation: 47 patients. *Neurology* 1985;35:725–728.
129. Keane JR. Ocular skew deviation. Analysis of 100 cases. *Arch Neurol* 1975;32:185–190.
130. Johkura K, Komiyama A, Tobita M, Hasegawa O. Saccadic ping-pong gaze. *J Neuroophthalmol* 1998;18:43–46.
131. Daroff RB, Hoyt WF. Supranuclear disorders of ocular control systems in man: clinical, anatomical, and physiological correlations. In: Bach-y Rita P, Collins CC; Hyde JE, eds. *The Control of Eye Movements*. New York: Academic Press; 1971:17–235.
132. Ochs AL, Stark L, Hoyt WF, D'Amico D. Opposed adducting saccades in convergence-retraction nystagmus: a patient with sylvian aqueduct syndrome. *Brain* 1979;102:497–508.
133. Fisher CM. Ocular bobbing. *Arch Neurol* 1964;11:543–546.
134. Rosenberg ML. Spontaneous vertical eye movements in coma. *Ann Neurol* 1986;20:635–637.
135. Herishanu YO, Abarbanel JM, Frisher S, Farkash P, Berginer J, Amir-Schechter D. Spontaneous vertical eye movements associated with pontine lesions. *Isr J Med Sci* 1991;27:320–324.
136. Lourie H. Seesaw nystagmus. case report elucidating the mechanism. *Arch Neurol* 1963;147:531–533.
137. Kim SH, Kim HJ, Oh SW, Kim JS. Visual and positional modulation of pendular seesaw nystagmus: implications for the mechanism [published online ahead of print, July 18, 2018]. *J Neuroophthalmol.* doi: 10.1097/WNO.0000000000000678
138. Sano K, Sekino H, Tsukamoto Y, Yoshimasu N, Ishijima B. Stimulation and destruction of the region of the interstitial nucleus in cases of torticollis and see-saw nystagmus. *Confin Neurol* 1972;34:331–338.
139. Keane JR. Intermittent see-saw eye movements. Report of a patient in coma after hyperextension head injury. *Arch Neurol* 1978;35:173–174.
140. Schott JM, Rossor MN. The grasp and other primitive reflexes. *J Neurol Neurosurg Psychiatry* 2003;74:558–560.
141. Jacobs L, Gossman MD. Three primitive reflexes in normal adults. *Neurology* 1980;30:184–188.
142. De Renzi E, Barbieri C. The incidence of the grasp reflex following hemispheric lesion and its relation to frontal damage. *Brain* 1992;115 Pt 1:293–313.
143. Nicolson SE, Chabon B, Larsen KA, Kelly SE, Potter AW, Stern TA. Primitive reflexes associated with delirium: a prospective trial. *Psychosomatics* 2011;52:507–512.
144. Cannon WB, Britton SW. Studies on the conditions of activity in endocrine glands. XV. Pseudoaffective medulloadrenal secretion. *Am J Physiol* 1925:283–294.
145. Sherrington CS. Decerebrate rigidity, and reflex co-ordination of movements. *J Physiol* 1898;22:319–332.
146. Greenberg DA, Simon RP. Flexor and extensor postures in sedative drug-induced coma. *Neurology* 1982;32:448–451.
147. Chen R, Bolton CF, Young B. Prediction of outcome in patients with anoxic coma: a clinical and electrophysiologic study. *Crit Care Med* 1996;24:672–678.
148. Kirk MM, Hoogwerf BJ, Stoller JK. Reversible decerebrate posturing after profound and prolonged hypoglycemia. *Cleve Clin J Med* 1991;58:361–363.
149. Conomy JP, Swash M. Reversible decerebrate and decorticate postures in hepatic coma. *N Engl J Med* 1968;278:878–879.
150. Passino C, Giannoni A, Mannucci F, et al. Abnormal hyperventilation in patients with hepatic cirrhosis: role of enhanced chemosensitivity to carbon dioxide. *Int J Cardiol* 2012;154:22–26.
151. Jimenez JV, Carrillo-Perez DL, Rosado-Canto R, et al. Electrolyte and acid-base disturbances in end-stage liver disease: a physiopathological approach. *Dig Dis Sci* 2017;62:1855–1871.
152. Szrama J, Smuszkiewicz P. An acid-base disorders analysis with the use of the Stewart approach in patients with sepsis treated in an intensive care unit. *Anaesthesiol Intensive Ther* 2016;48:180–184.
153. Frangiosa A, De Santo LS, Anastasio P, De Santo NG. Acid-base balance in heart failure. *J Nephrol* 2006;19(Suppl 9):S115–S120.
154. Spector RH, Davidoff RA, Schwartzman RJ. Phenytoin-induced ophthalmoplecpia. *Neurology* 1976;26:1031–1034.
155. Pulst SM, Lombroso CT. External ophthalmoplegia, alpha and spindle coma in imipramine overdose: case report and review of the literature. *Ann Neurol* 1983;14:587–590.
156. Odaka M, Yuki N, Yamada M, et al. Bickerstaff's brainstem encephalitis: clinical features of 62 cases and a subgroup associated with Guillain-Barre syndrome. *Brain* 2003;126:2279–2290.
157. Ragosta K. Miller Fisher syndrome, a brainstem encephalitis, mimics brain death. *Clin Pediatr (Phila)* 1993;32:685–687.
158. Dhiravibulya K, Ouvrier R, Johnston I, Procopis P, Antony J. Benign intracranial hypertension in

childhood: a review of 23 patients. *J Paediatr Child Health* 1991;27:304–307.

159. Thomke F, Mika-Gruttner A, Visbeck A, Bruhl K. The risk of abducens palsy after diagnostic lumbar puncture. *Neurology* 2000;54:768–769.

160. Speer C, Pearlman J, Phillips PH, Cooney M, Repka MX. Fourth cranial nerve palsy in pediatric patients with pseudotumor cerebri. *Am J Ophthalmol* 1999;127:236–237.

161. Malouf R, Brust JC. Hypoglycemia: causes, neurological manifestations, and outcome. *Ann Neurol* 1985;17:421–430.

162. Albayram S, Ozer H, Gokdemir S, Gulsen F, Kiziltan G, Kocer N, Islak C. Reversible reduction of apparent diffusion coefficient values in bilateral internal capsules in transient hypoglycemia-induced hemiparesis. *Amer J Neuroradiol* 2006; 27:1760–1762.

163. Lee MK, Cho YJ, Lee KS, Jung SK, Heo K. The effect of presymptomatic hypertension in posterior reversible encephalopathy syndrome. *Brain Behav* 2018; e01061.

164. Nelson SE, Sair HI, Stevens RD. Magnetic resonance imaging in aneurysmal subarachnoid hemorrhage: current evidence and future directions. *Neurocrit Care* 2018.

165. Oz G, Alger JR, Barker PB, et al. Clinical proton MR spectroscopy in central nervous system disorders. *Radiology* 2014;270:658–679.

166. Xu V, Chan H, Lin AP, et al. MR spectroscopy in diagnosis and neurological decision-making. *Semin Neurol* 2008;28:407–422.

167. Guillevin R, Vallee JN, Demeret S, et al. Cerebral fat embolism: usefulness of magnetic resonance spectroscopy. *Ann Neurol* 2005;57:434–439.

168. Viski S, Olah L. Use of transcranial Doppler in intensive care unit. *J Crit Care Med (Universitatea de Medicina si Farmacie din Targu-Mures)* 2017;3:99–104.

169. Droste DW, Metz RJ. Clinical utility of echocontrast agents in neurosonology. *Neurol Res* 2004;26:754–759.

170. Brenner RP. EEG in convulsive and nonconvulsive status epilepticus. *J Clin Neurophysiol* 2004; 21:319–331.

171. Brenner RP. The interpretation of the EEG in stupor and coma. *Neurologist* 2005;11:271–284.

172. Sutter R, Semmlack S, Kaplan PW. Nonconvulsive status epilepticus in adults—insights into the invisible. *Nat Rev Neurol* 2016;12:281–293.

173. Towne AR, Waterhouse EJ, Boggs JG, et al. Prevalence of nonconvulsive status epilepticus in comatose patients. *Neurology* 2000; 54:340–345.

174. Kaplan PW. The clinical features, diagnosis, and prognosis of nonconvulsive status epilepticus. *Neurologist* 2005;11:348–361.

175. Fischer C, Luaute J, Adeleine P, Morlet D. Predictive value of sensory and cognitive evoked potentials for awakening from coma. *Neurology* 2004;63:669–673.

Chapter 3

Structural Causes of Stupor and Coma

COMPRESSIVE LESIONS AS A CAUSE OF COMA

COMPRESSIVE LESIONS MAY DIRECTLY DISTORT THE AROUSAL SYSTEM
Compression at Different Levels of the Central Nervous System Presents in Distinct Ways
The Role of Increased Intracranial Pressure in Coma
The Role of Vascular Factors and Cerebral Edema in Mass Lesions

HERNIATION SYNDROMES: INTRACRANIAL SHIFTS IN THE PATHOGENESIS OF COMA
Anatomy of the Intracranial Compartments
Patterns of Brain Shifts that Contribute to Coma

Clinical Findings in Uncal Herniation Syndrome
Clinical Findings in Central Herniation Syndrome
Clinical Findings in Dorsal Midbrain Syndrome
Safety of Lumbar Puncture in Comatose Patients
False Localizing Signs in the Diagnosis of Structural Coma

DESTRUCTIVE LESIONS AS A CAUSE OF COMA
Diffuse, Bilateral Cortical Destruction
Destructive Disease of the Diencephalon
Destructive Lesions of the Brainstem

Two major classes of structural brain injuries cause coma (Table 3.1): (1) *Compressive lesions* may impair consciousness either by directly compressing the ascending arousal system or by distorting brain tissue so that it moves out of position and secondarily compresses components of the ascending arousal system or its forebrain targets (see *herniation syndromes*, page 99). These processes include a wide range of space-occupying lesions such as tumors,

hematomas, and abscesses. (2) *Destructive lesions* cause coma by direct damage to the ascending arousal system or its forebrain targets. To cause coma, lesions of the diencephalon or brainstem must be bilateral, but can be quite focal if they damage the ascending activating system near the midline in the midbrain or caudal diencephalon; cortical or subcortical damage must be both bilateral and diffuse. Processes that may cause these changes include tumor, hemorrhage, infarct, trauma, or infection. Both destructive and compressive lesions may cause additional compression by producing brain edema.

Most compressive lesions are treated surgically, whereas destructive lesions are generally treated medically. This chapter describes the pathophysiology and general approach to patients with structural lesions of the brain, first considering compressive and then destructive lesions. Chapter 4 deals with some of the specific causes of coma outlined in Table 3.1.

Chapter 2 described some of the physical findings that distinguish structural from nonstructural causes of stupor and coma. The physician must first decide whether the patient is indeed stuporous or comatose, distinguishing those patients who are not in coma but suffer from abulia, akinetic mutism, psychologic unresponsiveness, or the locked-in state from those truly stuporous or comatose (see Chapter 1). This is usually relatively easily done during the course of the initial examination. More difficult is distinguishing structural from metabolic causes of stupor or coma. As indicated in Chapter 2, if the structural cause of coma involves the ascending arousal system in the brainstem, the presence of focal findings usually makes the distinction between metabolic

Table 3.1 Sites and Representative Causes of Structural Lesions that can Cause Coma

Destructive	Compressive
Cerebral	*Cerebral*
Cortex (e.g., acute anoxic injury)	Bilateral subdural hematomas
Subcortical white matter (e.g., delayed anoxic injury)	
Diencephalon	*Diencephalon*
Thalamus (e.g., infarct)	Thalamus (e.g., hematoma)
	Hypothalamus (e.g., pituitary tumor)
Brainstem	*Brainstem*
Midbrain, pons (e.g., infarct)	Midbrain (e.g., uncal herniation)
	Pons, medulla (e.g., cerebellar tumor, hemorrhage, abscess)

and structural coma easy. However, when the structural disease involves the cerebral cortex diffusely or the diencephalon bilaterally, focal signs are often minimal or absent, and it may be difficult to distinguish structural from metabolic coma. Compressive lesions that initially do not cause focal signs eventually do so, but by then coma may be irreversible. Thus, if there is any question about the distinction between structural and metabolic coma, immediately after stabilizing the patient an imaging study must be obtained to rule out a mass lesion that may be surgically remediable. This is usually a computed tomography (CT) scan in an emergency situation, which is generally sufficient to rule out surgically correctable compressive causes of coma, or a CT angiogram if a stroke is suspected, to rule out a treatable vascular occlusion. However, a magnetic resonance imaging (MRI) scan, if available, will reveal many other types of pathology, including infarcts, infections, and other brain injuries. Identifying surgically remediable lesions that have not yet caused focal findings gives the physician time to stabilize the patient and investigate other additional nonstructural causes of coma. The time, however, is short and should be counted in minutes rather than hours or days. If focal findings are already present, efforts to decrease intracranial pressure (ICP), including hyperventilation, hyperosmolar agents and, in the case of brain tumors and certain other conditions (discussed in Chapters 4 and 8) administration of corticosteroids (Chapter 7), should be instituted before sending the patient for imaging.

COMPRESSIVE LESIONS AS A CAUSE OF COMA

Compressive lesions may impair consciousness in a number of critical ways: (1) by directly distorting the arousal system or its forebrain targets; (2) by increasing ICP diffusely to the point of impairing global cerebral blood flow; (3) by distorting tissue to the point of causing local ischemia; (4) by causing edema, thus further distorting neural tissue; or (5) by causing tissue shifts (herniations). Understanding the anatomy and pathophysiology of each of these processes is critical in evaluating patients in coma.

COMPRESSIVE LESIONS MAY DIRECTLY DISTORT THE AROUSAL SYSTEM

Compression at key levels of the brain may cause coma by exerting pressure on the structures of the arousal system. The mechanism by which local pressure may impair neuronal function is not entirely understood. However, neurons depend on axonal transport to supply critical proteins and mitochondria to their terminals and to transport used or damaged cellular components back to the cell body for destruction and disposal. Even a loose ligature around an axon causes damming of axon contents on both sides of the stricture, due to impairment of both anterograde and retrograde axonal flow, and results in axonal swelling and impairment of function. Perhaps the clearest example of this relationship is provided by patients with papilledema in whom the optic nerve behind the globe is surrounded by a sleeve of dura that exposes it to ICP (see section on "Increased ICP," page 96). The elevated ICP compresses the optic nerve, resulting in damming of axonal transport in the retinal ganglion cell axons and swelling of the nerve head. When a compressive lesion results in displacement of the structures of the arousal system, consciousness may become impaired, as described in the following sections.

Compression at Different Levels of the Central Nervous System Presents in Distinct Ways

When a *cerebral hemisphere is compressed by a lesion* such as a subdural hematoma, tumor, or abscess that grows slowly over a long period of time, it may reach a relatively large size with little in the way of local signs that can help identify the diagnosis. The tissue in the cerebral hemispheres can absorb a surprising amount of distortion and stretching as long as the growth of the mass can be compensated for by displacing cerebrospinal fluid (CSF) from the ventricles in that hemisphere. However, when there is no further room in the hemisphere to expand, even a small increase in the volume of the lesion can only be accommodated by compressing the diencephalon and midbrain either laterally across the midline or downward.

In such patients, the impairment of consciousness correlates with the displacement of the diencephalon and upper brainstem in a lateral or caudal direction.[1] Hence, when a patient with a hemispheric lesion reaches the point of impairment of consciousness, there is very little time left to intervene before the brain is irreparably injured.

The *diencephalon may also be compressed* by a mass lesion in the thalamus itself (generally a tumor or a hemorrhage) or a mass in the suprasellar cistern (typically a craniopharyngioma, a germ cell tumor, or suprasellar extension of a pituitary adenoma; see Chapter 4). In addition to causing impairment of consciousness, suprasellar tumors typically cause visual field deficits, classically a bitemporal hemianopsia, although a wide range of optic nerve or tract injuries may also occur. If a suprasellar tumor extends into the cavernous sinus, there may be injury to the cranial nerves that supply the ocular muscles (III, IV, VI) and the ophthalmic division of the trigeminal nerve (V1). On occasion, these tumors may also cause endocrine dysfunction. If they damage the pituitary stalk, they may cause diabetes insipidus or panhypopituitarism. In women, the presence of a pituitary tumor is often heralded by galactorrhea and amenorrhea, as prolactin is the sole anterior pituitary hormone under negative regulation, and it is typically elevated when the pituitary stalk is damaged.

The *dorsal midbrain* may be compressed by a tumor in the pineal region. Pineal mass lesions may be suprasellar germinomas or other germ cell tumors (embryonal cell carcinoma, teratocarcinoma) that occur along the midline, or pineal masses including pinealocytoma or pineal astrocytoma. Pineal masses compress the pretectal area as well. Thus, in addition to causing impairment of consciousness, they produce diagnostic neuro-ophthalmologic signs including fixed, slightly enlarged pupils; impairment of voluntary vertical eye movements (typically elevation is impaired earlier and more severely than depression) and convergence; and convergence nystagmus and sometimes retractory nystagmus (see dorsal midbrain syndrome, pp. 116–118).[2,3] Hemorrhage into the pulvinar of the thalamus, which overlies the pretectal area and dorsal midbrain, may sometimes produce a similar constellation of signs.

Posterior fossa compressive lesions most often originate in the cerebellum, including tumors, hemorrhages, infarctions, or abscesses, although occasionally extra-axial lesions, such as a subdural or epidural hematoma, may have a similar effect. Tumors of the cerebellum include the full range of primary and metastatic brain tumors (Chapter 4), as well as juvenile pilocytic astrocytomas and medulloblastomas in children and hemangioblastoma in patients with von Hippel-Lindau syndrome.[4]

A cerebellar mass causes coma by direct compression of the brainstem, which may also cause the brainstem to herniate upward through the tentorial notch. As the patient loses consciousness, there is a pattern of pontine level dysfunction, with small reactive pupils, impairment of vestibulo-ocular responses (which may be asymmetric), and decerebrate motor responses.[5] Because the base of the pons is farthest from the cerebellum, motor signs (e.g., upgoing toes) are usually a relatively late finding and suggest instead an intrinsic brainstem mass. With upward pressure on the midbrain, the pupils become asymmetric or unreactive.[6] If vestibulo-ocular responses were not previously impaired by pontine compression, vertical eye movements may be lost.

Cerebellar mass lesions may also cause coma by compressing the fourth ventricle to the point of impairment of CSF flow. This causes acute hydrocephalus and rapidly increasing ICP (see page 151). The onset of obstruction of the fourth ventricle is typically heralded by nausea and sometimes sudden, projectile vomiting. There may also be a history of ataxia, vertigo, neck stiffness, and eventually respiratory arrest as the cerebellar tonsils are impacted upon the lip of the foramen magnum. If the compression develops slowly (i.e., over more than 12 hours), there may also be papilledema. Because cerebellar masses may cause acute obstruction of the fourth ventricle by expanding by only a few millimeters in diameter, they are potentially very dangerous.

On occasion, impairment of consciousness may occur as a result of *a mass lesion directly compressing the brainstem*. These are more commonly intrinsic masses, such as an abscess or a hemorrhage, in which case it is difficult to determine how much of the impairment is due to compression as opposed to destruction. Occasionally, a mass lesion of the cerebellopontine angle, such as a vestibular schwannoma, meningioma, or cholesteatoma, may compress the brainstem. However, these are usually slow processes and the mass may reach a very large size and often causes signs of local injury before consciousness is impaired.

The Role of Increased Intracranial Pressure in Coma

A key and often misunderstood point is that increases in ICP are withstood remarkably well by the brain as long as they progress relatively slowly. In patients with chronic diffuse elevation of CSF pressure, such as those with pseudotumor cerebri, there is little evidence of brain dysfunction, even when CSF pressures reach 600 mm of water or greater. The chief problems induced by increased ICP are papilledema and headache until the pressure gets high enough to impair cerebral blood flow.

Papilledema is due to the pressure differential applied to the optic nerve by the increase in ICP. Retinal ganglion cells within the eye are subject to intraocular pressure, typically in the same range as normal CSF pressure. Their axons leave the eye through the optic disk and travel to the brain via the optic nerve. Axoplasm flows from the retinal ganglion cell bodies in the eye, down the axon, and through the optic disc. Similarly, the retinal veins within the eye are subject to intraocular pressure. They also leave through the optic disc and run along the optic nerve. The optic nerve in turn is surrounded by a dural and arachnoid sleeve, which contains CSF that communicates with the CSF in the subarachnoid space around the brain.[7,8] The optic disk itself is composed of a dense fibrous network forming a cribriform (from the Latin for *sieve*) plate that acts as a pressure fitting, so that the optic nerve and retinal vein are exposed to intraocular pressure on one side of the disk and to ICP on the other side.

In a healthy individual, these are both generally less than 20 cm of water pressure, so there is little differential between them, and axonal transport proceeds unimpeded, and the retinal veins show normal venous pulsations. As ICP rises above systemic venous pressure, retinal venous pulsations are damped or eliminated as an early feature of papilledema. The retinal veins become larger and more numerous appearing because increased venous pressure causes smaller veins to become more noticeable on funduscopy. Thus, the presence of retinal venous pulsations is a good but not invariable sign of normal ICP, and engorgement of retinal veins is a reliable early sign of increased ICP.[9,10] A second consequence of increased ICP is that axoplasmic flow is impaired (as if a loose ligature had been tied around the nerve), and there is buildup of axoplasm on the retinal side of the disk. The swollen optic axons obscure the disk margins, beginning at the superior and inferior poles, then extending laterally and finally medially.[11] The size of the optic disk increases, and this can be mapped as a larger "blind spot" in the visual field. Some patients even complain of a visual scotoma in this area. If ICP is increased sufficiently, the ganglion cells begin to fail from the periphery of the retina in toward the macula. This results in a concentric loss of vision.

Because papilledema reflects the back-pressure on the optic nerves from increased ICP, it is virtually always bilateral. A rare exception occurs when the optic nerve on one side is itself compressed by a mass lesion (such as an olfactory groove meningioma), thus resulting in optic atrophy in one eye and papilledema in the other eye (the Foster Kennedy syndrome). On the other hand, optic nerve injury at the level of the optic disk, either due to demyelinating disease or vascular infarct of the vasa nervorum (anterior ischemic optic neuropathy), can also block axonal transport and venous return due to retrobulbar swelling of the optic nerve.[7,8] The resulting papillitis can look identical to papilledema but is typically unilateral, or at least it does not involve the optic nerves simultaneously. In addition, papillitis is usually accompanied by the relatively rapid onset of visual loss, particularly focal loss called a scotoma, so the clinical distinction is usually clear.

The origin of *headache* in patients with increased ICP is not understood. CSF normally leaves the subarachnoid compartment mainly by resorption at the arachnoid villi.[12] These structures are located along the surface of the superior sagittal sinus, and they consist of invaginations of the arachnoid membrane into the wall of the sinus. CSF is taken up from the subarachnoid space by endocytosis into vesicles, the vesicles are transported across the arachnoid epithelial cells, and then their contents are released by exocytosis into the venous sinus. Imbalance in the process of secretion and resorption of CSF occurs in cases of CSF-secreting tumors as well as in pseudotumor cerebri (idiopathic intracranial hypertension). In both conditions, very high levels of CSF pressure, in excess of 600 mm of water, may be achieved, but rather little in the way of brain dysfunction occurs other than headache. Experimental infusion of artificial CSF into the subarachnoid space, to pressures as high as 800 or even 1,000 mm of water, also does not cause cerebral dysfunction and, curiously, often does not cause headache.[13,14] However, conditions that cause diffusely increased ICP such as pseudotumor cerebri usually do cause headache,[15] suggesting that they must cause some subtle distortion of pain receptors in the cerebral blood vessels or the meninges.[16]

Pseudotumor cerebri in association with tinnitus is thought to be due to partial obstruction of the transverse sinus.[15] Complete *obstruction of a cerebral venous sinus*, by contrast, typically causes increased ICP in association with signs of brain dysfunction as well as severe headache. The headache is localized to the venous sinus that is obstructed (superior sagittal sinus headache is typically at the vertex of the skull, whereas transverse sinus headache is usually behind the ear on the affected side). The headache in these conditions is thought to be due to irritation and local distortion of the sinus itself. Brain dysfunction is produced by back-pressure on the draining veins that feed into the sinus, thus reducing the perfusion pressure of the adjacent areas of the brain to the point of precipitating venous infarction (see page 160). Small capillaries may be damaged, producing local hemorrhage and focal or generalized seizures. Superior sagittal sinus thrombosis produces parasagittal ischemia in the hemispheres, causing lower extremity paresis. Lateral sinus thrombosis typically causes infarction in the inferior lateral temporal lobe, which may produce little in the way of signs other than seizures.

The most important mechanism by which diffusely raised ICP can cause symptoms is by *impairment of the cerebral arterial supply*. The brain usually compensates for the increased ICP by regulating its blood supply, as described in Chapter 2. However, as ICP reaches and exceeds 600 mm of water, the back-pressure on cerebral perfusion reaches 45–50 mm Hg, which becomes a major hemodynamic challenge. Typically, this is seen in severe acute liver failure,[17] with vasomotor paralysis following head injury, occasionally in acute encephalitis which can cause massive brain swelling, or in the course of acute hydrocephalus or leptomeningeal carcinomatosis where CSF resorption can be compromised. When perfusion pressure falls below the lower limit required for brain function, neurons fail to maintain their ionic gradients due to energy failure, resulting in additional swelling which further increases ICP and results in a downward spiral of reduced perfusion and further brain infarction.

Decreased perfusion pressure can also occur when systemic blood pressure drops, such as when assuming a standing position. Some patients with increased ICP develop brief bilateral visual loss when they stand, called *visual obscurations*, presumably due to failure to autoregulate the posterior cerebral blood flow. Failure of perfusion pressure can also occur focally (i.e., in a patient with an otherwise asymptomatic carotid occlusion who develops symptoms in the ipsilateral carotid distribution on standing because of the resulting small drop in blood pressure).

Patients with elevated ICP from mass lesions often suffer sudden rises in ICP precipitated by changes in posture, coughing, sneezing, or straining, or even during tracheal suctioning (plateau waves).[18] The sudden rises in ICP can reduce cerebral perfusion and produce a variety of neurologic symptoms including confusion, stupor, and coma (Table 3.2). In general, the symptoms last only a few minutes and then resolve, leading some observers to confuse these with seizures.[19]

Finally, the *loss of compliance of the intracranial system to further increases in volume and the rate of change in ICP* plays an important role in the response of the brain to increased ICP. Compliance is the change in pressure caused by an increase in volume. In a normal brain, increases in brain volume (e.g., due to a small intracerebral hemorrhage) can be compensated by displacement of an equal volume of CSF from the compartment. However, when a mass has increased in size to the point where there is little remaining CSF in the compartment, even a small further increase in volume can produce a large increase in compartmental pressure. This loss of compliance in cases where diffuse brain edema

Table 3.2 Paroxysmal Symptoms that may Result from a Sudden Increase in Intracranial Pressure

Impairment of consciousness	Opisthotonus, trismus
Trancelike state; unreality/warmth	Rigidity and tonic extension/flexion of the arms and legs
Confusion, disorientation	Bilateral extensor plantar responses
Restlessness, agitation	Sluggish/absent deep tendon reflexes
Disorganized motor activity, carphologia	Generalized muscular weakness
Sense of suffocation, air hunger	Facial twitching
Cardiovascular/ respiratory disturbances	Clonic movements of the arms and legs
Headache	Facial/limb paresthesias
Pain in the neck and shoulders	Rise in temperature
Nasal itch	Nausea, vomiting
Blurring of vision, amaurosis	Facial flushing
Mydriasis, pupillary areflexia	Pallor, cyanosis
Nystagmus	Sweating
Oculomotor/abducens paresis	Shivering and "goose flesh"
Conjugate deviation of the eyes	Thirst
External ophthalmoplegia	Salivation
Dysphagia, dysarthria	Yawning, hiccoughing
Nuchal rigidity	Urinary and fecal urgency/ incontinence
Retroflexion of the neck	

Adapted from Ingvar and Lundberg.[20]

has caused a critical increase in ICP can lead to the development of *plateau waves*. These are large, sustained increases in ICP, which may approach the mean arterial blood pressure and which occur at intervals as often as every 15–30 minutes.[21] They are thought to be due to episodic arterial vasodilation, which is due to systemic vasomotor rhythms, but a sudden increase in vascular volume in a compartment with limited compliance, even if very small, can dramatically increase ICP.[22] These sudden increases in ICP can thus cause a wide range of neurologic paroxysmal symptoms (see Table 3.2). When pressure in neighboring compartments is lower, this imbalance can cause herniation (see later discussion).[15]

Conversely, when a patient shows early signs of herniation, it is often possible to reverse the situation by restoring a small margin of compliance to the compartment containing the mass lesion. Hyperventilation causes a fall in arterial pCO_2, resulting in arterial and venous vasoconstriction. The small reduction in intracranial blood volume may reverse the herniation syndrome dramatically in just a few minutes.

The Role of Vascular Factors and Cerebral Edema in Mass Lesions

As indicated earlier, an important mechanism by which compressive lesions may cause symptoms is by inducing local tissue ischemia. Even in the absence of a diffuse impairment of cerebral blood flow, local increases in pressure and tissue distortion in the vicinity of a mass lesion may stretch small arteries and reduce their caliber to the point where they are no longer able to supply sufficient blood to their targets.

Many mass lesions, including tumors, inflammatory lesions, and the capsules of subdural hematomas, are able to induce the growth of new blood vessels (angiogenesis).[23] These blood vessels do not have the features that characterize normal cerebral capillaries (i.e., lack of fenestrations and tight junctions between endothelial cells) and that are the basis for the blood–brain barrier. Thus, the vessels leak; the leakage of contrast dyes during CT or MRI scanning provides the basis for contrast enhancement of a lesion that lacks a blood–brain barrier. The vascular leak also results in the extravasation of fluid into the extracellular space and *vasogenic edema* (see Figure 3.1B).[24] This edema further displaces surrounding tissues that are pushed progressively farther from the source of their own feeding arteries. Because the large arteries are tethered to the circle of Willis and small ones are tethered to the pial vascular system, they may not be able to be displaced as freely as the brain tissue they supply. Hence, the distensibility of the blood supply becomes the limiting factor to tissue perfusion and, in many cases, tissue survival.

Ischemia and consequent energy failure cause loss of the electrolyte gradient across the neuronal membranes. Neurons depolarize

but are no longer able to repolarize and so fail. As neurons take on more sodium, they swell (*cytotoxic edema*), thus further increasing the mass effect on adjacent sites (see Figure 3.1C). Increased intracellular calcium meanwhile results in the activation of apoptotic programs for neuronal cell death. This vicious cycle of swelling produces ischemia of adjacent tissue, which in turn causes further tissue swelling. Either cytotoxic or vasogenic edema may cause a patient with a chronic and slowly growing mass lesion to decompensate quite suddenly,[24] particularly if it causes a herniation syndrome with rapid onset of brain failure and coma when the lesion reaches a critical limit.

HERNIATION SYNDROMES: INTRACRANIAL SHIFTS IN THE PATHOGENESIS OF COMA

The Monro-Kellie doctrine states that because the contents of the skull are not compressible and are contained within an unyielding case of bone, the sum of the volume of the brain, CSF, and intracranial blood is constant at all times.[25] A corollary is that these same restrictions apply to each compartment (right vs. left supratentorial space, infratentorial space, spinal subarachnoid space). In a normal brain, increases in the size of a growing mass lesion can be compensated for by the displacement of an equal volume of CSF from the compartment. The displacement of CSF, and in some cases blood volume, by the mass lesion raises ICP. As the mass grows, there is less CSF to be displaced, and hence *the compliance of the intracranial contents decreases as the size of the compressive lesion increases.* When a mass has increased in size to the point where there is little remaining CSF in the compartment, even a small further increase in volume can produce a large increase in compartmental pressure. When pressure in neighboring compartments is lower, this imbalance causes the malleable brain tissue to herniate from the high pressure to the lower pressure compartment. These intracranial shifts are of key concern in the diagnosis of coma due to supratentorial mass lesions (Figure 3.2).

The pathogenesis of signs and symptoms of an expanding mass lesion that causes coma is

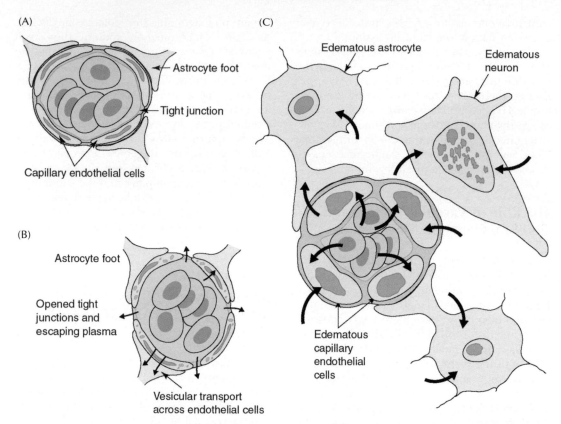

Figure 3.1 A schematic drawing illustrating cytotoxic versus vasogenic edema. (A) Under normal circumstances, the brain is protected from the circulation by a blood–brain barrier, consisting of tight junctions between cerebral capillary endothelial cells that do not permit small molecules to penetrate the brain, as well as a basal lamina surrounded by astrocytic end-feet. (B) When the blood–brain barrier is breached (e.g., by neovascularization in a tumor or the membranes of subdural hematoma), fluid transudates from fenestrated blood vessels into the brain. This results in an increase in fluid in the extracellular compartment, vasogenic edema. Vasogenic edema can usually be reduced by corticosteroids, which decrease capillary permeability. (C) When neurons are injured, they can no longer maintain ion gradients. The increased intracellular sodium causes a shift of fluid from the extracellular to the intracellular compartment, resulting in cytotoxic edema. Cytotoxic edema is not affected by corticosteroids.
Modified from Fishman RA. Brain edema. *N Engl J Med* 1975;293(14):706–711. By permission of Massachusetts Medical Society.

rarely a function of the increase in ICP itself, but usually results from imbalances of pressure between different compartments leading to tissue herniation.

To understand herniation syndromes, it is first necessary to review briefly the structure of the intracranial compartments between which herniations occur.

Anatomy of the Intracranial Compartments

The cranial sutures of babies close at about 18 months, encasing the intracranial contents

in a nondistensible box of finite volume. The intracranial contents include the brain tissue (approximately 87%, of which 77% is water), CSF (approximately 9%), blood vessels (approximately 4%), and the meninges (dura, arachnoid, and pia that occupy a negligible volume). The dural septa that divide the intracranial space into compartments play a key role in the herniation syndromes caused by supratentorial mass lesions.

The falx cerebri (Figures 3.2 and 3.3) separates the two cerebral hemispheres by a dense dural leaf that is tethered to the superior sagittal sinus along the midline of the cranial vault. The falx contains the inferior sagittal

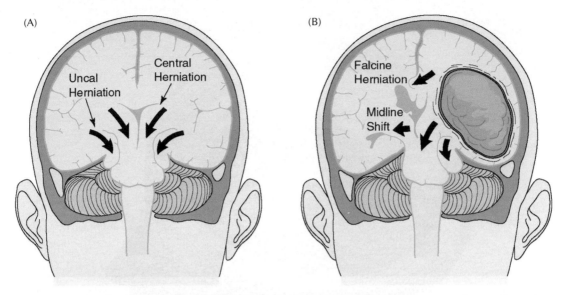

Figure 3.2 A schematic drawing to illustrate the different herniation syndromes seen with intracranial mass effect. When the increased mass is symmetric in the two hemispheres (A), there may be central herniation, as well as herniation of either or both medial temporal lobes, through the tentorial opening. Asymmetric compression (B), from a unilateral mass lesion, may cause herniation of the ipsilateral cingulate gyrus under the falx (falcine herniation). This type of compression may cause distortion of the diencephalon by either downward herniation or midline shift. The depression of consciousness is more closely related to the degree and rate of shift, rather than the direction. Finally, the medial temporal lobe (uncus) may herniate early in the clinical course.

sinus along its free edge. The free edge of the falx normally rests just above the corpus callosum. The pericallosal branch of the anterior cerebral artery also runs in close proximity to the free edge of the falx. Fragile brain tissues can be damaged by displacement against the unyielding falx. For example, during severe head injury, violent displacement of the brain can cause a contusion of the corpus callosum.[26] A mass lesion in one hemisphere can displace the cingulate gyrus under the falx. This herniation can cause stretching of branches of the pericallosal artery and result in ischemia or infarction of the cingulate gyrus (see *falcine herniation*, Figure 3.2).

The tentorium cerebelli (Figure 3.3) separates the cerebral hemispheres (supratentorial compartment) from the brainstem and cerebellum (infratentorial compartment/posterior fossa). The tentorium is less flexible than the falx because its fibrous dural lamina is stretched across the surface of the middle fossa and is tethered in position for about three-quarters of its extent (see Figure 3.3). It attaches anteriorly at the petrous ridges and posterior clinoid processes and laterally to the occipital bone along the lateral sinus.

Extending posteriorly into the center of the tentorium from the posterior clinoid processes is a large semioval opening, the incisura or tentorial notch, whose diameter is usually between 25 and 40 mm mediolaterally and 50 and 70 mm rostrocaudally.[27] The tentorium cerebelli also plays a key role in the pathophysiology of supratentorial mass lesions because when the tissue volume of a supratentorial compartment exceeds that compartment's capacity, there is no alternative but for tissue to herniate through the tentorial opening (see *uncal herniation*, Figure 3.2).

Tissue shifts in any direction can damage structures occupying the tentorial opening. The midbrain traverses the opening from the posterior fossa to attach to the diencephalon; the oculomotor nerves exit the midbrain to run into the cavernous sinus. The superior portion of the cerebellar vermis is typically applied closely to the surface of the midbrain and occupies the posterior portion of the tentorial opening. The quadrigeminal cistern, above the tectal plate of the midbrain, and the peduncular and interpeduncular cisterns along the base of the midbrain provide flexibility; there may be considerable tissue shift before symptoms

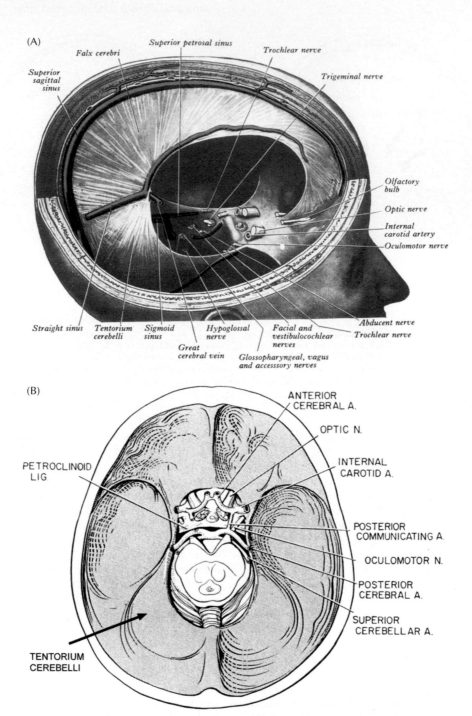

(A)

Falx cerebri   Superior petrosal sinus   Trochlear nerve

Superior sagittal sinus

Trigeminal nerve

Olfactory bulb

Optic nerve

Internal carotid artery

Oculomotor nerve

Straight sinus   Tentorium cerebelli   Sigmoid sinus   Hypoglossal nerve   Facial and vestibulocochlear nerves   Abducent nerve   Trochlear nerve

Great cerebral vein   Glossopharyngeal, vagus and accesssory nerves

(B)

ANTERIOR CEREBRAL A.

OPTIC N.

INTERNAL CAROTID A.

PETROCLINOID LIG

POSTERIOR COMMUNICATING A.

OCULOMOTOR N.

POSTERIOR CEREBRAL A.

SUPERIOR CEREBELLAR A.

TENTORIUM CEREBELLI

Figure 3.3 The intracranial compartments are separated by tough dural leaflets. (A) The falx cerebri separates the two cerebral hemispheres into separate compartments. Excess mass in one compartment can lead to herniation of the cingulate gyrus under the falx. (B) The midbrain occupies most of the tentorial opening, which separates the supratentorial from the infratentorial (posterior fossa) space. Note the vulnerability of the oculomotor nerve to both herniation of the medial temporal lobe and aneurysm of the posterior communicating artery.

Panel A from Williams PL, and Warwick R. *Functional Neuroanatomy of Man.* WB Saunders, Philadelphia, 1975, p. 986. By permission of Elsevier B.V.

are produced if a mass lesion expands slowly (Figure 3.2).

The basilar artery lies along the ventral surface of the midbrain. As it nears the tentorial opening, it gives off superior cerebellar arteries bilaterally, then branches into the posterior cerebral arteries (Figure 3.4). The posterior cerebral arteries give off a range of thalamoperforating branches that supply the posterior thalamus and pretectal area, followed by the posterior communicating arteries.[28] Each posterior cerebral artery then wraps around the lateral surface of the upper midbrain and reaches the ventral surface of the hippocampal gyrus, where it gives off a posterior choroidal artery.[29] The posterior choroidal artery anastomoses with the anterior choroidal artery, a branch of the internal carotid artery that runs along the choroid fissure on the medial surface of the temporal lobe. The posterior cerebral artery then runs caudally along the medial surface of the occipital lobe to supply the visual cortex. Either one or both posterior cerebral arteries are vulnerable to compression when tissue herniates through the tentorium. Unilateral compression causes a homonymous hemianopsia; bilateral compression causes cortical blindness (see Patient 3.1).

The oculomotor nerves leave the ventral surface of the midbrain between the superior cerebellar arteries and the diverging posterior cerebral arteries (Figure 3.3). The oculomotor nerves cross the posterior cerebral artery and run along the posterior communicating artery

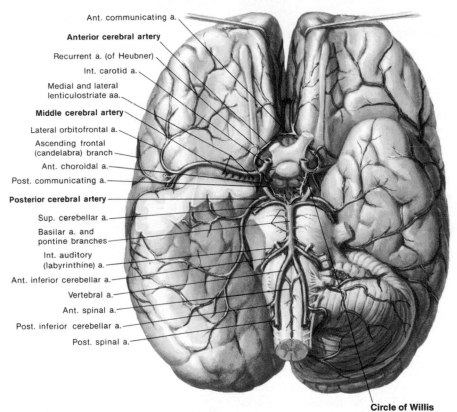

Arteries of Brain (basal views)

Ant. communicating a.
Anterior cerebral artery
Recurrent a. (of Heubner)
Int. carotid a.
Medial and lateral lenticulostriate aa.
Middle cerebral artery
Lateral orbitofrontal a.
Ascending frontal (candelabra) branch
Ant. choroidal a.
Post. communicating a.
Posterior cerebral artery
Sup. cerebellar a.
Basilar a. and pontine branches
Int. auditory (labyrinthine) a.
Ant. inferior cerebellar a.
Vertebral a.
Ant. spinal a.
Post. inferior cerebellar a.
Post. spinal a.

Circle of Willis

Figure 3.4 The basilar artery is tethered at the top to the posterior cerebral arteries, and at its lower end to the vertebral arteries. As a result, either upward or downward herniation of the brainstem puts at stretch the paramedian feeding vessels that leave the basilar at a right angle and supply the paramedian midbrain and pons. The posterior cerebral arteries can be compressed by the medial temporal lobes when they herniate through the tentorial notch.

From Netter FH. *The CIBA Collection of Medical Illustrations*. CIBA Pharmaceuticals, New Jersey, 1983, p. 46. By permission of CIBA Pharmaceuticals.

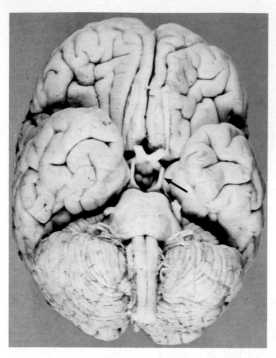

Figure 3.5 Relationship of the oculomotor nerve to the medial temporal lobe. Note that the course of the oculomotor nerve takes it along the medial aspect of the temporal lobe where uncal herniation can compress its dorsal surface.
From Williams PL, Warwick R. *Functional Neuroanatomy of Man.* WB Saunders, Philadelphia, 1975, p. 929. By permission of Elsevier B.V.

to penetrate through the dural edge at the petroclinoid ligament and enter the cavernous sinus. Along this course, the oculomotor nerves run along the medial edge of the temporal lobe (Figure 3.5). The uncus, which represents the bulging medial surface of the amygdala within the medial temporal lobe, usually sits over the tentorial opening, and its medial surface may even be grooved by the tentorium.

A key relationship in the pathophysiology of supratentorial mass lesions is the close proximity of the oculomotor nerve to the posterior communicating artery (Figure 3.4) and the medial temporal lobe (Figure 3.5). Compression of the oculomotor nerve by either of these structures results in early injury to the pupillodilator fibers that run along its dorsal surface[30]; hence, a unilateral dilated pupil frequently heralds a neurologic catastrophe (see Box 3.1).

The other ocular motor nerves are generally not involved in early transtentorial herniation.

The trochlear nerves emerge from the dorsal surface of the midbrain just caudal to the inferior colliculi. These slender fiber bundles wrap around the lateral surface of the midbrain and follow the third nerve through the petroclinoid ligament into the cavernous sinus. Because the free edge of the tentorium sits over the posterior edge of the inferior colliculi, trauma that displaces the brainstem back into the unyielding edge of the tentorium may injure the trochlear nerves as well as the underlying dorsolateral pons.[31,32] Trochlear nerve palsy is thus a common complication of even relatively mild closed head injury,[33] whereas head trauma severe enough to damage the dorsolateral pons is associated with coma.

The abducens nerves emerge from the ventral surface of the pons and run along the ventral surface of the midbrain to enter the cavernous sinus as well. Abducens paralysis is often a nonspecific sign of increased[15] or decreased[34] (e.g., after a lumbar puncture or CSF leak) ICP. However, the abducens nerves are rarely damaged by supratentorial or infratentorial mass lesions unless they invade the cavernous sinus or displace the entire brainstem downward.

The foramen magnum, at the lower end of the posterior fossa, is the only means by which brain tissue may exit from the skull. Hence, just as progressive enlargement of a supratentorial mass lesion inevitably results in herniation through the tentorial opening, continued downward displacement either from an expanding supratentorial or infratentorial mass lesion ultimately causes herniation of the cerebellum and the brainstem through the foramen magnum.[35] Here the medulla, the cerebellar tonsils, and the vertebral arteries are juxtaposed. Usually, a small portion of the cerebellar tonsils protrudes into the aperture (and may even be grooved by the posterior lip of the foramen magnum). However, when the cerebellar tonsils are jammed against the foramen magnum during tonsillar herniation, compression of the tissue may compromise its blood supply, causing tissue infarction and further swelling.

Patterns of Brain Shifts that Contribute to Coma

There are seven major patterns of brain shift: falcine herniation, mediolateral displacement

Box 3.1 Historical View of the Pathophysiology of Brain Herniation

In the nineteenth century, many neurologists thought that supratentorial lesions caused stupor or coma by impairing function of the cortical mantle, although the mechanism was not understood. Cushing proposed that the increase in intracranial pressure (ICP) caused impairment of blood flow, especially to the medulla.[36] He was able to show that translation of pressure waves from the supratentorial compartments to the lower brainstem may occur in experimental animals. Similarly, in young children, a supratentorial pressure wave may compress the medulla, causing an increase in blood pressure and fall in heart rate (the Cushing reflex). Such responses are rare in adults, who almost always show symptoms of more rostral brainstem failure before developing symptoms of lower brainstem dysfunction.

The role of temporal lobe herniation through the tentorial notch was appreciated by MacEwen in the 1880s, who froze and then serially cut sections through the heads of patients who died from temporal lobe abscesses.[37] His careful descriptions demonstrated that the displaced medial surface of the temporal uncus compressed the oculomotor nerve, causing a dilated pupil. In the 1920s, Meyer pointed out the importance of temporal lobe herniation into the tentorial gap in patients with brain tumors[38]; Kernohan and Woltman demonstrated the lateral compression of the brainstem produced by this process.[39] They noted that a lateral shift of the midbrain compressed the cerebral peduncle on the side opposite the tumor against the opposite tentorial edge, resulting in ipsilateral hemiparesis. In the following decade, the major features of the syndrome of temporal lobe herniation were clarified, and the role of the tentorial pressure cone was widely appreciated as a cause of symptoms in patients with coma.

In the 1980s, the role of lateral displacement of the diencephalon and upper brainstem versus downward displacement of the same structures in causing coma had received considerable attention.[40,41] Careful studies of the displacement of midline structures, such as the pineal gland, in patients with coma due to forebrain mass lesions demonstrate that the symptoms are due to distortion of the structures at the mesodiencephalic junction, with the rate of displacement being more important than the absolute value or direction of the movement.

of the diencephalon, uncal herniation, central transtentorial herniation, rostrocaudal brainstem herniation, tonsillar herniation, and upward brainstem herniation. The first five patterns are caused by supratentorial mass lesions, whereas tonsillar herniation and upward brainstem herniation usually result from infratentorial mass lesions, as described later.

Falcine herniation occurs when an expanding lesion presses the cerebral hemisphere medially against the falx (Figure 3.2A). The cingulate gyrus and the pericallosal and callosomarginal arteries are compressed against the falx and may be displaced under it. The compression of the pericallosal and callosomarginal arteries causes ischemia in the medial wall of the cerebral hemisphere that swells and further increases the compression. Eventually, the ischemia may advance to frank infarction, which increases the cerebral mass effect further.[42]

Mediolateral displacement of the diencephalon occurs when an expanding mass lesion, such as a basal ganglionic hemorrhage, pushes the diencephalon on that side medially across the midline (Figure 3.2B). This process may be monitored by displacement of the calcified pineal gland, which is adherent to the dorsal surface of the diencephalon and whose position with respect to the midline is easily seen on plain CT scanning.[40] This lateral displacement of the midline is roughly correlated with the degree of impairment of consciousness: 0–3 mm is associated with alertness, 3–5 mm with drowsiness, 6–8 mm with stupor, and 9–13 mm with coma.[1]

Uncal herniation occurs when an expanding mass lesion, usually located laterally in one cerebral hemisphere, forces the medial edge of the temporal lobe to herniate medially and downward over the free tentorial edge into the tentorial notch (Figure 3.2). In contrast to central herniation, in which the first signs are mainly those of diencephalic dysfunction, in uncal herniation the most prominent signs are due to pressure of the herniating temporal lobe on the structures that occupy the tentorial notch.

The key sign associated with uncal herniation is an ipsilateral fixed and dilated pupil due to compression of the dorsal surface of the oculomotor nerve. There usually is also evidence of some impairment of ocular motility by this stage, but it may be less apparent to the examiner as the patient may not be sufficiently awake either to complain about it or to follow commands on examination (i.e., to look to the side or up or down), and some degree of exophoria is present in most people when they are not completely awake. However, examining oculocephalic responses by rotating the head usually will disclose limitations of eye movement consistent with third-nerve compression.

A second key feature of uncal herniation that is sufficient to cause pupillary dilation is impaired level of consciousness. This may be due to the distortion of the ascending arousal systems as they pass through the midbrain, distortion of the adjacent diencephalon, or perhaps stretching of blood vessels perfusing the midbrain, thus causing parenchymal ischemia. Nevertheless, the impairment of arousal is so prominent a sign that, in a patient with a unilateral fixed and dilated pupil and normal level of consciousness, the examiner must look for another cause of pupillodilation. Pupillary dilation from uncal herniation with a preserved level of consciousness is rare enough to be the subject of case reports.[43]

Hemiparesis may also occur due to compression of the cerebral peduncle by the uncus. The paresis may be contralateral to the herniation (if the advancing uncus impinges on the adjacent cerebral peduncle) or ipsilateral (if the uncus pushes the midbrain so that the opposite cerebral peduncle is compressed against the incisural edge of Kernohan's notch).[44] Hence, the side of paresis is not helpful in localizing the lesion, but the side of the enlarged pupil accurately identifies the side of the herniation more than 90% of the time.[45]

Patient Vignette 3.1

A 30-year-old woman in the seventh month of pregnancy began to develop right frontal headaches. The headaches became more severe, and, toward the end of the eighth month, she sought medical assistance. A magnetic resonance imaging (MRI) scan revealed a large right frontal mass. Her physicians planned to admit her to hospital, perform an elective cesarean section, and then operate on the tumor. She was admitted to the hospital the day before the surgery. During the night she complained of a more severe headache and rapidly became lethargic and then stuporous. An emergency computed tomography (CT) scan disclosed hemorrhage into the tumor and transtentorial herniation. At craniotomy, a right frontal hemorrhagic oligodendroglioma was removed, and she rapidly recovered consciousness. Upon awakening she complained that she was unable to see. Examination revealed complete loss of vision including ability to appreciate light but with retained pupillary light reflexes. Repeat MRI scan showed an evolving infarct involving the occipital lobes bilaterally (see Figure 3.6). Over the following week, she gradually regained some central vision, after which it became clear that she had severe prosopagnosia (difficulty recognizing faces).[46] Many months after recovery of vision she was able to get around and read, but she was unable to recognize her own face in the mirror and could only distinguish between her husband and her brother by the fact that her brother was taller.

An additional problem in many patients with uncal herniation is compression of the posterior cerebral artery in the tentorial notch, which may give rise to infarction in the territory of its distribution.[47] The ensuing visual field cut is often overlooked at the time of the herniation, when the impairment of consciousness may make it impossible to test visual fields, but emerges as a concern after the crisis is past when the patient is unable to see on the side of space opposite the herniation. Bilateral compression of the posterior cerebral arteries can result in bilateral infarction of the occipital cortex and cortical blindness (see Patient Vignette 3.1, Figure 3.6).[48]

Central transtentorial herniation is due to pressure from an expanding mass lesion on the diencephalon. If the mass effect is medially located, the displacement may be primarily downward, in turn pressing downward on the midbrain, although the mass may also have a substantial lateral component shifting the diencephalon in the lateral direction.[40] The diencephalon is mainly supplied by small penetrating end arteries that arise directly from the vessels of the circle of Willis. Hence, even

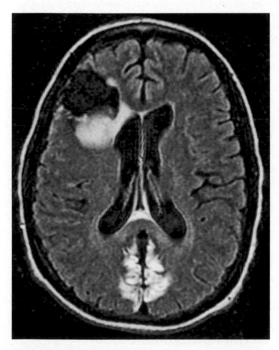

Figure 3.6 Bilateral occipital infarction in Patient 3.1. Hemorrhage into a large frontal lobe tumor caused transtentorial herniation, compressing both posterior cerebral arteries. The patient underwent emergency craniotomy to remove the tumor, but when she recovered from surgery she was cortically blind.

small degrees of displacement may stretch and compress important feeding vessels and reduce blood flow. In addition to accounting for the pathogenesis of coma (due to impairment of the ascending arousal system at the mesodiencephalic junction), the ischemia causes local swelling and eventually infarction, which causes further edema, thus contributing to gradually progressive downward displacement of the diencephalon. In severe cases, the pituitary stalk may even become partially avulsed, causing diabetes insipidus, and the diencephalon may buckle against the midbrain. The earliest and most subtle signs of impending central herniation due to compression of the diencephalon are sleepiness and small, reactive pupils, as well as diffusely increased in muscle tone.

Less commonly, the midbrain may be forced downward through the tentorial opening by a mass lesion impinging on it from the dorsal surface. Dorsal midbrain compression is usually due to a pineal mass, but occasionally may be seen due to a hemorrhage into the pulvinar nucleus of the thalamus. Dorsal midbrain pressure produces the characteristic dorsal midbrain or Parinaud's syndrome (large fixed pupils, loss of upgaze and convergence, and retractory nystagmus; see later discussion). It is also possible for the venous drainage of the brainstem to be compromised by compression of the great vein of Galen, which runs along the midline on the dorsal surface of the midbrain. However, in postmortem series, venous infarction is a rare contributor to brainstem injury.[49]

Rostrocaudal herniation of the brainstem may occur when the distortion of the brainstem compromises its vascular supply. Downward displacement of the midbrain or pons stretches the medial perforating branches of the basilar artery, which itself is tethered to the circle of Willis and cannot shift downward (Figure 3.4). The consequent paramedian ischemia may contribute to loss of consciousness. Postmortem study of the basilar artery demonstrates that the paramedian arteries are at risk of necrosis and extravasation during downward herniation. The characteristic slit-like hemorrhages seen in the area of brainstem displacement postmortem are called *Duret hemorrhages*[49,50] (Figure 3.7).

Tonsillar herniation occurs in cases in which the pressure gradient across the foramen magnum impacts the cerebellar tonsils

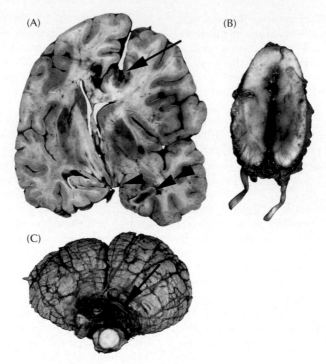

Figure 3.7 Neuropathology of herniation due to a large brain tumor. A large, right hemisphere brain tumor caused subfalcine herniation (arrow in A) and pushed the temporal lobe against the diencephalon (arrowhead). Herniation of the uncus caused hemorrhage into the hippocampus (double arrowhead). Downward displacement of the brainstem caused elongation of the brainstem and midline Duret hemorrhages (B). Downward displacement of the cerebellum impacted the cerebellar tonsils against the foramen magnum, infarcting the tonsillar tissue (arrow in C).

against the foramen magnum, closing off the fourth ventricular outflow and compressing the medulla (Figures 3.7 and 3.8). This may occur quite suddenly, as in cases of subarachnoid hemorrhage, when a large pressure wave drives the cerebellar tonsils against the foramen magnum, compressing the caudal medulla. The patient suddenly stops breathing, and blood pressure rapidly increases as the vascular reflex pathways in the lower brainstem attempt to perfuse the lower medulla against the intense local pressure. A similar syndrome is sometimes seen when lumbar puncture is performed on a patient whose intracranial mass lesion has exhausted the intracranial compliance.[51] In patients with sustained tonsillar herniation, the cerebellar tonsils are typically found to be necrotic due to their impaction against the unyielding edge of the foramen magnum. This problem is discussed further later.

Upward brainstem herniation may also occur through the tentorial notch in the presence of a rapidly expanding posterior fossa lesion.[6] The superior surface of the cerebellar vermis and the midbrain are pushed upward, compressing the dorsal mesencephalon as well as the adjacent blood vessels and the cerebral aqueduct (Figure 3.8).

The dorsal midbrain compression results in impairment of vertical eye movements as well as consciousness. The pineal gland is typically displaced upward on CT scan.[52] The compression of the cerebral aqueduct can cause acute hydrocephalus, and the superior cerebellar artery may be trapped against the tentorial edge, resulting in infarction and edema of the superior cerebellum and increasing the upward pressure.

Clinical Findings in Uncal Herniation Syndrome

EARLY THIRD-NERVE STAGE

The proximity of the dorsal surface of the oculomotor nerve to the medial edge of the temporal

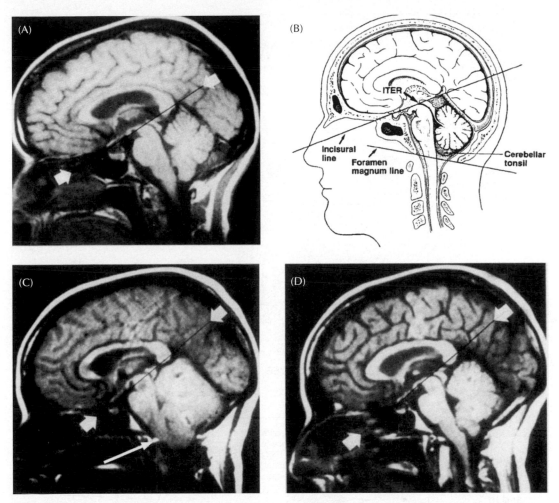

Figure 3.8 Herniation due to a cerebellar mass lesion. The incisural line (A, B) is defined by a line connecting the dorsum sellae with the inferior point of the confluence of the inferior sagittal and straight sinuses with the great vein of Galen, in a midline sagittal magnetic resonance imaging (MRI) scan, shown by a line in each panel. The iter, or anterior tip of the cerebral aqueduct, should lie along this line; upward herniation of the brainstem is defined by the iter being displaced above the line. The cerebellar tonsils should be above the foramen magnum line (B), connecting the most inferior tip of the clivus and the inferior tip of the occiput, in the midline sagittal plane. Panel (C) shows the MRI of a 31-year-old woman with metastatic thymoma to the cerebellum who developed stupor and loss of upgaze after placement of a ventriculoperitoneal shunt. The cerebellum is swollen, the fourth ventricle is effaced, and the brainstem is compressed. The iter is displaced 4.8 mm above the incisural line, and the anterior tip of the base of the pons is displaced upward toward the mammillary body, which also lies along the incisural line. The cerebellar tonsils have also been forced 11.1 mm below the foramen magnum line (demarcated by thin, long white arrow). Following treatment, the cerebellum and metastases shrank (D), and the iter returned to its normal location, although the cerebellar tonsils remained somewhat displaced.
Modified from Reich et al.,[53] with permission.

lobe (Figure 3.5) means that the earliest and most subtle sign of uncal herniation is often an increase in the diameter of the ipsilateral pupil. The pupil may respond sluggishly to light, and typically it dilates progressively as the herniation continues. Early on, there may be no other impairment of oculomotor function (i.e., no ptosis or ocular motor signs). Once the herniation advances to the point where the function of the brainstem is compromised, signs of brainstem deterioration may proceed rapidly, and the patient may slip from full consciousness to deep coma over a matter of minutes (Figure 3.9 and Patient Vignette 3.2).

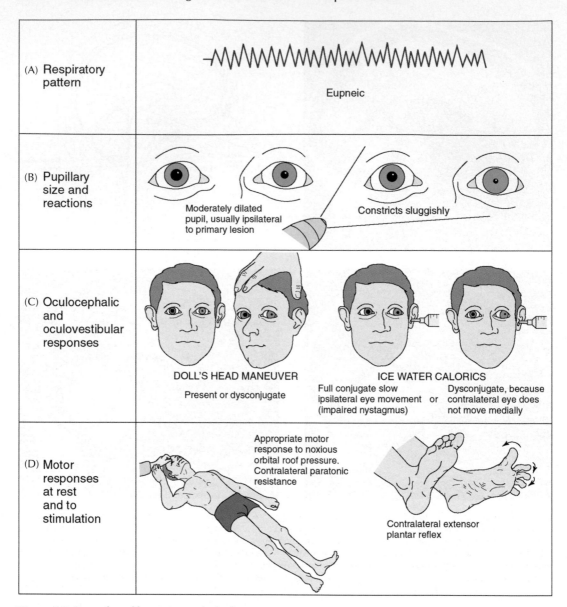

(A) Respiratory pattern	Eupneic
(B) Pupillary size and reactions	Moderately dilated pupil, usually ipsilateral to primary lesion · Constricts sluggishly
(C) Oculocephalic and oculovestibular responses	DOLL'S HEAD MANEUVER — Present or dysconjugate · ICE WATER CALORICS — Full conjugate slow ipsilateral eye movement (impaired nystagmus) or Dysconjugate, because contralateral eye does not move medially
(D) Motor responses at rest and to stimulation	Appropriate motor response to noxious orbital roof pressure. Contralateral paratonic resistance · Contralateral extensor plantar reflex

Figure 3.9 Signs of uncal herniation, early third-nerve stage.

Patient Vignette 3.2

A 22-year-old woman was admitted to the emergency room with the complaint of erratic behavior "since her boyfriend had hit her on the head with a gun." She was awake but behaved erratically in the emergency room and was sent for CT scanning while a neurology consult was called. The neurologist found the patient in the x-ray department; the technician noted that she had initially been uncooperative, but for the previous 10 minutes she had lain still while the study was completed.

Immediate examination on the radiology table showed that breathing was slow and regular and she was unresponsive except to deep pain, with localizing movements of the right but not the left extremities. The right pupil was 8 mm and unreactive to light, and there was no adduction, elevation, or depression of the right eye on oculocephalic testing. Muscle tone was increased on the left compared to the right, and the left plantar response was extensor.

She was immediately treated with hyperventilation and mannitol and awakened. The radiologist reported that there were fragments of metal embedded in the skull and that the underlying right frontal lobe was edematous. The patient confirmed that the boyfriend had actually tried to shoot her, but that the bullet had struck her skull with only a glancing blow, where it apparently had fragmented. The right frontal lobe was contused and swollen, and downward pressure had caused transtentorial herniation of the uncus. Following right frontal lobectomy to decompress her brain, she improved and was discharged.

LATE THIRD-NERVE STAGE

As the foregoing case illustrates, the signs of the late third-nerve stage are due to more complete impairment of the oculomotor nerve as well as compression of the midbrain. Pupillary dilation becomes complete and the pupil no longer reacts to light. Adduction, elevation, and depression of the affected eye are lost, and there is usually ptosis (if indeed the patient opens the eyes at all).

The lapse into coma may take place over just a few minutes, as occurred with the woman in Patient Vignette 3.2 who was uncooperative with the x-ray technician and 10 minutes later was found by the neurologist to be deeply comatose. Hemiparesis may be ipsilateral to the herniation (if the midbrain is compressed against the opposite tentorial edge) or may be contralateral (if the paresis is due to the lesion damaging the descending corticospinal tract or to a herniating temporal lobe compressing the ipsilateral cerebral peduncle). Breathing is typically normal, or the patient may lapse into a Cheyne-Stokes pattern of respiration (Figure 3.10).

MIDBRAIN-UPPER PONTINE STAGE

If treatment is delayed or unsuccessful, signs of midbrain damage appear and progress caudally, as in central herniation (see later discussion). Both pupils may be fixed at midposition, and neither eye elevates, depresses, or turns medially with oculocephalic or caloric vestibular testing. Either decorticate or decerebrate posturing may be seen.

Clinical Findings in Central Herniation Syndrome

DIENCEPHALIC STAGE

The first evidence that a supratentorial mass is beginning to impair the diencephalon is usually a change in alertness and behavior. Initially, subjects might find it difficult to concentrate and may be unable to retain the orderly details of recent events. As the compression of the diencephalon progresses, the patient lapses into torpid drowsiness, and finally stupor and coma.

Respiration in the *early diencephalic stage* of central herniation is commonly interrupted by sighs, yawns, and occasional pauses (Figure 3.11). As the sleepiness deepens, many patients lapse into the periodic breathing of Cheyne-Stokes respiration. The pupils are typically small (1–3 mm), and it may be difficult to identify their reaction to light without a bright light source or a magnifying glass. However, the pupils typically dilate briskly in response to a pinch of the skin over the neck (ciliospinal reflex).[54] The eyes are typically conjugate or slightly divergent if the patient is not awake, and there may be roving eye movements, with slow to-and-fro rolling conjugate displacement. Oculocephalic testing typically demonstrates brisk, normal responses. There is typically a diffuse, waxy increase in motor tone (paratonia or gegenhalten), and the toe signs may become bilaterally extensor.

The appearance of a patient in the early diencephalic stage of central herniation is quite similar to that in metabolic encephalopathy. This is a key problem, because one would like to identify patients in the earliest phase of central herniation to institute specific therapy, and yet these patients look most like patients who have no structural cause of coma. For this reason, every patient with the clinical appearance of metabolic encephalopathy requires careful serial examinations until a structural lesion can be ruled out with an imaging study and a metabolic cause of coma can be identified and corrected.

During the *late diencephalic stage* (Figure 3.12), the clinical appearance of the patient

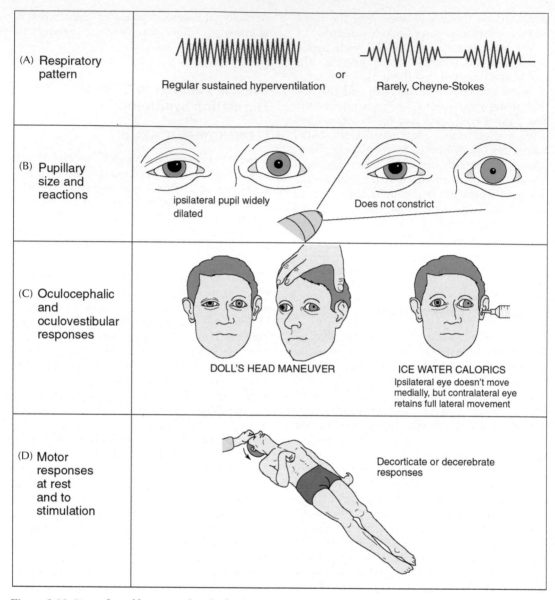

Figure 3.10 Signs of uncal herniation, late third-nerve stage.

becomes more distinctive. The patient becomes gradually more difficult to arouse, and eventually localizing motor responses to pain may disappear entirely or decorticate responses may appear. Initially, the upper extremity flexor and lower extremity extensor posturing tends to appear on the side contralateral to the lesion and only in response to noxious stimuli. Later, the response may become bilateral, and eventually the contralateral and then ipsilateral side may progress to full extensor (decerebrate) posturing.

The mechanism for brain impairment during the diencephalic stage of central herniation is not clear. Careful quantitative studies show that the depressed level of consciousness correlates with either lateral or vertical displacement of the pineal gland, which lies along the midline at the rostral extreme of the dorsal midbrain.[53,55] The diencephalic impairment may be due to the stretching of small penetrating vessels tethered to the posterior cerebral and communicating arteries that supply

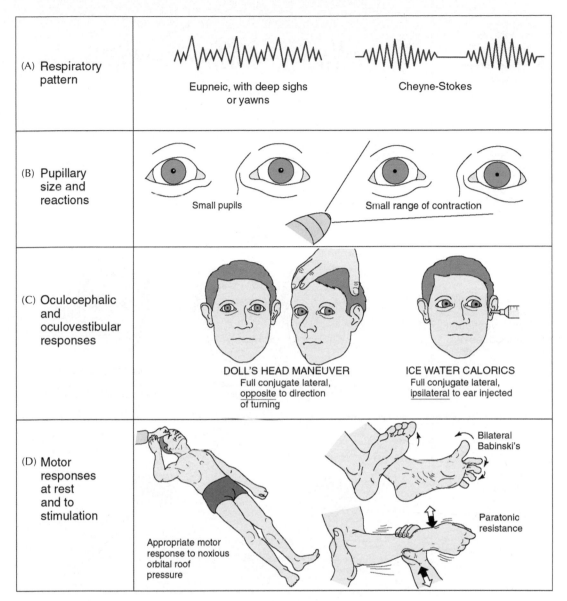

(A) Respiratory pattern	Eupneic, with deep sighs or yawns	Cheyne-Stokes
(B) Pupillary size and reactions	Small pupils	Small range of contraction
(C) Oculocephalic and oculovestibular responses	DOLL'S HEAD MANEUVER Full conjugate lateral, opposite to direction of turning	ICE WATER CALORICS Full conjugate lateral, ipsilateral to ear injected
(D) Motor responses at rest and to stimulation	Appropriate motor response to noxious orbital roof pressure	Bilateral Babinski's / Paratonic resistance

Figure 3.11 Signs of central transtentorial herniation or lateral displacement of the diencephalon, early diencephalic stage.

the caudal thalamus and hypothalamus. There is little evidence that either increases in ICP or changes in overall cerebral blood flow can account for these findings. As patients with diencephalic signs of the central herniation syndrome worsen, they tend to pass rapidly to the stage of midbrain damage, suggesting that the same pathologic process has merely extended to the next more caudal level.

The clinical importance, therefore, of the diencephalic stage of central herniation is that it warns of a potentially reversible lesion that is about to encroach on the brainstem and create irreversible damage. If the supratentorial process can be alleviated before the signs of midbrain injury emerge, chances for a recovery from the herniation are good. Once signs of lower diencephalic and midbrain dysfunction appear, it becomes increasingly likely that they will reflect infarction rather than compression and reversible ischemia, and the outlook for neurologic recovery rapidly becomes much poorer.

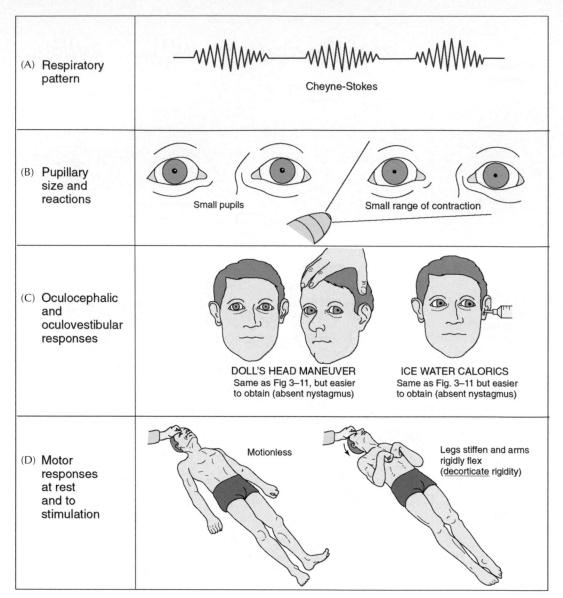

Figure 3.12 Signs of central transtentorial herniation, or lateral displacement of the diencephalon, late diencephalic stage.

As herniation progresses to the *midbrain stage* (Figure 3.13), signs of oculomotor failure appear. The pupils become irregular, then fixed at midposition. Oculocephalic movements become more difficult to elicit, and it may be necessary to examine cold water caloric responses to determine their full extent. Typically, there is limited and slower, and finally no medial movement of the eye contralateral to the cold water stimulus, and bilateral warm or cold water irrigation confirms lack of vertical eye movements. Motor responses are difficult to obtain or result in extensor posturing. In some cases, extensor posturing appears spontaneously or in response to internal stimuli. Motor tone and tendon reflexes may be heightened, and plantar responses are extensor.

After the midbrain stage becomes complete, it is rare for patients to recover fully.

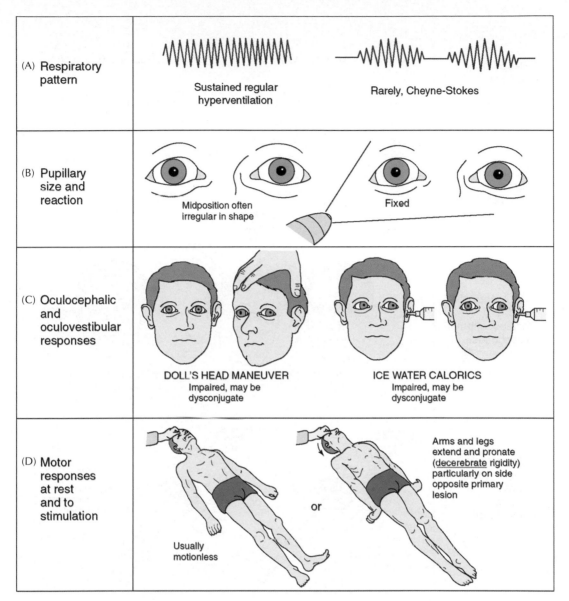

Figure 3.13 Signs of transtentorial herniation, midbrain–upper pons stage.

Most patients in whom the herniation can be reversed suffer chronic neurologic disability.[56,57] Hence, it is critical, if intervention is anticipated, that it begin as early as possible and that it be as vigorous as possible because the patient's life hangs in the balance.

As the patient enters the *pontine stage* (Figure 3.14) of rostrocaudal herniation, breathing becomes more shallow and irregular as the upper pontine structures that modulate breathing are lost. As the damage approaches the lower pons, the lateral eye movements produced by cold water caloric stimulation are also lost. Motor tone becomes flaccid, tendon reflexes may be difficult to obtain, and lower extremity posturing may become flexor.

The *medullary stage* is terminal. Breathing becomes irregular and slows, often assuming a gasping quality. As breathing fails, sympathetic reflexes may cause adrenalin release, and the

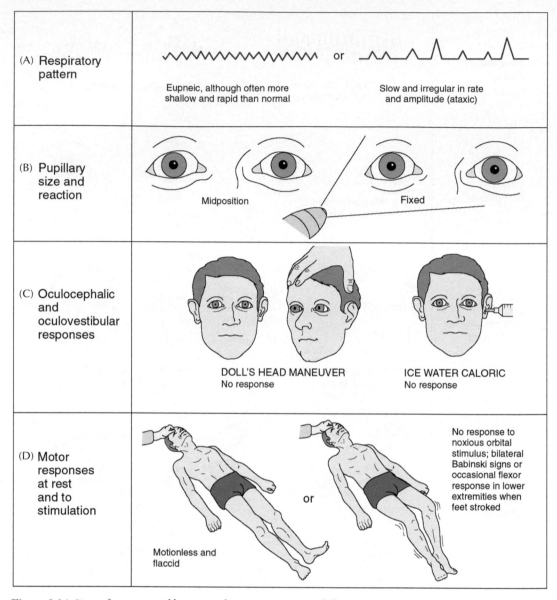

| (A) Respiratory pattern | Eupneic, although often more shallow and rapid than normal | or | Slow and irregular in rate and amplitude (ataxic) |

| (B) Pupillary size and reaction | Midposition | Fixed |

| (C) Oculocephalic and oculovestibular responses | DOLL'S HEAD MANEUVER No response | ICE WATER CALORIC No response |

| (D) Motor responses at rest and to stimulation | Motionless and flaccid | or | No response to noxious orbital stimulus; bilateral Babinski signs or occasional flexor response in lower extremities when feet stroked |

Figure 3.14 Signs of transtentorial herniation, lower pons–upper medulla stage.

pupils may transiently dilate. However, as cerebral hypoxic and baroreceptor reflexes also become impaired, autonomic reflexes fail and blood pressure drops to levels seen after high spinal transection (systolic pressures of 60–70 mm Hg).

At this point, intervening with artificial ventilation and pressor drugs may keep the body alive, but there is little chance of a useful recovery. Therefore, it is important to discuss the situation with the family of the patient as early as possible in the course of the illness and to make it clear that mechanical ventilation in this situation merely prolongs the process of dying.

Clinical Findings in Dorsal Midbrain Syndrome

The midbrain may be forced downward through the tentorial opening by a mass lesion impinging on it from the dorsal surface (Figure 3.15). The most common causes are masses in the pineal gland (pinealocytoma or germ cell line tumors)[58] or in the posterior thalamus (tumor or hemorrhage into the pulvinar, which normally overhangs the quadrigeminal plate at the posterior opening of the tentorial notch). Pressure from this direction produces the characteristic dorsal midbrain syndrome. A similar picture may be seen during upward transtentorial herniation, which kinks the midbrain (Figure 3.8).

Pressure on the olivary pretectal nucleus and the posterior commissure produces slightly enlarged (typically 4–6 mm in diameter) pupils that are fixed to light.[2] There is limitation of vertical eye movements, typically manifested first by limited upgaze. In severe cases, the eyes may be fixed in a forced, downward position. If the patient is awake, there may also

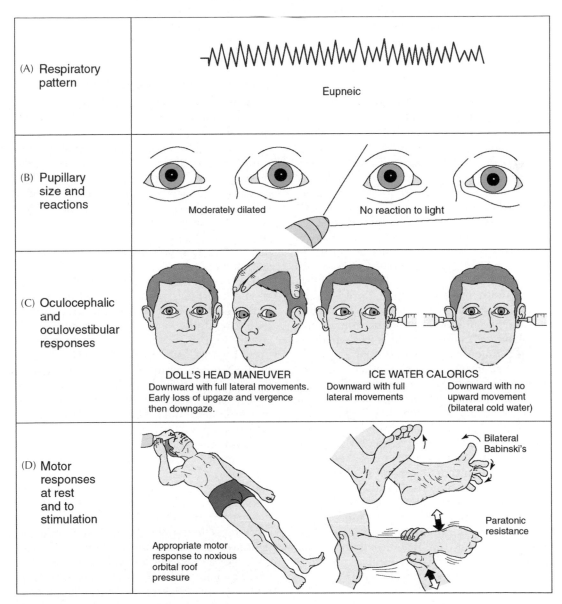

Figure 3.15 Signs of dorsal midbrain compression.

be a deficit of convergent eye movements and associated pupilloconstriction. The presence of retractory nystagmus, in which all of the eye muscles contract simultaneously to pull the globe back into the orbit, is characteristic. Retraction of the eyelids may produce a staring appearance.[59]

Deficits of arousal are present in only about 15% of patients with pineal region tumors, but these are due to early central herniation.[60] If the cerebral aqueduct is compressed sufficiently to cause hydrocephalus, however, an acute increase in supratentorial pressure may ensue. This may cause downward pressure on the midbrain, resulting in sudden lapse into deep coma.

Safety of Lumbar Puncture in Comatose Patients

A common question encountered clinically is, *"Under what circumstances is lumbar puncture safe in a patient with an intracranial mass lesion?"* There is often a large pressure gradient between the supratentorial compartment and the lumbar sac,[61] and lowering the lumbar pressure by removing CSF may increase the gradient. The actual frequency of cases in which this hypothetical risk causes transtentorial herniation is difficult to ascertain. Studies done during the pre-CT era, examining series of patients with brain tumors who underwent lumbar puncture, found complication rates in the range of 1–2% in patients with documented increased CSF pressure or papilledema.[62,63] On the other hand, of patients referred to a neurosurgical service because of complications following lumbar puncture, Duffy reported that 22 had focal neurologic signs before the lumbar puncture, but only one-half had increased CSF pressure and one-third had papilledema.[51] The experience of the authors supports the view that although lumbar puncture rarely precipitates transtentorial (or foramen magnum) herniation, even in patients who may be predisposed by an existing supratentorial mass lesion, neither the physical examination nor the evaluation of CSF pressure at lumbar puncture is sufficient to predict which patients will suffer complications. Hence, before any patient undergoes lumbar puncture, it is wise to obtain a CT (or MRI) scan of the cranial contents. If a patient has no evidence of compartmental shift on the study and the ventricular system is open as judged by CSF in the cisterns on CT, it is quite safe to obtain a lumbar puncture. On the other hand, if it is impossible to obtain an imaging study in a timely fashion and the neurologic examination shows no papilledema or focal signs, the risk of lumbar puncture is quite low (probably less than 1%). Under such circumstances, risk-benefit analysis may well favor proceeding with lumbar puncture if the examination of the CSF is needed to make potentially life-saving decisions about clinical care.

False Localizing Signs in the Diagnosis of Structural Coma

It is usually relatively easy for a skilled examiner to differentiate supratentorial from infratentorial signs, and the cranial nerve findings due to herniation syndromes are characteristic. However, there are a number of specific situations in which the neurologic signs may falsely cause the examiner to consider an infratentorial process or to mistake an infratentorial process for one that is supratentorial.

The most common false localizing sign is abducens palsy. This may be caused by increased ICP, or it may occur after lumbar puncture. In the latter case, the reduced CSF volume can cause the brain to lose its usual buoyant suspension in the CSF. The sagging of the brain in an upright posture is thought to cause traction on the abducens nerve. More rarely, impairment of the trochlear, oculomotor, or trigeminal nerves may occur post-lumbar puncture.

Differentiation of supratentorial from infratentorial causes of ataxia has presented a diagnostic dilemma since the earliest days of neurology.[64] In the days before imaging, despite highly developed clinical skills, it was not unusual for a neurosurgeon to explore the posterior fossa, find nothing, and then turn the patient over and remove a frontal tumor. The gait disorder that is associated with bilateral medial frontal compression or hydrocephalus can be replicated on occasion by cerebellar lesions. Similarly, unilateral ataxia of finger-nose-finger testing, which appears to be cerebellar in origin, may occasionally be seen with parietal lobe lesions.[65]

Another source of confusion is the differentiation of upper (supranuclear) versus lower motor neuron cranial nerve palsies. Acute supratentorial lesions can on rare occasion cause lower cranial nerve palsies (asymmetric palate, tongue weakness on one side). Bilateral supratentorial lesions can produce dysarthria, dysphagia, and bilateral facial weakness (pseudobulbar palsy, also called the opercular or Foix-Chavany-Marie syndrome).[66] Conversely, the well-known upper motor neuron facial palsy (weakness of the lower part of the face) can be seen with some posterior fossa lesions. The distinction between upper versus lower motor neuron cranial nerve weakness can often be made on the basis of reflex versus voluntary movement. For example, a patient with supranuclear bulbar weakness will often show intact, or even hyperactive, corneal or gag reflexes. A patient with an upper motor neuron facial palsy will typically show a much more symmetric smile on responding to a joke than when asked to smile voluntarily.

Fortunately, these classic problems with localization rarely intrude on interpretation of the examination of a patient with an impaired level of consciousness as the signs associated with herniation typically develop relatively rapidly as the patient loses consciousness. If the patient displays false localizing signs while awake, the progression of new signs that occur during the herniation process generally clarifies the matter. Patients with impaired consciousness and focal brainstem signs are generally treated as having structural causes of coma and receive immediate imaging studies, so any confusion about the source of the findings is short-lived.

DESTRUCTIVE LESIONS AS A CAUSE OF COMA

Destructive lesions of the ascending arousal system or its forebrain targets are paradoxically less of an immediate diagnostic concern for the examining neurologist. Unlike compressive lesions, which can often be reversed by removing a mass, destructive lesions typically cannot be reversed. Although it is important to recognize the hallmarks of a destructive, as opposed to a compressive lesion, the real value comes in distinguishing patients who may benefit from immediate therapeutic intervention from those who need mainly supportive care.

Diffuse, Bilateral Cortical Destruction

Diffuse, bilateral destruction of the cerebral cortex or its underlying white matter can occur as a result of deprivation of metabolic substrate (i.e., oxygen, glucose, or the blood that carries them) or as a consequence of certain metabolic or infectious diseases. This condition is often the consequence of prolonged cardiac arrest in a patient who is eventually resuscitated, but it may also occur in patients who have diffuse hypoxia due to pulmonary failure or occasionally in patients with severe and prolonged hypoglycemia. The lack of metabolic substrate causes neurons in layers III and V of the cerebral cortex, and in the CA1 and CA3 fields of the hippocampal formation, to be damaged,[67,68] presumably as a result of excitatory amino acid toxicity (see Figure 1.10). During periods of metabolic deprivation, there is a rundown of the ion gradients that support normal membrane polarization, resulting in depolarization of neurons and release of their neurotransmitters. Excess excitatory transmitter, particularly acting on N-methyl-D-aspartate (NMDA) receptors that allow the intracellular shift of calcium ions, results in activation of genetic neuronal death programs and the elimination of neurons that receive intense excitatory amino acid inputs.[69] Because excitatory amino acids are used extensively for corticocortical communication, the neurons that are at greatest risk are those that receive those connections, which in turn are the ones that are most responsible for cortical output as well. The remaining neurons are essentially cut off from one another and from their outputs and thus are unable to provide meaningful behavioral response.

Patients who have suffered from a period of hypoxia of somewhat lesser degree may appear to recover after brain oxygenation is restored. However, over the following week or so, there may be a progressive degeneration of the subcortical white matter, essentially isolating the cortex from its major inputs and outputs.[70,71] This condition is seen most commonly after carbon monoxide poisoning (see pp. 201–203), but also may occur after other sublethal episodes of hypoxia. The mechanism of white matter injury is not known, although it may be related to similar white matter injury that is seen in Leigh's disease, mitochondrial encephalopathy with "strokes," and other disorders of cerebral intermediary metabolism that leave the brain with inadequate but sublethal impairment of oxidative energy metabolism.[72]

Other metabolic leukoencephalopathies, such as metachromatic leukodystrophy and Canavan's disease, rarely occur in adults but are considerations when assessing infants or very young children. Adrenoleukodystrophy may cause mainly posterior hemispheric white matter disease but rarely affects the level of consciousness until very late in the disease.

Infectious causes of diffuse dysfunction of the cerebral cortex or subjacent white matter include prion infections (Creutzfeldt-Jakob disease, Gerstmann-Sträussler syndrome, etc.) and progressive multifocal leukoencephalopathy. These disorders typically begin with focal cortical signs and progress over a period of weeks to months, and so rarely present a diagnostic dilemma by the time global consciousness is impaired. Subacute sclerosing panencephalitis, due to slow viral infection with the measles virus, can also cause this picture, but it is rarely seen in populations in which measles vaccination is practiced.

Destructive Disease of the Diencephalon

Bilateral destructive lesions of the *diencephalon* are a rare cause of coma, in part because the diencephalon receives its blood supply directly from feeding vessels that take off from the major arteries of the circle of Willis. Hence, although vascular disease may affect the diencephalon when any one major arterial source is compromised, it is typically unilateral and does not impair consciousness. An exception occurs when there is occlusion of the tip of the basilar artery, which supplies the posterior cerebral and posterior communicating arteries bilaterally.[73] The posterior thalamic penetrating arteries may take their origin from a single artery of Percheron arising from these posterior components of the circle of Willis, and, as a consequence, there may be bilateral posterior thalamic infarction with a single site of vascular occlusion.[74] However, nearly all cases in which there is impairment of consciousness also have some paramedian midbrain ischemia as well (see *distal basilar occlusion* in Chapter 4, p. 157).

Occasional inflammatory and infectious disorders may have a predilection for the diencephalon. Fatal familial insomnia, a prion disorder, is reported to affect the thalamus selectively but is thought to be the cause of the hyperwakefulness in that disorder, rather than coma.[75] Behçet's disease may cause sterile abscess formation in the diencephalon, which may depress the level of consciousness.[76,77]

Autoimmune disorders may also affect the diencephalon. In patients with anti-Ma antitumor antibodies, there are often diencephalic lesions as well as excessive sleepiness and sometimes other symptoms of narcolepsy, such as cataplexy.[78] It is now recognized that, in most patients with narcolepsy, there is a progressive loss of neurons in the lateral hypothalamus that express the neurotransmitter orexin (also called hypocretin).[79–81] This selective loss of orexin neurons is believed to be autoimmune in origin, although this remains to be demonstrated definitively. Loss of orexin neurons results in excessive sleepiness, but patients can readily be awakened to a fully conscious state.

Rarely, primary brain tumors may arise in the diencephalon. These may be either astrocytomas or primary central nervous system lymphomas, and they can cause impairment of consciousness as an early sign. Suprasellar tumors such as craniopharyngioma or suprasellar germinoma, or suprasellar extension of a large pituitary adenoma, can compress the diencephalon, but this does not usually cause destruction unless attempts at surgical excision cause local vasospasm.[82]

Destructive Lesions of the Brainstem

In destructive disorders of the brainstem, acute loss of consciousness is typically accompanied by a distinctive pattern of pupillary, oculomotor, motor, and respiratory signs that indicate the level of the brainstem that has been damaged. Unlike rostrocaudal herniation, however, in which functions of the brainstem are progressively lost as the wave of herniation proceeds from the diencephalon downward, tegmental lesions of the brainstem are accompanied by more limited findings that pinpoint the level of the lesion.

Destructive lesions at the level of the *midbrain* tegmentum may destroy the oculomotor nuclei bilaterally, resulting in fixed midposition pupils and paresis of adduction, elevation, and depression of the eyes. At the same time, the abduction of the eyes with oculocephalic maneuvers is preserved. If the cerebral peduncles are also damaged, as with a basilar artery occlusion, there is bilateral flaccid paralysis.

A destructive lesion of the *rostral pontine* tegmentum spares the oculomotor nuclei, so that the pupils remain reactive to light. If the lateral pontine tegmentum is involved, the descending sympathetic and ascending pupillodilator pathways are both damaged, resulting in tiny pupils whose reaction to light may be discernible only by using a magnifying glass. Damage to the medial longitudinal fasciculus causes loss of adduction, elevation, and depression in response to vestibular stimulation, but abduction is preserved on oculovestibular testing. If the patient is sufficiently arousable, behaviorally directed vertical and vergence eye movements may be elicited. If the lesion extends somewhat caudally into the midpons, there may be gaze paresis toward the side of the lesion or slow vertical eye movements, called ocular bobbing, or its variants (Table 2.3). When the lesion involves the base of the pons, there may be bilateral flaccid paralysis. However, this is not necessarily seen if the lesion is confined to the pontine tegmentum, and, conversely, lesions of the base of the pons can cause bilateral

flaccid paralysis without loss of consciousness (the locked-in syndrome). Facial or trigeminal lower motor neuron paralysis can also be seen if the lesion extends into the more caudal pons. Involvement of the pons may also produce apneustic or ataxic breathing.

On the other hand, destructive lesions that are confined to the lower pons or medulla do not cause loss of consciousness.[83,84] Such patients may, however, have sufficient damage to the descending motor systems that they are locked-in (i.e., have quadriplegia and supranuclear impairment of facial and oropharyngeal motor function).[85] Motor responses may be limited to vertical eye movements and blinking.

Destructive lesions of the brainstem may occur as a result of vascular disease, tumor, infection, or trauma. The most common cause of brainstem destructive lesions is the occlusion of the vertebral or basilar arteries. Such occlusions typically produce signs that pinpoint the level of the infarction. Hemorrhagic lesions of the brainstem are most commonly intraparenchymal hemorrhages into the base of the pons, although arteriovenous malformations may occur at any level. Infections that have a predilection for the brainstem include *Listeria monocytogenes*, which tends to cause rhombencephalic abscesses[86] (see Figure 4.12). Trauma that penetrates the brainstem is usually not a problem diagnostically as it is almost always immediately fatal.

REFERENCES

1. Ropper AH. A preliminary MRI study of the geometry of brain displacement and level of consciousness with acute intracranial masses. *Neurology* 1989;39:622–627.
2. Baloh RW, Furman JM, Yee RD. Dorsal midbrain syndrome: clinical and oculographic findings. *Neurology* 1985;35:54–60.
3. Roper-Hall G. Historical vignette: Henri Parinaud (1844–1905): French ophthalmologist and pioneer in neuroophthalmology. *Am Orthopt J* 2014;64:126–133.
4. Chittiboina P, Lonser RR. Von Hippel-Lindau disease. *Handb Clin Neurol* 2015;132:139–156. doi:10.1016/B978-0-444-62702-5.00010-X.
5. van Loon J, Van Calenbergh F, Goffin J, Plets C. Controversies in the management of spontaneous cerebellar haemorrhage. A consecutive series of 49 cases and review of the literature. *Acta Neurochir (Wien)* 1993;122:187–193.

6. Cuneo RA, Caronna JJ, Pitts L, Townsend J, Winestock DP. Upward transtentorial herniation: seven cases and a literature review. *Arch Neurol* 1979;36:618–623.
7. Hayreh SS. The sheath of the optic nerve. *Ophthalmologica* 1984;189:54–63.
8. Hayreh SS. Pathogenesis of optic disc edema in raised intracranial pressure. *Prog Retin Eye Res* 2016;50:108–144.
9. Jacks AS, Miller NR. Spontaneous retinal venous pulsation: aetiology and significance. *J Neurol Neurosurg Psychiatry* 2003;74:7–9.
10. Van Uitert RL, Eisenstadt ML. Venous pulsations not always indicative of normal intracranial pressure. *Arch Neurol* 1978;35:550.
11. Hayreh SS. Optic disc edema in raised intracranial pressure. V. Pathogenesis. *Arch Ophthalmol* 1977;95:1553–1565.
12. d'Avella D, Baroni A, Mingrino S, Scanarini M. An electron microscope study of human arachnoid villi. *Surg Neurol* 1980;14:41–47.
13. Browder J, Meyers R. Behavior of the systemic blood pressure, pulse rate, and spinal fluid pressure associated with acute changes in intracranial pressure artificially produced. *Arch Surg* 1938;36:1–19.
14. Schumacher GA, Wolfe HG. Experimental studies on headache. *Arch Neurol Psychiatr* 1941;45:199–214.
15. Mollan SP, Ali F, Hassan-Smith G, Botfield H, Friedman DI, Sinclair AJ. Evolving evidence in adult idiopathic intracranial hypertension: pathophysiology and management. *J Neurol Neurosurg Psychiatry* 2016;87:982–992.
16. Goodwin J. Recent developments in idiopathic intracranial hypertension (IIH). *Semin Ophthalmol* 2003;18:181–189.
17. Ranjan P, Mishra AM, Kale R, Saraswat VA, Gupta RK. Cytotoxic edema is responsible for raised intracranial pressure in fulminant hepatic failure: in vivo demonstration using diffusion-weighted MRI in human subjects. *Metab Brain Dis* 2005;20:181–192.
18. Magnaes B. Body position and cerebrospinal fluid pressure. Part 1: clinical studies on the effect of rapid postural changes. *J Neurosurg* 1976;44:687–697.
19. Ingvar DH, Lundberg N. Paroxysmal systems in intracranial hypertension, studied with ventricular fluid pressure recording and electroencephalography. *Brain* 1961;84:446–459.
20. Ingvar DH, Lundberg N. Paroxysmal symptoms in intracranial hypertension, studied with ventricular fluid pressure recording and electroencephalography. *Brain* 1961;84:446–459.
21. Risberg J, Lundberg N, Ingvar DH. Regional cerebral blood volume during acute transient rises of the intracranial pressure (plateau waves). *J Neurosurg* 1969;31:303–310.
22. Kim MO, Adji A, O'Rourke MF, et al. Principles of cerebral hemodynamics when intracranial pressure is raised: lessons from the peripheral circulation. *J Hypertens* 2015;33:1233–1241.
23. Greenberg DA, Jin K. From angiogenesis to neuropathology. *Nature* 2005;438:954–959.
24. Leinonen V, Vanninen R, Rauramaa T. Raised intracranial pressure and brain edema. *Handb Clin Neurol* 2017;145:25–37.
25. Mokri B. The Monro-Kellie hypothesis: applications in CSF volume depletion. *Neurology* 2001;56:1746–1748.
26. Bigler ED, Maxwell WL. Neuroimaging and neuropathology of TBI. *NeuroRehabilitation* 2011;28:63–74.
27. Adler DE, Milhorat TH. The tentorial notch: Anatomical variation, morphometric analysis, and classification in 100 human autopsy cases. *J Neurosurg* 2002;96:1103–1112.
28. Schmahmann JD. Vascular syndromes of the thalamus. *Stroke* 2003;34:2264–2278.
29. Neau JP, Bogousslavsky J. The syndrome of posterior choroidal artery territory infarction. *Ann Neurol* 1996;39:779–788.
30. Kerr FW, Hollowell OW. Location of pupillomotor and accommodation fibres in the oculomotor nerve: experimental observations on paralytic mydriasis. *J Neurol Neurosurg Psychiatry* 1964;27:473–481.
31. Adams JH, Graham DI, Murray LS, Scott G. Diffuse axonal injury due to nonmissile head injury in humans: an analysis of 45 cases. *Ann Neurol* 1982;12:557–563.
32. Adams JH, Graham DI, Gennarelli TA, Maxwell WL. Diffuse axonal injury in non-missile head injury. *J Neurol Neurosurg Psychiatry* 1991;54:481–483.
33. Burgerman RS, Wolf AL, Kelman SE, Elsner H, Mirvis S, Sestokas AK. Traumatic trochlear nerve palsy diagnosed by magnetic resonance imaging: case report and review of the literature. *Neurosurgery* 1989;25:978–981.
34. Akal A, Goncu T, Boyaci N, Sarikaya S. Peculiar MRI findings of intracranial hypotension in patients with abducens nerve palsy. *BMJ Case Rep* 2013;2013.
35. Simonetti F, Pergami P, Ceroni M, Ropper AH, Viviani R. About the original description of cerebellar tonsil herniation by Pierre Marie. *J Neurol Neurosurg Psychiatry* 1997;63:412.
36. Cushing H. Some experimental and clinical observations concerning states of increased intracranial tension. *Am J Med Sci* 1902;1241:375–400.
37. Macewen W. Herniation of the brain. *Am J Med Sci* 1887;94:123–146.
38. Meyer A. Incisura of the crus due to contralateral brain tumor. *Arch Neurol Psychiatr* 1920;4:387–400.
39. Kernohan JW, Woltman HW. Incisura of the crus due to contralateral brain tumor. *Arch Neurol* 1929;21:274–287.
40. Ropper AH. Lateral displacement of the brain and level of consciousness in patients with an acute hemispheral mass. *N Engl J Med* 1986;314:953–958.
41. Fisher CM. Brain herniation: A revision of classical concepts. *Can J Neurol Sci* 1995;22:83–91.
42. Rothfus WE, Goldberg AL, Tabas JH, Deeb ZL. Callosomarginal infarction secondary to transfalcial herniation. *AJNR Am J Neuroradiol* 1987;8:1073–1076.
43. Weiner LP, Porro RS. Total third nerve paralysis: a case with hemorrhage in the oculomotor nerve in subdural hematoma. *Neurology* 1965;15:87–90.
44. Binder DK, Lyon R, Manley GT. Transcranial motor evoked potential recording in a case of Kernohan's notch syndrome: case report. *Neurosurgery* 2004;54:999–1002; discussion1003.
45. Marshman LA, Polkey CE, Penney CC. Unilateral fixed dilation of the pupil as a false-localizing sign with intracranial hemorrhage: case report and literature review. *Neurosurgery* 2001;49:1251–1255; discussion 1255–1256.

46. Corrow SL, Dalrymple KA, Barton JJ. Prosopagnosia: current perspectives. *Eye Brain* 2016;8:165–175.

47. Sato M, Tanaka S, Kohama A, Fujii C. Occipital lobe infarction caused by tentorial herniation. *Neurosurgery* 1986;18:300–305.

48. Keane JR. Blindness following tentorial herniation. *Ann Neurol* 1980;8:186–190.

49. Friede RL, Roessmann U. The pathogenesis of secondary midbrain hemorrhages. *Neurology* 1966;16:1210–1216.

50. Chew KL, Baber Y, Iles L, O'Donnell C. Duret hemorrhage: demonstration of ruptured paramedian pontine branches of the basilar artery on minimally invasive, whole body postmortem CT angiography. *Forensic Sci Med Pathol* 2012;8:436–440.

51. Duffy GP. Lumbar puncture in the presence of raised intracranial pressure. *Br Med J* 1969;1:407–409.

52. Osborn AG, Heaston DK, Wing SD. Diagnosis of ascending transtentorial herniation by cranial computed tomography. *AJR Am J Roentgenol* 1978;130:755–760.

53. Reich JB, Sierra J, Camp W, Zanzonico P, Deck MD, Plum F. Magnetic resonance imaging measurements and clinical changes accompanying transtentorial and foramen magnum brain herniation. *Ann Neurol* 1993;33:159–170.

54. Reeves AG, Posner JB. The ciliospinal response in man. *Neurology* 1969;19:1145–1152.

55. Wijdicks EF, Miller GM. MR imaging of progressive downward herniation of the diencephalon. *Neurology* 1997;48:1456–1459.

56. Zervas NT, Hedley-Whyte J. Successful treatment of cerebral herniation in five patients. *N Engl J Med* 1972;286:1075–1077.

57. Qureshi AI, Geocadin RG, Suarez JI, Ulatowski JA. Long-term outcome after medical reversal of transtentorial herniation in patients with supratentorial mass lesions. *Crit Care Med* 2000;28:1556–1564.

58. Schild SE, Scheithauer BW, Schomberg PJ, et al. Pineal parenchymal tumors. Clinical, pathologic, and therapeutic aspects. *Cancer* 1993;72:870–880.

59. Gaillard F, Jones J. Masses of the pineal region: clinical presentation and radiographic features. *Postgrad Med J* 2010;86:597–607.

60. Hoehn ME, Calderwood J, O'Donnell T, Armstrong GT, Gajjar A. Children with dorsal midbrain syndrome as a result of pineal tumors. *J AAPOS* 2017;21:34–38.

61. Kaufmann GE, Clark K. Continuous simultaneous monitoring of intraventricular and cervical subarachnoid cerebrospinal fluid pressure to indicate development of cerebral or tonsillar herniation. *J Neurosurg* 1970;33:145–150.

62. Lubic LG, Marotta JT. Brain tumor and lumbar puncture. *AMA Arch Neurol Psychiatry* 1954;72:568–572.

63. Korein J, Cravioto H, Leicach M. Reevaluation of lumbar puncture: a study of 129 patients with papilledema or intracranial hypertension. *Neurology* 1959;9:290–297.

64. Grant FC. Cerebellar symptoms produced by supratentorial tumors: a further report. *Arch Neurol Psychiat* 1928;20:292–309.

65. Battaglia-Mayer A, Caminiti R. Optic ataxia as a result of the breakdown of the global tuning fields of parietal neurones. *Brain* 2002;125:225–237.

66. Weller M. Anterior opercular cortex lesions cause dissociated lower cranial nerve palsies and anarthria but no aphasia: Foix-Chavany-Marie syndrome and "automatic voluntary dissociation" revisited. *J Neurol* 1993;240:199–208.

67. Adams JH. Hypoxic brain damage. *Br J Anaesth* 1975;47:121–129.

68. Zola-Morgan S, Squire LR, Amaral DG. Human amnesia and the medial temporal region: enduring memory impairment following a bilateral lesion limited to field CA1 of the hippocampus. *J Neurosci* 1986;6:2950–2967.

69. Snider BJ, Gottron FJ, Choi DW. Apoptosis and necrosis in cerebrovascular disease. *Ann N Y Acad Sci* 1999;893:243–253.

70. Peter L, Nighoghossian N, Jouvet A, et al. [Delayed post-anoxic leukoencephalopathy]. *Rev Neurol (Paris)* 2004;160:1085–1088.

71. Goedee S, van der Nat GA, Roks G. Temporary recovery after resuscitation: delayed postanoxic encephalopathy. *BMJ Case Rep* 2013;2013.

72. Lerman-Sagie T, Leshinsky-Silver E, Watemberg N, Luckman Y, Lev D. White matter involvement in mitochondrial diseases. *Mol Genet Metab* 2005;84:127–136.

73. Caplan LR. "Top of the basilar" syndrome. *Neurology* 1980;30:72–79.

74. Caruso P, Manganotti P, Moretti R. Complex neurological symptoms in bilateral thalamic stroke due to Percheron artery occlusion. *Vasc Health Risk Manag* 2017;13:11–14.

75. Montagna P, Gambetti P, Cortelli P, Lugaresi E. Familial and sporadic fatal insomnia. *Lancet Neurol* 2003;2:167–176.

76. Akman-Demir G, Bahar S, Coban O, Tasci B, Serdaroglu P. Cranial MRI in Behcet's disease: 134 examinations of 98 patients. *Neuroradiology* 2003;45:851–859.

77. Baumann CR, Bassetti CL, Hersberger M, Jung HH. Excessive daytime sleepiness in Behcet's disease with diencephalic lesions and hypocretin dysfunction. *Eur Neurol* 2010;63(3):190.

78. Rosenfeld MR, Eichen JG, Wade DF, Posner JB, Dalmau J. Molecular and clinical diversity in paraneoplastic immunity to Ma proteins. *Ann Neurol* 2001;50:339–348.

79. Peyron C, Faraco J, Rogers W, et al. A mutation in a case of early onset narcolepsy and a generalized absence of hypocretin peptides in human narcoleptic brains. *Nat Med* 2000;6:991–997.

80. Crocker AD, Espana RA, Papadopoulou M, et al. Concomitant loss of dynorphin, NARP, and orexin in human narcolepsy. *Neurology* 2005;65(8):1184–1188.

81. Thannickal TC, Moore RY, Nienhuis R, et al. Reduced number of hypocretin neurons in human narcolepsy. *Neuron* 2000;27:469–474.

82. Scammell TE, Nishino S, Mignot E, Saper CB. Narcolepsy and low CSF orexin (hypocretin) concentration after a diencephalic stroke. *Neurology* 2001;56:1751–1753.

83. Parvizi J, Damasio AR. Neuroanatomical correlates of brainstem coma. *Brain* 2003;126:1524–1536.

84. Fischer DB, Boes AD, Demertzi A, et al. A human brain network derived from coma-causing brainstem lesions. *Neurology* 2016;87:2427–2434.

85. Levy DE, Sidtis JJ, Rottenberg DA, et al. Differences in cerebral blood flow and glucose utilization in vegetative versus locked-in patients. *Ann Neurol* 1987;22:673–682.

86. Armstrong RW, Fung PC. Brainstem encephalitis (rhombencephalitis) due to Listeria monocytogenes: case report and review. *Clin Infect Dis* 1993;16:689–702.

Chapter 4

Specific Causes of Structural Coma

Delayed Encephalopathy After Head Injury

INFRATENTORIAL DESTRUCTIVE LESIONS

BRAINSTEM VASCULAR DESTRUCTIVE DISORDERS
Brainstem Hemorrhage
Basilar Migraine

Posterior Reversible Leukoencephalopathy Syndrome

INFRATENTORIAL INFLAMMATORY DISORDERS

INFRATENTORIAL TUMORS

CENTRAL PONTINE MYELINOLYSIS

INTRODUCTION

The previous chapter divided structural lesions causing coma into compressive and destructive lesions. It further indicated that lesions could be supratentorial, compressing or destroying the diencephalon and upper midbrain, or infratentorial, directly affecting the pons and cerebellum. A physician attempting to determine the cause of coma resulting from a structural lesion must establish, first, the site of the lesion, determining whether the lesion is supratentorial or infratentorial, and, second, whether the lesion is causing its symptoms by compression or destruction or both. Those considerations were the focus of Chapter 3. This chapter discusses, in turn, the specific causes of supratentorial and infratentorial compressive and destructive lesions that cause

coma. Meanwhile, Chapters 7 and 8 will provide detailed discussion of the treatment of many of these conditions. For that reason, we will give only brief descriptions of the approach to treatment in this chapter, and we refer the reader to those later chapters for details.

Although the designations of supratentorial and infratentorial lesions as either compressive or destructive are useful for rapid bedside diagnosis, it is of course possible for a lesion such as an intracerebral hemorrhage both to destroy and to compress normal tissues both above and below the tentorium. Extracerebral mass lesions can also cause sufficient compression to lead to infarction (i.e., tissue destruction). Thus, in some instances, the division is arbitrary. However, the types of conditions that cause the compression versus destruction of neural tissue tend to be distinct, and often they

Table 4.1 **Examples of Structural Causes of Coma**

Compressive lesions	Destructive lesions
Cerebral hemispheres	*Cerebral hemispheres*
Epidural and subdural hematomas, tumors, and abscesses	Hypoxia-ischemia
Subarachnoid hemorrhages, infections (meningitis), and tumors (leptomeningeal neoplasms)[a]	Hypoglycemia
Intracerebral hemorrhages, infarcts, tumors, and abscesses	Vasculitis
	Encephalitis
	Leukoencephalopathy
	Prion diseases
	Progressive multifocal leukoencephalopathy
Diencephalon	*Diencephalon*
Basal ganglia hemorrhages, tumors, infarcts, and abscesses [a]	Thalamic infarct
Pituitary tumor	Encephalitis
Pineal tumor	Fatal familial insomnia
	Paraneoplastic syndrome Tumor
Brainstem	*Brainstem*
Cerebellar tumor	Infarct
Cerebellar hemorrhage	Hemorrhage
Cerebellar abscess	Infection

[a] Both compressive and destructive.

have distinct clinical presentations as well. The guide provided in this chapter, while not exhaustive, is meant to cover the most commonly encountered causes and ones where understanding their pathophysiology can influence diagnosis and treatment (Table 4.1).

When any structural process impairs consciousness, the physician must find a way to halt the progression promptly or the patient will run the risk of irreversible brain damage or death. Beyond that generality, different structural lesions have distinct clinical properties that govern the rate of progression, hint at the diagnosis, and may dictate the treatment.

Structural causes of unconsciousness often result in focal signs that help localize the lesion, particularly when the lesion develops acutely. However, if the lesion has developed slowly over a period of many weeks or even months, it may attain a remarkably large size without causing focal neurologic signs. In those cases, the first evidence of a space-occupying lesion may be signs of increased intracranial pressure (ICP) (e.g., headache, nausea) or even herniation itself (see Patient Vignette 3.2).

SUPRATENTORIAL COMPRESSIVE LESIONS

The supratentorial compartments are dominated by the cerebral hemispheres. However, many of the most dangerous and difficult lesions to diagnose involve the overlying meninges. Within the hemisphere, a compressive lesion may originate in the gray matter or the white matter of the hemisphere, and it may directly compress the diencephalon from above or laterally (central herniation) or compress the midbrain by herniation of the temporal lobe through the tentorial notch (uncal herniation). In addition, there are a number of compressive lesions that affect mainly the diencephalon.

EPIDURAL, DURAL, AND SUBDURAL MASSES

Tumors, infections, and hematomas occupying the epidural, dural, and subdural spaces can cause compression of the underlying brain, and eventual herniation. Most epidural tumors result from extensions of skull lesions that grow into the epidural space. Dural tumors, by contrast, are usually primary tumors of the meninges, or occasionally metastases. The growth of both epidural and dural tumors is relatively slow; they mostly commonly cause focal signs and are discovered long before they affect consciousness. Epidural or subdural hematomas, on the other hand, may develop acutely or subacutely and can be a diagnostic problem.

Epidural Hematoma

Because the external leaf of the dura mater forms the periosteum of the inner table of the skull, the space between the dura and the skull is a potential space that accumulates blood only when there has been an injury to the skull itself. Epidural hematomas commonly result from a skull fracture that crosses the groove in the bone containing the middle meningeal artery (see Figure 4.1). Arterial bleeding is usually under high pressure, with the result that the vessel may not seal and blood continues to accumulate. Thus, instead of causing symptoms that develop slowly or wax and wane over days or weeks, a patient with an epidural hematoma may pass from having only a headache to impairment of consciousness and signs of herniation within a few hours after the initial trauma.

If the ruptured epidural vessel is a vein, the bleeding may develop more slowly and be self-limited, having a course more similar to subdural hematomas, which are discussed later. On rare occasions, epidural hematomas may result from bleeding into skull lesions, as from eosinophilic granuloma,[1] metastatic skull or dural tumors particularly from hepatocellular carcinoma,[2] or craniofacial infections such as sinusitis.[3]

Although epidural hematomas can occur frontally, occipitally, at the vertex,[4] or even on the side opposite the side of trauma (contrecoup),[5] the most common site is in the lateral temporal area as a result of laceration of the middle meningeal artery. Trauma sufficient to cause such a fracture may also fracture the skull base. For this reason, it is necessary for the examiner to be alert to signs of basal skull fracture on examination, such as blood behind the tympanic membrane or ecchymosis of the skin behind the ear (Battle's sign) or around the

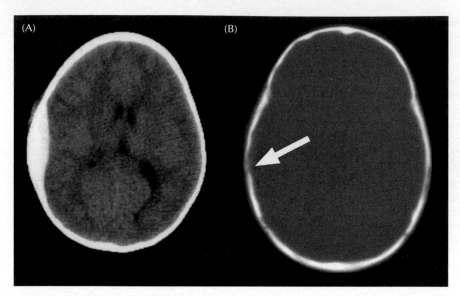

Figure 4.1 A pair of computed tomography scans showing an epidural hematoma. The image in (A) shows the lens shaped (biconvex), bright mass along the inner surface of the skull. In (B), the skull is imaged with bone windows, showing a fracture at the white arrow, crossing the middle meningeal groove.
Images courtesy of Dr. Jonathan Kleefield.

eyes (raccoon eyes). The epidural hemorrhage pushes the brain medially, and, in so doing stretches and tears pain-sensitive meninges and blood vessels at the base of the middle fossa, causing headache. However, the headache is often attributed to the original head injury, and unless the lesion causes sufficiently increased ICP to produce nausea and vomiting, the condition may not be recognized. Subsequently, the hematoma compresses the adjacent temporal lobe and causes uncal herniation with gradual impairment of consciousness. Early dilation of the ipsilateral pupil is often seen followed by complete ophthalmoparesis and then impairment of the opposite third nerve as the herniation progresses.[6] Motor signs often occur late in such cases.

In many patients, the degree of head trauma is less than one might expect to cause a fracture. Even in the pre-computed tomography (CT) era, several large series found that half or more of patients had mild symptoms without loss of consciousness initially.[7,8] In the modern imaging era, when CT scans are done for even mild degrees of concussion, most epidural hematomas are picked up on imaging with minimal symptoms, and only about 30% eventually require surgical intervention.[9] This is particularly true in children, one-half of whom

have suffered a fall of less than one-half meter, and many of whom complained of nonspecific symptoms.[10] Only 15–20% of patients have the "classic" history of traumatic loss of consciousness, followed by a lucid interval, and then a relapse into coma (patients who "talk and die").[11] Thus, even though most epidural hematomas are identified by CT scans performed acutely in emergency departments on trauma patients by using current evidence-based decision paradigms,[12,13] the examiner must remain alert to the possibility of an epidural hematoma that develops or rapidly enlarges after an apparently negative CT. It is therefore important to review the CT scan of trauma patients with attention directed to whether there is a skull fracture that crosses the middle meningeal groove. The hematoma appears as a hyperdense, lens-shaped mass between the skull and the brain (i.e., the hematoma is convex on both surfaces; subdural hematomas, by comparison, are concave on the surface facing the brain; see Figure 4.1). A vertex hematoma may be missed on a routine axial CT scan, but a coronal reconstruction should identify the lesion.[4] A magnetic resonance imaging (MRI) scan is not required for evaluation of an epidural hematoma, but it may be necessary to evaluate contusions and edema in the underlying brain. In addition, mass lesions outside the brain may cause hyperdensity of subarachnoid cisterns that may be mistaken for subarachnoid hemorrhage on CT but that is probably an artifact of partial volume averaging.[14] In these instances, MRI helps rule out subarachnoid hemorrhage.

In those circumstances where an immediate CT scan is not readily available, a plain skull film can often identify the fracture. Certainly, all patients with head trauma should be cautioned that it is important to remain under the supervision of a family member or friend who must awaken them periodically for the next 24 hours; the patient must be returned to the hospital immediately if he or she cannot be awakened. Careful follow-up is required even in patients in whom the original CT was negative, as occasionally the development of the hematoma is delayed.[15]

If an epidural hematoma causes sufficient brain displacement to cause impairment of consciousness, the treatment is surgical evacuation (see Chapter 8). The surgery is an emergency, as the duration from time of injury to treatment is an important determinant of the prognosis.[16] Other factors in determining outcome are age, depth of coma, degree of midline shift, and size of the hematoma. Most patients operated on promptly recover, even including about one-third of those with one pupil that is dilated and fixed before surgery.[16]

Subdural Hematoma

The unique anatomy of the subdural space also can produce much slower, chronic subdural hematomas in patients in whom the history of head trauma is remote or trivial. The potential space between the inner leaf of the dura mater and the arachnoid membrane (subdural space) is traversed by numerous small draining veins that bring venous blood from the brain to the dural sinus system that runs between the two leaves of the dura. These veins can be damaged with minimal head trauma, particularly in elderly individuals with cerebral atrophy in whom the veins are subject to considerable movement of the hemisphere that may occur with acceleration-deceleration injury. When focal signs are absent, these cases can be quite difficult to diagnose. A useful rule when faced with a comatose patient is that "it could always be a subdural," and hence imaging is needed even in cases where focal signs are absent.

Subdural bleeding is usually under low pressure, and it typically tamponades early unless there is a defect in coagulation. Acute subdural bleeding is particularly dangerous in patients who take anticoagulants for vascular thrombotic disease. Continued venous leakage over several hours can cause a mass large enough to produce herniation. Patients who are being treated with oral anticoagulants are especially high risk for continued venous leakage, and the anticoagulation should be reversed promptly. See Chapter 8, page 329 for discussion of this issue.

Acute subdural hematomas, which are usually the result of a severe head injury, are often associated with underlying cerebral contusions. Rarely, acute subdural hematomas may occur without substantial trauma, particularly in patients on anticoagulants. Rupture of an aneurysm into the subdural space, sparing the subarachnoid space, can also cause an acute subdural hematoma. The mass accumulates rapidly, causing underlying brain edema and herniation. Ischemic brain edema results when herniation compresses the anterior or posterior cerebral arteries and causes ischemic brain damage.[17] Patients with acute subdural hematomas usually present with coma, and such cases are surgical emergencies. Early evacuation of the mass probably improves outcome, but because of underlying brain damage, mortality remains significant. Prognostic factors include age, time from injury to treatment, presence of pupillary abnormalities, and immediate and persisting coma as opposed to the presence of a lucid interval or volume of the mass.[18]

Chronic subdural hematomas usually occur in elderly patients or those on anticoagulants. Chronic alcoholism, hemodialysis, and intracranial hypotension are also risk factors. A history of trauma can be elicited in only about one-half of patients, and then the trauma is usually minor. The pathogenesis of chronic subdural hematomas is controversial. One hypothesis is that minor trauma to an atrophic brain causes a small amount of bleeding. A membrane forms around the hematoma. Vessels of the membrane are quite friable and this, plus an increase of fibrinolytic products in the fluid, leads to repetitive bleeding, causing an enlarging hematoma.[19] Another hypothesis is that minor trauma leads to the accumulation of either serum or cerebrospinal fluid (CSF) in the subdural space. This subdural hygroma also causes membrane formation that leads to repetitive bleeding and an eventual mass lesion.[20] If the hemorrhage is small and no additional bleeding occurs, the hematoma may resorb spontaneously. However, if the hematoma is larger or it is enlarged gradually by recurrent bleeds, it may swell as the breakdown of the blood into small molecules causes the hematoma to take on additional water, thus further compressing the adjacent brain.[20] In addition, the membrane surrounding the hematoma contains luxuriant neovascularization that lacks a blood–brain barrier and may cause additional edema in the underlying brain. Chronic subdural hematomas are usually unilateral, overlying the lateral cerebral cortex, but may be subtemporal. They are bilateral in about 20% of patients, and occasionally are interhemispheric (i.e., within the falx cerebri), sometimes causing bilateral leg weakness by compression of the medial frontal lobes.

Table 4.2 lists the clinical features of the typical patient with a chronic subdural hematoma who presents with a fluctuating level of consciousness.

Table 4.2 Diagnostic Features of 73 Patients with Fluctuating Level of Consciousness due to Subdural Hematoma

Unilateral hematoma	62
Bilateral hematomas	11
Mortality	14
	(3 unoperated)
Number of patients in stupor or coma	27
Principal clinical diagnosis before hematoma discovered	
Intracranial mass lesion or subdural hematoma	24
Cerebral vascular disease, but subdural hematoma possible	17
Cerebral infarction or arteriosclerosis	12
Cerebral atrophy	5
Encephalitis	8
Meningitis	3
Metabolic encephalopathy secondary to systemic illness	3
Psychosis	1

A majority of patients, but no more than 70%, complain of headache. A fluctuating level of consciousness is common.[19,21] There may be tenderness to percussion of the skull at the site of the hematoma. About 15–30% of patients present with parenchymal signs such as seizures, hemiparesis, or visual field defects. Unusual focal signs such as parkinsonism, dystonia, or chorea occasionally confuse the clinical picture.[22] Focal signs such as hemiparesis or aphasia may fluctuate, giving an appearance similar to transient ischemic attacks.[23] Occasionally, patients may have unilateral asterixis. Because a subdural hematoma can appear identical to a metabolic encephalopathy (Chapter 5), imaging is required in any patient without an obvious cause of the impairment of consciousness.

The symptoms of subdural hematoma have a remarkable tendency to fluctuate from day to day or even from hour to hour, which may suggest the diagnosis. The pathophysiology of fluctuations is not clear. Some may reflect increases in ICP associated with plateau waves,[24] and careful clinical observations suggest that the level of consciousness reflects the patient moving in and out of diencephalic or uncal herniation. Given the breakdown in the blood–brain barrier along the margin of the hematoma, this fluctuation may be due to fluid shifts into and out of the brain, a situation from which the brain is normally protected. When the brain is critically balanced on the edge of herniation, such fluid shifts may rapidly make the difference between full consciousness and an obtunded state. Cerebral blood flow in the hemisphere underlying a subdural hematoma is reduced, perhaps accounting for some of the unusual clinical symptoms.[25]

In favor of the vasogenic edema hypothesis is the observation that oral administration of corticosteroids rapidly and effectively reverses the symptoms in subdural hematoma.[26] Corticosteroids reduce the leakage of fluid from capillaries,[27] and they are quite effective in minimizing the cerebral edema associated with subdural hematomas.

Subdural hematoma can usually be diagnosed by CT scanning. Depending on the age of the bleeding, the contents of the mass between the dura and the brain may be either hyperdense or isodense (Figure 4.2). Acute subdural hematomas are generally hyperdense, with the rare exception of those occurring in

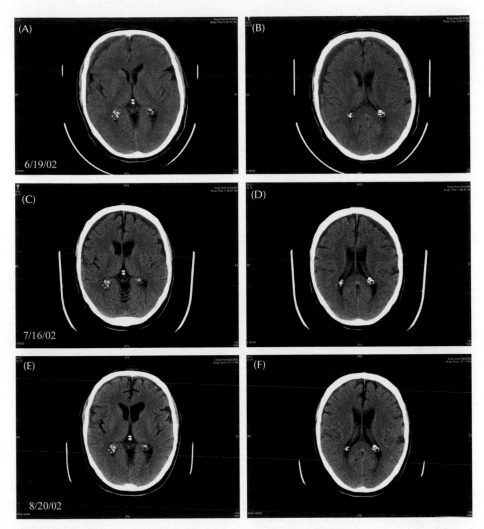

Figure 4.2 A series of magnetic resonance imaging scans through the brain of Patient 4.1 demonstrating bilateral subdural hematomas and their evolution over time. In the initial scan from 6/19/02 (A, B), there is an isodense subdural hematoma of 11.5 mm thickness on the right (left side of image) and 8 mm thickness on the left. The patient was treated conservatively with oral prednisone, and by the time of the second scan 1 month later (C, D), the subdural hematomas were smaller and hypodense and the underlying brain was less edematous. By the end of the second month (E, F), the subdural hematomas had been almost completely resorbed.

extremely anemic patients and occasionally in a hyperacute patient, when CSF may enter the subdural space, diluting the blood. In the latter case, the hematoma may even be isodense in the hyperacute period, immediately after it occurs. More often, though, the hematoma may become isodense with brain after 2–3 weeks as the blood products begin to break down. If the mass does not still contain areas of hyperdense fresh blood, and contrast is not given, the subdural hematoma may be difficult to distinguish from brain tissue, particularly if

the hematomas are bilaterally symmetric and do not cause the brain to shift. The lack of definable sulci in the area of the hematoma and a "supraphysiologic"-appearing brain in an elderly individual (i.e., a brain that lacks atrophy and deep sulci, usually seen with aging) are clues to the presence of bilateral isodense subdural hematomas. Chronic subdurals typically become hypodense. A CT scan with contrast clearly defines the hematoma as the membranes—with a luxuriant, leaky vascular supply—enhance profusely. MRI scanning can also define the hematoma, but the density is a complex function of the sequence used and age of the hemorrhage.

Lumbar puncture is potentially dangerous in a patient with a subdural hematoma. If the brain is balanced on the edge of herniation, the sudden relief of subarachnoid pressure from below may further enhance the pressure cone and lead to frank herniation. In such patients, the CSF pressure may be low due to the blockage at the foramen magnum, leading to a false sense of security. Hence, all patients who have an impaired level of consciousness require an imaging study of the brain prior to lumbar puncture, even if meningitis is a consideration.[28]

The treatment of subdural hematomas causing neurological impairment is covered in Chapter 8. However, many patients seen in the ED or office setting after mild head trauma have modest-sized subdural hematomas with minimal symptoms (typically only a headache) and considerable ventricular and cisternal space, so there is no danger of herniation. We have treated some of these patients with steroids only to resolve their headache, and followed with CT as the subdural hematoma was resorbed (see Patient Vignette 4.1). Several recent meta-analyses that have examined the effect of treating a chronic subdural hematoma with corticosteroids alone have found no evidence for surgery being superior to treatment with corticosteroids, although in the absence of a large randomized clinical trial, the evidence is weak.[29,30] An ongoing randomized trial (the SUCRE study) may provide a more definitive answer.[31,32]

Patient Vignette 4.1

A 73-year-old professor of art history developed chronic bifrontal, dull headache. He had no history of head trauma, but was taking 81 mg of aspirin daily for cardiovascular prophylaxis. He felt mentally dulled, but his neurologic examination was normal. Computed tomography (CT) scan of the brain disclosed bilateral chronic (low-density) subdural hematomas of 8 mm depth on the left and 11.5 mm on the right. He was started on 20 mg/day of prednisone with immediate resolution of the headaches, and, over a period of 2 months,

serial CT scans showed that the hematoma resolved spontaneously (see Figure 4.2). Repeat scan 3 months later showed no recurrence.

Epidural Abscess/Empyema

In developing countries, epidural infections are a feared complication of mastoid or sinus infection.[33] In developed countries, neurosurgical procedures,[34] particularly second or third craniotomies in the same area, and trauma are more likely causes.[35] Sinusitis and otitis, if inadequately treated, may extend into the epidural space, either along the base of the temporal lobe or along the surface of the frontal lobe. The causative organisms are usually aerobic and anaerobic streptococci if the lesion originates from the ear or the sinuses and *Staphylococcus aureus* if from trauma or surgery. The patient typically has local pain and fever. Vomiting is common; focal skull tenderness and meningismus suggest infection rather than hemorrhage.[33] The pathophysiology of impairment of consciousness is similar to that of an epidural hematoma, except that epidural empyema typically has a much slower course and is not associated with acute trauma. CT scan is characterized by a crescentic or lentiform mass between the skull and the brain with an enhanced rim. Diffusion is restricted on diffusion-weighted MRI, distinguishing it from hematomas or effusions where diffusion is normal or increased.[36,37] Antibiotics and surgical drainage are effective treatments.[34] If the patient has not been treated previously with partially effective antibiotics, the causal organisms can usually be cultured to allow appropriate selection of antibiotics. Some children whose epidural abscess originates from the sinuses can be treated conservatively with antibiotics and drainage of the sinus rather than the epidural mass.[38]

Dural and Subdural Tumors

A number of tumors and other mass lesions may invade the dura and compress the brain. These lesions include dural metastases,[39] primary tumors such as hemangiopericytoma, hematopoietic neoplasms (plasmacytoma, leukemia, lymphoma), and inflammatory diseases such as sarcoidosis.[40] These are often mistaken for the most common dural tumor, meningioma.[41]

Meningiomas can occur anywhere along the dural lining of the anterior and middle cranial fossas. The most common locations are over the convexities, along the falx, or along the base of the skull at the sphenoid wing or olfactory tubercle. The tumors typically present by compression of local structures. In some cases, this produces seizures, but a meningioma over the convexity may cause hemiparesis. Falcine meningiomas may present with hemiparesis and upper motor neuron signs in the contralateral lower extremity; the "textbook presentation" of paraparesis is quite rare. If the tumor occurs near the frontal pole, it may compress the medial prefrontal cortex, causing lapses in judgment, inconsistent behavior, and, in some cases, an apathetic, abulic state. Meningioma underlying the orbitofrontal cortex may similarly compress both frontal lobes and present with behavioral and cognitive dysfunction. When the tumor arises from the olfactory tubercle, ipsilateral loss of smell is a clue to the nature of the problem. Meningiomas of the sphenoid wing may invade the cavernous sinus and cause impairment of the oculomotor (III), trochlear (IV), and abducens nerves (VI) as well as the first division of the trigeminal nerve (V_1).

On rare occasions, a meningioma may first present symptoms of increased ICP or even impaired level of consciousness. Acute presentation with impairment of consciousness may also occur with hemorrhage into a meningioma. Fortunately, this condition is rare, involving only 1–2% of meningiomas, and may suggest a more malignant phenotype.[42] In such cases, the tumor typically has reached sufficient size to cause diencephalic compression or herniation. There is often considerable edema of the adjacent brain, which may be due in part to the leakage of blood vessels in the tumor or to production by the tumor of angiogenic factors.[43] Treatment with corticosteroids reduces the edema and may be life-saving while awaiting a definitive surgical procedure.

On CT scanning, meningiomas are typically isodense with brain, although they may have areas of calcification. On MRI scan, a typical meningioma is hypointense or isointense on T1-weighted MRI and usually hypointense on T2. In either imaging modality, the tumor often contains areas of calcification, and it uniformly and intensely enhances with contrast. The CT scan may also help in identifying bone erosion or hyperostosis, the latter being rather characteristic of meningiomas. Meningiomas typically have an enhancing dural tail that spreads from the body of the tumor along the dura, a finding less common in other dural tumors. The dural tail is not tumor, but a hypervascular response of the dura to the tumor.[44]

Dural malignant metastases and hematopoietic tumors grow more rapidly than meningiomas and cause more underlying brain edema. Thus, they are more likely to cause alterations of consciousness and, if not detected and treated early enough, cerebral herniation. Breast and prostate cancer and M4-type acute myelomonocytic leukemia have a particular predilection for the dura, which may be the only site of metastasis in an otherwise successfully treated patient.[40] CT and MRI scans may be similar to those of meningioma, the diagnosis being established only by surgery.

PITUITARY TUMORS

Tumors of the pituitary fossa are outside the brain and its coverings and typically are separated from the subarachnoid space by the diaphragma sellae, a portion of the dura that covers the pituitary fossa but that contains an opening for the pituitary stalk. Pituitary tumors that are confined to the sella turcica may precipitate alterations of consciousness by causing endocrine failure (see Chapter 5). If the tumor extends beyond the confines of the cavernous sinus, it may impair consciousness by compressing the overlying hypothalamus, especially if there is acute hemorrhage into the pituitary tumor, so-called *pituitary apoplexy*.

Pituitary adenomas that extend outside of the pituitary fossa may compress the overlying optic chiasm, causing bitemporal hemianopsia. If the tumor extends laterally through the wall of the sella turcica into the cavernous sinus, there may be impairment of cranial nerves III, IV, VI, or V_1. In some cases, pituitary tumors may achieve a very large size by suprasellar extension. These tumors compress the overlying hypothalamus and basal forebrain and may extend up between the frontal lobes or backward down the clivus. Such tumors may present primarily with prefrontal signs, or signs of increased ICP, but they occasionally present with impairment of consciousness.

The most common endocrine presentation in women is amenorrhea, often with galactorrhea due to high prolactin secretion. Prolactin is the only pituitary hormone under inhibitory control; if a pituitary tumor damages the pituitary stalk, other pituitary hormones fall to basal levels, but prolactin levels rise. Most pituitary adenomas are nonsecreting tumors, but some pituitary tumors may secrete anterior pituitary hormones, resulting in Cushing's syndrome (if the tumor secretes adrenocorticotropic hormone), hyperthyroidism (if it secretes thyroid-stimulating hormone), galactorrhea/amenorrhea (if it secretes prolactin), or acromegaly (if it secretes growth hormone).

Pituitary adenomas may outgrow their blood supply and undergo spontaneous infarction or hemorrhage. Pituitary apoplexy presents with the sudden onset of severe headache, signs of local compression of the optic chiasm and sometimes the nerves of the cavernous sinus.[45,46] There may be subarachnoid blood, and there often is impairment of consciousness. It is not clear if the depressed level of consciousness is due to the compression of the overlying hypothalamus, the release of subarachnoid blood (see later discussion), or the increase in ICP. If there are cranial nerve signs, pituitary apoplexy is often sufficiently characteristic to be diagnosed clinically, but if the main symptoms are due to subarachnoid hemorrhage, it may be confused with meningitis or meningoencephalitis[47]; the correct diagnosis is easily confirmed by MRI or CT scan (Figure 4.3). Treatment is a surgical emergency, and patients often require endocrine replacement therapy post-operatively.

Craniopharyngiomas are epithelial neoplasms that are thought to arise from a remnant of Rathke's pouch, the embryologic origin of the anterior pituitary gland.[48] The typical presentation is similar to that of a pituitary tumor, but craniopharyngiomas are often cystic and may rupture, releasing thick fluid into the subarachnoid space that may cause a chemical meningitis (see later discussion). Craniopharyngiomas are more common in childhood, but there is a second peak in the seventh decade of life.[49]

PINEAL TUMORS

The pineal gland is technically outside the brain, sitting in the subdural space overlying the pretectal area and rostral midbrain. Tumors of the pineal gland commonly compress the dorsal surface of the midbrain, causing Parinaud's dorsal midbrain syndrome (loss of upward gaze

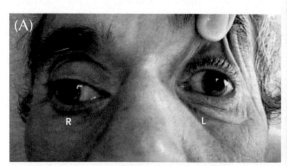
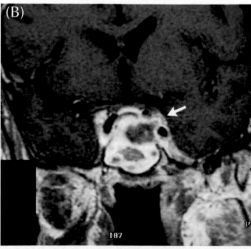

Figure 4.3 Images from a patient with pituitary apoplexy. This 63-year-old man had a severe headache with sudden onset of left III and IV nerve palsies. In A, the examiner is holding the left eye open because of ptosis, and the patient is trying to look to his right. A magnetic resonance imaging scan, B, shows a hemorrhage (bright white on T1 imaging) into a large pituitary tumor that is invading the left cavernous sinus (arrow). The tumor abuts the optic chiasm. In pituitary apoplexy, there may be sudden visual loss in either or both eyes if the optic nerves are compressed, or in a bitemporal pattern if the chiasm is compressed, as well as impairment of some combination of cranial nerves III, IV, VI, and V_1.
From Glass LC. Pituitary apoplexy. *N Engl J Med* 2003;349:20–34, with permission.

and convergence, large poorly reactive pupils, and retractory nystagmus), which points to the diagnosis. The tumor may also compress the cerebral aqueduct, causing hydrocephalus; typically, this only alters consciousness when increased ICP from hydrocephalus causes plateau waves (see page 98) or if there is sudden hemorrhage into the pineal tumor (pineal apoplexy).[50] In cases of pineal apoplexy, quite often the main symptoms at presentation is headache and depressed level of consciousness, raising suspicion for subarachnoid hemorrhage. CT or MRI will demonstrate both the tumor and the hydrocephalus and can detect hemorrhage into the tumor.

SUBARACHNOID LESIONS

Like epidural, dural, and subdural lesions, subarachnoid lesions are outside of the brain itself. Unlike epidural or dural lesions, alterations of consciousness resulting from subarachnoid lesions are not usually the result of a mass effect, but occur when hemorrhage, tumor, or infection either compress, infiltrate, or cause inflammation of blood vessels in the subarachnoid space that supply the brain, or alter CSF absorptive pathways, thus causing hydrocephalus. Thus, strictly speaking, in some cases the damage done by these lesions may be more "metabolic" than structural. On the other hand, subarachnoid hemorrhage and bacterial meningitis are among the most deadly emergencies encountered in evaluating comatose patients, and, for that reason, this class of disorders is considered here.

Subarachnoid Hemorrhage

Subarachnoid hemorrhage, in which there is little if any intraparenchymal component, is usually due to rupture of a saccular aneurysm, although it can also occur when a superficial arteriovenous malformation ruptures. Saccular aneurysms occur throughout life, generally at branch points of large cerebral arteries, such as the origin of the anterior communicating artery from the anterior cerebral artery; the origin of the posterior communicating artery from the posterior cerebral artery; the origin of the posterior cerebral artery from the basilar artery; or

the origin of the middle cerebral artery from the internal carotid artery. Microscopic examination discloses an incomplete elastic media, which results in an aneurysmal dilatation that may enlarge with time. Aneurysms are found with increasing frequency with age.

Aneurysms are typically silent until they hemorrhage. About 25% of ruptures are presaged by a severe headache, a so-called *sentinel headache*,[51,52] presumably resulting from sudden dilation or leakage of blood from the aneurysm. Giant aneurysms of the internal carotid artery sometimes occur in the region of the cavernous sinus, and these may present as a mass lesion causing impairment of the cranial nerves of the cavernous sinus (III, IV, VI, and V_1) or by compressing the frontal lobes. Occasionally an aneurysm of the posterior communicating artery compresses the adjacent third nerve causing ipsilateral pupillary dilation. For this reason, new onset of anisocoria even in an awake patient is considered a medical emergency until the possibility of a posterior communicating artery aneurysm is eliminated. Rarely, giant aneurysms present with embolic strokes downstream from the aneurysm caused by clot formation within the aneurysm.

Unfortunately, most aneurysms are not apparent until they bleed. The classic presentation of a subarachnoid hemorrhage is the sudden onset of the worst headache of the patient's life. However, many other types of headaches may present in this way (e.g., "thunderclap headache"),[53] so it is often necessary to rule out subarachnoid hemorrhage in the emergency department. Misdiagnosis of headache from aneurysmal bleeding may be fatal and even among survivors impacts long-term outcomes.[54] If the hemorrhage is sufficiently large, the sudden pressure wave, as ICP approximates arterial pressure, may result in impaired cerebral blood flow and loss of consciousness. About 20% of patients with subarachnoid hemorrhage die before reaching medical care.[55] At the other end of the spectrum, if the leak is small or seals rapidly, there may be little in the way of neurologic signs. The most salient finding in subarachnoid hemorrhage often is impairment of consciousness. The symptoms may vary from mild dullness to confusion to stupor or coma. The cause of continued behavioral impairment hours to days after subarachnoid hemorrhage, particularly if the initial increase in ICP is alleviated

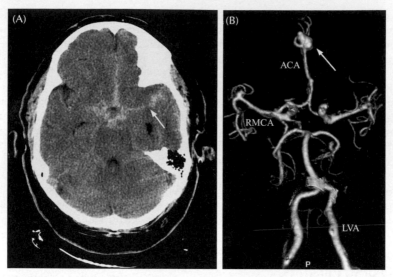

Figure 4.4 A 66-year-old man was brought to the emergency department after sudden onset of a severe global headache with nausea and vomiting. His legs collapsed under him. Computed tomography (CT) scan (A) showed blood in the cisterns surrounding the circle of Willis at the base of the brain, with blood extending into the interhemispheric fissure at the midline, and the right Sylvian fissure (arrow). A CT angiogram (B) showed that the anterior cerebral arteries were fused from the anterior communicating artery up to a bifurcation point, at which a large saccular aneurysm was noted (arrow). ACA, anterior cerebral artery; LVA, left vertebral artery; RMCA, right middle cerebral artery.

(see Chapter 7, p. 317) is not well understood. It is believed that the blood excites an inflammatory response with cytokine expression that may diffusely impair brain metabolism as well as cause brain edema. Microglial cells in the extravascular space may also be activated, which may contribute to vasospasm and reduced cerebral blood flow.[56] However, the encephalopathy often appears to be global and lacks focal signs unless a jet of blood from the ruptured aneurysm has damaged the brain or there is sufficient vasospasm to cause cerebral infarction.

Patient Vignette 4.2

An 18-year-old woman was brought to the emergency department by her sister because she had been confused and forgetful for 2 days. She did not offer a history of headache, but upon being asked, the patient did admit that she had one. On examination the neck was stiff, but the neurologic examination showed only lethargy and inattention. A computed tomography (CT) scan disclosed a subarachnoid hemorrhage, with blood collection around the circle of Willis on

the right side. Lumbar puncture yielded bloody fluid, with 23,000 red blood cells and 500 white blood cells. Cultures were negative. A cerebral angiogram demonstrated a saccular aneurysm at the junction of the internal carotid and middle cerebral arteries on the right.

CT scans are highly sensitive to subarachnoid blood, making the diagnosis in more than 99% of cases if done within 6 hours in patients who are asymptomatic other than headache,[57] but the accuracy drops to 95% if done within 12 hours of onset (Figure 4.4),[58] and MRI fluid-attenuated inversion recovery (FLAIR) sequences are of similar sensitivity.[57] Hence, in most cases (more than 6 hours delay after onset of headache, or presence of any other symptoms), even if CT is negative, a lumbar puncture is mandatory.[59,60] As lumbar puncture itself may introduce blood into the CSF, the analysis of blood in the CSF is of great importance. Signs that suggest that the blood was present before the tap include the persistence of the same number of red cells in tubes 1 and 4, or the presence of crenated red blood cells and/or xanthochromia if the hemorrhage is at least several hours old. Spectrophotometry of CSF for bilirubin may increase accuracy.[61,62] Another alternative is to centrifuge the CSF and test the supernate with a urine dipstick for blood. If the bleeding preceded the tap by at least 6 hours, it is likely that there will be blood breakdown products in the CSF, which can be visualized on the dipstick.

Treatment of subarachnoid hemorrhage is covered in Chapter 8.

Subarachnoid Tumors

Both benign and malignant tumors may invade the subarachnoid space, infiltrating the leptomeninges either diffusely or focally and sometimes invading roots or growing along the Virchow-Robin spaces to invade the brain. Leptomeningeal tumors include lymphomas and leukemias and solid tumors such as breast, renal cell, and lung cancers, as well as medulloblastomas and glial tumors.[63–65] The hallmark of meningeal neoplasms is multilevel dysfunction of the nervous system, including signs of damage to cranial or spinal nerves, spinal cord, brainstem, or cerebral hemispheres. Many patients with meningeal carcinoma have impairment of consciousness that is difficult to explain on the basis of the distribution of the tumor cells. The cause of

the depressed level of consciousness in these patients is not clear. Explanations have included hydrocephalus from obstruction of spinal fluid pathways,[66] invasion of the brain along the Virchow-Robin spaces accompanying penetrating pial vessels (the so-called encephalitic form of metastatic carcinoma),[67] nonconvulsive status epilepticus,[68] vasculitis causing cortical ischemia,[69,70] or an immunologic response to the tumor with production of cytokines and prostaglandins[71]; most patients also have some white blood cells in their CSF as well as tumor cells.

The diagnosis of subarachnoid tumor is challenging, particularly when the multilevel dysfunctions of the nervous system are the first signs of the tumor. The MRI scan may show tumor implants in the leptomeninges or on the surface of the brain, or it may demonstrate thickening or contrast enhancement of cranial nerve or spinal roots (Figure 4.5). If the scan is negative, the diagnosis is established by the presence of tumor cells[72] or tumor markers[73,74] in the spinal fluid. However, the clinician must think of the diagnosis to perform these tests. Fortunately, there are nearly always other abnormalities in the CSF (lymphocytes, low glucose, elevated protein) that give a clue to the diagnosis. Wasserstrom and colleagues found that in patients with pathologically demonstrated meningeal carcinoma or lymphoma, only 40% of the first CSF samples contained malignant cells.[75] Thus demonstration

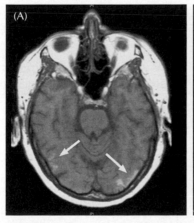 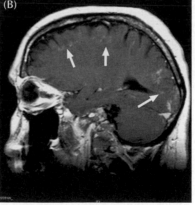

Figure 4.5 A pair of images from a magnetic resonance imaging (MRI) scan with contrast in a patient with meningeal lymphoma. This 52-year-old man presented with bilateral visual distortion and some left leg weakness. Both chronic lymphocytic leukemia and a non-Hodgkin's lymphoma had recently been diagnosed. The MRI scan showed superficial enhancement outlining the cortical sulci (arrows).

of the malignant cells may require repeated, large volume samples.

Although the diagnosis of meningeal cancer generally indicates a poor prognosis, there are occasional patients with leukemia, lymphoma, or breast cancer in whom vigorous treatment of the meningeal tumor may result in marked improvement or even complete remission. Treatment usually includes high-dose intravenous or intraventricular chemotherapy, as well as irradiation of areas of focal central nervous system (CNS) dysfunction (but not the entire neuraxis).[63,76]

Subarachnoid Infection

Subarachnoid infection (i.e., meningitis) is a common cause of impaired consciousness. Meningitis can be either acute or chronic and can be caused by a variety of different organisms including bacteria, fungi, rickettsiae, parasites, and viruses. Neurologic signs and symptoms caused by meningitis vary depending on the acuity of the infection and the nature of the infecting organisms, but certain aspects are common to all. For organisms to cause meningitis, they must first invade the meninges. This is usually done via the bloodstream, and for this reason blood cultures will often identify the organism. Less commonly, meningitis is a result of spread of organisms from structures adjacent to the brain (sinusitis, otitis). Meningitis can also occur in the absence of sepsis if there is communication between the meninges and the outside of the skull (CSF fistula, head injury, neurosurgery). Once in the meninges, organisms multiply, inducing the macrophage system that lines the meninges and superficial blood vessels in the brain to produce a variety of cytokines and other proinflammatory molecules that in turn attract other white cells to the meninges. The inflammatory reaction can disrupt the blood–brain barrier; obstruct spinal fluid absorptive pathways, causing hydrocephalus and cellular swelling; or cause a vasculitis of subarachnoid or penetrating cortical blood vessels with resulting cerebral ischemia or infarction. Inflammatory reactions also cause metabolic disturbances that lower the pH, promoting vasodilation and increasing cerebral blood volume, leading to increased ICP.[77] Thus, although the infection itself does not cause a supratentorial mass, the combination of vasogenic and cytotoxic edema caused by the inflammatory response may produce enough diffuse mass effect to cause herniation. Both transtentorial and tonsillar herniation may occur, although both are rare.

The major causes of community-acquired bacterial meningitis include *Streptococcus pneumoniae* (51%) and *Neisseria meningitis* (37%),[78] although this is modified by vaccination, which reduces the frequency of the serotypes included in the various vaccines.[79] *Neisseria* infections may occur in epidemics. It is typically spread by respiratory droplets in groups of susceptible individuals living at close quarters, as in university dormitories, military barracks, or prisons. In immunocompromised patients, *Listeria monocytogenes* meningitis accounts for about 4% of cases.[80] *Listeria* meningitis may be noticeably slower in its course but has a tendency to cause brainstem abscesses. *Staphylococcus aureus* and, since a vaccine became available, *Haemophilus influenzae* are uncommon causes of community-acquired meningitis.[78]

Acute bacterial meningitis is a medical emergency because untreated patients can die within hours of onset. Viral meningitis may clinically mimic bacterial meningitis, but most cases are self-limiting. The clinical signs of acute bacterial meningitis are headache, fever, stiff neck, photophobia, and an alteration of mental status. Focal neurologic signs can occur either from ischemia of underlying brain or from damage to cranial nerves as they pass through the subarachnoid space. In a series of adults with acute bacterial meningitis, 97%

Table 4.3 **Clinical Findings in 103 Patients with Acute Bacterial Meningitis**

Symptom	%
Fever	97 [a]
Nuchal rigidity	87
Headache	66
Nausea/vomiting	55
Confusion	56
Altered consciousness	51
Seizures	25
Focal signs	23
Papilledema	2

[a] Not all patients were examined for each finding.

Data from Hussein and Shafran.[81]

of patients had fever, 87% nuchal rigidity, and 84% headache.[81] Nausea or vomiting was present in 55%, confusion in 56%, and a decreased level of consciousness in 51%. Papilledema was identified in only 2% of patients, although it was not looked for in almost half. Seizure activity occurred in 25% of patients, but was always within 24 hours of the clinical diagnosis of acute meningitis. More than 40% of the patients had been partially treated before the diagnosis was established, so that in 30% of patients neither Gram stain nor cultures were positive. Eighteen percent of the patients died (Table 4.3).[82]

However, the classic triad of fever, nuchal rigidity, and alteration of mental status was present in only 44% of patients in a large series of community-acquired meningitis.[78] Focal neurologic signs were present in one-third and included cranial nerve palsies, aphasia, and hemiparesis; papilledema was found in only 3%.

Subacute or chronic meningitis runs an indolent course and may be accompanied by the same symptoms, but it also may occur in the absence of fever in debilitated or immune-suppressed patients. Both acute and chronic meningitis may be characterized only by lethargy, stupor, or coma in the absence of the other common signs. Chronic meningitis (e.g., with tuberculosis or cryptococcus) can also cause a local arteritis, resulting in cranial nerve dysfunction and focal areas of CNS infarction.[83] *Aspergillus* meningitis, which is typically seen only in patients who have been immune suppressed, causes a hemorrhagic arteritis, which may produce a combination of focal findings and impaired consciousness. However, the impairment of consciousness in each of these cases is primarily due to the immunologic processes concerned with the infection rather than structural causes (see Chapter 5).

The examination should include careful evaluation of nuchal rigidity even in patients who are stuporous. Attempting to flex the neck in a patient with meningitis may lead to grimacing and a rapid flexion of knees and hips (Brudzinski sign). Turning the head to the side, as in eliciting the doll's head eye signs, is not resisted. If one flexes the hip so the thigh forms a right angle with the axis of the trunk, the patient grimaces and resists

extension of the leg at the knee (Kernig sign). Pain with jolt accentuation (the patient is asked to turn the head to the side at two to three cycles per second) is a very sensitive sign of meningismus (positive in 97% of patients with meningitis) if the patient is sufficiently awake to cooperate, but is nonspecific (positive in 40% of patients with suspected meningitis, but no pleocytosis in the CSF).[84] Examination of the nose and ears for CSF discharge, and of the back for a CSF-to-skin sinus tract, may aid in the diagnosis. CSF can be distinguished from other clear fluid discharges at the bedside by its containing glucose. Measurement of beta-trace protein, a major component of CSF, in the discharge fluid is more accurate.[85]

Meningitis, particularly in children, can cause acute brain edema with transtentorial herniation as the initial sign. Clinically, such children rapidly lose consciousness and develop hyperpnea disproportionate to the degree of fever. The pupils dilate, at first moderately and then widely, then fix, and the child develops decerebrate motor signs. Urea, mannitol, or other hyperosmotic agents, if used properly, can prevent or reverse the full development of the ominous changes that are otherwise rapidly fatal.

In elderly patients, bacterial meningitis sometimes presents as insidiously developing stupor or coma in which there may be focal neurologic signs but little evidence of severe systemic illness or stiff neck. In one series, 50% of such patients with meningitis were admitted to the hospital with an incorrect diagnosis.[86] This error can be avoided by urgent spinal fluid examination in every patient who comes into the hospital with impaired consciousness without obvious cause.

If meningitis is suspected, the timing of a lumbar puncture (i.e., whether it should be performed before or after a CT scan) is controversial.[28,87] Some observers believe that the diagnostic value warrants the small but definite risk of an immediate lumbar puncture. Others argue that a CT scan cannot determine the safety of a lumbar puncture. Many patients with either supratentorial or infratentorial mass lesions tolerate lumbar puncture without complication; conversely, some patients with apparently normal CT may herniate. Most who want to perform CT first argue that when there

Table 4.4 **Typical Cerebrospinal Fluid (CSF) Findings in Bacterial versus Aseptic Meningitis**

CSF parameter	Bacterial meningitis	Aseptic meningitis
Opening pressure	>180 mm H_2O	Normal or slightly elevated
Glucose	<40 mg/dL	<45 mg/dL
CSF-to-serum glucose ratio	<0.31	>0.6
Protein	>50 mg/dL	Normal or elevated
White blood cells	>10 to <10,000/mm³—neutrophils predominate	50–2,000/mm³—lymphocytes predominate
Gram stain	Positive in 70–90% of untreated cases	Negative
Lactate	≥3.8 mmol/L	Normal
C-reactive protein	>100 ng/mL	Minimal
Limulus lysate assay	Positive indicates Gram-negative meningitis	Negative
Latex agglutination	Specific for antigens of *Streptococcus pneumoniae*, *Neisseria meningitidis* (not serogroup B), and Hib	Negative
Coagglutination	Same as above	Negative
Counterimmuno electrophoresis	Same as above	Negative

From Roos et al.,[88] with permission

is a strong suspicion of acute bacterial meningitis, one can begin antibiotics before the CT scan if the tap is done promptly after an emergent CT; Gram stain and cultures may still be positive. They further argue that the presence of a mass lesion suggests that the neurologic signs are not a result of meningitis alone and that lumbar puncture is probably unnecessary. Finally, even in the absence of a mass lesion, obliteration of the perimesencephalic cisterns or descent of the tonsils below the foramen magnum is a major risk factor for the development of herniation after a lumbar puncture. In such cases, lumbar puncture should be deferred until after hyperosmolar agents decrease the ICP (see Chapter 7, p. 317). Regardless of which approach is taken, blood cultures should be drawn immediately, followed by administration of appropriate antibiotics.

In acute bacterial meningitis, CSF pressure at lumbar puncture is usually elevated. A normal or low pressure raises the question of whether there has already been partial herniation of the cerebellar tonsils. The cell count and protein are elevated, and glucose may be depressed or normal. Examination of the spinal fluid helps one differentiate acute bacterial meningitis from acute aseptic

meningitis (Table 4.4). Testing for infectious agent antigens (e.g., cryptococcus, syphilis), antibodies (Borrelia, syphilis, various viruses) or DNA (by polymerase chain reaction, e.g., herpes simplex or zoster, tuberculosis) sometimes can provide a rapid diagnosis, but each of these has an appreciable false-negative rate. Hence, until there is a definitive cause, most patients are put on empiric broad-spectrum antibiotics. If definitive diagnosis continues to remain elusive, a repeat tap is indicated in a few days.

CT scans may show pus in the subarachnoid space as hypodense CSF with enlargement of sulci, but, in the absence of prior scans in the same patient, this is often difficult to interpret. Meningeal enhancement usually does not occur until several days after the onset of infection. Cortical infarction, which may be due to inflammation and occlusion either of penetrating arteries or cortical veins, also tends to occur late. The MRI scan is much more sensitive for showing the changes just indicated but may be entirely normal in patients with acute meningitis (Table 4.5).[89]

Initial treatment involves empiric antibiotics based on the most likely organisms. Adjuvant dexamethasone is recommended for children

Table 4.5 **Imaging Findings in Acute Meningitis**

Finding	CT [a]	MR [a]	Sensitivity
Sulcal dilation	Hypodense CSF; enlargement of sulci	T1WI: Hypointense CSF in sulci T2WI: Hyperintense CSF in sulci	MR>CT
Leptomeningeal enhancement	CE: Increase in density of subarachnoid space	T1WI, CE: Marked increase in signal intensity	MR>CT
Ischemic cortical infarction secondary to vasculitis	Hypodense cortical mass effect CE: Subacute increase in density (enhancement)	T1WI: Hypointense cortex; mass effect T2WI: Hyperintense cortex, mass effect FLAIR: Hyperintense cortex, mass effect CE: Subacute enhancement; hyperintense on T1WI DWI: Bright (white) ADC: Dark (black)	MR>CT
Subdural collections	Hypodense peripheral CSF plus density collection CE: Hygroma, no; empyema, yes	T1WI: Hypointense peripheral collection T2WI: Hyperintense peripheral collection FLAIR: hygroma, hypointense; empyema, variable CE: Hygroma, no; empyema, yes DWI: Hydroma, dark; empyema, bright ADC: Hygroma, bright; empyema, dark	MR>CT

ADC, apparent diffusion coefficient map; CE, contrast enhanced; CSF, cerebrospinal fluid; CT, computed tomography; DWI, diffusion-weighted imaging; FLAIR, fluid-attenuated inversion recovery; MR, magnetic resonance; T1WI, T1-weighted image; T2WI, T2-weighted image.

[a] Intensity relative to normal brain ±.

From Zimmerman et al.,[90] with permission.

and adults with *Haemophilus* meningitis or pneumococcal meningitis but is not currently recommended for the treatment of gram-negative meningitis. Nevertheless, if prompt antibiotic therapy is begun and the patient shows signs of increased ICP, it is probably wise to use dexamethasone.[91] Treatment will be covered in detail in Chapters 7 and 8.

INTRACEREBRAL MASSES

Intracerebral masses by nature tend to include both destructive and compressive elements.

However, in many cases, the damage from the mass effect far exceeds the damage from disruption of local neurons and white matter. Hence, we have included this class of lesions with compressive processes.

Intracerebral Hemorrhage

Intracerebral hemorrhage may result from a variety of pathologic processes that affect the blood vessels. These include rupture of deep cerebral end arteries, trauma, rupture of an arteriovenous malformation, rupture of

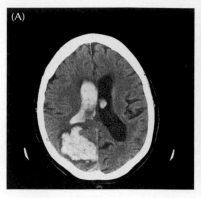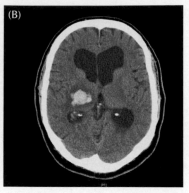

Figure 4.6 Computed tomography scans from two patients with intracerebral hemorrhages. (A) A large hemorrhage into the right parieto-occipital lobe in a 77-year-old woman who was previously healthy and presented with difficulty walking and a headache. Examination showed left-sided neglect. She took 325 mg aspirin at home on the advice of her primary care doctor because she suspected a stroke. The hematoma ruptured into the lateral ventricle. (B) A right thalamocapsular hemorrhage in a 60-year-old man with a history of hypertension who was not being treated at the time of the hemorrhage. He presented with headache, left-sided weakness and sensory loss, and some left-sided inattention.

a mycotic aneurysm, amyloid angiopathy, or hemorrhage into a tumor. Rupture of a saccular aneurysm can also cause an intraparenchymal hematoma, but the picture is generally dominated by the presence of subarachnoid blood. In contrast, despite their differing pathophysiology, the signs and symptoms of primary intracerebral hemorrhages are due to the compressive effects of the hematoma and thus are more alike than different, depending more on location than on the underlying pathologic process. Spontaneous supratentorial intracerebral hemorrhages are therefore usually classified as lobar or deep, with the latter sometimes extending intraventricularly.

Lobar hemorrhages can occur anywhere in the cerebral hemispheres and may involve one or multiple lobes (Figure 4.6A). As compared to deeper hemorrhages, patients with lobar hemorrhages are older, less likely to be male, and less likely to be hypertensive. Severe headache is a characteristic of lobar hemorrhages. Focal neurologic deficits occur in almost 90% of patients and vary somewhat depending on the site of the hemorrhage. About half the patients have a decreased level of consciousness, and 20% are in a coma when admitted.[92,93] Seizures are a common occurrence and may be nonconvulsive (see page 281), so that electroencephalographic (EEG) evaluation is valuable if there is impairment of consciousness.

Deep hemorrhages in the supratentorial region include those into the basal ganglia, internal capsule, and thalamus. Hemorrhages into the pons and cerebellum are discussed in the section on infratentorial hemorrhages. Chung and colleagues divided patients with striatocapsular hemorrhages into six groups with varying clinical findings and prognoses.[94] These included posterolateral (33%), affecting primarily the posterior portion of the putamen; massive (24%), involving the entire striatal capsular region but occasionally sparing the caudate nucleus and the anterior rim of the internal capsule; lateral (21%), located between the external capsule and insular cortex; anterior (11%), involving the caudate nucleus; middle (7%), involving the globus pallidus in the middle portion of the medial putamen; and posterior medial (4%), localized to the anterior half of the posterior rim of the internal capsule. Consciousness was only rarely impaired in anterior and posterior medial lesions, but was impaired in about one-third of patients with middle lesions. About half the patients with posterolateral lesions were drowsy, but not comatose, as were about one-half the patients with the lateral lesions who rarely become comatose. However, massive lesions usually cause severe impairment of consciousness including coma. Hemiparesis is common in posterolateral and massive lesions. Sensory deficits are relatively frequent in posterior and medial lesions. Prognosis is fair to good in patients with all of the lesions save the massive ones, where the fatality rate is about 50%. Eye deviation occurs usually toward the lesion site, but may be "wrong way" in those with posterolateral and massive lesions.

Thalamic hemorrhages can be categorized by size (smaller or larger than 2 cm in diameter) and by location (posterolateral, anterolateral, medial, and dorsal; Figure 4.6B). About one-fifth of patients with thalamic hemorrhages are stuporous or comatose at presentation.[95] The loss of consciousness is usually accompanied by ocular signs including skew deviation (the lower eye on the side of the lesion); gaze preference, which may either be toward or away (wrong-way eyes) from the side of the lesion; loss of vertical gaze; and miotic pupils. "Peering at the tip of the nose" is an almost pathognomonic sign.[96] Sensory and motor disturbances depend on the site and size of the lesion. About 25% of patients die,[95] and the outcome is related to the initial consciousness, nuchal rigidity, size of the hemorrhage, and whether the hemorrhage dissects into the lateral ventricle or causes hydrocephalus.

Intraventricular hemorrhages may be either primary or result from extension of an intracerebral hemorrhage. Intraventricular hemorrhages were once thought to be uniformly fatal but, since the advent of CT scanning, have been shown to run the gamut of symptoms from simple headache to coma and death.[97] *Primary intraventricular hemorrhages* can result from vascular anomalies within the ventricle, surgical procedures, or bleeding abnormalities.[98] Clinical findings include sudden onset of headache and vomiting sometimes followed by collapse and coma. If the hemorrhage finds its way into the subarachnoid space, nuchal rigidity occurs. The clinical findings of *secondary intraventricular hemorrhage* depend on the initial site of bleeding. Hemorrhage into the ventricle from a primary intracerebral hemorrhage worsens the prognosis.

The emergency treatment of intraventricular hemorrhage is generally aimed at stopping the bleeding and controlling ICP, and will be discussed in Chapter 8, p. 329. Most patients who have relatively small lesions and do not die make good recoveries; those with massive lesions typically either die or are left devastated. Herniation should be treated vigorously in

patients with relatively small hematomas because of the potential for good recovery.

Despite these similarities, the clinical setting in which one sees patients with intracerebral hemorrhage depends on the pathologic process involved. These include rupture of a deep cerebral end artery, amyloid angiopathy, mycotic aneurysm, arteriovenous malformation, or hemorrhage into a tumor, and each requires a different clinical approach.

Box 4.1 summarizes the major points that differentiate clinically between acute cerebral vascular lesions potentially causing stupor or coma.

Rupture of deep cerebral end arteries usually occurs in patients with long-term, poorly treated hypertension; it can also complicate diabetes or other forms of atherosclerotic arteriopathy. The blood vessels that are most likely to hemorrhage are the same ones that cause lacunar strokes (i.e., end arteries that arise at a right angle from a major cerebral artery): the *striatocapsular arteries*, which give rise to *capsular and basal ganglionic bleeds*; the *thalamic perforating arteries*, which give rise to *thalamic hemorrhages*; the midline *perforating arteries of the pons*, which give rise to *pontine hemorrhages*; and the *penetrating branches of the cerebellar long circumferential arteries*, which cause *cerebellar hemorrhages*. We will deal with the first two, which cause supratentorial masses, in this section, and the latter two in the section on infratentorial masses.

The focal neurologic findings in each case are characteristic of the part of the brain that is injured. Capsular or basal ganglionic hemorrhages typically present with the acute onset of hemiplegia. Thalamic hemorrhage may present with sensory phenomena, but often the hemorrhage compresses ascending arousal systems early so that loss of consciousness is the primary presentation.[95] When the hemorrhage is into the caudal part of the thalamus, such as the putamen, which overlies the posterior commissure, the initial signs may be due to dorsal midbrain compression or injury (see page 116), with some combination of forced downgaze and convergence ("peering at the tip of the nose"), fixed pupils, and retractory nystagmus.[96] Another neuro-ophthalmologic presentation of thalamic hemorrhage was described by Miller Fisher as "wrong-way

Box 4.1 Typical Clinical Profiles of Acute Cerebrovascular Lesions Affecting Consciousness

Acute Massive Cerebral Infarction with or without Hypotension

Distribution: Internal carotid-proximal middle cerebral artery or middle cerebral plus anterior cerebral arteries. Onset during wakefulness or sleep. Massive hemiplegia with aphasia, hemisensory defect. Obtundation is from swelling of the infarcted tissue, progressing to stupor in 12–24 hours, coma usually in 36–96 hours. Convulsions rare. Pupils small and reactive, or constricted ipsilateral to lesion (Horner's), or moderately dilated ipsilateral to lesion (III nerve). Conjugate gaze paresis to side of motor weakness; contralateral oculovestibular responses can be suppressed for 12 hours or so. Contralateral hemiplegia, usually with extensor plantar response and paratonia ipsilateral to lesion. Cheyne-Stokes breathing 10–20%. Signs of progressive rostral caudal deterioration begin in 12–24 hours. Spinal fluid usually unremarkable or with mildly elevated pressure and cells.

Frontoparietal Hemorrhage

Onset during wakefulness. Sudden-onset headache, followed by more or less rapidly evolving aphasia, hemiparesis to hemiplegia, conjugate ocular deviation away from hemiparesis. Convulsions at onset in approximately one-fifth. Pupils small and reactive, or ipsilateral Horner's with excessive contralateral sweating, or stupor to coma and bilateral motor signs within hours of onset. Bloody spinal fluid.

Thalamic Hemorrhage

Hypertensive, onset during wakefulness. Clinical picture similar to frontoparietal hemorrhage but seizures rare, vomiting frequent, eyes characteristically deviated down and laterally to either side. Pupils small and reactive. Conscious state ranges from awake to coma. Bloody spinal fluid.

Bilateral Thalamic Infarction in the Paramedian Regions

Sudden onset of coma, akinetic mutism, hypersomnolence, or altered mental status may accompany bland infarcts of the paramedian thalamus arising bilaterally as a result of a "top of the basilar" syndrome or a branch occlusion of a thalamopeduncular artery (Percheron's artery) providing vascular supply to both thalami as well as the midline mesencephalon.

Pontine Hemorrhage

Hypertensive. Sudden onset of coma or speechlessness, pinpoint pupils, ophthalmoplegia with absent or impaired oculovestibular responses, quadriplegia, irregular breathing, hyperthermia. Bloody spinal fluid.

Cerebellar Hemorrhage

Hypertensive and awake at onset. Acute and rapid onset and worsening within hours of occipital headache, nausea and vomiting, dizziness or vertigo, unsteadiness, dysarthria, and drowsiness. Small and reactive pupils, nystagmus, or horizontal gaze paralysis toward the side of the lesion. Midline and ipsilateral ataxia, ipsilateral peripheral facial palsy, and contralateral extensor plantar response. Occasionally, course may proceed for 1–2 weeks. Spinal fluid bloody.

Box 4.1 Typical Clinical Profiles of Acute Cerebrovascular Lesions Affecting Consciousness (cont.)

Acute Cerebellar Infarction

Mostly hypertensive, mostly males. Onset at any time. Vertigo, ataxia, nausea, dull headache, nystagmus, dysarthria, ipsilateral dysmetria; 24–96 hours later: drowsiness, miosis, ipsilateral gaze paresis and facial paresis, worsening ataxia, extensor plantar responses. Coma, quadriplegia, and death may follow if not decompressed. Spinal fluid sometimes microscopically bloody.

Acute Subarachnoid Hemorrhage

Awake at onset, sometimes hypertensive, sudden headache, often followed within minutes by unconsciousness. Pupils small or unilaterally dilated. Subhyaloid hemorrhages, hemiparesis or aphasia may or may not be present, hemisensory changes rare. Neck stiff within 24 hours. Bloody spinal fluid.

eyes."[99] Whereas frontal lobe insults usually result in deviation of the eyes toward the side of the lesion (i.e., paresis of gaze to the opposite side of space), after thalamic hemorrhage there may be a paresis of gaze toward the side of the lesion (see Chapter 3).

PATHOPHYSIOLOGY

Hemorrhages of the end artery type are often called hypertensive hemorrhages, although they may occur in other clinical settings. The reason for the predilection of this class of artery for both occlusion (lacunar infarction) and hemorrhage is not known. Miller Fisher attempted to identify the arteries that had caused lacunar infarctions in postmortem examination of the brain.[100] He found eosinophilic degeneration of the wall of small penetrating arteries in the region of the infarct and proposed that this "lipohyalinosis" was the cause of the infarction. However, this description was based on a small number of samples and did not give any insight into the nature of the pathologic process. Given the fact that such vessels typically take off at a right angle from large cerebral arteries, one might expect high shearing forces at the vessel origin, so that high blood pressure or other atherosclerotic risk factors might cause earlier or more severe damage. However, the mechanism for this phenomenon remains unclear.

End artery hemorrhages typically produce a large hematoma with considerable local tissue destruction and edema. Because much of the clinical appearance is due to the mass effect of the blood, which eventually is resorbed, the patient may initially be much more neurologically impaired than would be caused by a comparably sized infarct. However, if the patient can be supported through the initial event, recovery is often much greater than might be initially anticipated, and the hematoma is resorbed, leaving a slit-like defect in the brain.

Amyloid angiopathy results from deposition of beta-amyloid peptide in the walls of cerebral blood vessels.[101] These deposits disrupt the arterial elastic media resulting in predisposition to bleeding. Because amyloid deposits occur along blood vessels as they penetrate the cerebral cortex, the hemorrhages are typically lobar (i.e., into a specific lobe of the cerebral cortex).[102] The arteries that hemorrhage tend to be small vessels that seal spontaneously so that the patient usually survives but may have multiple recurrences in later years.[103] Acute onset of focal hemispheric signs and a headache are the most common presentation. As with end artery hemorrhages, the severity of the initial presentation often is misleading, and, as the hemorrhage is resorbed, there may be much greater return of function than in a patient with a similarly placed infarction. Gradient echo MRI may reveal additional areas of small, subclinical cortical and subcortical hemorrhage.[104] In addition, some patients mount an autoimmune attack on the amyloid deposits in blood vessels, resulting in more aggressive vasculitis.[105]

Mycotic aneurysms are typically seen in the setting of a patient who has subacute bacterial endocarditis.[106] Infected emboli that reach the brain lodge in small penetrating arteries in the white matter just deep to the cerebral cortex. The wall of the blood vessel is colonized by bacteria, resulting in aneurysmal dilation several millimeters in diameter. These aneurysms, which may be visualized on cerebral angiography, may be multiple. Because there may be multiple mycotic aneurysms, and to eliminate an arteriovenous malformation or saccular aneurysm as the source, an angiogram is generally necessary. Unruptured mycotic aneurysms are treated by antibiotics, but ruptured aneurysms may require endovascular or open surgical intervention.[107,108] The details of treatment are considered in Chapter 8, page 333.

Vascular malformations may occur in any location in the brain. They range from small cavernous angiomas to large arteriovenous malformations that are life-threatening. MRI identifies many more cavernous angiomas than are seen on conventional arteriography or CT scanning. The abnormal vessels in these malformations are thin-walled, low-pressure, and low-flow venous channels. As a result, cavernous angiomas bleed easily, but rarely are life-threatening. Cavernous angiomas of the brainstem may cause coma if they hemorrhage; the patient usually recovers, but these angiomas have a tendency to rebleed.[109] They can often be removed successfully.[110] Radiosurgery may also reduce the risk of hemorrhage, but can cause local edema or even hemorrhage acutely.[111] Treatment of vascular malformation is discussed in detail in Chapter 8.

Complex arteriovenous malformations (AVMs) contain large arterial feeding vessels and are often devastating when they bleed.[112,113] Although somewhat less likely to cause immediate death than are saccular aneurysms, arteriovenous malformations may be much harder to treat, and bleeding may recur multiple times with gradually worsening outcome. AVMs may also cause symptoms by inducing epilepsy or by causing a vascular steal from surrounding brain. AVMs that come to attention without hemorrhage have about a 2–4% per year chance of bleeding, but those that have previously bled have a much higher risk. AVMs are typically treated by a combination of endovascular occlusion of the arterial supply followed, if necessary, by surgery, although radiosurgery may also shrink AVMs in inaccessible regions (see Chapter 8).

Hemorrhage into a tumor typically occurs in the setting of a patient with known metastatic cancer. However, in some cases, the hemorrhage may be the first sign of the tumor. A higher percentage of metastatic melanoma, thyroid carcinoma, renal cell carcinoma, and germ cell tumors hemorrhage than is true for other tumor types, but lung cancer is so much more common than these tumors that it is the single most common cause of hemorrhage into a tumor.[65] Primary brain tumors, particularly oligodendrogliomas, may also present with a hemorrhage into the tumor. Because it is often difficult to see contrast enhancement of the tumor amid the initial blood on MRI or CT scan, it is generally necessary to reimage the brain several weeks later, when the acute blood has been resorbed, if no cause of the hemorrhage is seen on initial imaging.

Intracerebral Tumors

Both primary and metastatic tumors may invade the brain, resulting in impairment of consciousness.[65,114] Primary tumors are typically either gliomas or primary CNS lymphomas, whereas metastatic tumors may come from many types of systemic cancer. Certain principles apply broadly across these classes of tumors.

Gliomas include both astrocytic tumors and oligodendrogliomas.[114] Astrocytic tumors typically invade the substance of the brain and, in extreme cases (gliomatosis cerebri), may diffusely infiltrate the entire brain. Oligodendrogliomas typically are slower growing and may contain calcifications visible on CT or MRI. They more often present as seizures than as mass lesions.[115] Astrocytomas typically present either with seizures or as a mass lesion, with headache and increased ICP. In other cases, the patients may present with focal or multifocal signs of cerebral dysfunction. As they enlarge, astrocytomas may outgrow their blood supply, resulting in internal areas of necrosis or hemorrhage and formation of cystic components. Impairment of consciousness is usually due to compression or infiltration of the diencephalon or herniation. Surprisingly, primary brainstem astrocytomas, which are typically seen in adolescents and young adults, cause mainly impairment of cranial motor nerves while leaving sensory function and consciousness intact until very late in the course.[116]

Primary CNS lymphoma (PCNSL) was once considered to be a rare tumor that was seen mainly in patients who were immune suppressed; however, PCNSL has increased in frequency in recent years in patients who are not immune compromised.[114,117] The reason for the increased incidence is not known. PCNSL behaves quite differently from systemic lymphomas. The tumors invade the brain much like astrocytic tumors. They often occur along the ventricular surfaces and may infiltrate along white matter tracts. In this respect, primary CNS lymphomas present in ways that are similar to astrocytic tumors. However, it is unusual for a primary CNS lymphoma to reach so large a size, or to present by impairment of consciousness, unless it begins in the diencephalon.

Metastatic tumors are most often from lung, breast, or renal cell cancers or melanoma.[65] Tumors arising below the diaphragm usually do not invade the brain unless they first cause pulmonary metastases. Unlike primary brain tumors, metastases rarely infiltrate the brain and can often be shelled out at surgery. Metastatic tumors often enlarge quite rapidly and can present as mass lesions. This tendency also results in tumors outgrowing their blood supply, resulting in infarction and hemorrhage (see previous section).

Other patients with brain tumors present with seizures, which require treatment. However, some antiepileptic drugs, such as phenytoin or phenobarbital, can cause erythema multiforme in patients receiving cranial radiation, so are best avoided. Prophylactic administration of anticonvulsants to brain tumor patients who have not yet had seizures has not been found to be of value.[118] Treatment of brain tumors is considered in Chapter 8.

Brain Abscess and Granuloma

A wide range of microorganisms, including viruses, bacteria, fungi, and parasites, can invade the brain parenchyma, producing an acute destructive encephalitis (see page 156). However, if the immune response is successful in containing the invader, a more chronic abscess or granuloma may result, which may act more as a compressive mass.

A brain abscess is a focal collection of pus within the parenchyma of the brain. The infective agents reach the brain hematogenously or by direct extension from an infected contiguous organ (paranasal sinus, middle ear).[119] Most bacterial brain abscesses occur in the cerebral hemispheres, particularly in the frontal or temporal lobes. In many countries in Central and South America, cysticercosis is the most common cause of infectious mass lesions in the cerebral hemispheres. However, cysticercosis typically presents as seizures and only occasionally as a mass lesion.[120] In countries in which sheep herding is a major activity, echinococcal (hydatid) cyst must also be considered, although these can usually be recognized because they are more cystic in appearance than abscesses on CT or MRI scan.[121,122] Patients with HIV-AIDS who are not adequately treated with retroviral drugs present a special challenge in the diagnosis of coma as they may have a much wider array of cerebral infectious lesions and are also disposed to primary CNS lymphoma. However, toxoplasmosis is so common in this group of patients that most clinicians begin with 2 weeks of therapy for that organism.[123] When the appearance on scan is unusual, though, early biopsy is often indicated to establish the cause of the lesion(s) and optimal mode of treatment.

Other organisms may cause chronic infection resulting in formation of granulomas that may reach sufficient size to act as a mass lesion. These include tuberculomas in tuberculosis, torulomas in cryptococcal infection, and gummas in syphilis.

Because the symptoms are mainly due to brain compression, the clinical symptoms of brain abscess are similar to those of brain neoplasms, except they usually evolve more rapidly (Table 4.6).[119]

Headache, focal neurologic signs, and seizures are relatively common. Fever and nuchal rigidity are generally present only during the early encephalitic phase of the infection and are uncommon in encapsulated brain abscesses. The diagnosis may be suspected in a patient with a known source of infection or an immunosuppressed patient.

Table 4.6 **Presenting Signs and Symptoms in 968 Patients with Brain Abscess**

Sign or symptom	Frequency range	Mean
Headache	55–97%	77%
Depressed consciousness	28–91%	53%
Fever	32–62%	53%
Nausea with vomiting	35–85%	51%
Papilledema	9–56%	39%
Hemiparesis	23–44%	36%
Seizures	13–35%	24%
Neck stiffness	5–41%	23%

From Kastenbauer et al.,[124] with permission.

On imaging with either CT or MRI, the enhanced rim of an abscess is usually thinner and more regular than that of a tumor and may be very thin where it abuts the ventricle, sometimes leading to ventricular rupture (Figure 4.7). The infective nidus is often surrounded by more vasogenic edema than usually surrounds brain neoplasms. Diffusion-weighted images indicate restricted diffusion within the abscess, which can be distinguished

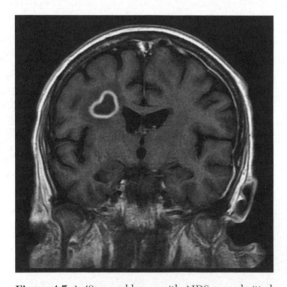

Figure 4.7 A 49-year-old man with AIDS was admitted for evaluation of headache, nausea, and bilateral weakness and intermittent focal motor seizures. Magnetic resonance imaging showed multiple ring-enhancing lesions. Note that the smooth, contrast-enhancing wall of this right parietal lesion is typical of an abscess. He was treated with broad spectrum antibiotics and improved.

from the cystic areas within tumors, which represent areas of infarction. The presence of higher levels of amino acids within the abscess on magnetic resonance spectroscopy (MRS) may also be helpful in differentiating the pathologies (Table 4.7).

If the lesion is small and the organism can be identified, antibiotics can treat the abscess successfully. Larger lesions require drainage or excision.

INFRATENTORIAL COMPRESSIVE LESIONS

The same mass lesions that affect the supratentorial space can also occur infratentorially (i.e., in the posterior fossa). Hence, while both the focal symptoms caused by posterior fossa masses and the symptoms of herniation differ substantially from those of supratentorial masses, the pathophysiologic mechanisms are similar. For that reason, we will focus in this section on the ways in which posterior fossa compressive lesions differ from those that occur supratentorially. Depending on the site of the lesion, compressive lesions of the posterior fossa are more likely to cause cerebellar signs and eye movement disorders and less likely to cause isolated hemiplegia. Herniation may be either downward as the cerebellar tonsils are forced through the foramen magnum or upward as the cerebellar vermis pushes the upper brainstem through the tentorium, or usually both.

EPIDURAL AND DURAL MASSES

Epidural Hematoma

Epidural hematomas of the posterior fossa are much less common than their supratentorial counterparts, representing about 10% of all epidural hematomas.[125,126] Posterior fossa epidural hematomas typically follow fracture of the occipital bone; they are usually arterial, but may occasionally result from venous bleeding. The hematomas are bilateral in about one-third of cases.

Patients present with headache, nausea and vomiting, and loss of consciousness.[127,128] Neuro-ophthalmologic signs are relatively uncommon, usually consisting of abducens

Table 4.7 Imaging Findings in Brain Abscess

Finding	CT	MR [a]	Sensitivity
Capsule	Isodense	T1WI: Isointense to hyperintense Enhances T2WI: Hypointense to hyperintense	Plain: MR>CT CE: MR>CT
Vasogenic edema	Hypodense	T1WI: Hypointense T2WI: Hyperintense	Plain: MR>CT
Abscess contents	Hypodense	T1WI: Hypointense T2WI: Hyperintense MRS: Amino acid, lactate, acetate, succinate, and pyruvate peaks DWI: Bright (white) ADC: Dark (black)	Plain: MR = CT

ADC, apparent diffusion coefficient map; CE, contrast enhanced; CT, computed tomography; DWI, diffusion-weighted image; MR, magnetic resonance spectroscopy; T1WI, T1-weighted image; T2WI, T2-weighted image.

[a] Intensity relative to normal brain.

From Zimmerman et al.,[90] with permission.

paresis due to the increased ICP. Occasionally a stiff neck is seen as an early sign of tonsillar herniation.

A typical lucid interval occurs in only a minority of patients: after initial injury, those patients either continue to be alert or rapidly recover after a brief loss of consciousness only to subsequently, after minutes to days, first become lethargic and then lapse into coma. Without treatment, death ensues from acute respiratory failure (tonsillar herniation). Even those patients with a lucid interval suffer headache and often cerebellar ataxia after the injury. If not treated, symptoms progress to vertigo, stiff neck, ataxia, nausea, and drowsiness.

It is important to identify an occipital fracture even in the absence of a hematoma because of the possibility of delayed development of an epidural hematoma.[125] If a fracture crosses the transverse sinus, it may cause thrombosis of that vessel, causing a supratentorial hemorrhagic infarct or increased ICP. Because of the small amount of space in the posterior fossa and the narrow exit foramina of CSF (Sylvian aqueduct and fourth ventricle), obstructive hydrocephalus is often an early problem that may require emergent therapy.[129] About one-half of patients have evidence of other injury, such as cerebellar hemorrhage or supratentorial bleeding.[130]

Treatment of epidural hematomas will be considered in Chapter 8.

Epidural Abscess

Epidural abscesses in the posterior fossa are rare, representing only 9 out of almost 4,000 patients with intracranial infections in one series.[131] Most were complications of ear infections and mastoiditis. Unlike epidural hematomas, fever and meningismus, as well as evidence of a chronic draining ear, are common. Focal neurologic signs are similar to those of epidural hematomas but develop over days to weeks rather than hours. Cerebellar signs occur in a minority of patients. The CT scan demonstrates a hypodense or isodense extraaxial mass with a contrast-enhancing rim. Hydrocephalus is common. Diffusion-weighted MRI identifies restricted diffusion, as in supratentorial empyemas and abscesses.[37] The prognosis is generally good with evacuation of the abscess and treatment with antimicrobials, except in those patients suffering venous sinus thrombosis as a result of the infection.

Dural and Epidural Tumors

As with supratentorial lesions, both primary and metastatic tumors can involve the dura of the posterior fossa. *Meningioma* is the most common primary tumor.[132] Meningiomas usually arise from the tentorium or other dural structures, but can occur in the posterior fossa without dural attachment.[133] Meningiomas produce their symptoms both by direct compression and by causing hydrocephalus. However, because they grow slowly, focal neurologic symptoms are common and the diagnosis is generally made long before they cause alterations of consciousness. Dural *metastases* from myelocytic leukemia, so-called chloromas or granulocytic sarcomas, have a particular predilection for the posterior fossa.[134,135] Although more rapidly growing than primary tumors, these tumors rarely cause alterations of consciousness. Other metastatic tumors to the posterior fossa meninges may cause symptoms by involving cranial nerves.

SUBDURAL POSTERIOR FOSSA COMPRESSIVE LESIONS

Subdural hematomas of the posterior fossa are rare. Only 1% of traumatic acute subdural hematomas are found in the posterior fossa.[136,137] Chronic subdural hematomas in the posterior fossa, without a clear history of head trauma, are even rarer. A review in 2002 reported only 15 previous cases, including those patients taking anticoagulants.[138] Patients with acute subdural hematomas can be divided into those who are stuporous or comatose on admission and those who are alert. Patients with chronic subdural hematomas, many of whom had been on anticoagulation therapy or have sustained very mild head trauma, usually present with headache, vomiting, and cerebellar signs. The diagnosis is made by CT or MRI, and treatment is usually surgical. Stupor or coma portends a poor outcome, as do the CT findings of obliterated basal cisterns and fourth ventricle with resultant hydrocephalus.[137]

Subdural Empyema

Posterior fossa subdural empyemas are rare.[139] They constitute less than 2% of all subdural empyemas.[131] Like their epidural counterparts, ear infections and mastoiditis are the major cause. Headache, lethargy, and meningismus are common symptoms. Ataxia and nystagmus are less common.[131] The diagnosis is made by CT, which reveals a hypo- or isodense extra-axial collection with enhancement. On MRI, diffusion is restricted,[37] unlike tumors or hemorrhage. Treatment with drainage and antibiotics is usually successful.

Subdural Tumors

Isolated subdural tumors are exceedingly rare. Meningioma and other tumors of the dura may invade the subdural space. Subdural metastases from leukemia or solid tumors rarely occur in isolation. They can be differentiated from hematomas and infection on scans by their uniform contrast enhancement.

SUBARACHNOID POSTERIOR FOSSA LESIONS

Subarachnoid blood, infection, or tumor usually occurs in the posterior fossa in association with similar supratentorial lesions. Exceptions include subdural or parenchymal posterior fossa lesions that rupture into the subarachnoid space and posterior fossa subarachnoid hemorrhage.[140] *Posterior fossa subarachnoid hemorrhages* are caused either by aneurysms or dissection of vertebral or basilar arteries or their branches. Unruptured aneurysms of the basilar and vertebral arteries sometimes grow to a size of several centimeters and act like posterior fossa extramedullary tumors. However, they generally do not cause coma unless they rupture. When a vertebrobasilar aneurysm ruptures, the event is characteristically abrupt and frequently is marked by the complaint of sudden weak legs, collapse, and coma. Most patients also have sudden occipital headache, but—in contrast with anterior fossa aneurysms in which the history of coma, if present, is usually clear-cut—it sometimes is difficult to be certain whether a patient with a ruptured posterior fossa aneurysm had briefly lost consciousness or merely collapsed because of paralysis of the lower extremities. In the pre-CT era, ruptured vertebrobasilar aneurysms were notorious for presenting relatively few clinical signs that clearly localized the source of the subarachnoid bleeding to the posterior fossa.[141-143] Although, in our own experience, six of eight patients with rupture of confirmed vertebrobasilar aneurysms had pupillary, motor, or oculomotor signs of a posterior fossa lesion

Table 4.8 Localizing Signs in Six Cases of Ruptured Vertebrobasilar Aneurysms

Occipital headache	5
Skew deviation of the eyes	3
Third nerve paralysis	2
Cerebellar signs	3
Acute paraplegia before loss of consciousness	2

(see Table 4.8), it is still important to maintain a low threshold for imaging in patients with initial collapse and sudden onset of a severe occipital headache, even if the patient is awake by the time he or she reaches medical attention. The diagnosis is usually obvious on CT. Blood isolated to the fourth ventricle suggests a ruptured posterior inferior cerebellar artery aneurysm.[140]

Perimesencephalic hemorrhage is characterized by subarachnoid blood accumulating around the midbrain. While this often presents with a headache and loss of consciousness, it has a relatively benign prognosis.[144] Unlike most subarachnoid hemorrhage, the bleeding is usually venous in origin; cerebral angiograms do not reveal an aneurysm but may demonstrate a primitive basal vein of Rosenthal drainage pattern in at least one hemisphere.[145]

INTRAPARENCHYMAL POSTERIOR FOSSA MASS LESIONS

Intraparenchymal mass lesions in the posterior fossa that cause coma by compression usually are located in the cerebellum. In part, this is because the cerebellum occupies a large portion of this compartment, but in part it is because the brainstem is so small that an expanding mass lesion often does more damage by tissue destruction than as a compressive lesion.

Cerebellar Hemorrhage

About 10% of intraparenchymal intracranial hemorrhages occur in the cerebellum. A cerebellar hemorrhage can cause coma and death by compressing the brainstem. Increasing numbers of reports in recent years indicate that if the diagnosis is made promptly, many patients

can be treated successfully by evacuating the clot or removing an associated angioma.[146] However, for those patients who are comatose, mortality is high despite prompt surgical intervention. Approximately three-quarters of patients with cerebellar hemorrhage have hypertension; most of the remaining ones have cerebellar angiomas or are receiving anticoagulant drugs. In elderly patients, amyloid angiopathy may be the culprit, especially if the hemorrhage is superficial.[147] Hemorrhages in hypertensive patients arise in the neighborhood of the dentate nuclei; those coming from angiomas tend to lie more superficially. Both types usually rupture into the subarachnoid space or fourth ventricle and cause coma chiefly by compressing the brainstem.

Table 4.9 lists the most frequent early physical signs as recorded in a series of 72 patients.[148] Subsequent reports from several large centers have increasingly emphasized that early diagnosis is critical for satisfactory treatment of cerebellar hemorrhage and that once patients become stuporous or comatose, the outcome after surgical drainage is much worse.[149] The most common initial symptoms of cerebellar hemorrhage are headaches (most often occipital), nausea and vomiting, dizziness or vertiginous sensations, unsteadiness or an inability to walk, dysarthria, and, less often, drowsiness. The man in Patient Vignette 4.3 is a typical example.

Patient Vignette 4.3

A 55-year-old man with hypertension and a history of poor medication compliance had sudden onset of severe occipital headache and nausea when sitting down with his family to Christmas dinner. He noticed that he was uncoordinated when he tried to carve the turkey. When he arrived in the hospital emergency department, he was unable to sit or stand unaided, and he had severe bilateral ataxia in both upper extremities. He was a bit drowsy but had full eye movements with end gaze nystagmus to either side. There was no weakness or change in muscle tone, but tendon reflexes were brisk, and toes were downgoing. He was sent for a computed tomography (CT) scan, but by the time the scan was finished the CT technician could no longer arouse him.

The CT scan showed a 5-cm egg-shaped hemorrhage into the left cerebellar

Table 4.9 Presenting Clinical Findings in 72 Patients with Cerebellar Hemorrhage

Symptoms	No. patients (%)	Signs	No. patients (%)
Vomiting	58 (81)	Anisocoria	10 (14)
Headache	48 (67)	Pinpoint pupils	4 (6)
Dizziness/vertigo	43 (60)	Abnormal OCR or EOM	23 (32)
Truncal/gait ataxia	40 (56)	Skew deviation	6 (8)
Dysarthria	30 (42)	Nystagmus	24 (33)
Drowsiness	30 (42)	Absent/asymmetric CR	9 (13)
Confusion	8 (11)	Facial paresis	13 (18)
		Dysarthria	18 (25)
		Limb ataxia	32 (44)
		Hemiparesis	8 (11)
		Babinski sign	36 (50)

CR, corneal reflex; EOM, extraocular movements; OCR, oculocephalic reflex.
Modified from Fisher et al.[150]

hemisphere, compressing the fourth ventricle, with hydrocephalus. By the time the patient returned to the emergency department, he had no oculocephalic responses and breathing was ataxic. Shortly afterward, he had a respiratory arrest and died before the neurosurgical team could take him to the operating room.

As the patient in Patient Vignette 4.3 illustrates, deterioration from alertness or drowsiness to stupor often occurs over a few minutes, and even brief delays to carry out radiographic procedures can prove fatal. Mutism, a finding encountered in children after operations that split the inferior vermis of the cerebellum, occasionally occurs in adults with cerebellar hemorrhage.[151] Although usually not tested during the rush of the initial examination, cognitive dysfunction, including impairment of executive functions, difficulty with spatial cognition, and language deficits, as well as affective disorders including blunting of affect or disinhibited or inappropriate behavior, called the "cerebellar cognitive affective syndrome,"[152] are sometimes present (see also page 306, Chapter 6). Similar abnormalities may persist if there is damage to the posterior hemisphere of the cerebellum, even following successful treatment of cerebellar mass lesions.[153]

All patients who present to the emergency room with acute cerebellar signs, particularly when associated with headache and vomiting, require an urgent CT. The scan identifies the hemorrhage and permits assessment of the

degree of compression of the fourth ventricle and whether there is any complicating hydrocephalus. Our experience with acute cerebellar hemorrhage points to a gradation in severity that can be divided roughly into four relatively distinct clinical patterns. The least serious form occurs with small hemorrhages, usually less than 1.5–2 cm in diameter by CT, and includes self-limited, acute unilateral cerebellar dysfunction accompanied by headache. Without imaging, this disorder undoubtedly would go undiagnosed. With larger hematomas, occipital headache is more prominent, and signs of cerebellar or oculomotor dysfunction develop gradually or episodically over 1 to several days. There may be some associated drowsiness or lethargy. Patients with this degree of impairment have been reported to recover spontaneously, particularly from hemorrhages measuring less than 3 cm in diameter by CT. However, the condition requires extremely careful observation until one is sure that there is no progression due to edema formation, as patients almost always do poorly if one waits until coma develops to initiate surgical treatment. The most characteristic and therapeutically important syndrome of cerebellar hemorrhages occurs in individuals who develop acute or subacute occipital headache, vomiting, and progressive neurologic impairment including ipsilateral ataxia, nausea, vertigo, and nystagmus. Parenchymal brainstem signs, such as gaze paresis or facial weakness on the side of the hematoma, or pyramidal motor signs, develop as a result of brainstem compression, and hence usually are not seen until after drowsiness or obtundation is apparent. The appearance of impairment of consciousness mandates emergency intervention and surgical decompression that can be life-saving. About one-fifth of patients with cerebellar hemorrhage develop early pontine compression with sudden loss of consciousness, respiratory irregularity, pinpoint pupils, absent oculovestibular responses, and quadriplegia; the picture is clinically indistinguishable from primary pontine hemorrhage and is almost always fatal.

Clinical predictors of neurologic deterioration are a systolic blood pressure of greater than 200 mm Hg, pinpoint pupils, and abnormal corneal or oculocephalic reflexes. Imaging predictors are hemorrhage extending into the vermis, a hematoma greater than 3 cm in diameter, brainstem distortion, interventricular hemorrhage, upward herniation, or acute hydrocephalus. Hemorrhages in the vermis and acute hydrocephalus on admission independently predict deterioration.[148]

Treatment of cerebellar hemorrhages is aimed at reducing ICP, either by lateral ventricular drain or by removing the hematoma and infarcted brain tissue. Algorithms for deciding on the approach, as well as the outcomes, are covered in Chapter 8.

Cerebellar Infarction

Cerebellar infarction can act as a mass lesion if there is cerebellar edema. In these cases, as in cerebellar hemorrhage, the mass effect can cause stupor or coma by compression of the brainstem and death by herniation. Cerebellar infarction represents 2% of strokes.[154,155] Most victims are men. Hypertension, atrial fibrillation, hypercholesterolemia, and diabetes are important risk factors in the elderly; vertebral artery dissection should be considered in younger patients. The neurologic symptoms are similar to those of cerebellar hemorrhage, but they progress more slowly as they are typically due to edema that develops gradually over 2–3 days after the onset of the infarct rather than acutely (Table 4.10).

The onset is characteristically marked by acute or subacute dizziness, vertigo, unsteadiness, and, less often, dull headache. Most of the patients examined within hours of onset are ataxic, have nystagmus with gaze in either direction but predominantly toward the infarct, and have dysmetria ipsilateral to the infarct. Dysarthria and dysphagia are present in some patients and presumably reflect associated lateral medullary infarction. Only a minority of patients are lethargic, stuporous, or comatose on admission, which suggests additional injury to the brainstem.[155]

Initial CT rules out a cerebellar hemorrhage, but it is often difficult to demonstrate an infarct. Even if a hypodense lesion is not seen, asymmetric compression of the fourth ventricle may indicate the development of acute edema. A diffusion-weighted MRI is usually positive on initial examination.

Table 4.10 **Symptoms, Signs, and Consciousness Levels on Admission in 293 Patients with Cerebellar Infarction**

Symptoms	No. (%)	Signs	No. (%)	Consciousness levels on admission	No. (%)
Vertigo/dizziness	206 (70)	Limb ataxia	172 (59)	Clear	195 (67)
Nausea/vomiting	165 (56)	Truncal ataxia	133 (45)	Confused	73 (25)
Gait disturbance	116 (40)	Dysarthria	123 (42)	Obtunded	20 (7)
Headache	94 (32)	Nystagmus	111 (38)	Comatose	5 (2)
Dysarthria	59 (20)	Hemiparesis	59 (20)		
Tinnitus	14 (5)	Facial palsy	23 (8)		
		Anisocoria	17 (6)		
		Conjugate deviation	18 (6)		
		Horner's syndrome	15 (5)		
		Upward gaze palsy	12 (4)		
		Loss of light reflex	11 (4)		

From Tohgi et al.,[155] with permission.

In most instances, further progression, if it is to occur, develops by the third day and may progress to coma within 24 hours.[154] Progression is characterized by more intense ipsilateral dysmetria followed by increasing drowsiness leading to stupor, and then miotic and poorly reactive pupils, conjugate gaze paralysis ipsilateral to the lesion, ipsilateral peripheral facial paralysis, and extensor plantar responses. Once the symptoms of brainstem compression appear, unless surgical decompression is conducted promptly, the illness progresses rapidly to coma, quadriplegia, and death.

Only the evaluation of clinical signs can determine whether the swelling is resolving or the enlarging mass must be surgically treated (by ventricular shunt or evacuation of infarcted tissue).[154,156] The principles of management of a patient with a space-occupying cerebellar infarct are similar to those in cerebellar hemorrhage and are covered in Chapter 8.

Cerebellar Abscess

About 10% of all brain abscesses occur in the cerebellum.[157] Cerebellar abscesses represent about 2% of all intracranial infections. Most arise from chronic ear infections, but some occur after trauma (head injury or neurosurgery) and others are hematogenous in origin.[157,158] If untreated, they enlarge, compress the brainstem, and cause herniation and death. If successfully recognized and treated, the outcome is usually good. The clinical symptoms of a cerebellar abscess differ little from those of other cerebellar masses (Table 4.11).

Headache and vomiting are very common. Patients may or may not be febrile or have nuchal rigidity.[159] If the patient does not have an obvious source of infection, is not febrile, and has a supple neck, a cerebellar abscess is often mistaken for a tumor, with the correct diagnosis being made only by surgery.[157] The diagnosis is made by imaging, with scans revealing a mass with a contrast-enhancing rim and usually an impressive amount of edema. Restricted diffusion on diffusion-weighted MRI helps distinguish the abscess from tumor or hematoma. Hydrocephalus is a common complication and is treated with CSF diversion or drainage. As with other cerebellar masses, the treatment, covered in more detail in Chapter 8, is surgical, either primary excision or aspiration.[157]

Table 4.11 Clinical Features of Cerebellar Abscesses

	Cases before 1975 (N = 47) [a]		Cases after 1975 (N = 77) [b]	
	No.	%	No.	%
Symptoms				
Headache	47	100	74	96
Vomiting	39	83		
Drowsiness	32	66		
Unsteadiness	23	49		
Confusion	16	34		
Ipsilateral limb weakness	6	13		
Visual disturbances	4	8		
Blackout	3	6		
Signs				
Nystagmus	35	74		
Meningismus	31	66	59	77
Cerebellar signs	27	57	40	52
Papilledema	21	45		
Fever	16	34	70	90
Sixth-nerve palsy	2	4	7	15
Depressed consciousness	32	66	44	57

[a] Data from Shaw and Russell. [159]

[b] Data from Nadvi et al.[160]

Cerebellar Tumor

Most cerebellar tumors of adults are metastases.[65,161] The common cerebellar primary tumors of children, medulloblastoma and pilocytic astrocytoma, are rare in adults. Cerebellar hemangioblastomas may occur in adults, but they are uncommon.[162] The symptoms of cerebellar tumors are the same as those of any cerebellar mass, but because their growth is relatively slow, they rarely cause significant alterations of consciousness unless there is a sudden hemorrhage in the tumor. Patients present with headache, dizziness, and ataxia. Because the symptoms are rarely acute, MRI scanning can usually be obtained. The contrast-enhanced image will not only identify the enhancing cerebellar tumor, but will also inform the physician whether there are other metastatic lesions and whether hydrocephalus is present. The treatment of a single metastasis in the cerebellum is generally surgical or, in some instances, by radiosurgery.[65] Multiple metastases are treated with radiation therapy. Treatment is covered in Chapter 8.

Pontine Hemorrhage

Although pontine hemorrhage compresses the brainstem, it causes damage as much by tissue destruction as by mass effect (Figures 4.8 and 4.9). Hemorrhage into the pons typically produces the characteristic pattern of sudden onset of unconsciousness with tiny but reactive pupils (although it may require a magnifying glass or the plus-20 lens of the ophthalmoscope to visualize the light response). Most patients have impairment of oculocephalic responses, and eyes may show skew deviation, ocular bobbing, or one of its variants. Patients may have decerebrate rigidity, or they may demonstrate flaccid quadriplegia. We have seen one patient in whom a hematoma dissected along the medial longitudinal fasciculus and caused initial vertical and adduction ophthalmoparesis, which was followed about an hour later by loss of consciousness (see Patient Vignette 2.1). However, in most patients, the onset of coma is so sudden that there is not even a history of a complaint of headache.[163]

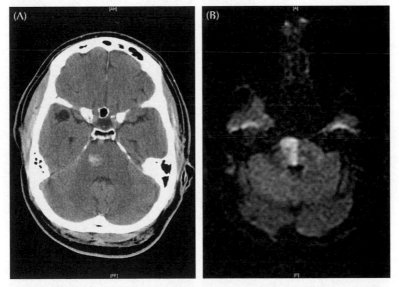

Figure 4.8 A pair of scans without contrast from two patients with pontine strokes. (A) A noncontrast computed tomography scan demonstrating a small hemorrhage into the right pontine base and tegmentum in a 55-year-old man with hypertension, who presented with left hemiparesis and dysarthria. He was treated by blood pressure control and improved markedly. (B) A diffusion-weighted magnetic resonance imaging (MRI) scan of a medial pontine infarct in a 77-year-old man with hypertension, hyperlipidemia, and prior history of coronary artery disease. He presented with left hemiparesis, dysarthria, and diplopia. On examination, there was right lateral gaze paresis and inability to adduct either eye on lateral gaze (one-and-a-half syndrome). There was extensive irregularity of the vertebrobasilar vessels on MR angiogram. He was treated with anticoagulants and improved slowly, although with significant residual diplopia and left hemiparesis at discharge.

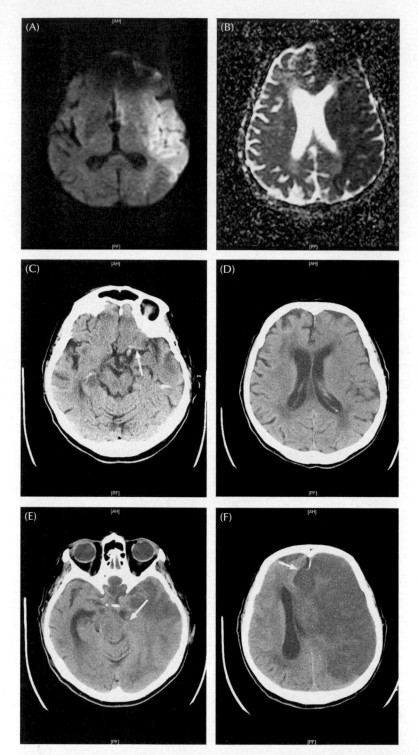

Figure 4.9 Development of cerebral edema and herniation in a patient with a left middle cerebral artery infarct. A 90-year-old woman with hypertension and diabetes had sudden onset of global aphasia, right hemiparesis, and left gaze preference. (A) A diffusion-weighted magnetic resonance imaging scan and (B) an apparent diffusion coefficient (ADC) map, which identify the area of acute infarction as including both the anterior and middle cerebral artery territories. The initial computed tomography scan (C, D) identified a dense left middle cerebral artery (arrow), indicating thrombosis, and swelling of the sulci on the left compared to the right, consistent with the region of restricted diffusion shown on the ADC map. By 48 hours after admission, there was massive left cerebral edema, with the medial temporal lobe herniation compressing the brainstem (arrow E) and subfalcine herniation of the left cingulate gyrus (arrow in F) and massive midline shift and compression of the left lateral ventricle. The patient died shortly after this scan.

SUPRATENTORIAL DESTRUCTIVE LESIONS CAUSING COMA

The most common supratentorial destructive lesions causing coma result from either anoxia or ischemia, although the damage may occur due to trauma, infection, or the associated immune response. To cause coma, a supratentorial lesion must either involve bilateral cortical or subcortical structures multifocally or diffusely or affect the diencephalon bilaterally. Following recovery from the initial insult, the coma is usually short-lived, the patient either awakening, entering a persistent vegetative state within a few days or weeks, or dying (see Chapter 9).

VASCULAR CAUSES OF SUPRATENTORIAL DESTRUCTIVE LESIONS

Diffuse anoxia and ischemia, including carbon monoxide poisoning and multiple cerebral emboli from fat embolism[164] or cardiac surgery,[165] are discussed in detail in Chapter 5. We will concentrate here on focal ischemic lesions that can cause coma.

Carotid Ischemic Lesions

Unilateral hemispheric infarcts due to *carotid or middle cerebral occlusion* may cause a quiet, apathetic, or even confused appearance, as the remaining cognitive systems in the patient's functional hemisphere attempt to deal with the sudden change in cognitive perspective on the world. This appearance is also seen in patients during a Wada test, when a barbiturate is injected into one carotid artery to determine the lateralization of language function prior to surgery. The appearance of the patient may be deceptive to the uninitiated examiner; acute loss of language with a dominant hemisphere lesion may make the patient unresponsive to verbal command, and acute lesions of the nondominant hemisphere often cause an "eye-opening apraxia," in which the patient keeps his or her eyes closed even though awake. However, a careful neurologic examination demonstrates that, despite the appearance

of reduced responsiveness, true coma rarely occurs in such cases.[166]

In the rare cases where unilateral carotid occlusion does cause loss of consciousness, there is nearly always an underlying vascular abnormality that explains the observation. For example, there may be a preexisting vascular anomaly or an occlusion of the contralateral carotid artery so that both cerebral hemispheres may be supplied, across the anterior communicating artery, by one carotid. In the absence of such a situation, unilateral carotid occlusion does not cause acute loss of consciousness.

Patients with large hemispheric infarcts are nearly always hemiplegic at onset, and if in the dominant hemisphere, aphasic as well. The lesion can be differentiated from a cerebral hemorrhage by CT scan that, in the case of infarct, may initially appear normal or show only slight edema with loss of gray–white matter distinction (Figure 4.9). MRI scans, however, show marked hyperintensity on the diffusion-weighted image, indicating ischemia. With the rapid evolution of more accurate imaging, intravenous and intra-arterial thrombolytics, and clot retrieval technology, it is often possible to intervene and reperfuse ischemic tissue as much as 24 hours after onset of symptoms.[167,168] Treatment will be covered in detail in Chapter 8. Although impairment of consciousness is rare as an immediate result of unilateral carotid occlusion, it may occur several days after acute infarction in the carotid territory, as edema of the infarcted hemisphere causes compression of the other hemisphere and the diencephalon, and can result in uncal or central herniation.[169] This problem is presaged by increasing lethargy and pupillary changes suggesting either central or uncal herniation. Many patients who survive the initial infarct succumb during this period. The swelling does not respond to corticosteroids, but may be treated with decompressive craniectomy, as discussed in Chapters 7 and 8.

Distal Basilar Occlusion

Distal basilar occlusion typically presents with a characteristic set of findings (the "top of the basilar syndrome") that can include impairment of consciousness.[170,171] The basilar

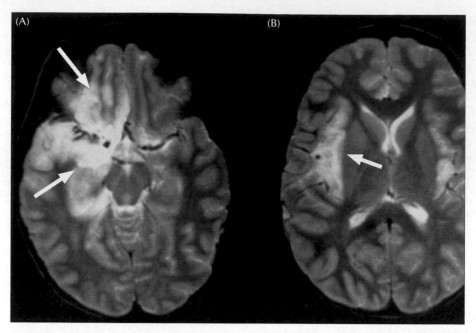

Figure 4.10 A pair of magnetic resonance images from the brain of a patient with herpes simplex 1 encephalitis. Note the preferential involvement of the medial temporal lobe and orbitofrontal cortex (arrows in A) and insular cortex (arrow in B). There is milder involvement of the contralateral side.
Images courtesy of Dr. Jonathan Kleefield.

arteries give rise to the posterior cerebral arteries, which perfuse the caudal medial part of the hemispheres. The posterior cerebral arteries also give rise to posterior choroidal arteries, which perfuse the caudal part of the hippocampal formation, the globus pallidus, and the lateral geniculate nucleus.[172] In addition, thalamo-perforating arteries originating from the basilar tip, posterior cerebral arteries, and posterior communicating arteries supply the caudal paramedian part of the thalamus and the adjacent paramedian midbrain.[171] Occlusion of the distal posterior cerebral arteries causes bilateral blindness, paresis, and memory loss. Some patients who are blind deny their condition (Anton syndrome). However, the infarction does not cause loss of consciousness. On the other hand, more proximal occlusion of the basilar artery that reduces perfusion of the junction of the midbrain with the posterior thalamus and hypothalamus bilaterally can cause profound coma.[170]

Isolated *thalamic infarction* can cause a wide variety of cognitive problems depending on which feeding vessels are occluded (Table 4.14). Several careful studies examining postmortem pathology[173] or MRI verification of thalamic lesions[174] have provided a comprehensive analysis of clinical syndromes related to occlusion of each vessel (Table 4.12). While about 90% of patients with paramedian thalamic infarcts have impairment of consciousness, the paramedian thalamus and paramedian midbrain reticular formation are both within the territory of the paramedian thalamic feeders, including the artery of Percheron, so the paramedian midbrain is generally involved in most paramedian thalamic infarcts. Castaigne's series, for example included only two cases of isolated paramedian thalamic stroke (without apparent midbrain involvement), and neither caused loss of consciousness.[173] A recent study of thalamic infarcts associated with impairment of consciousness found that isolated bilateral thalamic injuries are typically not associated with a depressed level of consciousness.[175] Infarcts that include the rostral midbrain reticular formation initially producing coma, which often gives way to a sleepy but arousable state within a few days.[173,174] However, patients with substantial damage to the paramedian thalamus bilaterally can have prolonged cognitive deficits.[176,177]

Table 4.12 Thalamic Arterial Supply and Principal Clinical Features of Focal Infarction

Thalamic blood vessel	Nuclei irrigated	Clinical features reported
Tuberothalamic artery (arises from middle third of posterior communicating artery)	Reticular, intralaminar, VA, rostral VL, ventral pole of MD, anterior nuclei (AD, AM, AV), ventral internal medullary lamina, ventral amygdalofugal pathway, mamillothalamic tract	Fluctuating arousal and orientation Impaired learning, memory, autobiographic memory Superimposition of temporally unrelated information Personality changes, apathy, abulia Executive failure, perseveration True to hemisphere: language if VL involved on left; hemispatial neglect if right-sided Emotional expression, acalculia, apraxia
Paramedian artery (arises from P1 segment of posterior cerebral artery)	MD, intralaminar (CM, Pf, CL), posteromedial VL, ventromedial pulvinar, paraventricular, LD, dorsal internal medullary lamina	Decreased arousal (coma vigil if bilateral) Impaired learning and memory, confabulation, temporal disorientation, poor autobiographic memory Aphasia if left-sided, spatial deficits if right-sided Altered social skills and personality, including apathy, aggression, agitation
Inferolateral artery (arises from P2 segment of posterior cerebral artery)		
Principal inferolateral branches	Ventroposterior complexes: VPM, VPL, VP1 Ventral lateral nucleus, ventral (motor) part	Sensory loss (variable extent, all modalities) Hemiataxia Hemiparesis Postlesion pain syndrome (Dejerine-Roussy): right hemisphere predominant
Medial branches	Medial geniculate	Auditory consequences
Inferolateral pulvinar branches	Rostral and lateral pulvinar, LD nucleus	Behavioral
Posterior choroidal artery (arises from P2 segment of posterior cerebral artery)		
Lateral branches	LGN, LD, LP, inferolateral parts of pulvinar	Visual field loss (hemianopsia, quadrantanopsia)
Medial branches	MGN, posterior parts of CM and CL, pulvinar	Variable sensory loss, weakness, aphasia, memory impairment, dystonia, hand tremor

Modified from Schmahmann,[171] with permission. Abbreviations of thalamic nuclei: AD, anterodorsal; AM, anteromedial; AV, anteroventral; CL, centrolateral CM, centromedial; LD, laterodorsal; LGN, lateral geniculate; LP, lateroposterior; MD, mediodorsal; MGN, medial geniculate;Pf, parafascicular; VA, ventroanterior; VL, ventrolateral; VPI, ventroposteroinferior; VPL, ventroposterolateral; VMP, ventroposteromedial.

Venous Sinus Thrombosis

The venous drainage of the brain is susceptible to thrombosis in the same way as other
venous circulations.[178] Most often, this occurs
during a hypercoagulable state related either
to dehydration, infection, or childbirth or associated with a systemic neoplasm. The thrombosis may begin in a draining cerebral vein, or
it may involve mainly one or more of the dural
sinuses. The most common of these conditions
is thrombosis of the superior sagittal sinus.[179]
Such patients complain of a vertex headache, which is usually quite severe. There is
increased ICP, which may be as high as 60 cm
of water on lumbar puncture and often causes
papilledema. The CSF pressure may be sufficiently high to impair brain perfusion. There
is also an increase in venous back-pressure in
the brain (due to poor venous drainage), and
so the arteriovenous pressure gradient is further reduced, and cerebral perfusion is at
risk. This causes local edema and sometimes
frank infarction. For example, in sagittal sinus
thrombosis, the impaired venous outflow from
the paramedian walls of the cerebral hemisphere may result in bilateral lower extremity
hyperreflexia and extensor plantar responses,
and sometimes even paraparesis. Extravasation
into the infarcted tissue, due to continued high
perfusion pressure, causes local hemorrhage,
hemorrhagic CSF, and seizures.

Thrombosis of the lateral sinus causes pain in
the region behind the ipsilateral ear. The thrombosis may be associated with mastoiditis, in
which case the pain due to the sinus thrombosis
may be overlooked. If the outflow through the
other lateral sinus remains patent, there may be
little or no change in CSF pressure. However,
the lateral sinuses are often asymmetric, and if
the dominant one is occluded, there may not
be sufficient venous outflow from the intracranial space. This may cause impairment of CSF
outflow as well, a condition that is sometimes
known as "otitic hydrocephalus." Lateral sinus
thrombosis also causes venous stasis in the adjacent ventrolateral wall of the temporal lobe.
Infarction in this area may produce little in the
way of focal signs, but hemorrhage into the
infarcted tissue may produce seizures or herniation from mass effect.

Thrombosis of superficial cortical veins may
be associated with local cortical dysfunction,
but more often may present with seizures and
focal headache.[180] Thrombosis of deep cerebral veins, such as the internal cerebral veins
or vein of Galen, or even in the straight sinus,
generally presents as a rapidly progressive syndrome with headache, nausea and vomiting,
and then impaired consciousness progressing
to coma.[181] Impaired blood flow in the thalamus and upper midbrain may lead to venous
infarction, hemorrhage, and coma. Venous
thrombosis associated with coma generally
has a poor prognosis, whereas awake and alert
patients usually do well.[179]

Venous occlusion is suggested when the pattern of infarction does not match an arterial
distribution, especially if the infarct contains a
region of hemorrhage. However, in many cases
of venous sinus thrombosis, there will be little,
if any, evidence of focal brain injury. In those
cases, the main clues will often be elevated
pressure with or without red cells in the CSF.
Sometimes lack of blood flow in the venous
sinus system will be apparent even on routine
CT or MRI scan, although often it is not clearly
evident. Either CT or MR venogram can easily
make the diagnosis, but unless the examining
physician thinks of the diagnosis and asks for
the study, the diagnosis may be overlooked.
Although no controlled trials prove efficacy,
anticoagulation and thrombolytic therapy
are believed to be effective; some thrombi
recanalize spontaneously.[179,180,182]

Vasculitis

Vasculitis affecting the brain either can occur as
part of a systemic disorder[183] (e.g., polyarteritis
nodosa, granulomatosis with polyangiitis, giant
cell arteritis) or can be restricted to the nervous
system (e.g., CNS granulomatous angiitis).[184,185]
Vasculitis causes impairment of consciousness
by ischemia or infarction that either affects the
hemispheres diffusely or the brainstem arousal
systems. The diagnosis can be suspected in
a patient with headache, fluctuating consciousness, and focal neurologic signs (Table
4.13). The systemic vasculitides are generally
diagnosed based on their involvement of other
organ systems.[183]

Granulomatous angiitis, also known as primary CNS vasculitis, is the most common
CNS vasculitis. The CSF may contain an
increased number of lymphocytes or may
be normal. The CT scan may likewise be
normal, but MRI usually demonstrates areas
of ischemia or infarction. Magnetic resonance
angiography (MRA) may demonstrate multifocal narrowing of small blood vessels or may
be normal. High-resolution arteriography
is more likely to demonstrate small vessel

Table 4.13 **Symptoms and Signs in 78 Reported Cases of Patients with Documented Central Nervous System Granulomatous Angitis**

Symptom/Sign	No. at onset	Total no. recorded during the course of the disease
Mental changes	45	61
Headache	42	42
Coma	0	42
Focal weakness	12	33
Seizure	9	18
Fever	16	16
Ataxia	7	11
Aphasia	4	10
Visual changes (diplopia, amaurosis, and blurring)	7	9
Tetraparesis	0	9
Flaccid or spastic paraparesis (with back pain, sensory level, and urinary incontinence)	7	8

From Younger et al.[196] with permission.

abnormalities. A definitive diagnosis can be made only by biopsy. Even then, because of sampling error, biopsy may not establish the diagnosis. The treatment depends on the cause of vasculitis; most of the disorders are immune-mediated and are treated by immunosuppression, usually with corticosteroids and cyclophosphamide.[184,185]

INFECTIONS AND INFLAMMATORY CAUSES OF SUPRATENTORIAL DESTRUCTIVE LESIONS

Viral Encephalitis

Although bacteria, fungi, and parasites can all invade the brain (encephalitis) with or without involvement of the meninges (meningoencephalitis), they tend to form localized infections. Viral encephalitis, by distinction, is often widespread and bilateral, and hence coma is a common feature. The organisms destroy tissue both by direct invasion and as a result of the immune response to the infectious agent. They may further impair neurologic function as toxins produced by the organisms, or cytokines or prostaglandins in response to the presence of the organisms, may interfere with neuronal function.

Although many different organisms can cause encephalitis, including a number of arthropod-borne viruses (so-called arboviruses)

with regional variations in prevalence (eastern and western equine, St. Louis, Japanese, and West Nile viruses), by far the most common and serious cause of sporadic encephalitis is herpes simplex type I.[187] Herpes encephalitis accounts for 10–20% of all viral infections of the CNS. Patients characteristically have fever, headache, and alteration of consciousness that culminate in coma (Table 4.14). Personality changes, memory impairment, or seizures focus attention on the medial temporal, frontal, and insular areas, where the infection usually begins and is most severe.[187,188]

Routine examination of CSF is not very helpful. There is usually a pleocytosis with a white count of as many as 100 cells and a protein concentration averaging 100 mg/dL. Red cells may or may not be present. As many as 10% of patients may have a normal CSF examination when initially seen. Polymerase chain reaction (PCR) detection of herpes simplex virus in CSF is diagnostic, but there is a small percentage of false-negative PCR so that a full course of antiviral treatment is recommended in typical cases, even if the initial PCR is negative. The EEG may be helpful if it shows slowing or epileptiform activity arising from the temporal lobe. CT and MRI are very helpful, showing edema and then destruction predominantly in the temporal and frontal lobes and often in the insular cortex (Figure 4.11). The destruction can initially be unilateral but usually rapidly becomes bilateral. The differential diagnosis includes other forms of encephalitis including bacterial and viral, and even

Table 4.14 Findings in 113 Patients with Herpes Simplex Encephalitis

	No. (%) of patients		No. (%) of patients
Historic Findings		*Clinical Findings at*	
Alteration of	109/112 (97)	*Presentation*	
consciousness		Fever	101/110 (92)
Cerebrospinal fluid	107/110 (97)	Personality change	69/81 (85)
pleocytosis		Dysphasia	58/76 (76)
Fever	101/112 (90)	Autonomic dysfunction	53/88 (60)
Headache	89/110 (81)	Ataxia	22/55 (40)
Personality change	62/87 (71)	Hemiparesis	41/107 (38)
Seizures	73/109 (67)	Seizures	43/112 (38)
Vomiting	51/111 (46)	Focal	28
Hemiparesis	33/100 (33)	Generalized	10
Memory loss	14/59 (24)	Both	5
Cranial nerve defects	34/105 (32)	Visual field loss	8/58 (14)
		Papilledema	16/111(14)

From Whitley et al. with permission.[189]

low-grade astrocytomas of the medial temporal lobe, which may present with seizures and a subtle low-density lesion.

It is very important to begin treatment as early as possible with an antiviral agent such as acyclovir.[180,181] Details of treatment are provided in Chapter 8. Most patients who are treated promptly at an early stage of the infection, before there is extensive tissue damage, make a full recovery, although an occasional patient is left with severe memory loss.

Acute Disseminated Encephalomyelitis

Acute disseminated encephalomyelitis (ADEM) is an allergic, presumably autoimmune, encephalitis that is seen during or after an infectious illness, but which may also be caused by vaccination. Spontaneous sporadic cases are believed to result from a subclinical infectious illness.[190] Patients develop multifocal neurologic symptoms, usually over a period of several days, about 1–2 weeks after a febrile illness. Neurologic signs may include a wide variety of sensory and motor complaints, as they do in patients with multiple sclerosis, but a key differentiating point is that a much larger percentage of patients with ADEM present with behavioral disturbances, whereas this is rare early in multiple sclerosis.[191] Occasionally patients

with ADEM may become stuporous or comatose (see Patient Vignette 4.4), findings that are also rare in early multiple sclerosis. CT or MRI scan shows multifocal enhancing lesions in the white matter, but these may appear late in the illness (see Patient Vignette 4.4). Although the pathology is distinct from multiple sclerosis, showing mainly perivascular infiltration and demyelination, the appearance of the lesions on MRI scan is essentially identical in the two illnesses. CSF may show 100 or more white blood cells and an elevation of protein, but may show no changes at all; oligoclonal bands are often absent.

In most cases, it is difficult to distinguish ADEM from the first onset of multiple sclerosis. The likelihood of ADEM is increased if the patient has recently had a febrile illness, if the illness is dominated by behavioral or cognitive problems or impairment of consciousness, or if there are large plaques in the hemispheric white matter. However, the proof of the diagnosis is established by the course of the illness. Although ADEM can fluctuate, and new symptoms and plaques can continue to appear for up to several weeks, it is essentially a monotonic illness, whereas new lesions appearing after 1 or more months generally portend the diagnosis of multiple sclerosis. Overall, in various series, approximately one-third of patients initially diagnosed with ADEM go on to develop multiple sclerosis.

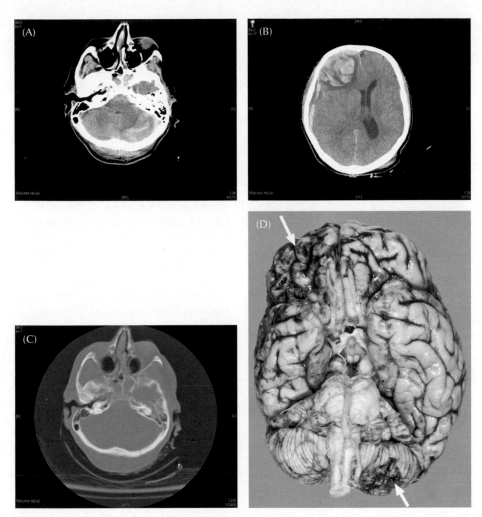

Figure 4.11 A series of computed tomography (CT) scans, and postmortem brain examination, of a 74-year-old woman who fell down a flight of stairs. She was initially alert and confused, but rapidly slipped into coma, which progressed to complete loss of brainstem reflexes by the time she arrived at the hospital. CT scan showed left cerebellar contusion (A) underlying an occipital fracture (C). There was a right frontal intraparenchymal hematoma and subdural hematoma (B). The cerebellar and frontal contusions could be seen from the surface of the brain at autopsy to demonstrate a coup (occipital injury) and contrecoup (frontal contusion from impact against the inside of the skull) injury pattern (arrows in D). Pathology image provided by Dr. Jeffrey Joseph.

Patient Vignette 4.4

A 42-year-old secretary had pharyngitis, fever, nausea, and vomiting, followed 3 days later by confusion and progressive leg weakness. She came to the emergency department, where she was found to have a stiff neck, left abducens palsy, and moderate leg weakness, with a sensory level at around T8 to pin. She rapidly became stuporous, then comatose, with flaccid quadriplegia.

Spinal fluid showed 81 white blood cells/mm^3, with 87% lymphocytes, protein 66 mg/dL, and glucose 66 mg/dL. A magnetic resonance imaging (MRI) scan of the brain and the spinal cord, including contrast, at the time of onset of impaired consciousness and then again 2 days later did not show any abnormalities. She required intubation and mechanical ventilation. A repeat MRI scan on day 8 demonstrated patchy, poorly marginated areas of T2 signal hyperintensity in the white matter of both cerebral hemispheres, the brainstem, and the cerebellum, consistent with ADEM. She was treated with corticosteroids and, over a period of 3 months, recovered, finished rehabilitation, and was able to resume her career and playing tennis.

Although there have been no controlled, randomized trials, treatment of ADEM generally differs from multiple sclerosis. Although most patients are treated initially with high-dose intravenous corticosteroids, this is usually followed by a prolonged, slowly tapering course of corticosteroids which may require several months to avoid recrudescence, rather than the more rapid steroid taper usually employed in treating multiple sclerosis.[191] Details of treatment are given in Chapter 8.

CONCUSSION AND OTHER TRAUMATIC BRAIN INJURIES

Traumatic brain injury, a common cause of coma, is usually easily established because there is a history or external signs of head injury at the time of presentation. Nevertheless, because so many traumatic events occur in individuals who are already impaired by drug ingestion or comorbid illnesses (e.g., hypoglycemia in a diabetic), other causes of loss of consciousness must always be considered. The nature of the traumatic intracranial process that produces impairment of consciousness requires rapid evaluation, as compressive processes such as epidural or subdural hematoma may need immediate surgical intervention. Once these have been ruled out, however, the underlying traumatic brain injury may itself be sufficient to cause coma.

Traumatic brain injury that causes coma falls into two broad classes: closed head trauma and direct brain injury as a result of penetrating head trauma. Penetrating head trauma may directly injure the ascending arousal system, or it may lead to hemorrhage or edema that further impairs brain function. These issues have been discussed in Chapter 3. An additional consideration is that trauma sufficient to cause head injury may also involve the neck, with dissection of a carotid or vertebral artery. These considerations are covered in the sections on vascular occlusions. The discussion that follows will focus primarily on the injuries that occur to the brain as a result of closed head trauma.

Mechanism of Brain Injury During Closed Head Trauma

During closed head trauma, several physical forces may act on the brain to cause injury. If the injuring force is applied focally, the skull is briefly distorted and a shock wave is transmitted to the underlying brain. This shock wave can be particularly intense when the skull is struck a glancing blow by a high-speed projectile, such as a bullet. As demonstrated in Patient Vignette 3.2, the bullet need not penetrate the skull or even fracture the bone to transmit enough kinetic energy to injure the underlying brain.

A second mechanism of injury occurs when the initial blow causes the head to snap backward or forward, to the point where it is stopped either by the limits of neck movement or by another solid object (a wall or floor, a head restraint in a car, etc.). The initial blow causes the skull to accelerate against the underlying brain, which floats semi-independently in a pool of CSF. When it is impelled by the inner table of the skull, the brain then accelerates to the same speed as the skull, but when the skull's trajectory is suddenly stopped, the brain continues onward to strike the inner table of the skull opposite the original site of the blow (Figure 4.11). This *coup-contrecoup injury* model was first described by Courville[192] and then documented in the pioneering studies by Gurdjian,[193] who used high-speed motion pictures to capture the brain and skull movements during concussion in monkeys in whom the calvaria had been replaced by a plastic dome. If the initial blow is occipital, frontal and temporal lobe damage may be worse than the damage at the site of the blow because of the conformation of the skull, which is smoothly curved at the occipital pole but comes to a narrow angle at the frontal and temporal poles. As a result of this anatomy, it is not unusual for the greatest damage to the brain to occur at these poles, regardless of where the head is hit. Even in the absence of parenchymal brain damage, movement of the brain may shear off the delicate olfactory nerve fibers exiting the skull through the cribriform plate, causing anosmia.

Brain injury as a result of closed head trauma may be either a contusion (an area of brain edema visualized on CT or MRI) or focal hemorrhage. Even when no hemorrhage is seen initially on scan, it is not unusual for CSF to show some blood if a lumbar puncture is done. The hemorrhage itself is typically not large enough to cause brain injury or dysfunction. However, the blood may incite seizure activity. Seizures occurring at the time of the head injury do not necessarily herald a subsequent seizure disorder, although the presence of hemorrhage does increase the risk of a long-term seizure disorder.[194] In addition, seizures themselves and the following postictal state may complicate the evaluation of the degree of brain injury.

A third mechanism of brain injury is due to shearing force on long axonal tracts. Because the long axis of the brainstem is located at about an 80-degree angle with respect to the long axis of the forebrain, the long tracts connecting the forebrain with the brainstem and spinal cord take an abrupt turn at the mesodiencephalic junction. In addition, because the head is tethered to the neck, which is not displaced by a blow to the head, there is an additional rotational displacement of the head depending on the angle of the blow. These movements of the forebrain with respect to the brainstem produce a transverse shearing force at the mesodiencephalic junction, resulting in diffuse axonal injury to the long tracts that run between the forebrain and brainstem.[195–198]

Mechanism of Loss of Consciousness in Concussion

The term *concussion* refers to transient alteration in mental status that may or may not involve loss of consciousness, resulting from trauma to the brain.[199,200] Although the most dramatic symptom of concussion is transient loss of consciousness, the hallmarks of the disorder are amnesia and confusion; other symptoms may include headache, visual disturbances, and dizziness.

The mechanism of loss of consciousness with a blow to the head is not completely understood. However, in experiments by Gennarelli and colleagues, using an apparatus to accelerate the heads of monkeys without skull impact, rotational acceleration in the sagittal plane typically produced only brief loss of consciousness,

whereas acceleration from the lateral direction caused mainly prolonged and severe coma.[196] Brief loss of consciousness, which in humans is usually not associated with any changes on CT or MRI scan, may be due to the shearing forces transiently applied to the ascending arousal system at the mesodiencephalic junction. Physiologically, the concussion causes abrupt neuronal depolarization and promotes release of excitatory neurotransmitters. There is increased glutamate release, which results in efflux of potassium from cells as well as calcium influx into cells, and spreading depression, which may account for some concussive symptoms. There are also alterations in cerebral blood flow and glucose metabolism, all of which impair neuronal and axonal function.[201]

Longer term loss of consciousness may be due to mechanical injury to the brain, a condition that Adams and colleagues termed *diffuse axonal injury*.[195] Examination of the brains of animals with prolonged unconsciousness in the Gennarelli experiments was associated with diffuse axonal injury (axonal retraction balls and microglial clusters in the white matter, indicating a site of injury) and with hemorrhagic injury to the corpus callosum and to the dorsal surface of the mesopontine junction. These latter sites underlie the free edge of the falx and the tentorium, respectively. Hence, in these cases, the brain displacement is presumably severe enough to hammer the free dural edges against the underlying brain with sufficient force to cause local tissue necrosis and hemorrhage. Similar pathology was seen in 45 human cases of traumatic closed head injury, all of whom died without awakening after the injury.[195] Contusion or hemorrhage into the corpus callosum or dorsolateral mesopontine tegmentum may be visible on MRI scan. Diffuse axonal injury may cause reduced white matter integrity detected by lower fractional anisotropy and higher mean diffusivity on diffusion tensor imaging MRI or by MRS, which typically shows a reduction in N-acetylaspartate as well as elevation of choline/creatinine ratios.[202–204]

Delayed Encephalopathy After Head Injury

In some cases after an initial period of unconsciousness after a closed head injury, the patient may awaken and the CT scan may be normal, but then the patient may show cognitive deterioration and lapse into coma hours to several days later. This pattern was characterized by Reilly and colleagues as patients who "talk and die."[11,205] Repeat CT scan typically shows areas of intraparenchymal edema and perhaps hemorrhage, which may have shown only minimal injury at the time of initial presentation. However, with the evolution of brain edema over the next few hours and days, the mass effect may reach a critical level at which it impairs cerebral perfusion or causes brain herniation.

This condition occurs most commonly in children and young adults in whom the brain usually fully occupies the intracranial space, so that even minimal swelling may put the brain at risk of injury. Elderly individuals, in whom there has been some cerebral atrophy, may have enough excess intracranial capacity to avoid reaching this crossroad. On the other hand, older individuals may be more likely to deteriorate later due to subdural or epidural hemorrhage or to injuries outside the nervous system.[11] Hence, any patient with deterioration of wakefulness in the days following head injury requires repeat and urgent scanning, even if the original scan was normal.

More common is the so-called postconcussion syndrome. This disorder is characterized by headache, dizziness, irritability, and difficulty with memory and attention after mild concussion and particularly after repeated concussions.[206] Because it often follows mild head injury, psychologic factors have been imputed by some, but the syndrome clearly appears to result from mild although not anatomically identifiable brain damage.

More disturbing is chronic traumatic encephalopathy, a neurodegenerative disorder seen in individuals with repeated head trauma, often due to high-impact sports or combat injuries. The distinctive distribution of tau deposition in the cerebral cortex, often in the depths of sulci, is associated with dementia and psychiatric disease.[207–209] MRI shows findings similar to more recent traumatic brain injury on diffusion tensor or MRS, suggesting that the changes that occur acutely may persist indefinitely.[210] However, the onset of the neurodegeneration is gradual and progressive, generally years after the original head injury, so that it is not a concern in acute disorders of consciousness.

INFRATENTORIAL DESTRUCTIVE LESIONS

Infratentorial destructive lesions causing coma include hemorrhage, tumors, infections, and infarcts in the brainstem. Although hemorrhage into tumors, infections, or masses also compress normal tissue, they appear to have their major effect in the brainstem through direct destruction of arousal systems.

If the lesion is large enough, patients with destructive infratentorial lesions often lose consciousness immediately, and the ensuing coma is accompanied by distinctive patterns of respiratory, pupillary, oculovestibular, and motor signs that clearly indicate whether it is the tegmentum of the midbrain, the rostral pons, or the caudal pons that initially is most severely damaged. The brainstem arousal system lies so close to nuclei and pathways influencing the pupils, eye movements, and other major functions that primary brainstem destructive lesions that cause coma characteristically cause focal neurologic signs that can precisely localize the lesion anatomically. This restricted, discrete localization is unlike metabolic lesions causing coma, where the signs commonly indicate incomplete but symmetric dysfunction and few, if any, focal signs of brainstem dysfunction (see Chapter 2). Primary brainstem injury also is unlike the secondary brainstem dysfunction that follows supratentorial herniation, in which *all* functions above a given brainstem level tend to be lost as the process descends from rostral to caudal along the neuraxis.

Certain combinations of signs stand out prominently in patients with infratentorial destructive lesions causing coma. At the *midbrain* level, centrally placed brainstem lesions interrupt the pathway for the pupillary light reflex and often damage the oculomotor nuclei as well. The resulting deep coma commonly is accompanied by pupils that are fixed at midposition or slightly wider, by abnormalities of eye movements due to damage to the third or fourth nerves or their nuclei, and by long-tract motor signs. These last-mentioned signs result from involvement of the cerebral peduncles and commonly are bilateral, although asymmetric.

Destructive lesions of the *rostral pons* commonly spare the oculomotor nuclei but interrupt the medial longitudinal fasciculus and the adjacent ocular sympathetic pathways. Patients typically have tiny pupils, internuclear ophthalmoplegia (only lateral movements of the eyes on vestibulo-ocular testing), and, in many instances, cranial nerve signs of trigeminal or facial dysfunction, betraying pontine destruction.

Severe *midpontine destruction* can cause a functional transection with physiologic effects that may be difficult to differentiate from metabolic coma. The pupils of such patients are miotic but may react minimally to light since midbrain parasympathetic oculomotor fibers are spared. Reflex lateral eye movements are absent because the pontine structures for lateral conjugate eye movements are destroyed. However, upward and downward ocular deviation occasionally is retained either spontaneously or in response to vestibulo-ocular testing, and, if present, this dissociation between lateral and vertical movement clearly identifies pontine destruction. Ocular bobbing sometimes accompanies such acute destructive lesions and, when present, usually, but not always, indicates primary posterior fossa disease. The motor signs of severe pontine destruction are not the same in every patient and can include flaccid quadriplegia, less often extensor posturing, or occasionally extensor posturing responses in the arms with flexor responses or flaccidity in the legs. Respiration may show any of the patterns characteristic of low brainstem dysfunction described in Chapter 1, but cluster breathing, apneusis, gasping, and ataxic breathing are characteristic.

As discussed in Chapter 2, patients with destructive lesions confined to the lower pons or medulla do not show loss of consciousness, although they may be locked-in, in which case only the preservation of voluntary vertical eye and eyelid movements may indicate the wakeful state.

BRAINSTEM VASCULAR DESTRUCTIVE DISORDERS

In contrast to the carotid circulation, occlusion of the vertebrobasilar system is frequently associated with coma. Although lesions confined to the lower brainstem do not cause coma, impairment of blood flow in the vertebral or low basilar arteries may reduce blood flow distally in the basilar artery to a level that is below the critical minimum necessary to maintain normal function. The classic presentation of ischemic coma of brainstem origin is produced by occlusion of the basilar artery. The patient falls acutely into a comatose state, and the pupils may initially be large, usually indicating intense adrenal outflow at the time of the initial onset, but eventually become either miotic (pontine level occlusion) or fixed and midposition (midbrain level occlusion). Oculovestibular eye movements may be absent, asymmetric, or skewed (pontine level), or vertical and adduction movements may be absent with preserved abduction (midbrain level). There may be hemiplegia, quadriplegia, or decerebrate posturing. Respiration may be apneustic or ataxic in pattern if the lesion also involves the pons.

Occlusion of the basilar artery either by thrombosis or embolism is a relatively common cause of coma. The occlusions are usually the result of atherosclerotic or hypertensive disease. Emboli to the basilar artery usually result from valvular heart disease or artery-to-artery embolization.[211] Cranial arteritis involving the vertebral arteries in the neck also can lead to secondary basilar artery ischemia with brainstem infarction and coma.[212] Vertebrobasilar artery dissection, either from trauma such as whiplash injury or chiropractic manipulation,[213,214] or occurring spontaneously, is becoming increasingly recognized as a common cause of brainstem infarction due to the ease of identifying it on MRA.

Most patients in coma from brainstem infarction are over 50 years of age, but this is not an exclusive limit. One of our patients was only 34 years old. The onset can be sudden coma or progressive neurologic symptoms culminating in coma. In some patients, characteristic transient symptoms and signs owing to brief ischemia of the brainstem precede coma by days or weeks.[215] These transient attacks typically change from episode to episode but always reflect infratentorial CNS dysfunction and include headaches (mainly occipital), diplopia, vertigo (usually with nausea), dysarthria, dysphagia, bilateral or alternating motor or sensory symptoms, or drop attacks (sudden spontaneous falls while standing or walking, without loss of consciousness and with complete recovery in seconds). The attacks usually last for as short a period as 10 seconds or as long as several minutes. Seldom are they more prolonged, although we have seen recurrent transient attacks of otherwise unexplained akinetic coma lasting 20–30 minutes in a patient who later died from pontine infarction caused by basilar occlusion. Except in patients who additionally have recurrent asystole or other severe cardiac arrhythmias, transient ischemic attacks caused by vertebrobasilar artery insufficiency nearly always occur in the erect or sitting position. Some patients with a critical stenosis may have positional symptoms that are present while sitting but improve when lying down.

Patient Vignette 4.5

A 78-year-old architect with hypertension and diabetes was returning on an airplane from Europe to the United States when he complained of dizziness, double vision, and nausea, then collapsed back into his seat unconscious. His seat was laid back and he gradually regained consciousness. A neurologist was present on the airplane and was called to his side. Limited neurologic examination found that he was drowsy, with small but reactive pupils and lateral gaze nystagmus to either side. There was dysmetria with both hands.

On taking a history, he was returning from a vacation in Germany where he had similar symptoms and had been hospitalized for several weeks. Magnetic resonance imaging (MRI) scans, which he was carrying with him back to his doctors at home, showed severe stenosis of the midportion of the basilar artery. He had been kept at bedrest with the head of the bed initially down, but gradually raised to 30 degrees while in the hospital, and then discharged when he could sit without symptoms. His chair back was kept as low as possible for the remainder of the flight, and he was taken from the airplane to a tertiary care hospital where he was treated with anticoagulants and gradual readjustment to an upright posture.

Table 4.15 **Symptoms and Signs of Basilar Artery Occlusion in 85 Patients**

Symptom	No. of patients	Supranuclear oculomotor disturbances	No. of patients
Vertigo, nausea	39	Horizontal gaze paresis	22
Headache, neckache	22	Gaze-paretic, gaze-induced nystagmus	15
Dysarthria	23	Oculocephalic reflex lost	6
Ataxia, dysdiadochokinesia	27	Vestibular nystagmus	5
Cranial nerve palsy		Vertical gaze palsy	4
III	13	Downbeat nystagmus	4
IV, VI, VII	30	Internuclear ophthalmoplegia	4
VIII (acoustic)	5	Ocular bobbing	3
IX–XII	24	One-and-a-half syndrome	2
Occipital lobe signs	11	Other/not classifiable	16
Respiration	9		
Central Horner's syndrome	4	**Long-tract signs**	**No. of patients**
Seizures	4		
Sweating	5	Hemiparesis	21
Myoclonus	6	Tetraparesis	31
		Tetraplegia	15
Consciousness	**No. of patients**	Locked-in syndrome	9
		Hemihypesthesia	11
Awake	31		
Psychosis, disturbed memory	5		
Somnolence	20		
Stupor	5		
Coma	26		

Modified from Ferbert et al. [215]

In some cases, segmental thrombi can occlude the vertebral or basilar arteries while producing only limited and temporary symptoms of brainstem dysfunction.[215] In one series, only 31 of 85 patients with angiographically proved basilar or bilateral vertebral artery occlusion were stuporous or comatose.[215] The degree of impairment of consciousness presumably depends on how much the collateral vascular supply protects the central brainstem structures contributing to the arousal system. The clinical signs of basilar artery occlusion are listed in Table 4.15. Most unconscious patients have respiratory abnormalities, which may include periodic breathing or various types of irregular or ataxic respiration. The pupils are almost always abnormal and may be small (pontine), midposition (midbrain), or dilated (third-nerve outflow in midbrain). Most patients have divergent or skewed eyes reflecting direct nuclear and internuclear damage (Table 4.15). Patients with basilar occlusion who become comatose have a nearly uniformly fatal outcome in the absence of thrombolytic or endovascular intervention.[216]

Historical Patient Vignette 4.6

A 56-year-old woman was admitted in coma. She had been an accountant and in good health except for known hypertension treated with hydrochlorothiazide. She suddenly collapsed at her desk and was rushed to the emergency department, where her blood pressure was 180/100 mm Hg. She had sighing respirations, which shortly changed to a Cheyne-Stokes pattern. The pupils were 4 mm in diameter and unreactive to light. The oculocephalic responses were absent, but cold caloric irrigation induced abduction of the eye only on the side being irrigated. She responded to noxious stimuli with extensor posturing and occasionally was racked by spontaneous waves of extensor rigidity.

A computed tomography (CT) scan was initially read as normal. A basilar artery embolus was suspected clinically, but as this occurred prior to the era of magnetic resonance imaging (MRI) scanning, intravenous thrombolysis, or endovascular intervention, she was brought to the neurology intensive

care unit for supportive care. The cerebrospinal fluid pressure on lumbar puncture was 140 mm of water; the fluid was clear, without cells, and contained 35 mg/dL of protein. Two days later, the patient continued in coma with extensor responses to noxious stimulation; the pupils remained fixed in midposition, and there was no ocular response to cold caloric irrigation. Respirations were eupneic. Repeat CT scan showed lucency in the medial pons and midbrain. She died the following day, and the brain was examined postmortem. The basilar artery was occluded in its midportion by a recent thrombus 1 cm in length. There was extensive infarction of the rostral portion of the base of the pons, as well as the medial pontine and midbrain tegmentum. The lower portion of the pons and the medulla were intact.

Comment

This woman suffered an acute brainstem infarction with unusually symmetric neurologic signs. She was initially diagnosed with an infarct at the midbrain level based on her clinical picture. Other considerations included a thalamic hemorrhage with sudden acute transtentorial herniation producing a picture of acute midbrain transection. However, such rapid progression to a midbrain level almost never occurs in patients with supratentorial intracerebral hemorrhages. The CT scan and the absence of red blood cells on the lumbar puncture ruled out subarachnoid hemorrhage as well. Finally, the neurologic signs of midbrain damage in this patient remained nearly constant from onset, whereas transtentorial herniation would rapidly have produced further rostral-caudal deterioration.

The diagnosis can usually be made on the basis of clinical signs alone, and eye movement signs are particularly helpful in determining the brainstem level of the dysfunction (Table 4.16). However, the nature of the problem must be confirmed by imaging.

Acutely, the CT scan may not reveal a parenchymal lesion, although hyperintensity within the basilar artery on CT may suggest

Table 4.16 Eye Movement Disorders in Brainstem Infarcts

Midbrain syndromes	Pons syndromes
Upper midbrain syndromes	**Paramedian syndromes**
Conjugate vertical gaze palsy: upgaze palsy, downgaze, palsy, combined upgaze and downgaze	Conjugate disorders
	Ipsilateral gaze paralysis
Dorsal midbrain syndrome	Complete gaze paralysis
Slowness of smooth pursuit movements	Loss of ipsilateral horizontal saccades
Torsional nystagmus	Loss of both horizontal and vertical saccadic gaze movements
Pseudoabducens palsy	
Convergence-retraction nystagmus	Primary-position downbeating nystagmus
Disconjugate vertical gaze palsy: monocular elevation palsy, prenuclear syndrome of the oculomotor nucleus, crossed vertical gaze paresis, and vertical one-and-a half syndrome	Tonic conjugate eye deviation away from lesion
	Disconjugate disorders
	Unilateral internuclear ophthalmoplegia
	Bilateral internuclear ophthalmoplegia
Skew deviation with alternating appearance	Internuclear ophthalmoplegia and skew deviation
Ocular tilt reaction	One-and-a-half syndrome
See-saw nystagmus	Paralytic pontine exotropia
Middle midbrain syndrome	Ocular bobbing: typical, atypical, and paretic
Nuclear third-nerve palsy	**Lateral pontine syndrome**
Fascicular third-nerve palsy: isolated or associated with crossed hemiplegia, ipsilateral or contralateral hemiataxia, and abnormal movements	Horizontal gaze palsy
	Horizontal and rotatory nystagmus
	Skew deviation
	Internuclear ophthalmoplegia
	Ocular bobbing
Lower midbrain syndrome	One-and-a-half syndrome
Internuclear ophthalmoplegia: isolated or associated with fourth-nerve palsy, bilateral ataxia, and dissociated vertical nystagmus	
Superior oblique myokymia	

Modified from Moncayo and Bogousslavsky.[217]

basilar occlusion.[218] An MRI scan with diffusion-weighted imaging is the most sensitive way to identify the area of infarction (see Figure 4.8B), although in the early stages the basilar artery may show "blooming" artifact on susceptibility-weighted images.[219] Early diagnosis may allow effective treatment with thrombolysis, angioplasty, or embolectomy.[220,221] The differential diagnosis of acute brainstem infarction can usually be made from clinical clues alone. With brainstem infarction, the fact that signs of midbrain or pontine damage accompany the *onset* of coma immediately places the site of the lesion as infratentorial. The illness is maximal at onset or evolves rapidly and in a series of steps, as would be expected with ischemic vascular disease. Supratentorial ischemic vascular lesions, by contrast, with rare exceptions pointed out on page 152, are not likely to cause coma at onset, and they do not begin with pupillary abnormalities or other signs of

direct brain-stem injury (unless the mesencephalon is also involved, e.g., as in the top of the basilar syndrome). Pontine and cerebellar hemorrhages, since they also compress the brainstem, sometimes resemble brainstem infarction in their manifestations. However, most such hemorrhages have a distinctive picture (see earlier discussion). Furthermore, they nearly always arise in hypertensive patients and often are more likely to cause occipital headache (which is unusual with infarction).

Brainstem Hemorrhage

Relatively discrete brainstem hemorrhage can affect the midbrain,[222] the pons,[223] or the medulla.[224] The causes of brainstem hemorrhage include hypertension, vascular malformations, clotting disorders, or trauma. Hypertensive brainstem hemorrhages tend to lie deep

Table 4.17 **Clinical Findings in Patients with Spontaneous Midbrain Hemorrhage**

Findings	Literature cases (N = 66)	Mayo cases (N = 7)	Combined series (N = 73)
Cranial nerve III or IV paresis	58	6	64
Disturbance of consciousness	33	6	39
Headache	34	4	38
Corticospinal tract deficits	32	4	36
Corticobulbar deficits	22 [a]	2	24
Hemisensory deficits	21	3	24
Gait ataxia	22	2	24
Visual hallucinations	3	0	3
Tinnitus or hyperacusis	3	2	5

[a] One patient had corticobulbar deficit without a corticospinal deficit.

From Link et al.,[222] with permission.

within the brainstem substance, are rather diffuse, frequently rupture into the fourth ventricle, occur in elderly persons, and have a poor prognosis for recovery.[225] Brainstem hematomas caused by cavernous angiomas occur in younger individuals, are usually subependymal in location, tend to be more discrete, do not rupture into the ventricle, and have a good prognosis for recovery, but tend to rebleed at a later time.[226] Surgery generally does not have a place in treating brainstem hypertensive hemorrhages, but it is sometimes used to remove superficially located cavernous angiomas.

Primary *midbrain hemorrhages*, which may be of either hypertensive or angiomatous type, are rare. Most patients present acutely with headache, alterations of consciousness, and abnormal eye signs (Table 4.17). The diagnosis is obvious on imaging. Most patients recover completely from bleeds from cavernous angiomas; some remain with mild neurologic deficits.

Hemorrhage into the pons typically arises from the paramedian arterioles, beginning at the base of the tegmentum and usually dissecting in all directions in a relatively symmetric fashion (Figure 4.8A). Rupture into the fourth ventricle is frequent, but dissection into the medulla is rare. Although most patients lose consciousness immediately, in a few cases (as in Patient Vignette 2.1) this is delayed, and in others when the hematoma is small, and particularly when it is confined to the base of the pons, consciousness can be retained. However, such patients often have other focal signs (e.g., a bleed into the base of the pons can present with an acute locked-in state). Such patients, however, often have considerable recovery.[227]

Coma caused by pontine hemorrhage begins abruptly, usually during the hours when patients are awake and active and often without a prodrome. When the onset is witnessed, only a few patients complain of symptoms such as sudden occipital headache, vomiting, dyscoordination, or slurred speech before losing consciousness. Almost every patient with pontine hemorrhage has respiratory abnormalities of the brainstem type: Cheyne-Stokes breathing, apneustic or gasping breathing, and progressive slowing of respiration or apnea (Table 4.18).[223]

In patients who present in coma, the pupils are nearly always abnormal and usually pinpoint. The pupils are often thought to be fixed to light on initial examination, but close examination with a magnifying glass usually demonstrates further constriction. The ciliospinal response disappears. If the hemorrhage extends into the midbrain, pupils may become asymmetric or dilate to midposition. About one-third of patients suffer from oculomotor abnormalities such as skewed or lateral ocular deviations or ocular bobbing (or one of its variants), and the oculocephalic responses disappear. Motor signs vary according to the extent of the hemorrhage. Some subjects become diffusely rigid, tremble, and suffer repeated waves of decerebrate rigidity. More frequently, however, patients are quadriplegic and flaccid with flexor responses at the hip, knee, and great

Table 4.18 **Clinical Findings in 80 Patients with Pontine Hemorrhage**

Level of consciousness	
Alert	15 (0)
Drowsy	21 (3)
Stuporous	4 (3)
Coma	40 (32)
Respiratory disturbance	
Yes	37 (29)
Brachycardia	
Yes	34 (23)
Hyperthermia	
Yes	32 (30)
Pupils	
Normal	29 (1)
Anisocoria	29 (11)
Pinpoint	23 (17)
Mydriasis	9 (9)
Motor disturbance	
Hemiplegia	34 (4)
Tetraplegia	22 (17)
Decerebrate posture [a]	16 (14)

[a] Number who died in parentheses.

Modified from Murata et al.[223]

toe to plantar stimulation, a reflex combination characteristic of acute low brainstem damage when it accompanies acute coma. Nearly all patients with pontine hemorrhage who survive more than a few hours develop fever with body temperatures of 38.5°C to 40°C.[228]

The diagnosis of pontine hemorrhage is usually straightforward. Almost no other lesion, except an occasional cerebellar hemorrhage with secondary dissection into the brainstem, produces sudden coma with periodic or ataxic breathing, pinpoint pupils, absence of oculovestibular responses, and quadriplegia. The pinpoint pupils may suggest an opiate overdose, but the other eye signs and the flaccid quadriplegia are not seen in that condition. If there is any question in an ambiguous case, naloxone can be administered to reverse any opiate intoxication.

Patient Vignette 4.7

A 54-year-old man with poorly treated hypertension was playing tennis when he suddenly collapsed on the court. The blood pressure was 170/90 mm Hg; the pulse was 84 per minute; respirations were Cheyne-Stokes in character and 16 per minute. The pupils were pinpoint but reacted equally to light; eyes were slightly dysconjugate with no spontaneous movement, and vestibulo-ocular responses were absent. The patient was flaccid with symmetric stretch reflexes of normal amplitude and bilateral flexor withdrawal responses in the lower extremities to plantar stimulation. A computed tomography (CT) scan showed a hemorrhage into the pontine tegmentum. The next morning he was still in deep coma, but now was diffusely flaccid except for flexor responses to noxious stimuli in the legs. He had slow, shallow, eupneic respiration; small, equally reactive pupils; and eyes in the neutral position. Shortly thereafter, breathing became irregular and he died. A 3-cm primary hemorrhage destroying the central pons and its tegmentum was found at autopsy.

The clinical features in Patient Vignette 4.7, including coma in the absence of motor responses, corneal reflexes, and oculocephalic responses, predicted the poor outcome.[229] In addition, if CT scanning shows a hematoma greater than 4 mL, hemorrhage in a ventral location, evidence of extension into the midbrain and thalamus, or hydrocephalus on admission, the prognosis is poor.[229,230]

Primary *hemorrhage into the medulla* is rare.[231] Patients present with vertigo, nausea, ataxia, dysphagia, dysarthria, and nystagmus. The combination of impaired elevation of the palate, with weakness of the tongue or the limbs is characteristic. Consciousness is usually preserved unless the hematoma dissects up into the pons.

Basilar Migraine

Altered states of consciousness are an uncommon but distinct aspect of what Bickerstaff called basilar artery migraine, associated with prodromal symptoms that suggest brainstem dysfunction.[232] The alteration in consciousness can take any of four major forms: confusional states, brief syncope, stupor, and unarousable coma. Although not technically a destructive lesion, and with a pathophysiology that is not understood, basilar migraine clearly causes parenchymal dysfunction of the brainstem that is often mistaken for a brainstem ischemic attack.

Alterations in consciousness often last longer than the usual sensorimotor auras seen with migraine. Encephalopathy and coma in migraine occur in patients with familial hemiplegic migraine associated with mutations in a calcium channel[233] and in patients with cerebral autosomal dominant arteriopathy with subcortical infarcts and leukoencephalopathy (CADASIL).[234] The former often have fixed cerebellar signs and the latter multiple hyperintensities of the white matter on MR scanning. Blood flow studies concurrent with migraine aura have demonstrated both diffuse and focal cerebral vasoconstriction, but this is an insufficient explanation for the striking focal symptoms in basilar migraine; however, some clinical lesions suggestive of infarction can be found in patients with migraine significantly more often than in controls.[235]

Selby and Lance in their classic study of 500 consecutive patients with migraine found that 6.8% had prodromal episodes of confusion, automatic behavior, or transient amnesia, while 4.6% actually fainted.[236] The confusional and stuporous attacks can last from minutes to as long as 24 hours or, rarely, more. They range in content from quiet disorientation through agitated delirium to unresponsiveness in which the patient is barely arousable. Transient vertigo, ataxia, diplopia, hemianopsia, hemisensory changes, or hemiparetic changes may immediately precede the mental changes. During attacks, most observers have found few somatic neurologic abnormalities, although occasional patients are reported as having oculomotor palsies, pupillary dilation, or an extensor plantar response. A few patients, at least briefly, have appeared to be in unarousable coma that in rare reportable cases may be prolonged; EEG is typically diffusely slow in the delta or theta range.[237,238]

Posterior Reversible Leukoencephalopathy Syndrome

Once believed to be associated only with malignant hypertension (hypertensive encephalopathy),[239] posterior reversible leukoencephalopathy syndrome (PRES) is known to be caused by several illnesses that affect endothelial cells, particularly in the posterior cerebral circulation.[240] Among the illnesses other than hypertension, pre-eclampsia and immunosuppressive and cytotoxic agents (e.g., cyclosporin, cisplatin) are probably the most common causes. Vasculitis, porphyria, and thrombotic thrombocytopenic purpura are also reported causes, as is occasionally migraine. Posterior leukoencephalopathy is characterized by vasogenic edema of white matter of the posterior circulation, particularly the occipital lobes, but sometimes including the brainstem. Clinically, patients acutely develop headache, confusion, seizures, and cortical blindness; coma is rare. The MRI reveals vasogenic edema primarily affecting the occipital and posterior parietal lobes. Brainstem and cerebellum may also be affected. With appropriate treatment (controlling hypertension or discontinuing drugs), symptoms resolve. In patients with pre-eclampsia who are pregnant, intravenous infusion of magnesium sulfate followed by delivery of the fetus has a similar effect. If PRES due to pre-eclampsia occurs in the postpartum period, immediate administration of magnesium sulfate followed by treatment for several weeks with verapamil is often effective in our experience. The differential diagnosis includes posterior circulation infarction, venous thrombosis, and metabolic coma (see Table 4.19 and Patient Vignette 5.8).

INFRATENTORIAL INFLAMMATORY DISORDERS

The same infective agents that affect the cerebral hemispheres can also affect the brainstem and cerebellum. Encephalitis, meningitis, and abscess formation may either be part of a more generalized infective process or be restricted to the brainstem.[241] Organisms that have a particular predilection for the brainstem include *L. monocytogenes*, which often causes brainstem abscesses (Figure 4.12).[242] Occasionally herpes zoster or simplex infection that begins in one of the sensory cranial nerves may cause a segmental brainstem encephalitis.[243] Behçet's disease may also cause brainstem inflammatory lesions.[244] These disorders usually cause headache with or without nuchal rigidity, fever, and lethargy, but rarely coma. In a minority of instances, the CT scan may show brainstem swelling. The MR scan

Table 4.19 Common Differential Diagnoses of Posterior Leukoencephalopathy Syndrome

	Posterior leukoencephalopathy	Central venous thrombosis	Top of basilar syndrome
Predisposing factors	Eclampsia, renal failure, cytotoxic and immunosuppressive agents, hypertension	Pregnancy, puerperium, dehydration	Risk factors for stroke, cardiac disorders
Onset and progression	Acute, evolves in days	Acute, evolves in days	Sudden, evolves in hours
Clinical features	Seizures precede all other manifestations, visual aura, cortical blindness, confusion, headache, rarely focal deficit	Headaches, seizures, stupor or coma, focal neurologic deficits (monoparesis or hemiparesis), papilledema, evidence of venous thrombosis elsewhere, infrequently hypertensive	Cortical blindness, hemianopia, confusional state, brainstem signs, cerebral signs, rarely seizures
Imaging features	Predominantly white matter edema in bilateral occipital and posterior parietal regions, usually spares paramedian brain parenchyma	Hemorrhage and ischemic infarcts, small ventricles, "cord sign" caused by hyperdense thrombosed vein, evidence of major venous sinus thrombosis on MRI	Infarcts of bilateral paracalcarine cortex, thalamus, inferior medial temporal lobe, and brainstem
Prognosis	Completely resolves after rapid control of BP and removal of offending drug	Intensive management is needed; mortality high in severe cases	No recovery or only partial eventual recovery

BP, blood pressure; MRI, magnetic resonance imaging.

From Garg,[245] with permission.

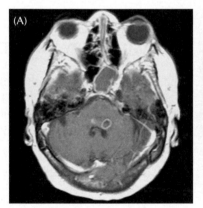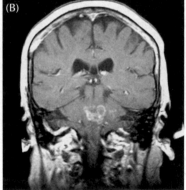

Figure 4.12 A pair of magnetic resonance images demonstrating a multiloculated pontine abscess in a 73-year-old woman (Patient Vignette 2.2) who had been taking chronic prednisone for ulcerative colitis. She developed a fever, nausea and vomiting, left facial numbness, left gaze paresis, left lower motor neuron facial weakness, and left-sided ataxia. Lumbar puncture showed 47 white blood cells/mm³, but culture was negative. She was treated for suspected *Listeria monocytogenes* and recovered slowly, but had residual facial and oropharyngeal weakness requiring chronic tracheostomy.

is usually more sensitive. CSF usually contains an increased number of cells. In bacterial infections, cultures are usually positive; in viral infections, PCR may establish the diagnosis. Stereotactic drainage of a brain abscess often identifies the organisms; appropriate antimicrobial therapy is usually successful.[246]

A peculiar form of brainstem encephalitis, chronic lymphocytic inflammation with pontine perivascular enhancement responsive to steroids (CLIPPERS), was reported in 2010 and may have accounted for some cases thought to represent "sarcoidosis" or "demyelination" of the brainstem in the past.[247,248] The clinical picture is usually one of predominantly motor symptoms (ataxia, diplopia, quadriparesis) rather than affecting level of consciousness.

A brainstem disorder often confused with infection is Bickerstaff's brainstem encephalitis.[249] Patients with this disorder have often had a preceding systemic viral infection, then acutely develop ataxia, ophthalmoplegia, long-tract signs, and alterations of consciousness including coma. In some patients, MRI reveals brainstem swelling and increased T2 signal; in others, the scan is normal. The CSF protein may be elevated, but there are no cells. The disease is believed to be autoimmune in origin related to postinfectious polyneuropathy (the Guillain-Barré syndrome) and the related Miller Fisher syndrome. The diagnosis can be established by the identification of anti-GQ1b ganglioside antibodies in serum.[250] Patients are generally treated as for other forms of the Guillain-Barré syndrome, with either intravenous immune globulin or by plasmapheresis.

INFRATENTORIAL TUMORS

Tumors within the brainstem cause their symptoms by a combination of compression and destruction. Although relatively common in children, primary tumors of the brainstem (brainstem glioma) are rare in adults. Metastatic tumors are more common, but with both primary and metastatic tumors, slowly or subacutely evolving brainstem signs typically establish the diagnosis long before impairment of consciousness occurs. An exception is the rare instance of an acute hemorrhage into the tumor causing the abrupt onset of paralysis and sometimes coma, in which case the signs and treatment are similar to other brainstem hemorrhages.

CENTRAL PONTINE MYELINOLYSIS

This is an uncommon disorder in which the myelin sheaths in the central basal pons are destroyed in a single confluent and symmetric lesion. Similar lesions may be found in the corpus callosum or cerebral hemispheres.[251] Lesions vary from a few millimeters across to ones that encompass almost the entire base of the pons, sparing only a rim of peripheral myelin. The typical clinical picture is one of quadriparesis, with varying degrees of supranuclear paresis of lower motor cranial nerves and impairment of oculomotor or pupillary responses. A majority of patients become "locked-in." Approximately one-quarter of patients demonstrate impairment of level of consciousness, reflecting extension of the lesion into the more dorsal and rostral regions of the pons.

It is now recognized that most cases of central pontine myelinolysis are due to overly vigorous correction of hyponatremia, giving rise to the "osmotic demyelination syndrome." Since the adoption of current regimens that recommend that hyponatremia be reversed at a rate no greater than 10 mEq/day, the frequency of this once-feared complication has decreased dramatically. On the other hand, a similar syndrome is seen in patients with liver transplantation, possibly due to the use of cyclosporine. As liver transplant has become more common, this population is increasing.

REFERENCES

1. Sadashiva N, Baruah S, Rao S, et al. Eosinophilic granuloma of skull with fluid level and epidural hematoma: a case report and review of the literature. *Pediatr Neurosurg* 2017;52:41–45.
2. Kanai R, Kubota H, Terada T, Hata T, Tawaraya E, Fujii K. Spontaneous epidural hematoma due to skull metastasis of hepatocellular carcinoma. *J Clin Neurosci* 2009;16:137–140.
3. Griffiths SJ, Jatavallabhula NS, Mitchell RD. Spontaneous extradural haematoma associated with craniofacial infections: case report and review of the literature. *Br J Neurosurg* 2002;16:188–191.
4. Ben-Israel D, Isaacs AM, Morrish W, Gallagher NC. Acute vertex epidural hematoma. *Surg Neurol Int* 2017;8:219.
5. Shamji MF, Lesiuk H. Traumatic coronal suture diastasis and contre-coup epidural hematoma. *Can J Neurol Sci* 2010;37:906–908.
6. Sunderland S, Bradley KC. Disturbances of oculomotor function accompanying extradural haemorrhage. *J Neurol Neurosurg Psychiatry* 1953;16:35–46.

7. Jamieson KG, Yelland JD. Extradural hematoma. Report of 167 cases. *J Neurosurg* 1968;29:13–23.
8. Gallagher JP, Browder EJ. Extradural hematoma. Experience with 167 patients. *J Neurosurg* 1968;29:1–12.
9. Zangbar B, Serack B, Rhee P, et al. Outcomes in trauma patients with isolated epidural hemorrhage: a single-institution retrospective cohort study. *Am Surg* 2016;82:1209–1214.
10. Browne GJ, Lam LT. Isolated extradural hematoma in children presenting to an emergency department in Australia. *Pediatr Emerg Care* 2002;18:86–90.
11. Dunn LT, Fitzpatrick MO, Beard D, Henry JM. Patients with a head injury who "talk and die" in the 1990s. *J Trauma* 2003;54:497–502.
12. Mower WR, Hoffman JR, Herbert M, Wolfson AB, Pollack CV Jr, Zucker MI. Developing a decision instrument to guide computed tomographic imaging of blunt head injury patients. *J Trauma* 2005;59:954–959.
13. Stiell IG, Clement CM, Rowe BH, et al. Comparison of the Canadian CT Head Rule and the New Orleans Criteria in patients with minor head injury. *JAMA* 2005;294:1511–1518.
14. Shimizu S, Endo M, Kan S, Kitahara T, Ohwada T, Fujii K. Tight sylvian cisterns associated with hyperdense areas mimicking subarachnoid hemorrhage on computed tomography—four case reports. *Neurol Med Chir (Tokyo)* 2001;41:536–540.
15. Servadei F, Teasdale G, Merry G. Defining acute mild head injury in adults: a proposal based on prognostic factors, diagnosis, and management. *J Neurotrauma* 2001;18:657–664.
16. Servadei F. Prognostic factors in severe head injured adult patients with epidural hematomas. *Acta Neurochir (Wien)* 1997;139:273–278.
17. Abe M, Udono H, Tabuchi K, Uchino A, Yoshikai T, Taki K. Analysis of ischemic brain damage in cases of acute subdural hematomas. *Surg Neurol* 2003;59:464–472; discussion 472.
18. Servadei F. Prognostic factors in severely head injured adult patients with acute subdural haematoma's. *Acta Neurochir (Wien)* 1997;139:279–285.
19. Adhiyaman V, Asghar M, Ganeshram KN, Bhowmick BK. Chronic subdural haematoma in the elderly. *Postgrad Med J* 2002;78:71–75.
20. Lee KS. Natural history of chronic subdural haematoma. *Brain Inj* 2004;18:351–358.
21. Jones S, Kafetz K. A prospective study of chronic subdural haematomas in elderly patients. *Age Ageing* 1999;28:519–521.
22. Nobbe FA, Krauss JK. Subdural hematoma as a cause of contralateral dystonia. *Clin Neurol Neurosurg* 1997;99:37–39.
23. Moster ML, Johnston DE, Reinmuth OM. Chronic subdural hematoma with transient neurological deficits: a review of 15 cases. *Ann Neurol* 1983;14:539–542.
24. Ingvar DH, Lundberg N. Paroxysmal systems in intracranial hypertension, studied with ventricular fluid pressure recording and electroencephalography. *Brain* 1961;84:446–459.
25. Inao S, Kawai T, Kabeya R, et al. Relation between brain displacement and local cerebral blood flow in patients with chronic subdural haematoma. *J Neurol Neurosurg Psychiatry* 2001;71:741–746.
26. Voelker JL. Nonoperative treatment of chronic subdural hematoma. *Neurosurg Clin N Am* 2000;11:507–513.
27. Olson JJ, Poor MM Jr, Beck DW. Methylprednisolone reduces the bulk flow of water across an in vitro blood-brain barrier. *Brain Res* 1988;439:259–265.
28. Hasbun R, Abrahams J, Jekel J, Quagliarello VJ. Computed tomography of the head before lumbar puncture in adults with suspected meningitis. *N Engl J Med* 2001;345:1727–1733.
29. Almenawer SA, Farrokhyar F, Hong C, et al. Chronic subdural hematoma management: a systematic review and meta-analysis of 34,829 patients. *Ann Surg* 2014;259:449–457.
30. Yao Z, Hu X, Ma L, You C. Dexamethasone for chronic subdural haematoma: a systematic review and meta-analysis. *Acta Neurochir (Wien)* 2017;159:2037–2044.
31. Henaux PL, Le Reste PJ, Laviolle B, Morandi X. Steroids in chronic subdural hematomas (SUCRE trial): study protocol for a randomized controlled trial. *Trials* 2017;18:252.
32. Roh D, Reznik M, Claassen J. Chronic subdural medical management. *Neurosurg Clin N Am* 2017;28:211–217.
33. Nathoo N, Nadvi SS, van Dellen JR, Gouws E. Intracranial subdural empyemas in the era of computed tomography: a review of 699 cases. *Neurosurgery* 1999;44:529–535.
34. Hlavin ML, Kaminski HJ, Fenstermaker RA, White RJ. Intracranial suppuration: a modern decade of postoperative subdural empyema and epidural abscess. *Neurosurgery* 1994;34:974–980; discussion 80–81.
35. Nathoo N, Nadvi SS, Van Dellen JR. Traumatic cranial empyemas: a review of 55 patients. *Br J Neurosurg* 2000;14:326–330.
36. Tamaki T, Eguchi T, Sakamoto M, Teramoto A. Use of diffusion-weighted magnetic resonance imaging in empyema after cranioplasty. *Br J Neurosurg* 2004;18:40–44.
37. Tsuchiya K, Osawa A, Katase S, Fujikawa A, Hachiya J, Aoki S. Diffusion-weighted MRI of subdural and epidural empyemas. *Neuroradiology* 2003;45:220–223.
38. Heran NS, Steinbok P, Cochrane DD. Conservative neurosurgical management of intracranial epidural abscesses in children. *Neurosurgery* 2003;53:893–897; discussion 7–8.
39. Harrison RA, Nam JY, Weathers SP, DeMonte F. Intracranial dural, calvarial, and skull base metastases. *Handb Clin Neurol* 2018;149:205–225.
40. Chourmouzi D, Potsi S, Moumtzouoglou A, et al. Dural lesions mimicking meningiomas: a pictorial essay. *World J Radiol* 2012;4:75–82.
41. Whittle IR, Smith C, Navoo P, Collie D. Meningiomas. *Lancet* 2004;363:1535–1543.
42. Bosnjak R, Derham C, Popovic M, Ravnik J. Spontaneous intracranial meningioma bleeding: clinicopathological features and outcome. *J Neurosurg* 2005;103:473–484.
43. Pistolesi S, Fontanini G, Camacci T, et al. Meningioma-associated brain oedema: the role of angiogenic factors and pial blood supply. *J Neurooncol* 2002;60:159–164.

44. Engelhard HH. Progress in the diagnosis and treatment of patients with meningiomas. Part I: diagnostic imaging, preoperative embolization. *Surg Neurol* 2001;55:89–101.
45. Wildemberg LE, Glezer A, Bronstein MD, Gadelha MR. Apoplexy in nonfunctioning pituitary adenomas. *Pituitary* 2018;21:138–144.
46. Sibal L, Ball SG, Connolly V, et al. Pituitary apoplexy: a review of clinical presentation, management and outcome in 45 cases. *Pituitary* 2004;7:157–163.
47. Jassal DS, McGinn G, Embil JM. Pituitary apoplexy masquerading as meningoencephalitis. *Headache* 2004;44:75–78.
48. Prabhu VC, Brown HG. The pathogenesis of craniopharyngiomas. *Childs Nerv Syst* 2005;21:622–627.
49. Haupt R, Magnani C, Pavanello M, Caruso S, Dama E, Garre ML. Epidemiological aspects of craniopharyngioma. *J Pediatr Endocrinol Metab* 2006;19(Suppl 1):289–293.
50. Patel AJ, Fuller GN, Wildrick DM, Sawaya R. Pineal cyst apoplexy: case report and review of the literature. *Neurosurgery* 2005;57:E1066; discussion E1066.
51. Joswig H, Fournier JY, Hildebrandt G, Stienen MN. Sentinel headache: A warning sign preceding every fourth aneurysmal subarachnoid hemorrhage. *AJNR Am J Neuroradiol* 2015;36:E62–E63.
52. Pereira JL, de Albuquerque LA, Dellaretti M, et al. Importance of recognizing sentinel headache. *Surg Neurol Int* 2012;3:162.
53. Malhotra A, Wu X, Gandhi D, Sanelli P. The patient with thunderclap headache. *Neuroimaging Clin N Am* 2018;28:335–351.
54. Kowalski RG, Claassen J, Kreiter KT, et al. Initial misdiagnosis and outcome after subarachnoid hemorrhage. *JAMA* 2004;291:866–869.
55. Lindbohm JV, Kaprio J, Jousilahti P, Salomaa V, Korja M. Risk factors of sudden death from subarachnoid hemorrhage. *Stroke* 2017;48:2399–2404.
56. Hanafy KA. The role of microglia and the TLR4 pathway in neuronal apoptosis and vasospasm after subarachnoid hemorrhage. *J Neuroinflammation* 2013;10:83.
57. Blok KM, Rinkel GJ, Majoie CB, et al. CT within 6 hours of headache onset to rule out subarachnoid hemorrhage in nonacademic hospitals. *Neurology* 2015; 84:1927–1932.
58. Stewart H, Reuben A, McDonald J. LP or not LP, htat is the question: Gold standard or unnecessary procedure in subarachnoid hemorrhage. *Emerg Med J* 2014; 31:720–723.
59. Mohamed M, Heasly DC, Yagmurlu B, Yousem DM. Fluid-attenuated inversion recovery MR imaging and subarachnoid hemorrhage: not a panacea. *AJNR Am J Neuroradiol* 2004;25:545–550.
60. Edlow JA, Caplan LR. Avoiding pitfalls in the diagnosis of subarachnoid hemorrhage. *N Engl J Med* 2000;342:29–36.
61. McCarron MO, Lynch M, McCarron P, et al. Clinical and diagnostic findings in patients with elevated cerebrospinal bilirubin. *Postgrad Med J* 2015;91:675–680.
62. Petzold A, Keir G, Sharpe TL. Why human color vision cannot reliably detect cerebrospinal fluid xanthochromia. *Stroke* 2005;36:1295–1297.
63. Nayar G, Ejikeme T, Chongsathidkiet P, et al. Leptomeningeal disease: current diagnostic and therapeutic strategies. *Oncotarget* 2017;8:73312–73328.
64. Narayan V, Savardekar A, Mohammed N, Patra DP, Georgescu MM, Nanda A. Primary focal intracranial leptomeningeal glioma: case report and review of the literature. *World Neurosurg* 2018;116:163–168.
65. DeAngelis LM, Posner JB. *Neurologic Complications of Cancer*. New York: Oxford University Press; 2009.
66. Chen HS, Shen MC, Tien HF, Su IJ, Wang CH. Leptomeningeal seeding with acute hydrocephalus— unusual central nervous system presentation during chemotherapy in Ki-1-positive anaplastic large-cell lymphoma. *Acta Haematol* 1996;95:135–139.
67. Floeter MK, So YT, Ross DA, Greenberg D. Miliary metastasis to the brain: clinical and radiologic features. *Neurology* 1987;37:1817–1818.
68. Broderick JP, Cascino TL. Nonconvulsive status epilepticus in a patient with leptomeningeal cancer. *Mayo Clin Proc* 1987;62:835–837.
69. Klein P, Haley EC, Wooten GF, VandenBerg SR. Focal cerebral infarctions associated with perivascular tumor infiltrates in carcinomatous leptomeningeal metastases. *Arch Neurol* 1989;46:1149–1152.
70. Herman C, Kupsky WJ, Rogers L, Duman R, Moore P. Leptomeningeal dissemination of malignant glioma simulating cerebral vasculitis. Case report with angiographic and pathological studies. *Stroke* 1995;26:2366–2370.
71. Weller M, Stevens A, Sommer N, Schabet M, Wietholter H. Tumor cell dissemination triggers an intrathecal immune response in neoplastic meningitis. *Cancer* 1992;69:1475–1480.
72. Glantz MJ, Cole BF, Glantz LK, et al. Cerebrospinal fluid cytology in patients with cancer: minimizing false-negative results. *Cancer* 1998;82:733–739.
73. Shi Q, Pu CQ, Huang XS, Tian CL, Cao XT. Optimal cut-off values for tumor markers in cerebrospinal fluid with ROC curve analysis. *Front Biosci (Elite edition)* 2011;3:1259–1264.
74. Corsini E, Bernardi G, Gaviani P, et al. Intrathecal synthesis of tumor markers is a highly sensitive test in the diagnosis of leptomeningeal metastasis from solid cancers. *Clin Chem Lab Med* 2009;47:874–879.
75. Wasserstrom WR, Glass JP, Posner JB. Diagnosis and treatment of leptomeningeal metastases from solid tumors: experience with 90 patients. *Cancer* 1982;49:759–772.
76. DeAngelis LM, Boutros D. Leptomeningeal metastasis. *Cancer Invest* 2005;23:145–154.
77. Scheld WM, Koedel U, Nathan B, Pfister HW. Pathophysiology of bacterial meningitis: mechanism(s) of neuronal injury. *J Infect Dis* 2002;186(Suppl 2):S225–S233.
78. van de Beek D, de Gans J, Spanjaard L, Weisfelt M, Reitsma JB, Vermeulen M. Clinical features and prognostic factors in adults with bacterial meningitis. *N Engl J Med* 2004;351:1849–1859.
79. Brouwer MC, van de Beek D. Epidemiology of community-acquired bacterial meningitis. *Curr Opin Infect Dis* 2018;31:78–84.
80. Gerner-Smidt P, Ethelberg S, Schiellerup P, et al. Invasive listeriosis in Denmark 1994–2003: a review of 299 cases with special emphasis on risk factors for mortality. *Clin Microbiol Infect* 2005;11:618–624.

81. Hussein AS, Shafran SD. Acute bacterial meningitis in adults. A 12-year review. *Medicine (Baltimore)* 2000;79:360–368.
82. Flores-Cordero JM, Amaya-Villar R, Rincón-Ferrari MD, Leal-Noval SR, Garnacho-Montero J, Llanos-Rodríguez AC, Murillo-Cabezas F. Acute community-acquired bacterial meningitis in adults admitted to the intensive care unit: Clinical manifestations, management and prognostic factors. *Intensive Care Med* 2003 Nov;29(11):1967–1973. Epub 2003 Aug 6.
83. Podlecka A, Dziewulska D, Rafalowska J. Vascular changes in tuberculous meningoencephalitis. *Folia Neuropathol* 1998;36:235–237.
84. Attia J, Hatala R, Cook DJ, Wong JG. Does this adult patient have acute meningitis? *JAMA* 1999;282:175–181.
85. Risch L, Lisec I, Jutzi M, Podvinec M, Landolt H, Huber AR. Rapid, accurate and non-invasive detection of cerebrospinal fluid leakage using combined determination of beta-trace protein in secretion and serum. *Clin Chim Acta* 2005;351:169–176.
86. Romer FK. Difficulties in the diagnosis of bacterial meningitis. Evaluation of antibiotic pretreatment and causes of admission to hospital. *Lancet* 1977;2:345–347.
87. Clark T, Duffell E, Stuart JM, Heyderman RS. Lumbar puncture in the management of adults with suspected bacterial meningitis—a survey of practice. *J Infect* 2006;52:315–319.
88. Roos KL, Tunkel AR, Scheld WM. Acute bacterial meningitis. In: Scheld WM, Whitley RJ, Marra CM, eds. *Infections of the Central Nervous System.* 3rd ed. Philadelphia: Lippincott; 2004:347–422.
89. Saberi A, Roudbary SA, Ghayeghran A, Kazemi S, Hosseininezhad M. Diagnosis of meningitis caused by pathogenic microorganisms using magnetic resonance imaging: a systematic review. *Basic Clin Neurosci* 2018;9:73–86.
90. Zimmerman RA, Wong AM, Girard N. Imaging of intracranial infections. In: Scheld WM, Whitley RJ, Marra CM, eds. *Infections of the Central Nervous System.* 3rd ed. Philadelphia: Lippincott; 2004:31–55.
91. Chaudhuri A. Adjunctive dexamethasone treatment in acute bacterial meningitis. *Lancet Neurol* 2004;3:54–62.
92. Massaro AR, Sacco RL, Mohr JP, et al. Clinical discriminators of lobar and deep hemorrhages: the Stroke Data Bank. *Neurology* 1991;41:1881–1885.
93. Sreekrishnan A, Dearborn JL, Greer DM, et al. Intracerebral hemorrhage location and functional outcomes of patients: a systematic literature review and meta-analysis. *Neurocrit Care* 2016;25:384–391.
94. Chung CS, Caplan LR, Yamamoto Y, et al. Striatocapsular haemorrhage. *Brain* 2000;123 (Pt 9):1850–1862.
95. Kumral E, Kocaer T, Ertubey NC, Kumral K. Thalamic hemorrhage—A prospective study of 100 patients. *Stroke* 1995;26:964–970.
96. Choi KD, Jung DS, Kim JS. Specificity of "peering at the tip of the nose" for a diagnosis of thalamic hemorrhage. *Arch Neurol* 2004;61:417–422.
97. Darby DG, Donnan GA, Saling MA, Walsh KW, Bladin PF. Primary intraventricular hemorrhage: clinical and neuropsychological findings in a prospective stroke series. *Neurology* 1988;38:68–75.
98. Engelhard HH, Andrews CO, Slavin KV, Charbel FT. Current management of intraventricular hemorrhage. *Surg Neurol* 2003;60:15–21.
99. Fisher CM. Some neuro-ophthalmological observations. *J Neurol Neurosurg Psychiatry* 1967;30:383–392.
100. Fisher CM. Lacunes: small, deep cerebral infarcts. *Neurology* 1965;15:774–784.
101. Greenberg SM, Gurol ME, Rosand J, Smith EE. Amyloid angiopathy-related vascular cognitive impairment. *Stroke* 2004;35:2616–2619.
102. Yamada M. Cerebral amyloid angiopathy: an overview. *Neuropathology* 2000;20:8–22.
103. Miller JH, Wardlaw JM, Lammie GA. Intracerebral haemorrhage and cerebral amyloid angiopathy: CT features with pathological correlation. *Clin Radiol* 1999;54:422–429.
104. Koennecke HC. Cerebral microbleeds on MRI: prevalence, associations, and potential clinical implications. *Neurology* 2006;66:165–171.
105. Auriel E, Charidimou A, Gurol ME, et al. Validation of clinicoradiological criteria for the diagnosis of cerebral amyloid angiopathy-related inflammation. *JAMA Neurol* 2016;73:197–202.
106. Barami K, Ko K. Ruptured mycotic aneurysm presenting as an intraparenchymal hemorrhage and nonadjacent acute subdural hematoma: case report and review of the literature. *Surg Neurol* 1994;41:290–293.
107. Flores BC, Patel AR, Braga BP, Weprin BE, Batjer HH. Management of infectious intracranial aneurysms in the pediatric population. *Childs Nerv Syst* 2016;32:1205–1217.
108. Ferro JM, Fonseca AC. Infective endocarditis. *Handb Clin Neurol* 2014;119:75–91.
109. Kivelev J, Niemela M, Hernesniemi J. Characteristics of cavernomas of the brain and spine. *J Clin Neurosci* 2012;19:643–648.
110. Kivelev J, Niemela M, Hernesniemi J. Treatment strategies in cavernomas of the brain and spine. *J Clin Neurosci* 2012;19:491–497.
111. Poorthuis MH, Klijn CJ, Algra A, Rinkel GJ, Al-Shahi Salman R. Treatment of cerebral cavernous malformations: a systematic review and meta-regression analysis. *J Neurol Neurosurg Psychiatry* 2014;85:1319–1323.
112. Choi JH, Mohr JP. Brain arteriovenous malformations in adults. *Lancet Neurol* 2005;4:299–308.
113. Lawton MT, Rutledge WC, Kim H, et al. Brain arteriovenous malformations. *Nat Rev Dis Primers* 2015;1:15008.
114. Behin A, Hoang-Xuan K, Carpentier AF, Delattre JY. Primary brain tumours in adults. *Lancet* 2003;361:323–331.
115. Engelhard HH. Current diagnosis and treatment of oligodendroglioma. *Neurosurg Focus* 2002;12:E2.
116. Grimm SA, Chamberlain MC. Brainstem glioma: a review. *Curr Neurol Neurosci Rep* 2013;13:346.
117. Grommes C, DeAngelis LM. Primary CNS lymphoma. *J Clin Oncol* 2017;35:2410–2418.
118. de Oliveira JA, Santana IA, Caires IQ, et al. Antiepileptic drug prophylaxis in primary brain tumor patients: is current practice in agreement to the consensus? *J Neurooncol* 2014;120:399–403.

119. Brouwer MC, Tunkel AR, McKhann GM 2nd, van de Beek D. Brain abscess. *N Engl J Med* 2014;371:447–456.
120. Zammarchi L, Strohmeyer M, Bartalesi F, et al. Epidemiology and management of cysticercosis and Taenia solium taeniasis in Europe, systematic review 1990–2011. *PloS One* 2013;8:e69537.
121. Lightowlers MW. Cysticercosis and echinococcosis. *Curr Top Microbiol Immunol* 2013;365:315–335.
122. Cemil B, Tun K, Gurcay AG, Uygur A, Kaptanoglu E. Cranial epidural hydatid cysts: clinical report and review of the literature. *Acta Neurochir (Wien)* 2009;151:659–662.
123. Collazos J. Opportunistic infections of the CNS in patients with AIDS: diagnosis and management. *CNS Drugs* 2003;17:869–887.
124. Kastenbauer S, Pfister HW, Wispelwey B. Brain abscess. In: Scheld WM, Whitley RJ, Marra CM, eds. *Infections of the Central Nervous System.* 3 ed. Philadelphia: Lippincott; 2004:479–507.
125. Winter RC. Posterior fossa epidural hematoma. *Pediatr Emerg Care* 2015;31:808–809.
126. Khwaja HA, Hormbrey PJ. Posterior cranial fossa venous extradural haematoma: an uncommon form of intracranial injury. *Emerg Med J* 2001;18:496–497.
127. Berker M, Cataltepe O, Ozcan OE. Traumatic epidural haematoma of the posterior fossa in childhood: 16 new cases and a review of the literature. *Br J Neurosurg* 2003;17:226–229.
128. Bor-Seng-Shu E, Aguiar PH, Almeida Leme RJ, Mandel M, Andrade AF, Marino R Jr. Epidural hematomas of the posterior cranial fossa. *Neurosurg Focus* 2004;16:ECP1.
129. Karasawa H, Furuya H, Naito H, Sugiyama K, Ueno J, Kin H. Acute hydrocephalus in posterior fossa injury. *J Neurosurg* 1997;86:629–632.
130. Pozzati E, Tognetti F, Cavallo M, Acciarri N. Extradural hematomas of the posterior cranial fossa. Observations on a series of 32 consecutive cases treated after the introduction of computed tomography scanning. *Surg Neurol* 1989;32:300–303.
131. Nathoo N, Nadvi SS, van Dellen JR. Infratentorial empyema: analysis of 22 cases. *Neurosurgery* 1997;41:1263–1268; discussion 1268–1269.
132. Roberti F, Sekhar LN, Kalavakonda C, Wright DC. Posterior fossa meningiomas: surgical experience in 161 cases. *Surg Neurol* 2001;56:8–20; discussion 21.
133. Ishigaki D, Arai H, Sasoh M, et al. Meningioma in the posterior fossa without dural attachment. *Neurol Med Chir (Tokyo)* 2007;47:364–366.
134. Saper CB, Jarowski CI. Leukemic infiltration of the cerebellum in acute myelomonocytic leukemia. *Neurology* 1982;32:77–80.
135. Cho SF, Liu TC, Chang CS. Isolated central nervous system relapse presenting as myeloid sarcoma of acute myeloid leukemia after allogeneic peripheral blood stem cell transplantation. *Ann Hematol* 2013;92:133–135.
136. Takemoto Y, Matsumoto J, Ohta K, Hasegawa S, Miura M, Kuratsu J. Bilateral posterior fossa chronic subdural hematoma treated with craniectomy: case report and review of the literature. *Surg Neurol Int* 2016;7:S255–S258.
137. d'Avella D, Servadei F, Scerrati M, et al. Traumatic acute subdural haematomas of the posterior fossa: clinicoradiological analysis of 24 patients. *Acta Neurochir (Wien)* 2003;145:1037–1044; discussion 44.
138. Stendel R, Schulte T, Pietila TA, Suess O, Brock M. Spontaneous bilateral chronic subdural haematoma of the posterior fossa. Case report and review of the literature. *Acta Neurochir (Wien)* 2002;144:497–500.
139. van de Beek D, Campeau NG, Wijdicks EF. The clinical challenge of recognizing infratentorial empyema. *Neurology* 2007;69:477–481.
140. Sadato N, Numaguchi Y, Rigamonti D, Salcman M, Gellad FE, Kishikawa T. Bleeding patterns in ruptured posterior fossa aneurysms: a CT study. *J Comput Assist Tomogr* 1991;15:612–617.
141. Logue V. Posterior fossa aneurysms. *Clin Neurosurg* 1964;11:183–219.
142. Duvoisin RC, Yahr MD. Posterior fossa aneurysms. *Neurology* 1965;15:231–241.
143. Jamieson KG. Aneurysms of the vertebrobasilar system. Further experience with nine cases. *J Neurosurg* 1968;28:544–555.
144. Mensing LA, Vergouwen MDI, Laban KG, et al. Perimesencephalic hemorrhage: a review of epidemiology, risk factors, presumed cause, clinical course, and outcome. *Stroke* 2018;49:1363–1370.
145. Rouchaud A, Lehman VT, Murad MH, et al. Nonaneurysmal perimesencephalic hemorrhage is associated with deep cerebral venous drainage anomalies: a systematic literature review and meta-analysis. *AJNR Am J Neuroradiol* 2016;37:1657–1663.
146. Datar S, Rabinstein AA. Cerebellar hemorrhage. *Neurol Clin* 2014;32:993–1007.
147. Pasi M, Marini S, Morotti A, et al. Cerebellar hematoma location: implications for the underlying microangiopathy. *Stroke* 2018;49:207–210.
148. St Louis EK, Wijdicks EF, Li H. Predicting neurologic deterioration in patients with cerebellar hematomas. *Neurology* 1998;51:1364–1369.
149. Kirollos RW, Tyagi AK, Ross SA, van Hille PT, Marks PV. Management of spontaneous cerebellar hematomas: a prospective treatment protocol. *Neurosurgery* 2001;49:1378–1386; discussion 1386–1387.
150. Fisher CM, Picard EH, Polak A, Dalal P, Pojemann RG. Acute hypertensive cerebellar hemorrhage: diagnosis and surgical treatment. *J Nerv Ment Dis* 1965;140:38–57.
151. Coplin WM, Kim DK, Kliot M, Bird TD. Mutism in an adult following hypertensive cerebellar hemorrhage: nosological discussion and illustrative case. *Brain Lang* 1997;59:473–493.
152. Hoche F, Guell X, Vangel MG, Sherman JC, Schmahmann JD. The cerebellar cognitive affective/Schmahmann syndrome scale. *Brain* 2018;141:248–270.
153. Stoodley CJ, MacMore JP, Makris N, Sherman JC, Schmahmann JD. Location of lesion determines motor vs. cognitive consequences in patients with cerebellar stroke. *Neuroimage Clin* 2016;12:765–775.
154. Datar S, Rabinstein AA. Cerebellar infarction. *Neurol Clin* 2014;32:979–991.
155. Tohgi H, Takahashi S, Chiba K, Hirata Y. Cerebellar infarction—Clinical and neuroimaging analysis in 293 patients. *Stroke* 1993;24:1697–1701.
156. Hornig CR, Rust DS, Busse O, Jauss M, Laun A. Space-occupying cerebellar infarction—Clinical course and prognosis. *Stroke* 1994;25:372–374.

157. Nathoo N, Nadvi SS, Narotam PK, van Dellen JR. Brain abscess: management and outcome analysis of a computed tomography era experience with 973 patients. *World Neurosurg* 2011;75:716–726; discussion 612–617.
158. Sennaroglu L, Sozeri B. Otogenic brain abscess: review of 41 cases. *Otolaryngol Head Neck Surg* 2000;123:751–755.
159. Shaw MD, Russell JA. Cerebellar abscess. A review of 47 cases. *J Neurol Neurosurg Psychiatry* 1975;38:429–435.
160. Nadvi SS, Parboosing R, van Dellen JR. Cerebellar abscess: the significance of cerebrospinal fluid diversion. *Neurosurgery* 1997;41:61–66.
161. Fadul C, Misulis KE, Wiley RG. Cerebellar metastases: diagnostic and management considerations. *J Clin Oncol* 1987;5:1107–1115.
162. Slater A, Moore NR, Huson SM. The natural history of cerebellar hemangioblastomas in von Hippel-Lindau disease. *AJNR Am J Neuroradiol* 2003;24:1570–1574.
163. Haines SJ, Mollman HD. Primary pontine hemorrhagic events. Hemorrhage or hematoma? Surgical or conservative management? *Neurosurg Clin N Am* 1993;4:481–495.
164. Takahashi M, Suzuki R, Osakabe Y, et al. Magnetic resonance imaging findings in cerebral fat embolism: correlation with clinical manifestations. *J Trauma* 1999;46:324–327.
165. Wityk RJ, Goldsborough MA, Hillis A, et al. Diffusion- and perfusion-weighted brain magnetic resonance imaging in patients with neurologic complications after cardiac surgery. *Arch Neurol* 2001;58:571–576.
166. Meador KJ, Loring DW, Lee GP, Nichols ME, Moore EE, Figueroa RE. Level of consciousness and memory during the intracarotid sodium amobarbital procedure. *Brain Cogn* 1997;33:178–188.
167. Nogueira RG, Jadhav AP, Haussen DC, et al. Thrombectomy 6 to 24 hours after stroke with a mismatch between deficit and infarct. *N Engl J Med* 2018;378:11–21.
168. Ducroux C, Khoury N, Lecler A, et al. Application of the DAWN clinical imaging mismatch and DEFUSE 3 selection criteria: benefit seems similar but restrictive volume cut-offs might omit potential responders. *Eur J Neurol* 2018;25:1093–1099.
169. Qureshi AI, Suarez JI, Yahia AM, et al. Timing of neurologic deterioration in massive middle cerebral artery infarction: a multicenter review. *Crit Care Med* 2003;31:272–277.
170. Caplan LR. "Top of the basilar" syndrome. *Neurology* 1980;30:72–79.
171. Schmahmann JD. Vascular syndromes of the thalamus. *Stroke* 2003;34:2264–2278.
172. Neau JP, Bogousslavsky J. The syndrome of posterior choroidal artery territory infarction. *Ann Neurol* 1996;39:779–788.
173. Castaigne P, Lhermitte F, Buge A, Escourolle R, Hauw JJ, Lyon-Caen O. Paramedian thalamic and midbrain infarct: clinical and neuropathological study. *Ann Neurol* 1981;10:127–148.
174. Weidauer S, Nichtweiss M, Zanella FE, Lanfermann H. Assessment of paramedian thalamic infarcts: MR imaging, clinical features and prognosis. *Eur Radiol* 2004;14:1615–1626.
175. Hindman J, Bowren MA, Bruss J, Wright B, Geerling JC, Boes AD. Thalamic coma? The neuroanatomic correlates of impaired arousal in humans. *Ann Neurol*. 2018;84(6):926–930.
176. Krolak-Salmon P, Croisile B, Setiey A, Girard-Madoux P, Vighetto A. Total recovery after bilateral paramedian thalamic infarct. *Eur Neurol* 2000;44:216–218.
177. van Domburg PH, ten Donkelaar HJ, Notermans SL. *J Neurol Sci* 1996;139:58–65.
178. Capecchi M, Abbattista M, Martinelli I. Cerebral venous sinus thrombosis. *J Thromb Haemost* 2018;16:1918–1931.
179. Masuhr F, Mehraein S, Einhaupl K. Cerebral venous and sinus thrombosis. *J Neurol* 2004;251:11–23.
180. Coutinho JM, Gerritsma JJ, Zuurbier SM, Stam J. Isolated cortical vein thrombosis: systematic review of case reports and case series. *Stroke* 2014;45:1836–1838.
181. Caplan LR, Wang Q. Thalamic lesions caused by deep cerebral venous thrombosis: a retrospective study. *Eur Neurol* 2015;74:118–126.
182. Patel SI, Obeid H, Matti L, Ramakrishna H, Shamoun FE. Cerebral venous thrombosis: current and newer anticoagulant treatment options. *Neurologist* 2015;20:80–88.
183. Nadeau SE. Neurologic manifestations of systemic vasculitis. *Neurol Clin* 2002;20:123–150, vi.
184. Twilt M, Benseler SM. Central nervous system vasculitis in adults and children. *Handb Clin Neurol* 2016;133:283–300.
185. Limaye K, Samaniego EA, Adams HP Jr. Diagnosis and treatment of primary central nervous system angiitis. *Curr Treat Options Neurol* 2018;20:38.
186. Younger DS, Hays AP, Brust JC, Rowland LP. Granulomatous angiitis of the brain. An inflammatory reaction of diverse etiology. *Arch Neurol* 1988;45:514–518.
187. Tyler KL. Acute viral encephalitis. *N Engl J Med* 2018;379:557–566.
188. Rabinstein AA. Herpes virus encephalitis in adults: current knowledge and old myths. *Neurol Clin* 2017;35:695–705.
189. Whitley RJ, Soong SJ, Linneman C Jr, Liu C, Pazin G, Alford CA. Herpes simplex encephalitis. *Clinical Assessment. JAMA* 1982;247:317–320.
190. Pohl D, Alper G, Van Haren K, et al. Acute disseminated encephalomyelitis: updates on an inflammatory CNS syndrome. *Neurology* 2016;87:S38–S45.
191. Javed A, Khan O. Acute disseminated encephalomyelitis. *Handb Clin Neurol* 2014;123:705–717.
192. Courville CB. The mechanism of coup-contrecoup injuries of the brain: a critical review of recent experimental studies in the light of clinical observations. *Bull Los Angel Neuro Soc* 1950;15:72–86.
193. Gurdjian ES. Re-evaluation of the biomechanics of blunt impact injury of the head. *Surg Gynecol Obstet* 1975;140:845–850.
194. Tubi MA, Lutkenhoff E, Blanco MB, et al. Early seizures and temporal lobe trauma predict post-traumatic epilepsy: A longitudinal study. *Neurobiol Dis* 2019 Mar;123:115–121.

195. Adams JH, Graham DI, Murray LS, Scott G. Diffuse axonal injury due to nonmissile head injury in humans: an analysis of 45 cases. *Ann Neurol* 1982;12:557–563.
196. Gennarelli TA, Thibault LE, Adams JH, Graham DI, Thompson CJ, Marcincin RP. Diffuse axonal injury and traumatic coma in the primate. *Ann Neurol* 1982;12:564–574.
197. Meythaler JM, Peduzzi JD, Eleftheriou E, Novack TA. Current concepts: diffuse axonal injury-associated traumatic brain injury. *Arch Phys Med Rehabil* 2001;82:1461–1471.
198. Golabek-Dropiewska K, Marks W, Brockhuis B, et al. Diffuse axonal injury: a brief review and examples of the use of neurofunctional imaging (Tc-99m HMPAO SPECT) in diagnosis and follow-up. *Neuroradiol J* 2010;23:301–306.
199. Shaw NA. The neurophysiology of concussion. *Prog Neurobiol* 2002;67:281–344.
200. Giza CC, Kutcher JS, Ashwal S, et al. Summary of evidence-based guideline update: evaluation and management of concussion in sports: report of the Guideline Development Subcommittee of the American Academy of Neurology. *Neurology* 2013;80:2250–2257.
201. Giza CC, Hovda DA. The new neurometabolic cascade of concussion. *Neurosurgery* 2014;75(Suppl 4):S24–S33.
202. Douglas DB, Muldermans JL, Wintermark M. Neuroimaging of brain trauma. *Curr Opin Neurol* 2018;31:362–370.
203. Dennis EL, Babikian T, Alger J, Rashid F, et al. Magnetic resonance spectroscopy of fiber tracts in children with traumatic brain injury. *Hum Brain Map* 2018; 39:3759–3768.
204. Croal I, Smith FE, Blamire AM. Magnetic resonance spectroscopy for traumatic brain injury. *Top Magn Reson Imaging* 2015;24:267–274.
205. Reilly PL, Graham DI, Adams JH, Jennett B. Patients with head injury who talk and die. *Lancet* 1975;2:375–377.
206. Ellis MJ, Leddy J, Willer B. Multi-disciplinary management of athletes with post-concussion syndrome: an evolving pathophysiological approach. *Front Neurol* 2016;7:136.
207. Hay J, Johnson VE, Smith DH, Stewart W. Chronic traumatic encephalopathy: the neuropathological legacy of traumatic brain injury. *Annu Rev Pathol* 2016;11:21–45.
208. Iverson GL, Gardner AJ, McCrory P, Zafonte R, Castellani RJ. A critical review of chronic traumatic encephalopathy. *Neurosci Biobehav Rev* 2015;56:276–293.
209. McKee AC, Stein TD, Kiernan PT, Alvarez VE. The neuropathology of chronic traumatic encephalopathy. *Brain Pathol* 2015;25:350–364.
210. Ruprecht R, Scheurer E, Lenz C. Systematic review on the characterization of chronic traumatic encephalopathy by MRI and MRS. *J Magn Reson Imaging* 2019 Jan;49(1):212–228.
211. Schwarz S, Egelhof T, Schwab S, Hacke W. Basilar artery embolism. Clinical syndrome and neuroradiologic patterns in patients without permanent occlusion of the basilar artery. *Neurology* 1997;49:1346–1352.
212. Zenone T, Puget M. Characteristics of cerebrovascular accidents at time of diagnosis in a series of 98 patients with giant cell arteritis. *Rheumatol Int* 2013;33:3017–3023.
213. Kennell KA, Daghfal MM, Patel SG, DeSanto JR, Waterman GS, Bertino RE. Cervical artery dissection related to chiropractic manipulation: One institution's experience. *J Fam Pract* 2017;66:556–562.
214. Hauser V, Zangger P, Winter Y, Oertel W, Kesselring J. Late sequelae of whiplash injury with dissection of cervical arteries. *Eur Neurol* 2010;64:214–218.
215. Ferbert A, Bruckmann H, Drummen R. Clinical features of proven basilar artery occlusion. *Stroke* 1990;21:1135–1142.
216. Devuyst G, Bogousslavsky J, Meuli R, Moncayo J, de Freitas G, van Melle G. Stroke or transient ischemic attacks with basilar artery stenosis or occlusion: clinical patterns and outcome. *Arch Neurol* 2002;59:567–573.
217. Moncayo J, Bogousslavsky J. Vertebro-basilar syndromes causing oculo-motor disorders. *Curr Opin Neurol* 2003;16:45–50.
218. Ehsan T, Hayat G, Malkoff MD, Selhorst JB, Martin D, Manepalli A. Hyperdense basilar artery. An early computed tomography sign of thrombosis. *J Neuroimaging* 1994;4:200–205.
219. Lingegowda D, Thomas B, Vaghela V, Hingwala DR, Kesavadas C, Sylaja PN. 'Susceptibility sign' on susceptibility-weighted imaging in acute ischemic stroke. *Neurol India* 2012;60:160–164.
220. Ausman JI, Liebeskind DS, Gonzalez N, et al. A review of the diagnosis and management of vertebral basilar (posterior) circulation disease. *Surg Neurol Int* 2018;9:106.
221. Schulz UG, Fischer U. Posterior circulation cerebrovascular syndromes: diagnosis and management. *J Neurol Neurosurg Psychiatry* 2017;88:45–53.
222. Link MJ, Bartleson JD, Forbes G, Meyer FB. Spontaneous midbrain hemorrhage: report of seven new cases. *Surg Neurol* 1993;39:58–65.
223. Murata Y, Yamaguchi S, Kajikawa H, Yamamura K, Sumioka S, Nakamura S. Relationship between the clinical manifestations, computed tomographic findings and the outcome in 80 patients with primary pontine hemorrhage. *J Neurol Sci* 1999;167:107–111.
224. Barinagarrementeria F, Cantu C. Primary medullary hemorrhage. Report of four cases and review of the literature. *Stroke* 1994;25:1684–1687.
225. Posadas G, Vaquero J, Herrero J, Bravo G. Brainstem haematomas: early and late prognosis. *Acta Neurochir (Wien)* 1994;131:189–195.
226. Xie MG, Li D, Guo FZ, et al. Brainstem cavernous malformations: surgical indications based on natural history and surgical outcomes. *World Neurosurg* 2018;110:55–63.
227. Jang JH, Song YG, Kim YZ. Predictors of 30-day mortality and 90-day functional recovery after primary pontine hemorrhage. *J Korean Med Sci* 2011;26:100–107.
228. Sung CY, Lee TH, Chu NS. Central hyperthermia in acute stroke. *Eur Neurol* 2009;62:86–92.
229. Wijdicks EF, St Louis E. Clinical profiles predictive of outcome in pontine hemorrhage. *Neurology* 1997;49:1342–1346.

230. Matsukawa H, Shinoda M, Fujii M, Takahashi O, Murakata A. Risk factors for mortality in patients with non-traumatic pontine hemorrhage. *Acta Neurol Scand* 2015;131:240–245.

231. Baringaarrementeria F, Cantu C. Primary medullary hemorrhage. Report of four cases and review of the literature. *Stroke* 1994;25:1684–1687.

232. Kaniecki RG. Basilar-type migraine. *Curr Pain Headache Rep* 2009;13:217–220.

233. Ducros A, Denier C, Joutel A, et al. The clinical spectrum of familial hemiplegic migraine associated with mutations in a neuronal calcium channel. *N Engl J Med* 2001;345:17–24.

234. Schon F, Martin RJ, Prevett M, Clough C, Enevoldson TP, Markus HS. "CADASIL coma": an underdiagnosed acute encephalopathy. *J Neurol Neurosurg Psychiatry* 2003;74:249–252.

235. Palm-Meinders IH, Koppen H, Terwindt GM, et al. Structural brain changes in migraine. *JAMA* 2012;308:1889–1897.

236. Selby G, Lance JW. Observations on 500 cases of migraine and allied vascular headache. *J Neurol Neurosurg Psychiatry* 1960;23:23–32.

237. Frequin ST, Linssen WH, Pasman JW, Hommes OR, Merx HL. Recurrent prolonged coma due to basilar artery migraine. A case report. *Headache* 1991;31:75–81.

238. Muellbacher W, Mamoli B. Prolonged impaired consciousness in basilar artery migraine. *Headache* 1994;34:282–285.

239. Thambisetty M, Biousse V, Newman NJ. Hypertensive brainstem encephalopathy: clinical and radiographic features. *J Neurol Sci* 2003;208:93–99.

240. Willard N, Honce JM, Kleinschmidt-DeMasters BK. PRES: Review of histological features. *J Neuropathol Exp Neurol* 2018;77:100–118.

241. Hall WA. Infectious lesions of the brain stem. *Neurosurg Clin N Am* 1993;4:543–551.

242. O'Callaghan M, Mok T, Lefter S, Harrington H. Clues to diagnosing culture negative Listeria rhombencephalitis. *BMJ Case Rep* 2012;2012.

243. Tyler KL, Tedder DG, Yamamoto LJ, et al. Recurrent brainstem encephalitis associated with herpes simplex virus type 1 DNA in cerebrospinal fluid. *Neurology* 1995;45:2246–2250.

244. Kidd DP. Neurological complications of Behcet's syndrome. *J Neurol* 2017;264:2178–2183.

245. Garg RK. Posterior leukoencephalopathy syndrome. *Postgrad Med J* 2001;77:24–28.

246. Fuentes S, Bouillot P, Regis J, Lena G, Choux M. Management of brain stem abscess. *Br J Neurosurg* 2001;15:57–62.

247. Kerrn-Jespersen BM, Lindelof M, Illes Z, et al. CLIPPERS among patients diagnosed with non-specific CNS neuroinflammatory diseases. *J Neurol Sci* 2014;343:224–227.

248. Tobin WO, Guo Y, Krecke KN, et al. Diagnostic criteria for chronic lymphocytic inflammation with pontine perivascular enhancement responsive to steroids (CLIPPERS). *Brain* 2017;140:2415–2425.

249. Odaka M, Yuki N, Yamada M, et al. Bickerstaff's brainstem encephalitis: clinical features of 62 cases and a subgroup associated with Guillain-Barre syndrome. *Brain* 2003;126:2279–2290.

250. Shahrizaila N, Yuki N. Bickerstaff brainstem encephalitis and Fisher syndrome: anti-GQ1b antibody syndrome. *J Neurol Neurosurg Psychiatry* 2013;84:576–583.

251. Singh TD, Fugate JE, Rabinstein AA. Central pontine and extrapontine myelinolysis: a systematic review. *Eur J Neurol* 2014;21:1443–1450.

Chapter 5

Metabolic and Diffuse Encephalopathies: Disruption of the Internal Milieu

PART 1: DISTINGUISHING METABOLIC FROM STRUCTURAL COMA

The key feature distinguishing diffuse or metabolic impairment of consciousness is that it is generally not associated with focal neurological findings that would suggest a structural lesion of the brain. However, there are some features of the neurological examination of patients with metabolic encephalopathies that can help to pinpoint the cause of the disturbance. In addition, there are some findings on examination that may appear to be due to focal lesions, but which can be due to diffuse or metabolic disease. In this chapter, we will first consider the diagnostic features of metabolic encephalopathies, then the internal metabolic milieu in which the brain functions normally, and then specific types of metabolic and diffuse disturbances of that internal milieu that can cause encephalopathy. Finally, we will consider various endogenous and exogenous toxins that produce toxic encephalopathies.

The very term "encephalopathy" is worthy of some discussion. This is a very general term, simply meaning that the brain is not working properly, and not necessarily implying that the main problem is one of level of consciousness. Other terms are often used, including "altered state of consciousness" or "altered

mental status." Neither of these is quite right, as an altered state of consciousness (e.g., sleep) is not necessarily pathological, and altered mental state could mean any of a wide range of cognitive disturbances. In fact, one of the chief jobs of a neurologist when faced with a patient who has a pathologically altered state of consciousness is to determine whether the disorder could be due to a focal cognitive deficit. This may be difficult to do if the patient tends to fall asleep or is awake but inattentive.

The tendency to be sleepy is the hallmark of a metabolic encephalopathy. If due to a structural lesion of the ascending arousal system, there is generally evidence of that consisting of focal findings on the neurological exam, as reviewed in Chapter 2. However, on rare occasion, patients may have a nonfocal exam and be encephalopathic due to a diffuse or multifocal structural process. Examples of this include plugging of widely distributed small blood vessels in the brain during disseminated intravascular coagulation or with fat emboli after fracture of a long bone. These are almost impossible to distinguish from a metabolic encephalopathy without careful testing, and thus will be discussed later. Alternatively, bilateral diffuse cerebral compression from bilateral subdural hematomas can occasionally present without focal signs and be indistinguishable from a metabolic encephalopathy. Because of these rare, diffuse, bilateral structural hemispheric lesions, it is always necessary to get brain imaging on metabolic encephalopathy patients for whom a metabolic cause does not become apparent.

The other source for error in diagnosing an encephalopathic patient occurs when the patient is "inattentive." Such patients may be wakeful, or even hypervigilant, or they may fluctuate in level of consciousness depending upon how they perceive or misperceive events going on around them. They are often described as "delirious," and clinical delirium rating scales typically focus mainly on inattention (e.g., see Box 5.1 for the Confusion Assessment Method for the Intensive Care Unit, or CAM-ICU). In general, delirious patients tend to have a metabolic encephalopathy underlying their acute onset of inattentiveness. However, in some cases, they may have acute injury (often vascular) to the posterior parietal lobe in the nondominant hemisphere. Particularly if the lesion involves the parieto-temporo-occipital junction, the patient may have active multimodal sensory hallucinations that appear to be very real to the patient.

It is also not uncommon for a patient to be referred to a neurologist for "confusion" who actually has a much more restricted cognitive deficit. For example, acutely aphasic patients, particularly those with a posterior hemisphere (Wernicke) type aphasia, can appear to be speaking gibberish, are unable to participate in verbal requests, and often are very agitated (because they do not realize why other people cannot understand them). Patients with bilateral parietal injuries can have difficulty putting together the elements of a visual scene (simultanagnosia) and cannot find things in space although they apparently can see (optic ataxia and psychic paralysis of gaze), which a skilled examiner will recognize as the elements of Balint's syndrome. Other patients, who may claim to have vision, may consistently confabulate about what they see due to bilateral occipito-temporal infarcts causing Anton's syndrome (denial of blindness). Such patients often are classified as "confused" by nonneurologists, and only a careful neurological examination will reveal the focality of the neurological deficit.

Finally, when confronted by a new patient who appears to be confused, it is important to determine the tempo of the cognitive impairment. If it can be determined that the confusion has acute or subacute onset and lacks focal features, then it is very likely to be due to a metabolic encephalopathy. On the other hand, if it can be established that the confusion is chronic, the patient may be suffering from dementia or even a developmental cognitive deficit. See Patient Vignette 5.1.

Patient Vignette 5.1

A 55-year-old woman was referred from the gastroenterology clinic because of confusion. She had been doing well until earlier that year when her primary care doctor noted that she had lost 15 pounds since her last physical exam. He referred her to gastroenterology for evaluation of the cause of her weight loss. After extensive evaluation including upper and lower endoscopy, they could not find a reason for her weight loss, but did notice that she was easily confused and had difficulty finding her away around the hospital, so she was referred to neurology.

On examination, she was alert and oriented, but not sure of the date. Spoken language was normal, but with a limited vocabulary, and she could read simple words and numbers, but not do arithmetic. Praxis was normal, and she could follow simple, but not complex commands. She was not aware of current events, but registered and remembered three of three objects at 5 minutes. Her neurological examination did not disclose any focal features.

On further history, it turned out that her husband had died the previous year. She had never been able to progress in school beyond the primary grades because she could not keep up with the other children. She had married her husband as a teenager, and he had done all the cooking and interactions with the outside world, while she mainly did housekeeping tasks and took care of their children. When he died, she only knew how to open cans, so had been eating beans almost exclusively since his death, which accounted for her weight loss. She found her way to the hospital by waiting at a bus stop near her house and asking each bus driver if they went to the hospital. She found her way home the same way. Her IQ was estimated at around 50, a finding that her previous physicians had not been aware of.

Box 5.1 The Confusion Assessment Method for the Intensive Care Unit (CAM-ICU)

Delirium is diagnosed when both features 1 and 2 are positive, along with either feature 3 or feature 4.

Feature 1. Acute Onset of Mental Status Changes or Fluctuating Course

- Is there evidence of an acute change in mental status from the baseline?
- Did the (abnormal) behavior fluctuate during the past 24 hours; that is, tend to come and go or increase and decrease in severity?

Sources of information: Serial Glasgow Coma Scale or sedation score ratings over 24 hours as well as readily available input from the patient's bedside critical care nurse or family

Feature 2. Inattention

- Did the patient have difficulty focusing attention?
- Is there a reduced ability to maintain and shift attention?

Sources of information: Attention screening examinations by using either picture recognition or Vigilance A random letter test (see Ely et al.[1] for description of attention screening examinations). Neither of these tests requires verbal response, and thus they are ideally suited for mechanically ventilated patients.

Feature 3. Disorganized Thinking

- Was the patient's thinking disorganized or incoherent, such as rambling or irrelevant conversation, unclear or illogical flow of ideas, or unpredictable switching from subject to subject?
- Was the patient able to follow questions and commands throughout the assessment?

  1. "Are you having any unclear thinking?"
  2. "Hold up this many fingers." (Examiner holds two fingers in front of the patient.)
  3. "Now, do the same thing with the other hand." (Not repeating the number of fingers.)

Feature 4. Altered Level of Consciousness

- Any level of consciousness other than "alert."
- Alert—normal, spontaneously fully aware of environment and interacts appropriately
- Vigilant—hyperalert
- Lethargic—drowsy but easily aroused, unaware of some elements in the environment, or not spontaneously interacting appropriately with the interview; becomes fully aware and appropriately interactive when prodded minimally
- Stupor—difficult to arouse, unaware of some or all elements in the environment, or not spontaneously interacting with the interviewer; becomes incompletely aware and inappropriately interactive when prodded strongly
- Coma—unarousable, unaware of all elements in the environment, with no spontaneous interaction or awareness of the interviewer, so that the interview is difficult or impossible even with maximum prodding

From Ely et al.,[1] with permission.

In summary, the key features of the neurological examination that identify a patient who appears to be confused due to a focal brain injury rather than a diffuse or metabolic encephalopathy are basically ones that provide evidence for damage to the multimodal areas of the cerebral cortex. Injuries to the posterior temporo-parietal area for convergence of information from individual sensory modalities cause focal loss of attention to the opposite side of space, aphasia, apraxia, or difficulty coordinating hand or eye movements with vision. Damage to the frontal lobe may also cause contralateral inattention, as well as perseveration, impersistence, and poor judgment. Medial temporal lobe injury may appear as anterograde amnesia, and occipito-temporo-parietal damage can cause formed and complex multimodal hallucinations (i.e., combined visual, auditory, somatosensory). If the examiner keeps this in mind, looks for those syndromes, and is alert to obtain early imaging in such cases, most cases of encephalopathy due to a focal lesion can be identified early on.

Key Features of the Neurological Examination in Metabolic Encephalopathies

RESPIRATION

While metabolic diseases generally do not cause the unusual respiratory patterns that are characteristic of brainstem injury, such as apneusis or ataxic respiration (see Chapter 2), they often result in changes in the rate and depth of respiration. There are three main reasons for this.

First, diffuse depression of forebrain activity results in the *loss of the descending signal from the frontal lobes that causes continuous to-and-fro breathing*, even when there is no metabolic need to breathe. As noted in Chapter 2, this can be demonstrated in the lethargic or slightly obtunded patient by testing for posthyperventilation apnea. If asked to take five deep breaths and given no further instructions, an intact subject will start breathing again within about 10 seconds.[2] A patient who is obtunded (or one who has a cortically based dementia such as Alzheimer's disease) will not breathe for up to 20 or 30 seconds, until the increase in pCO_2 in his or her blood engages brainstem circuits that promote breathing.[2]

In patients who have prolonged circulation time (i.e., for whom it takes a longer than normal time for the reduction of pCO_2 in the lungs after breathing is initiated to reach the brainstem), this will cause waxing and waning breathing, known as Cheyne-Stokes respiration.[3] Cheyne-Stokes respiration is common in patients who have prolonged circulatory times when they are sleeping, and in patients with metabolic encephalopathy. In all cases, this is a normal set of brainstem respiratory responses and does not imply any focal abnormality in the brainstem.

Second, many types of metabolic encephalopathies upset acid–base balance in the bloodstream. The brain recognizes elevated pCO_2 in the blood mainly because the carbon dioxide (CO_2) dissolved in the blood combines with water to form bicarbonate ion and ionic hydrogen, or acid. It is the elevated H^+ that is recognized by neurons in the carotid body and in the brainstem as elevated CO_2.[4] Thus, any metabolic derangement that produces excess H^+ causes the same symptoms as if CO_2 is elevated (i.e., hyperventilation). In diabetic ketoacidosis or in renal failure, the deep, labored breathing is often called Kussmaul respiration. This drives down CO_2 and bicarbonate, causing a compensatory respiratory alkalosis. The combination of a *metabolic acidosis and a compensatory respiratory alkalosis* is recognized clinically as hyperventilation, with decreased pH and pCO_2 in the blood gases and decreased serum bicarbonate.

The sum of sodium + potassium ion levels in the blood (in meq/L) minus the sum of chloride and bicarbonate ions is called the *anion gap*. The anion gap estimates unmeasured negatively charged ions in the blood, and it is typically less than 20 meq/L. If the anion gap exceeds this level in a patient with a metabolic acidosis, this is generally due to unknown negatively charged substances in the bloodstream. Causes of *metabolic acidosis with or without an anion gap* that also can cause a metabolic encephalopathy are included in Box 5.2.

The third type of respiratory metabolic encephalopathy is hypoxemia. Hypoxemia may occur in a patient who has pulmonary compromise (e.g., pneumonia or pulmonary embolus resulting in shunting; i.e., much of the blood from the pulmonary artery is passing through the lung with inadequate opportunity for gas exchange) or in a patient in whom the oxygen

Box 5.2 Some Causes of Abnormal Ventilation in Unresponsive Patients

I. *Hyperventilation*
  A. *Primary metabolic acidosis*
    1. *With an anion gap*
      Diabetic ketoacidosis[a]
      Diabetic hyperosmolar coma[a]
      Lactic acidosis
      Uremia[a]
      Alcoholic ketoacidosis
      Acidic poisons[a]
      Ethylene glycol
      Propylene glycol
      Methyl alcohol
      Paraldehyde
      Salicylism (primarily in children)
    2. *Without an anion gap*
      Diarrhea
      Pancreatic drainage
      Carbonic anhydrase inhibitors
      NH_4Cl ingestion
      Renal tubular acidosis
      Ureteroenterostomy
  B. *Primary respiratory alkalosis*
      Hepatic failure[a]
      Sepsis[a]
      Pneumonia
      Pulmonary embolus
      Anxiety (hyperventilation syndrome)
  C. *Mixed acid–base disorders (metabolic acidosis with respiratory alkalosis)*
      Salicylism
      Sepsis[a]
      Hepatic failure[a]
II. *Hypoventilation*
  A. *Respiratory acidosis*
    1. *Acute (uncompensated) respiratory failure*
      Sedative drugs[a]
      Brainstem injury
      Neuromuscular disorders
      Chest injury
      Acute pulmonary disease
    2. *Chronic respiratory insufficiency with metabolic compensation[a]*
      Chronic obstructive lung disease with respiratory failure
      Neurological respiratory failure (e.g., ALS, GBS)
  B. *Metabolic alkalosis*
      Vomiting or gastric drainage
      Diuretic therapy
      Adrenal steroid excess (Cushing's syndrome)
      Primary aldosteronism
      Bartter's syndrome

[a]Common causes of stupor or coma.

carrying capacity of the blood is compromised (e.g., severe anemia or carbon monoxide poisoning). In such patients, there will be a primary respiratory alkalosis (high pH, low pCO_2, low pO_2), potentially with a compensatory metabolic acidosis. Alternatively, in patients with chronic obstructive lung disease, the chronic hypoventilation may cause a primary respiratory acidosis, with metabolic compensation. The blood gases show low pH, high pCO_2, and low pO_2, and serum bicarbonate is high. When pCO_2 becomes elevated above 50, it may cause CO_2 narcosis. This further depresses the level of consciousness and may prevent the hyperventilation that would otherwise be caused by hypoxemia.

PUPILS

Among patients in deep coma, the state of the pupils becomes the single most important criterion that clinically distinguishes between metabolic and structural disease. The presence of preserved pupillary light reflexes despite concomitant respiratory depression, vestibulo-ocular caloric unresponsiveness, decerebrate rigidity, or motor flaccidity suggests metabolic coma. Conversely, if poisoning with anticholinergic drugs or preexisting pupillary disease can be ruled out, the absence of pupillary light reflexes strongly implies that the disease is structural rather than metabolic.

Pupils cannot be considered conclusively nonreactive to a light stimulus unless care has been taken to examine them with magnification using a very bright light and maintaining the stimulus for several seconds. Infrared pupillometry is more reliable than the flashlight.[5]

Ciliospinal reflexes (see Chapter 2) are less reliable than light reflexes but, like them, are usually preserved in metabolic coma even when motor and respiratory signs signify lower brainstem dysfunction.[6]

EYE MOVEMENTS

The eyes usually rove randomly with mild metabolic coma and come to rest in the forward position as coma deepens. The depressed level of consciousness often brings out a latent exophoria. Although almost any eye position or random movement can be observed transiently when brainstem function is changing rapidly, a maintained conjugate lateral deviation or dysconjugate positioning of the eyes at rest,

particularly skew deviation, suggests structural disease. Conjugate downward gaze, or occasionally upward gaze, can occur in metabolic as well as in structural disease and by itself is not helpful in the differential diagnosis.[7]

Historical Patient Vignette 5.2

A 63-year-old woman with severe hepatic cirrhosis and a portacaval shunt was found in coma. She groaned spontaneously but otherwise was unresponsive. Her respirations were 18 per minute and deep. The pupillary diameters were 4 mm on the right and 3 mm on the left, and both reacted to light. Her eyes were deviated conjugately downward and slightly to the right. Oculocephalic responses were conjugate in all directions. Her muscles were flaccid, but her stretch reflexes were brisk and more active on the right with bilateral extensor plantar responses. No decorticate or decerebrate responses could be elicited. Her arterial blood pH was 7.58, and her $PaCO_2$ was 21 mm Hg. Two days later she awoke, at which time her eye movements were normal. Four days later, she again drifted into coma, this time with the eyes in the physiologic position and with sluggish but full oculocephalic responses. She died on the sixth hospital day with severe hepatic cirrhosis. No structural central nervous system (CNS) lesion was found at autopsy.

Comment

This patient was seen prior to the availability of computed tomography (CT) scanning, but the later autopsy confirmed the clinical impression that these focal abnormalities were due to her liver failure, not a structural lesion. The initial conjugate deviation of the eyes downward and slightly to the right had suggested a deep, right-sided cerebral hemispheric mass lesion. But the return of gaze to normal with awakening within 24 hours and the fact that the downward deviation did not recur when the coma deepened ruled out a structural lesion. At autopsy, no intrinsic cerebral pathologic lesion was found to explain the abnormal eye movements. We have observed transient downward as well as transient upward deviation of the eyes in other patients in metabolic coma.

Because reflex oculocephalic eye movements are particularly sensitive to depressant drugs, cold caloric stimulation often provides valuable information about the depth of coma in patients with metabolic disease (see Historical Patient Vignette 5.2). Cold caloric stimulation produces tonic conjugate deviation toward the irrigated ear in patients in light coma and little or no response in those in deep coma (see Chapter 2). If caloric stimulation evokes nystagmus, cerebral regulation of eye movements is intact and the impairment of consciousness is either very mild or the "coma" is psychogenic. If the eyes spontaneously deviate downward following lateral deviation, one should suspect drug-induced coma (see Patient Vignette 5.3).[7] Finally, if caloric stimulation repeatedly produces dysconjugate eye movements, structural brainstem disease should be suspected (but see Chapter 2).

Patient Vignette 5.3

A 20-year-old woman became unresponsive while riding in the back seat of her parents' car. There was no history of previous illness, but her parents stated that she had severe emotional problems. On examination, her vital signs and general physical examination were normal. She appeared to be asleep when left alone, with quiet shallow respiration and no spontaneous movements. Her pupils were 3 mm and reactive. Oculocephalic responses were absent. She lay motionless to noxious stimuli but appeared to resist passive elevation of her eyelids. Cold caloric testing elicited tonic deviation of the eyes with no nystagmus. Blood and urine toxicology screens were positive for barbiturates, and she awoke the next morning and admitted ingesting a mixture of sedative drugs to frighten her mother.

Comment

The coma in this patient initially appeared light or even simulated. However, tonic deviation of the eyes in response to cold caloric irrigation signified that normal cerebral control of eye movements was impaired and indicated that her unresponsiveness was the result of organic, but probably toxic or metabolic, and not structural brain dysfunction. Toxicology screening

discovered at least one cause, but drug overdosages are often mixed, and not all of the components may be picked up on screening.

MOTOR ACTIVITY

Patients with metabolic brain disease generally present two types of motor abnormalities: (1) nonspecific disorders of strength, tone, and reflexes, as well as focal or generalized seizures, and (2) certain characteristic adventitious movements that are almost diagnostic of metabolic brain disease (see Patient Vignette 5.4).

Patient Vignette 5.4

A 60-year-old man was found in the street, stuporous, with an odor of wine on his breath. No other history was obtainable. His blood pressure was 120/80 mm Hg, pulse rate 100 per minute, and respirations 26 per minute and deep. After assessing radiographically for cervical spine injury, his neck was found to be supple. There was fetor hepaticus, and the skin was jaundiced. The liver was palpably enlarged. He responded to noxious stimuli only by groaning. There was no response to visual threat. His left pupil was 5 mm, the right pupil was 3 mm, and both reacted to light. The eyes diverged at rest, but passive head movement elicited full conjugate ocular movements. The corneal reflexes were decreased but present bilaterally. There was a left facial droop. The gag reflex was present. He did not move spontaneously, but grimaced and demonstrated extensor responses to noxious stimuli. The limb muscles were symmetrically rigid, and stretch reflexes were hyperactive. The plantar responses were extensor. An emergency computed tomography (CT) scan was normal. The lumbar spinal fluid pressure was 120 mm, and the cerebrospinal fluid (CSF) contained 30 mg/dL protein and one white blood cell. The serum bicarbonate was 16 mEq/L, chloride 104 mEq/L, sodium 147 mEq/L, and potassium 3.9 mEq/L. Liver function studies were grossly abnormal.

The following morning he responded appropriately to noxious stimulation. Hyperventilation had decreased, and the extensor posturing had disappeared. Diffuse rigidity, increased deep tendon reflexes, and bilateral extensor plantar responses remained. Improvement was rapid, and, by the fourth hospital day, he was awake and had normal findings on neurologic examination. However, on the seventh hospital day, his blood pressure declined and his jaundice increased. He became hypotensive on the ninth hospital day and died. The general autopsy disclosed severe hepatic cirrhosis. An examination of the brain revealed old infarcts in the frontal lobes and the left inferior cerebellum. There were no other lesions.

Comment

In this patient, the signs of liver disease suggested the diagnosis of hepatic coma. At first, anisocoria and decerebrate rigidity hinted at a supratentorial mass lesion such as a subdural hematoma. However, the hyperventilation (which is characteristic of hepatic encephalopathy) and normal pupillary and oculocephalic reactions favored metabolic disease, and the subsequent CT scan and absence of further signs of brainstem injury supported that diagnosis.

NONSPECIFIC MOTOR ABNORMALITIES

Diffuse motor abnormalities are frequent in metabolic coma and reflect the degree and distribution of central nervous system (CNS) depression (Chapter 1). Paratonia and snout, suck, or grasp reflexes may be seen in dementia as well as in patients in light coma. With increasing brainstem depression, flexor and extensor rigidity and sometimes flaccidity appear. The rigid states are sometimes asymmetric.

Focal weakness is surprisingly common with metabolic brain disease. Several of our patients with hypoglycemia or hepatic coma were transiently hemiplegic, and several patients with uremia or hyponatremia had focal weakness of upper motor neuron origin. Others have reported similar findings (see Historical Patient Vignette 5.5).[8–10]

Historical Patient Vignette 5.5

A 37-year-old man had been diabetic for 8 years. He received 35 units of protamine zinc insulin each morning in addition to 5 units of regular insulin when he believed he needed it. One week before admission he lost consciousness transiently upon arising, and, when he awoke, he had a left hemiparesis, which disappeared within seconds. The evening before admission, the patient had received 35 units of protamine zinc and 5 units of regular insulin. He awoke at 6 A.M. on the floor and was soiled with feces. His entire left side was numb and paralyzed. His pulse was 80 per minute, respirations 12, and blood pressure 130/80 mm Hg. The general physical examination was unremarkable. He was lethargic but oriented. His speech was slurred. There was supranuclear left facial paralysis and left flaccid hemiplegia with weakness of the tongue and the trapezius muscles. There was a left extensor plantar response but no sensory impairment. The blood sugar was 31 mg/dL. Electroencephalogram (EEG) was normal with no slow-wave focus. He was given 25 g of glucose intravenously and recovered fully in 3 minutes.

Comment

This patient, who was seen prior to the availability of computed tomography (CT) scanning, provides a closer look at the range of physical signs and EEG phenomena that may occur in hypoglycemia. Today, fingerstick glucose testing would have occurred much earlier, often before reaching the hospital, and the physician rarely gets to see such cases. In this man, the occurrence of a similar brief attack of left hemiparesis a week previously suggested right carotid distribution infarction initially. However, the patient was a little drowsier than expected, with an uncomplicated unilateral carotid stroke in which the damage was apparently rather limited. The fact that his attack might have begun with unconsciousness and the fecal staining made his physicians suspect a seizure. However, hypoglycemia also can cause unconsciousness as well as focal signs in conscious patients. After treatment of the low glucose, the hemiplegia cleared rapidly.

Patients with metabolic brain disease may have either focal or generalized seizures that can be indistinguishable from the seizures of structural brain disease. However, when metabolic encephalopathy causes focal seizures, the focus tends to shift from attack to attack, something that rarely happens with structural seizures. Such migratory seizures are especially common and hard to control in uremia.

MOTOR ABNORMALITIES CHARACTERISTIC OF METABOLIC COMA

Tremor, asterixis, and multifocal myoclonus are prominent manifestations of metabolic brain disease; they are less commonly seen with focal structural lesions unless these latter have a toxic or infectious component. The tremor of metabolic encephalopathy is coarse and irregular and has a rate of 8–10 per second. Usually these tremors are absent at rest and, when present, are most evident in the fingers of the outstretched hands. Severe tremors may spread to the face, tongue, and lower extremities and frequently interfere with purposeful movements in agitated patients, such as those with delirium tremens. The physiologic mechanism responsible for this type of tremor is unknown. It is not seen in patients with unilateral hemispheric or focal brainstem lesions.

First described by Adams and Foley in patients with hepatic coma, *asterixis* is now known to accompany a wide variety of metabolic brain diseases and even some structural lesions.[11,12] Asterixis is very closely related to myoclonus, which is a brief contraction (20–250 ms) or sudden cessation of muscle activity.[13] The contraction produces a jerking movement, while the cessation (negative myoclonus) causes a brief failure of muscle tone, which is seen in asterixis when the muscle is active. Asterixis was originally described as a sudden palmar flapping movement of the outstretched hands at the wrists.[14] It is most easily elicited in lethargic but awake patients by directing them to hold their arms outstretched with hands dorsiflexed at the wrist and fingers extended and abducted (i.e., "stopping traffic"). Incipient asterixis comprises a slight irregular tremor of the fingers, beginning after a latent period of 2–30 seconds that is difficult to distinguish from the tremor of metabolic encephalopathy.

Leavitt and Tyler have described the two separate components of this tremulousness.[15] One is an irregular oscillation of the fingers, usually in the anterior-posterior direction but with a rotary component at the wrist. The second consists of random movements of the fingers at the metacarpal-phalangeal joints. This second pattern becomes increasingly marked as the patient holds his or her wrist dorsiflexed until finally the fingers lead the hand into a sudden downward jerk followed by a slower return to the original dorsiflexed position. Both hands are affected, but asynchronously, and as the abnormal movement intensifies, it spreads to the feet, tongue, and face (dorsiflexion of the feet is often an easier posture for obtunded patients to maintain). Indeed, with severe metabolic tremors, it sometimes becomes difficult to distinguish between intense asterixis and myoclonus, and there is some evidence that the two types of movements represent the same underlying phenomena (sudden and transient loss of muscle tone followed by sudden compensation). Asterixis is generally seen in awake but lethargic patients and generally disappears with the advent of stupor or coma, although occasionally one can evoke the arrhythmic contraction in such subjects by passively dorsiflexing the wrist. Asterixis can also be elicited in stuporous patients by passively flexing and abducting the hips.[16] Flapping abduction-adduction movements occurring either synchronously or asynchronously suggest metabolic brain disease (Figure 5.1).

Unilateral, or less commonly bilateral, asterixis has been described in patients with focal brain lesions.[12] Electromyograms (EMGs) recorded during asterixis show a brief absence of muscular activity during the downward jerk followed by a sudden muscular compensatory contraction, much like the sudden bobbing of the head that normally accompanies drowsiness. The sudden electrical silence is unexplained and not accompanied by electroencephalographic (EEG) changes.[17,18]

Multifocal myoclonus consists of sudden, nonrhythmic, nonpatterned gross twitching or jerking involving parts of muscles or groups of muscles first in one part of the body, then another, and particularly affecting the face and proximal limb musculature. Multifocal myoclonus most commonly accompanies uremic encephalopathy, a large dose of intravenous penicillin, CO_2 narcosis,

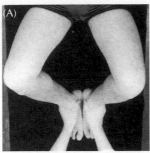

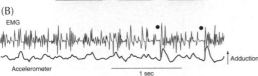

Figure 5.1 (A) Technique of hip flexion-abduction. (B) Electromyographic (EMG) recording from the hip adductors (upper trace) and accelerometric recording from the patella (lower trace). Brief periods of EMG silence (black dots) are followed by a burst of high-voltage electrical activity and a striking change in acceleration. From Noda et al.[16] with permission.

posthypoxic encephalopathy, and hyperosmotic-hyperglycemic encephalopathy. Multifocal myoclonus in a patient who is stuporous or in coma is indicative of severe metabolic disturbance. However, it may be seen in some waking patients with neurodegenerative disorders (e.g., Lewy body dementia or Alzheimer's disease) or prion disorders (Creutzfeldt-Jakob disease and related disorders). Its physiology is unknown; the motor twitchings are not always reflected by a specific EEG abnormality and have, in fact, been reported in a patient with electrocerebral silence.[19]

PART 2: THE INTERNAL MILIEU: AN OVERVIEW OF CEREBRAL METABOLISM AND THE ENVIRONMENT NECESSARY TO MAINTAIN NORMAL NEURONAL FUNCTION

The physiologic principles of cerebral metabolism and blood flow are highly interdependent although we artificially separate them for discussion here. Decreases in blood flow will, among many other changes, result in an alteration of the ionic environment, which may lead to cortical spreading depolarization and abnormal synaptic activity of neurons. Here we illustrate some fundamental physiologic principles that underlie normal neuronal activity. We do not suggest that any of these functions should be understood in isolation, but the intention is rather to provide the reader with the basic building blocks that are necessary to understand normal brain function.

Cerebral Blood Flow, Oxygen, and Glucose Utilization

CEREBRAL BLOOD FLOW

Under normal resting conditions, the total cerebral blood flow (CBF) in man is about 55 mL/100 g/minute, an amount that equals 15–20% of the resting cardiac output. A number of studies have found that the overall CBF remains relatively constant during the states of wakefulness or slow-wave sleep, as well as in the course of various mental and physical activities. Positron emission tomography (PET) and functional magnetic resonance imaging (MRI) scanning reveal that this apparent uniformity masks a regionally varying and dynamically fluctuating CBF which is closely adjusted to meet the metabolic requirements posed by local physiologic changes in the brain. Overall flow in gray matter, for example, is normally three to four times higher than in white matter.[20] When neural activity increases within a region, cerebral metabolism increases to meet the increased demand.[21] Cerebral metabolic rates for glucose and CBF each increase about 50% in the active area, whereas the metabolic rate for oxygen increases only about 5%.[21] See Figures 5.2 and 5.3.

Thus, the oxygen extraction falls, increasing the concentration of oxyhemoglobin in venous blood. This is the basis for the blood oxygenation level detection (BOLD) signal obtained using functional MRI. The increase in glucose metabolism over oxygen metabolism results in increased lactate production, possibly the substrate for the increased demand of neurons (Figure 5.4).[22] The stimulus for the increase in regional CBF is complex.[23] Arteriolar dilation is promoted by astrocytic release of calcium (Ca(2+)) that triggers the release of a number of vasoactive substances by neurons and glia during increased neural activity.[24] Important among these are adenosine, nitric oxide,

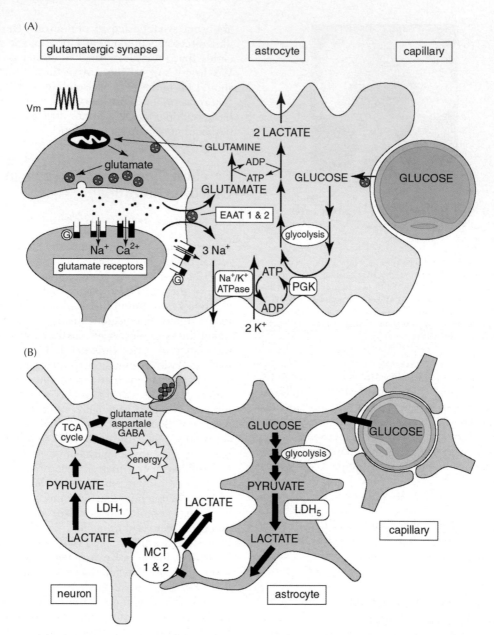

Figure 5.2 (A) Schematic representation of the mechanism for glutamate-induced glycolysis in astrocytes during physiologic activation. At glutamatergic synapses, presynaptically released glutamate depolarizes postsynaptic neurons by acting at specific receptor subtypes. The action of glutamate is terminated by an efficient glutamate uptake system located primarily in astrocytes. Glutamate is cotransported with Na+, resulting in an increase in8 the intra-astrocytic concentration of Na+, leading to an activation of the astrocyte Na+/K+-ATPase. Activation of the Na+/K+-ATPase stimulates glycolysis (i.e., glucose use and lactate production). Lactate, once released by astrocytes, can be taken up by neurons and serves them as an adequate energy substrate. (For graphic clarity, only lactate uptake into presynaptic terminals is indicated. However, this process could also occur at the postsynaptic neuron.) This model, which summarizes in vitro experimental evidence indicating glutamate-induced glycolysis, is taken to reflect cellular and molecular events occurring during activation of a given cortical area. (B) Schematic representation of the proposed astrocyte–neuron lactate shuttle. Following neuronal activation and synaptic glutamate release, glutamate reuptake into astrocytes triggers increased glucose uptake from capillaries via activation of an isoform of the Na+/K+-ATPase, which is highly sensitive to ouabain, possibly the alpha-2 isoform.[25–27] Glucose is then processed glycolytically to lactate by astrocytes that are enriched in the muscle form of lactate dehydrogenase (LDH$_5$). The exchange of lactate between astrocytes and neurons is operated by monocarboxylate transporters (MCTs). Lactate is then converted to pyruvate since neurons contain the heart form of LDH (LDH$_1$). Pyruvate, via the formation of acetyl-CoA by pyruvate dehydrogenase (PDH), enters the tricarboxylic acid (TCA) cycle, thus generating 17 adenosine triphosphate (ATP) molecules per lactate molecule. ADP, adenosine diphosphate.
From Magistretti and Pellerin,[25] with permission.

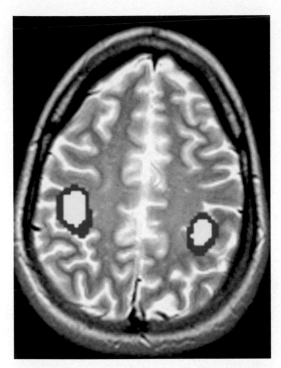

Figure 5.3 A functional magnetic resonance imaging scan of the normal individual flexing and extending his fingers. Blood flow increases to a greater degree than oxygen consumption in the motor areas, leading to an increase in oxyhemoglobin. The paramagnetic oxyhemoglobin causes an increased blood oxygen level-dependent signal in the motor cortex bilaterally.
Image courtesy Dr. Andrei Holodny.

dopamine, acetylcholine, neuropeptide Y, vasoactive intestinal polypeptide, and arachidonic acid metabolites.[23,28]

Several pathologic states of brain are marked by a disproportionately high or low rates of local blood flow in relation to metabolism. Examples of reactive hyperemia or "uncoupling" of flow and metabolism occur in areas of traumatic or postischemic tissue injury, as well as in regions of inflammation or in the regions surrounding certain brain tumors.

Primary reductions in CBF can be regional or general (global). *Regional impairments of CBF* result from intrinsic diseases of the cervical and cerebral arteries (atherosclerosis, thrombosis, and, rarely, inflammation), from arterial embolism, and from the extrinsic pressure on individual cerebral arteries produced by compartmental herniation. *General or global reductions in CBF* result from systemic hypotension, complete

or functional cardiac arrest (e.g., ventricular arrhythmias in which output falls below requirements of brain perfusion), and increased intracranial pressure (ICP). As noted earlier in this volume, however, unless some primary abnormality of brain tissue acts to increase regional vascular resistance, an increase in the ICP must approach the systemic systolic pressure before the CBF declines sufficiently to cause recognizable changes in neurologic functions.

Cessation of blood flow to the brain (*ischemia*), as discussed in subsequent paragraphs, appears to cause a greater risk of irreversible tissue damage than does even a profound reduction in the arterial oxygen tension (*anoxemia*). The precise lower level of arterial perfusion required to maintain the vitality of the tissue in man is not known. Extrapolations based on animal experiments suggest that the CBF of 20 mL/100 g of brain per minute causes loss of consciousness but not permanent damage. If the flow falls to 10 mL/100 g/minute, membrane integrity is lost and calcium influx into the cells leads to irreversible damage. Time is also an important factor. Flows of 18 mL can be tolerated for several hours without leading to infarction, whereas flows of 5 mL lasting for more than 30 minutes will cause infarction.[29]

Several factors may explain why ischemia so severely threatens tissue structure. A change in pH or lactic acid concentration is one factor. Anaerobic metabolism produces large amounts of lactic acid and lowers the pH. The increased concentration of hydrogen ions leads to cell death[30] by increasing brain edema, interfering with mitochondrial adenosine triphosphate (ATP) generation, and increasing calcium levels and the formation of free radicals, all of which can cause cellular death.[31] Hypoglycemia (see later discussion), by increasing lactate production, contributes to the brain damage.

Several other factors play a role in helping regulate CBF, the most important of which is PCO_2 or, more accurately, cerebral pH. Cerebral acidosis is a potent vasodilator, as is potassium, which leaks into the brain extracellular space during hypoxia. Other factors that serve to increase CBF include nitric oxide (which in older literature was referred to as endothelial-derived relaxing factor), adenosine (probably working through nitric oxide), and

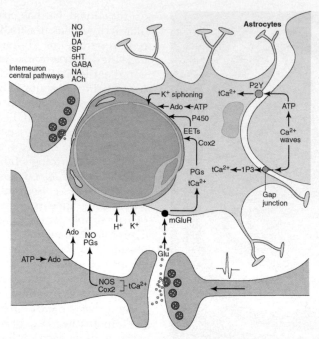

Figure 5.4 Vasoactive mediators released from neurons and glia by neural activity. Ions (H⁺ and K⁺) contribute to the extracellular currents that are associated with synaptic transmission. Adenosine (Ado) is produced through adenosine triphosphate (ATP) catabolism. Glutamate (Glu)-induced increases in the intracellular concentration of Ca^{2+} in neurons and glia activate the synthesis of nitric oxide (NO), of the cyclooxygenase-2 (Cox2) products prostaglandins (PGs), and of the cytochrome P450 epoxygenase products epoxyeicosatrienoic acids (EETs). In astrocytes, the [Ca^{2+}] increase is produced by activation of metabotropic glutamate receptors (mGluRs) and by propagation of Ca^{2+} waves from neigh-boring astrocytes through activation of purinergic receptors (P2Y) or entry of 1P3 (inositol (1,4,5)-triphosphate) through gap junctions. Astrocytic lipoxygenase products could also produce vasodilation by inducing NO release from endothelial cells. Spatial buffering currents in astrocytes release K⁺ from perivascular end-feet, where K⁺ conductance is greatest (K⁺ siphoning). Interneurons and projecting neurons with perivascular contacts release vasoactive neurotransmitters and neuropeptides, including NO, vasoactive intestinal polypeptide (VIP), dopamine (DA), substance P (SP), serotonin (5HT), gamma-aminobutyric acid (GABA), noradrenaline (NA), and acetylcholine (ACh).
From Iadecola,[23] with permission.

prostaglandins (for a review see Iadecola[23] and Zauner et al.[32]).

OXYGEN

Sufficient availability of oxygen is fundamental for maintaining aerobic metabolism, the primary pathway for energy generation in the brain. While isolated hypoxia is better tolerated than hypoxia coupled with ischemia, oxygen at higher concentration is cytotoxic.[33]

GLUCOSE METABOLISM

Glucose is the overwhelmingly predominant blood-borne substrate for brain metabolism. One might question why this is so since it is

known that slices of cerebral cortex in vitro can utilize a variety of substrates, including fatty acids and other compounds, to synthesize acetoacetate for entry into the citric acid cycle. The answer appears to lie in the specialized properties of the blood–brain barrier, which, by rigorously limiting or facilitating the entry or egress of substances to and from the brain, guards the narrow homeostasis of that organ. Glucose is transported across the blood–brain barrier by a carrier-mediated glucose transporter (Glut-1). The uptake of glucose into neurons is also facilitated by a glucose transporter (Glut-3), and glucose uptake into astrocytes is facilitated by Glut-1. Under normal circumstances, brain glucose concentration is approximately 30% of that of plasma. Insulin is not required for the entry of glucose into brain or for its metabolism by brain cells.

In net metabolic terms, each 100 g of brain in a normal human being utilizes about 0.31 mol (5.5 mg) of glucose per minute so that, in the basal, prolonged fasting state, the brain's consumption of glucose almost equals the total amount that the liver produces. This net figure, however, hides the fact that glucose consumption in local regions of the brain varies widely according to local functional changes. Because of its rapid transfer into brain, glucose represents essentially the organ's only substrate under normal physiologic conditions. However, neurons probably utilize lactate produced from glucose by astrocytes when stimulated with glutamate.[34,35]

Ketone bodies can diffuse into brain and also are transported across the blood–brain barrier. These substances provide increased fuel to the brain when beta-hydroxybutyrate, acetoacetate, and other ketones increase in the blood during states such as starvation, the ingestion of high-fat diets, or ketoacidosis. During starvation, in fact, liver gluconeogenesis may fall below the level required to meet cerebral substrate needs; at such times ketone utilization can contribute as much as 30% of the brain's fuel for oxidative metabolism. For unknown reasons, however, the brain does not appear able to subsist entirely on ketone bodies, and as mentioned later, some investigators believe that ketones contribute to the neurologic toxicity of diabetic ketoacidosis.

Under normal circumstances, all but about 15% of glucose uptake in the brain is accounted for by combustion with O_2 to produce H_2O and energy, the remainder going to lactate production. The brain contains about 1 mmol/kg of free glucose in reserve and a considerable amount of glycogen, perhaps as high as 10 mg/L, which is present in astrocytes.[36,37] With the addition of either increased metabolic demand or decreased metabolic supply, glycogen in astrocytes can break down to lactate to support neuronal function. Despite this, deprivation of glucose and oxygen to the brain rapidly results in loss of consciousness, with normal cerebral function being maintained for only a matter of seconds.

The energy balance of the brain is influenced both by its supply of energy precursors (i.e., its input) and by the work the organ does (i.e., its output). Just as intrinsic mechanisms appropriately increase or decrease the rate of metabolism in different regions of the brain during periods of locally increased or decreased functional activity, intrinsic mechanisms appear able to "turn down" general cerebral metabolic activity and produce stupor or coma when circumstances threaten to deplete blood-borne substrate.

Several metabolic disorders are known to cause a decrease in the brain's rate of metabolism and physiologic function without initially resulting in any encroachment on the energy reserves of the tissue. For example, metabolic rate is reversibly reduced during anesthesia, hypothermia, and sleep.[37,38] The reversible hypometabolism that accompanies other causes of metabolic encephalopathy, such as hypoglycemia, hypoxemia, reduced states of CBF, and hyperammonemia is less well understood than what occurs under anesthesia. The response appears to be important in protecting the brain against irreversible damage, as both hypoglycemia and hyperglycemia can damage the brain.

Ionic Environment in the Brain and Cortical Spreading Depolarization

IONIC ENVIRONMENT

The ionic environment, acid–base status, carbon dioxide tension, and osmolarity are physiologically and pathophysiologically linked processes. Major ions like sodium, potassium, and calcium must be kept in a very tight range to ensure normal neurological function. Ionic concentration in the CSF and interstitial fluid are therefore kept stable in order to allow proper functioning of brain neurons and glia.[39,40] Sodium is the most abundant serum cation, and, for practical purposes, systemic alterations of osmolarity are related to changes in serum sodium or glucose. As sodium is functionally an impermeable solute, hypo- and hypernatremia will at least transiently cause movement of water across the vascular membrane. Intra- and extracellular changes in sodium and water concentration together account for much of the encountered clinical symptoms in these disorders.

ACID–BASE BALANCE

Acid–base status is determined by the concentration of hydrogen ions in a given fluid. It is reported as pH, with the pH of blood and brain in a healthy human ranging between 7.35 to 7.45 and 7.35 to 7.40, respectively.[41] In blood, a pH of lower than 7.37 or of higher than 7.46 is called acidotic or alkalotic, respectively.[42] Abnormalities in CSF pH affect neuronal function, and localized brain pH changes have been linked to electrical brain activity.[43] Acid–base status is closely linked to respiratory status. As such, acidosis or alkalosis may develop due to changes in respiration, or hyper- or hypoventilation may be triggered to compensate for acid–base derangements. Chemoreceptors located in the carotid, as well as in the lower brainstem, quickly respond to alterations in the blood of either hydrogen ion concentration or PCO_2. Hypoxia sensitizes peripheral chemoreceptors and activates central chemoreceptors, but, under most circumstances, CO_2 levels, which are linked to blood pH, are more important in determining respiration.

OSMOLALITY

The term *osmolality* refers to the number of solute particles dissolved in a solvent. Osmolality is usually expressed as milliosmoles per liter of water (mOsm/L). It can either be measured directly in the serum by the freezing point depression method or, for clinical purposes, calculated from the concentrations of sodium, potassium, glucose, and urea (the predominant solutes) in the serum (assuming that there is no intoxication). The formula here gives a rough but clinically useful approximation of the serum osmolality:

$$mOsm/kg = 2(Na + K) + \frac{glucose}{18} + \frac{BUN}{2.8}$$

Sodium and potassium are expressed in mEq/L, and the divisors convert glucose and blood urea nitrogen (BUN) expressed in mg/dL to mEq/L. If the glucose and BUN are normal, the serum osmolality can be approximated by doubling the serum Na^+ and adding 10. Normal serum osmolality is 290 ± 5 mOsm/kg.

A measured osmolality higher than the calculated osmolality indicates a substantial concentration of an unmeasured osmolar substance, usually a toxin. Hypo-osmolality leads to an increased cellular water content and tissue swelling. Only a few agents are equally and rapidly distributed throughout the body water (e.g., alcohol); therefore, hyperosmolality due to excess ethanol does not affect water distribution within the brain. However, the blood–brain barrier prevents most agents from entering the CNS. As a result, hyperosmolality due to these agents results in redistribution of water from within the CNS to the circulation. This property is used clinically when mannitol (a nonmetabolizable sugar) is injected intravenously to draw fluid out of the brain and temporarily decrease cerebral edema. However, the brain has protective mechanisms against osmolar shifts, including slow redistribution of solutes, so that while the rapid changes in serum osmolality may produce more improvement in neurologic symptoms, the slow changes will ultimately result in the edema returning.[44,45] Direct measurement of osmolar substances using magnetic resonance spectroscopy can demonstrate decreases in myoinositol, choline, creatine, phosphocreatine, and probably glutamate/glutamine. As expected (see Figure 5.5), in patients with chronic hyponatremia (mean serum sodium 120 mEq/L), water content of brain was not different from controls.[46] Because the brain adapts to long-term hypo- or hypernatremia, it is not possible to give exact values of serum sodium or osmolality above or below normal at which symptoms will develop. However, subacute changes in serum osmolalities below about 260 mEq/L or above about 330 mEq/L over hours or a few days are likely to produce cerebral symptoms. In addition, cerebral symptoms can be produced by sudden restorations of osmolality toward normal when an illness has produced a sustained osmolar shift away from normal. In extreme cases, this can cause central pontine myelinolysis.

CORTICAL SPREADING DEPOLARIZATION

Brain homeostasis is actively maintained in a fine balance by an energy-consuming number of interconnected physiological processes

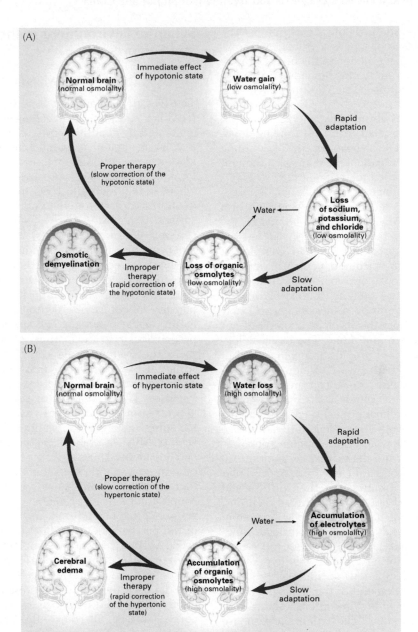

Figure 5.5 Effects of hypo- and hypernatremia on the brain. (A) When blood osmolality becomes hypotonic compared to brain, there is rapid brain swelling as water enter the brain to maintain isotonicity with blood. The brain adapts over the next few hours by rapid loss of electrolytes. Over the next few days, there is slower loss of organic osmolytes in the brain. If blood osmolality is corrected too quickly, there can be osmotic demyelination, usually most prominent in the pons and corpus callosum. (B) When blood osmolality becomes hypertonic relative to brain, there is rapid water loss (an effect that is exploited to reduce cerebral edema during brain herniation). Over the next few hours, the brain adapts by electrolytes entering the brain. During the next few days, the brain adapts by intracellular accumulation of organic osmolytes. Overly aggressive lowering of blood osmolality may then produce cerebral edema.

Panel A from Adrogue and Madias[44] and Panel B from Androgue HJ, Madias NE. Hypernatremia. *N Engl J Med* 2000;342:1493–1499, with permission.

such as the sodium-potassium pump. The created balance of ions is a crucial prerequisite for neuronal function in the healthy brain. In acute brain injury, this homeostasis may be disturbed resulting in brain dysfunction, which is reflected in intracortical EEG recordings. These waves of abrupt, sustained mass depolarization are labeled cortical spreading depolarization (CSD).[47] These waves are common in brain-injured patients and are also thought to be the basis for migraine auras.[48–50] CSDs are slow, sustained waves of mass depolarization and the electrical representation of a breakdown of the brain's ionic homeostasis.[52] Ionic gradients between the neuron and the extracellular space break down completely, associated with sustained neuronal depolarization, shutdown of membrane resistance, loss of electrical activity, and swelling and distortion of dendritic spines. The waves may propagate across the brain at a speed of approximately 2–6 mm min^{-1}. The exact biological mechanism of propagation is unclear, but it is associated with a wave of increased extracellular potassium concentration from about 2.5 mM up to as much as 35 mM.[53] As this wave of extracellular potassium diffuses across the cortex, it would be sufficient to depolarize neurons, which would cause opening of potassium channels and the extrusion of additional intracellular potassium into the extracellular space, where it could also then diffuse and cause depolarization of additional neurons. These waves of high extracellular potassium appear to be independent of astrocyte function.[54] Regional CBF increases of more than 100% occur during CSD.[55] This hyperemia, however, is insufficient to adequately match the increased demand of the hypermetabolic tissue, thus creating low-energy states with local lactic acidosis.[56] The hyperemic response allows clearance of metabolites, which is fundamental to restore the homeostatic balance but may break down under a number of pathological conditions. Here, the hyperemia is replaced by an ischemic response secondary to severe arteriolar vasoconstriction in response to the CSD. Recovery of involved brain regions depends on the ability to adequately recruit sodium pump activity to repolarize affected neurons. If this fails, neuronal death occurs, a condition labeled as *terminal depolarization*.[57]

Synaptic Environment in the Brain and Seizures

SYNAPTIC ENVIRONMENT

The electrical signal that is recorded by the EEG is a measure of the extracellular current generated by dendritic postsynaptic potentials in a large number of parallel aligned pyramidal cells in the cerebral cortex.[58,59] While local field potentials can be measured anywhere in the brain, the EEG that is most frequently recorded from the skull or the cortical surface is almost entirely generated by the cerebral cortex (in rodents, the underlying hippocampus; in human brains, the hippocampus is deep in the medial temporal surface and not accessible to surface recordings). While there are other cortical neurons (particularly inhibitory interneurons), the parallel nature of the pyramidal cell apical dendrites, perpendicular to the cortical surface, makes them the overwhelming contributors to the surface EEG. Cortical neurons communicate with each other via excitatory and inhibitory synapses. These synapses release a variety of neurotransmitters from presynaptic terminals, including glutamate, gamma-aminobutyric acid (GABA), acetylcholine, norepinephrine, and dopamine. These signaling molecules then bind to postsynaptic receptors that activate either ligand-gated ion channels or are G-protein coupled and activate a sequence of intracellular responses that may alter the membrane voltage of the postsynaptic cell, affect its intracellular cyclic AMP or calcium levels, or have metabolic consequences. The dendritic depolarizations caused by these inputs (not the firing of the pyramidal cells themselves) represent the basis for the EEG field potentials measured at the cortical surface. Of course, the integration of synaptic inputs from many neurons underlies information processing in the cerebral cortex, and this synaptic communication is the foundation for proper brain function; both normal function and many types of dysfunction are reflected in the spatially distributed electrical oscillations recorded in the EEG.[60]

SEIZURES

Synchronized discharging groups of neurons with spread of the activity may manifest clinically as seizures. The underlying pathophysiological processes involve increased excitability of a group of neurons (seizure focus), an excitable network of neurons (glutamatergic spread of the seizure), and reduced activity of normally inhibitory projections (GABAergic). Neurons within the penumbral area surrounding a seizure focus are typically hyperpolarized and release the inhibitory neurotransmitter GABA.[61] The migrating edge of a seizing brain area triggers traveling waves of synaptic activity into adjacent cortical areas followed by induced slow dynamics as the seizure subsides.[62]

Seizures are characterized by intense, repetitive neuronal discharge followed by postictal metabolic cerebral depression of varying degrees and duration. In general, this requires re-entrant neuronal circuits that mainly occur in the forebrain when lesions involve the structures of the cortical mantle. In the experimental animal, one can demonstrate that major seizures produce a 200–300% increase in cerebral metabolic demand, a substantial degree of systemic hypertension, and an enormously increased CBF.[63] Repetitive convulsions result in a progressive, abnormal increase in the permeability of the blood–brain barrier.[61] If substrate depletion or a relative decline in blood flow occurs during seizures, the brain maintains its metabolism by the consumption of endogenous substrates. With sustained status epilepticus (SE) in such animals, progressive hypoxic-ischemic structural neuronal damage results soon after. Similar but necessarily less comprehensive analyses indicate that seizures cause comparable changes in the human brain.

PART 3: DISORDERS OF THE INTERNAL MILIEU: LACK OF SUBSTRATE

Cerebral Hypoxia and Ischemia

In understanding how cerebral hypoxia leads to impairment of consciousness, it is important first to dissociate hypoxia from ischemia. This is not easy, because the most common causes of cerebral hypoxia are due to inadequate blood flow (ischemic hypoxia). In addition, severe systemic hypoxia (e.g., due to ventilatory failure, hypoxic hypoxia) inevitably leads to cardiovascular collapse and secondary ischemia. On the other hand, there are conditions of pure hypoxia with adequate or even increased CBF, such as anemic hypoxia (low oxygen carrying capacity in the blood), in which metabolic demands of critical brain regions required for intact consciousness are not adequately met.

Surprisingly, unlike ischemia and hypoglycemia, pure hypoxia alone is rarely responsible for brain injuries such as laminar necrosis.[65] In fact, in individuals with chronic hypoxemia, such as seen in chronic lung disease, hypoxic preconditioning may act to limit the damage caused by acute exacerbations of hypoxia. For example, in experimental animals exposure to moderate hypoxia of 8% to 10% oxygen for 3 hours protects against cerebral ischemia delivered 1 or 2 days later.[66] Miyamoto and Auer exposed rats to an arterial PO_2 of 25 torr for 15 minutes and failed to find necrotic neurons.[65] On the other hand, unilateral carotid ligation (ischemia) causes neuronal necrosis even in animals exposed to an arterial O_2 of 100 torr. In these experiments, hypoxia exacerbated the effects of ischemia. Thus, ischemic hypoxia, the most common cause of hypoxia in humans, is really a mixture of hypoxic and ischemic mechanisms of injury and their effects on each other.

Pure hypoxia, such as occurs in carbon monoxide poisoning or a pure respiratory arrest, is more likely to lead to delayed injury to the subcortical structures of the hemispheres. Typically, the damage will occur one to several days after the patient awakens from the hypoxic episode and involves a characteristic distribution, including the posterior hemispheric white matter and basal ganglia, often leaving the patient blind and with a choreic movement disorder. A similar pattern of brain injury is seen with a variety of mitochondrial encephalopathies and deficits in carbohydrate metabolism, suggesting that the injury is due to failure of intracellular oxidative metabolism. The reason that the injury has a predilection for these sites is unknown, although neurons in the globus pallidus have a particularly high constitutive firing rate, and this may predispose them to hypoxic injury. See Patient Vignette 5.6.

Patient Vignette 5.6

A 38-year-old electrical engineer who had a history of hypokalemic periodic paralysis decided to exercise in a gym after eating a donut for breakfast. Within minutes, he became progressively weaker and experienced difficulty breathing. He lost consciousness, stopped breathing, and was resuscitated by nonmedical bystanders for about 10 minutes before emergency medical technicians arrived and intubated him. In the hospital emergency department, he initially was unresponsive, with pupils that were 5 mm and reacted to light sluggishly, and he had no eye movements spontaneously or with oculocephalic maneuvers. He was flaccid, with depressed reflexes, and had no toe movement with attempted Babinski testing. He recovered spontaneous respiration and awoke over the next 6 hours. The following day, his neurological examination was normal, and he was permitted to return home. On the fifth day following the collapse at the gym, he began to develop difficulty seeing, initially with graying of his vision and then complete loss of vision from both eyes. Over the next few days, he also developed choreic and athetotic movements of his neck, trunk, and upper limbs. Magnetic resonance imaging (MRI) scan revealed hyperintensity of the deep white matter, particularly posteriorly in the both hemispheres, as well as in the globus pallidus bilaterally.

Comment

Elevated blood sugar plus exercise is known to cause a fall in serum potassium as the sugar is taken up and metabolized. This resulted, in this patient with known hypokalemic periodic paralysis, in a period of flaccid paralysis, including of his respiratory muscles. This would cause pure hypoxic hypoxia, and the resuscitative attempts by the bystanders were apparently sufficient to prevent sufficient ischemia to cause immediate brain injury. The posthypoxic injury to the deep white matter and basal ganglia in this case is typical of that condition.

DIFFERENT TYPES OF HYPOXIA HAVE DIFFERENT CAUSES AND CONSEQUENCES

Hypoxia of the brain almost always arises as part of a larger problem in oxygen supply, either because the ambient pressure of the gas falls or systemic abnormalities in the individual interrupt its delivery to the tissues. Although there are many causes of tissue hypoxia, disturbances in oxygen supply to the brain in most instances can be divided into four main types: *hypoxic hypoxia, anemic hypoxia, histotoxic hypoxia,* and *ischemic hypoxia.*[67] Though caused by different conditions and diseases, all four categories share equally the potential for depriving brain tissue of its critical oxygen supply. The main differences between the hypoxic, anemic, and ischemic forms are on the arterial side. Hypoxic, anemic, and ischemic hypoxia all share the common effect of producing cerebral venous hypoxia, while normal blood oxygen measurements may be recorded in patients with histotoxic hypoxia.

Following acute brain injury, invasive and noninvasive measurements of venous and arterial oxygenation have been used. These include measures of oxygen saturation in the venous blood leaving the brain (e.g., invasive jugular venous oxygen saturation) and partial brain tissue oxygenation utilizing a polarographic oxygen electrode (e.g., parenchymal Clark electrode, usually inserted into the cerebral cortex), as well as optical systems based on oxygen quenching that allow direct measurements of cerebral oxygenation.[68] Noninvasive measures of cerebral oxygenation (i.e., near infrared spectroscopy) are desirable but currently still not accurate enough to reliably guide therapy. While noninvasive technologies are steadily being improved, support for invasive parenchymal oxygen monitoring is increasing. This is particularly true in comatose patients with traumatic brain injury (TBI) to complement parenchymal ICP monitoring in an effort to provide individualized targets for cerebral perfusion pressure, ventilator parameters, and transfusions.[69] Differentiation of these processes is best achieved when oxygen levels for the arterial input, utilization, and venous output are established. One approach to approximate this at the bedside is by utilizing both partial brain tissue oxygen monitors with jugular vein oxygen measurements. This comprehensive approach, which may only be applicable to a small number of patients, ideally allows the estimation of oxygen utilization and may guide therapeutic interventions.[70] Management purely guided by peripheral or cerebral oxygen targets has not improved patients' clinical outcomes.[71] Interventions aimed at augmenting oxygen delivery via augmentation of perfusion appear to be more promising.[72] Interestingly, studies have shown that brain tissue oxygen levels are more indicative of oxygen diffusion than oxygen delivery and metabolism in TBI patients.[73]

In *hypoxic hypoxia,* insufficient oxygen reaches the blood so that both the arterial oxygen content and tension are low. This situation results either from a low oxygen tension in the environment (e.g., high altitude or displacement of oxygen by an inert gas such as nitrogen or methane)[74] or from an inability of oxygen to reach and cross the alveolar capillary membrane (pulmonary disease, hypoventilation). With mild or moderate hypoxia, the CBF increases to maintain the cerebral oxygen delivery and no symptoms occur. However, clinical evidence suggests that even in chronic hypoxic conditions, the CBF can only increase to about twice normal. When the increase is insufficient to compensate for the degree of hypoxia, the cerebral metabolic rate of oxygen ($CMRO_2$) begins to fall and symptoms of cerebral hypoxia occur. Because hypoxic hypoxia affects the entire organism, all energy-intensive tissues are affected, and, eventually, if the oxygen delivery is sufficiently impaired, the myocardium fails, the blood pressure drops and the brain becomes ischemic. Most of the pathologic changes in patients who die after an episode of hypoxic hypoxia are related to ischemia[65]; therefore, it is difficult to define the actual damage done by hypoxic hypoxia alone.[75] These compensatory mechanisms to increase CBF rely on autoregulatory responses that are impaired in patients with acute brain injury such as TBI or subarachnoid hemorrhage (SAH).[75–79] This potentially augmented impact of hypoxia may also affect acute brain injury patients with other types of hypoxia such as anemic hypoxia, rendering these patients particularly vulnerable to episodes of hypoxia. Loss of consciousness due to hypoxic hypoxia before blood pressure drops may be a result of enhanced spontaneous transmitter release, which probably disrupts normal neural circuitry.[80]

In *anemic hypoxia,* sufficient oxygen reaches the blood, but the amount of hemoglobin available to bind and transport it is decreased. Under such circumstances, the blood oxygen content is decreased even though oxygen tension in the arterial blood is normal. Either low hemoglobin content (anemia) or chemical changes in hemoglobin that interfere with oxygen binding (e.g., carbon monoxyhemoglobin, methemoglobin) can be responsible. Coma occurs if the oxygen content drops so low that the brain's metabolic needs are not met even by an increased CBF. The lowered blood viscosity that occurs in anemia makes it somewhat easier for the CBF to increase than in carbon monoxide poisoning. Most of the toxicity from carbon monoxide poisoning is not due to hemoglobin binding but is histotoxic, a result of its binding to cytochromes,[81] as outlined later.

In *ischemic hypoxia,* the blood may or may not carry sufficient oxygen, but the CBF is insufficient to supply cerebral tissues. The usual causes are diseases that greatly reduce the cardiac output, such as myocardial infarction, arrhythmia, shock, and vasovagal syncope, or diseases that increase the cerebral vascular resistance by arterial occlusion (e.g., stroke) or spasm (e.g., migraine).

Histotoxic hypoxia results from agents that poison the electron transport chain. Such agents include cyanide and carbon monoxide. Carbon monoxide intoxication is by far the most common; smoke from house fires can cause both carbon monoxide and cyanide poisoning. Because the electron transport chain is impaired, glycolysis is increased leading to increased lactic acid; thus, high levels of lactic acid (greater than 7 mmol/L) in the blood are encountered in patients with severe cyanide poisoning. Some cyanide antidotes increase methemoglobin, which may add to the anemic hypoxic burden of patients who have also been poisoned with carbon monoxide[82]; hydroxycobalamin treatment does not help under such conditions.

The development of neurologic signs in most patients with ischemia or hypoxia depends more on the severity and duration of the process than on its specific cause. Ischemia (vascular failure) is generally more dangerous than hypoxia alone, in part because potentially toxic products of cerebral metabolism such as lactic acid are not removed. The clinical categories of hypoxic and ischemic brain damage can be subdivided into acute, chronic, and multifocal.

ACUTE, DIFFUSE (OR GLOBAL) HYPOXIA OR ISCHEMIA

This circumstance occurs with conditions that rapidly reduce the oxygen content of the blood or cause a sudden reduction in the brain's overall blood flow. The major causes include obstruction of the airways, such as occurs with drowning, choking, or suffocation; massive obstruction to the cerebral arteries, such as occurs with hanging or strangulation; and conditions causing a sudden decrease in cardiac output, such as asystole, severe arrhythmias, vasodepressor syncope, pulmonary embolism, or massive systemic hemorrhage. Embolic or thrombotic disorders, including thrombotic thrombocytopenic purpura, disseminated intravascular coagulation, acute bacterial endocarditis, falciparum malaria, and fat embolism, can all cause such widespread multifocal ischemia that they can give the clinical appearance of acute diffuse cerebral ischemia. If the cerebral circulation stops completely, consciousness is lost rapidly, within 6–8 seconds. It takes a few seconds longer if blood flow continues but oxygen is no longer supplied. Fleeting lightheadedness and blindness sometimes precede unconsciousness. Generalized convulsions, pupillary dilation (due to massive adrenal and sympathetic release of catecholamines as part of the emergency stress response), and bilateral extensor plantar responses quickly follow if anoxia is complete or lasts longer than a few seconds. If tissue oxygenation is restored immediately, consciousness returns in seconds or minutes without sequelae. If, however, the oxygen deprivation lasts longer than 1 or 2 minutes, or if it is superimposed upon preexisting cerebral vascular disease, then stupor, confusion, and signs of motor dysfunction may persist for a variable time (from several hours to permanently). Under clinical circumstances, total ischemic anoxia lasting longer than 4 minutes starts to kill brain cells, with the neurons of the cerebral cortex (especially the hippocampus) and cerebellum (the Purkinje cells) dying first. In humans, severe diffuse ischemic anoxia lasting 10 minutes or more begins to destroy the brain, with cortical pyramidal cells being most sensitive (resulting in laminar necrosis of the cortex).

In rare instances, particularly drowning, in which cold water rapidly lowers brain temperature, recovery of brain function has been noted despite more prolonged periods of anoxia, although such instances are more common in children than adults. Thus, resuscitation efforts after drowning (particularly in children) should not be abandoned just because the patient has been immersed for more than 10 minutes, particularly if the water was cold enough also to cause hypothermia.

As noted earlier, much experimental evidence indicates that the initial mechanism of anoxia's rapidly lethal effect on the brain may, to some degree, lie in the inability of the heart and the cerebral vascular bed to recover from severe ischemia or oxygen deprivation. Along those lines, guidelines for single-provider cardiopulmonary resuscitation now emphasize the need for uninterrupted chest compressions instead of interrupting for administering mouth-to-mouth ventilation.[83] New data suggest that supplying nasal oxygen but no ventilation may be preferred over bag-mask ventilation or mouth-to-mouth ventilation by allowing adequate oxygen supply without lowering the partial pressure of carbon dioxide that often accompanies Ambu bag ventilation with resultant cerebral vasoconstriction and other unwanted consequences (e.g., inflation of the stomach).[84–86]

It has been reported that if one makes meticulous efforts to maintain the circulation, the brains of experimental animals can recover from as long as 30 minutes of very severe hypoxemia with arterial PO_2 tensions of 20 mm Hg or less. Equally low arterial blood oxygen tensions have been reported in conscious humans (particularly those who have experienced chronic hypoxemia) and who recovered without sequelae. These laboratory findings suggest that guaranteeing the integrity of the systemic circulation offers the strongest chance of effectively treating or preventing hypoxic brain damage. Interestingly, previous episodes of hypoxia may protect against ischemic brain injury by inducing hypoxia inducible factor (HIF-1) that in turn induces vascular endothelial growth factor, erythropoietin, glucose transporters, glycolytic enzymes, heat shock proteins, and other genes that may protect against ischemia.[87]

Vigorous and prolonged attempts at cardiac resuscitation are justified, particularly in young and previously healthy individuals in whom recovery of cardiac function is more likely to occur. Acute, short-lived hypoxic-ischemic attacks causing unconsciousness are most often the result of transient global ischemia caused by syncope. Much less frequently, transient attacks of vertebrobasilar ischemia can cause unconsciousness. Such attacks may be accompanied by brief seizures, which often present problems in differential diagnosis as seizures themselves cause loss of consciousness.

Syncope or *fainting* results when cerebral perfusion falls below the level required to supply sufficient oxygen and substrate to maintain tissue metabolism. If the CBF falls below about 20 mL/100 g/minute, there is a rapid failure of cerebral function. Syncope has many causes. Among young persons, most syncope results from dysfunction of autonomic reflexes producing vasodepressor hypotension, so-called neurocardiogenic, vasovagal, or reflex syncope.[88] These events are typically driven by a beta-adrenergic vasodilation in response to increased blood norepinephrine, often during an episode of pain involving tissue invasion (e.g., having blood drawn) or even witnessing such an event in another person. Vasodepressor responses remain the predominant cause of syncope in older persons as well, but, with advancing age, syncopal attacks are more likely to occur as a result of cardiac arrhythmia or hyperactive baroreceptor reflexes due to peripheral, CNS, or cardiac disease.

Adequate, timely cardiopulmonary resuscitation ideally prevents permanent brain injury but typically does not restore sufficient circulation for complete restoration of the brain's function.[88] Rarely (fewer than 1% of out of hospital cardiac arrest cases) the phenomenon of cardiopulmonary resuscitation-induced consciousness has been described.[90] In these studies, the authors considered the occurrence of spontaneous eye opening, jaw tone, speech, or body movements in pulseless patients undergoing active cardiopulmonary resuscitation as an indicator of the presence of some conscious processing.[91] Considering these phenomena as evidence of consciousness is highly controversial, but, interestingly, the authors found that this rare observation was associated with better outcomes.

INTERMITTENT OR SUSTAINED HYPOXIA

Intermittent hypoxia can cause diminished cognitive function and sometimes acute delirium, such as in patients suffering from obstructive sleep apnea.[92] Sustained hypoxia such as occurs in young people at altitudes above 10,000 feet (3,000 meters)[93] can cause delirium and sometimes focal neurologic signs. These disorders are fully reversible. In addition, extreme degrees of anemia or low arterial oxygenation, which can be due to myocardial infarction, congestive heart failure, or pulmonary disease can, under appropriate circumstances, produce delirium, stupor, or coma. This is particularly true when more than one cause of hypoxia is present. For example, a myocardial infarct may cause encephalopathy in moderately anemic elderly subjects who also have chronic pulmonary disease.

Multifocal cerebral ischemia occurs in a number of conditions affecting the arterial bed or its contents. Hypertensive encephalopathy,[94] also referred to as hyperperfusion encephalopathy[95] or posterior reversible leukoencephalopathy (PRES),[96] is relatively rare but often misdiagnosed. Its importance lies in the fact that if the disorder is appropriately identified and treated, it is usually (but not always) reversible. Formerly associated only with acute hypertensive emergencies, particularly eclampsia, the illness is now seen in a variety of settings including after the administration of cyclosporin or tacrolimus, as well as after several cancer chemotherapeutic agents.[97,98] It is also seen in a slightly different form after carotid endarterectomy and in a variety of small vessel diseases including systemic lupus erythematosus, scleroderma, and cryoglobulinemia. In one series of 110 patients, 30 suffered from preeclampsia or eclampsia and 24 from cyclosporin or tacrolimus neurotoxicity.[95] Most but not all of the patients in whom the disorder is induced by chemotherapy are also hypertensive, although the hypertension may be quite transitory and missed unless the patient's blood pressure is being monitored.

Typically the patient, previously neurologically normal, complains of severe headache and may become agitated, leading to progressive confusion, delirium, stupor, or coma. Many patients suffer from focal or generalized seizures and multifocal neurologic signs, especially cortical blindness, but also hemi-plegia or other focal signs. On neurologic ex-amination, one clue is retinal artery spasm and papilloretinal edema; retinal exudates may also be present. The signs and symptoms of PRES may be more varied than traditionally reported.[99]

The imaging findings are characteristic and best seen on MRI[97] (CT scans may be normal or may show hypodensity in the parietal-occipital areas bilaterally). The MRI shows increased intensity on T2 and fluid-attenuated inversion recovery (FLAIR) images bilaterally and often symmetrically involving mainly the subcortical white matter but sometimes also the cortex in the posterior hemispheres and, less com-monly, the cerebellum, thalamus, brainstem, and splenium of the corpus callosum. Rarely, more frontal areas may be involved as well. T1 images may show hypointensity in the same areas and occasionally contrast enhancement. Diffusion-weighted images are usually normal, but in its more severe form, may indicate re-stricted diffusion. Perfusion studies demon-strate hyperperfusion in the areas of abnormal signal. These MR findings are characteristic of vasogenic cerebral edema. Abnormal diffusion images indicate cerebral ischemia or infarction and suggest a poorer prognosis. Hemorrhage, vasoconstriction, and contrast enhancement may be seen.[99]

It is not clear whether the white matter changes and encephalopathy are due to acute hypertension damaging cerebral blood vessels, or whether the encephalopathy represents areas of ischemia due to local vasoconstriction in disorders that cause diffuse systemic vaso-constriction, which also raises blood pressure. The first hypothesis suggests that the disorder is due to breakdown of the blood–brain bar-rier resulting from damage to endothelial cells when hypertension exceeds the boundaries of autoregulation and small vessels dilate, opening the blood–brain barrier. Other factors that also play a role include upregulation of aquaporin-4 (a water channel in cerebral blood vessels that is also up-regulated in normal pregnancy),[100] interleukin-6 (an inflammatory cytokine that opens the blood–brain barrier), and nitric oxide, which induces vasodilation, particularly when intravascular flow rates are high, thus overcoming autoregulation.[94]

However, given that PRES occurs so fre-quently in women with pre-eclampsia, in whom there is a known systemic vasoconstric-tive condition, and that many of these women and patients treated with chemotherapy do not have particularly high systemic pressure, others have proposed that the damage is due to a vasoconstrictive diathesis in which there is local reversible vasoconstriction in the poste-rior cerebral hemispheres. Once the area has become ischemic, then relief of the vasocon-striction would cause a reflex increase in perfu-sion. The posterior distribution of the changes is not understood. In hypertensive encephalop-athy, this has been explained as the tendency for swelling of the medial temporal lobes to compress the posterior cerebral arteries, which may cause occipital ischemia. However, the posterior predisposition is found even in cases with no hypertension.

In less severe cases neuropathologic findings only reveal edema of white matter,[101] and if treated (e.g., for preeclampsia), the MRI changes and functional impairment may be entirely reversible. In more severe cases, microangiopathy with endothelial swelling and fibrinoid necrosis of small vessels and some-times frank infarction occurs.[102]

The treatment consists first of recognizing the syndrome and, in cases with elevated blood pressure, lowering the blood pressure. Blood pressure lowering should be done judiciously, preferably in an intensive care unit (ICU) with an arterial line in place. Most authorities rec-ommend reduction of mean arterial pressure by no more than 20-25% within a period of minutes to a couple of hours; more rapid re-duction may lead to cerebral infarction.[103] In patients with eclampsia or pre-eclampsia, in-travenous magnesium sulfate has been shown in controlled trials to improve outcome, per-haps by its action as a vascular calcium channel blocker.[104]

SEQUELAE OF HYPOXIA

Shortly following cardiac arrest, patients lose consciousness, and the vast majority of cardiac arrest patients do not survive to hospital ad-mission.[105] Although 40–66% of patients with this hypoxic ischemic injury have return of spontaneous circulation,[106–108] in the field, im-pairment of consciousness persists to hospital admission. Most patients who do not imme-diately recover consciousness will not regain the ability to follow commands during the acute ICU stay.[109] Data from the large study of post-arrest patients by Levy and Plum provided a framework for predicting long-term outcome based on recovery of function in the first 4 days. Those data were generated in the era before hypothermia was commonly used for post-arrest patients. However, more recent studies have indicated that when hypothermia is applied for the first day, similar principles apply to recovery thereafter. In addition, patients who have hypothermia to 33°C appear not to do better than those who are simply maintained at normothermia throughout, but this is still a topic of ongoing debate.[110] Hypoxic ischemic injury frequently affects cortical and deep gray matter[111] but may, in some patients treated with hypothermia, spare thalamic and anterior frontal brain regions, resulting in an isolation syndrome.[112] Patients with isolation syndrome suffer from blindness and motor paralysis, preventing communication with the outside world despite retained cognitive function. The prevalence of this extreme form of cognitive motor dissociation is unknown.

DELAYED POSTANOXIC ENCEPHALOPATHY

Following initial recovery from a pure hypoxic insult, about 3% of patients relapse into a severe delayed postanoxic encephalopathy.[113] In our own experience with this disorder (e.g., Patient Vignette 1.1), the onset has been as early as 4 days and as late as 14 days after the initial hypoxia; reports from other authors give an even longer interval.[114] The clinical picture includes an initial hypoxic insult that usually is sufficiently severe that patients are in deep coma when first found but awaken within 24–48 hours. Occasionally, however, relapse has been reported after a mild hypoxic insult that was sufficient only to daze the patient and not to cause full unconsciousness.[114] In either event, nearly all patients resume full activity within 4 or 5 days after the initial insult and then enjoy a clear and seemingly normal interval of 2–40 days. Then, abruptly, affected subjects become irritable, apathetic, and confused. Some are agitated or develop mania. Walking changes to a halting shuffle, and diffuse spasticity or rigidity appears. The deterioration may progress to coma or death or may arrest itself at any point. Most patients have a second recovery period that leads to full health

within a year,[113] although some remain permanently impaired. Hyperbaric oxygen given at the initial insult does not appear to prevent the development of this neurologic problem.[115] The MRI reveals a low apparent diffusion coefficient, which recovers over several months to a year. The typical distribution of lesions includes the deep white matter, particularly in the posterior part of the hemisphere, and the basal ganglia. This pattern is similar to the distribution of infarcts seen in patients with mitochondrial encephalopathies and may be due to the impairment of cellular oxidative metabolism in both cases. The serial changes are consistent with cytotoxic edema, perhaps from apoptosis triggered by the initial hypoxia.[116] However, the pathogenesis of this delayed neurologic deterioration is not known.

Delayed coma after hypoxia has been reported most often after carbon monoxide or asphyxial gas poisoning, but as shown in Patient Vignette 5.8, cases are known in which other injuries, including hypoglycemia, cardiac arrest, strangulation, or a complication of surgical anesthesia, have provided the antecedent insult. Often, the neurologic changes are at first mistaken for a psychiatric disorder or even a subdural hematoma because of the lucid interval. Mental status examination clarifies the first of these errors, and the diffuse distribution of the neurologic changes, the lack of headache, and the absence of signs of rostral caudal deterioration, as well as the typical appearance of deep white matter lesions on head CT or MRI eliminate the second.

Pathologically, the brains of patients dying of delayed postanoxic deterioration contain diffuse, severe, and bilateral leukoencephalopathy of the cerebral hemispheres with sparing of the immediate subcortical connecting fibers and, usually, of the brainstem.[117] Demyelination is prominent and axons appear reduced in number. The basal ganglia are sometimes infarcted,[118] but the nerve cells of the cerebral hemispheres and the brainstem remain mostly intact. The mechanism of the unusual white matter response is unknown. A few patients have been reported to have had arylsulfatase-A pseudodeficiency. This genetic defect is not known to cause cerebral disease, and its relationship to the demyelination is unclear.[119] The diagnosis of coma caused by postanoxic encephalopathy is made from the history of the initial insult and by recognizing the characteristic signs and symptoms of metabolic coma. There is no specific treatment, but bedrest for patients with acute hypoxia may prevent the complication.

MYOCLONUS

Another sequela of severe diffuse hypoxia is myoclonus, which should be divided into one group with early development of cortical or subcortical myoclonus often associated with seizures or SE (sometimes erroneously called myoclonic seizures or myoclonic SE) and a second group in which there is late onset of the syndrome of *intention* or *action myoclonus* (also known as the Lance-Adams syndrome).[120,121] The early form of postanoxic myoclonus is encountered in up to every fifth patient who remains comatose after resuscitation.[122–124] Electrographic seizures are much more common in those with cortical myoclonus[125] but must be differentiated from myoclonic epilepsies, which are a class of developmental seizure disorders occurring early in life. Historically, myoclonus developing early after cardiac arrest, particularly if associated with SE, has been interpreted as an indicator of poor outcome.[120,126,127] Increasingly, cases of good outcome in patients with early postanoxic myoclonus are being reported,[123,128–130] and, like other prognostic findings following cardiac arrest, the prognostic significance of myoclonus has been called into question[131] as all forms of myoclonus may be compatible with good outcomes.[125] Digital EEG recordings with a dedicated EMG channel should be obtained and back-averaging performed on the recording to allow differentiation between cortical and subcortically generated myoclonus. Treatment of both cortical and subcortical myoclonus includes valproic acid, levetiracetam, and benzodiazepines.[132]

DELAYED MYOCLONUS (LANCE-ADAMS SYNDROME)

Myoclonus may also develop in a delayed fashion in patients who recover full consciousness.[133,134] These patients, upon awakening from posthypoxic coma, usually are dysarthric, and attempted voluntary movements are marked by myoclonic jerks of trunk and limb muscles. This intention myoclonus is distinctive and disabling. The pathophysiologic basis

of this disorder has not been established. The disorder may be managed similar to early postanoxic myoclonus.[135]

Hyperoxia

Oxygen can be toxic to cells,[136] and several observational studies have associated brief episodes of arterial hyperoxia with poor outcomes in brain-injured and critically ill patients.[137,138] Several studies have suggested the potential benefits[139] as well as the risks[138,140] of hyperoxic management of brain-injured patients.[141] Following TBI, improved metabolism based on multimodality monitoring has been reported,[142,143] and the potential for hyperbaric oxygen therapy has been discussed.[144] However, supra-physiologic oxygen concentrations may result in production of reactive oxygen species which have been linked to inflammation, reduced CBF, and necrosis.[145,146] If there is a potential for hyperoxia improving a patient's condition, the therapeutic window appears to be extremely narrow.[147]

Hypoglycemia

Glucose is the main substrate of energy metabolism in the brain under normal conditions, and, for that reason, hypoglycemia might be expected to interfere with cerebral metabolism by reducing the brain's energy supply in a manner similar to that caused by hypoxia. With very severe and prolonged hypoglycemia, this turns out to be true, but with less severe or transient reductions in glucose availability, brain functions often return with little injury after glucose levels are repleted. This curious paradox became clear soon after insulin was introduced into clinical use. It was realized that hypoglycemic coma due to insulin overdose could last for up to an hour or so without necessarily leaving any residual neurological effects or structural brain damage. It is now recognized that the brain has several additional sources of energy available beyond blood glucose. These are now known to include intrinsic ATP and phosphocreatine, as well as intrinsic energy substrates, including glycogen (stored in astrocytes) and lactate, and exogenous ketone bodies from the bloodstream that are formed by the liver as a result of oxidizing lipids during low availability of glucose. As a result, as blood glucose levels fall into the range of 31–46 mg/dL (1.7–2.6 mM/dL), cerebral glucose consumption declines moderately, but cerebral oxygen consumption remains normal. At this level, despite the preservation of consciousness, the latency of the P300 readiness potential increases, as does reaction time, suggesting a decrement in ability to make decisions. Below these levels, energy reserves collapse, and, by 1.0 mM/dL of glucose, the EEG becomes isoelectric.

Hypoglycemia is a common and serious cause of metabolic coma and one capable of remarkably varied combinations of signs and symptoms.[148] Among patients with severe hypoglycemic coma, most have been caused by excessive doses of insulin or oral hypoglycemic agents for the treatment of diabetes. In one series of 51 patients admitted to the hospital for hypoglycemia, 41 were diabetics, 36 being treated with insulin and 5 with sulfonylurea drugs. In nondiabetic patients, the hypoglycemia had been induced by excessive alcohol, and one patient had injected herself with insulin in a suicide attempt.[149] Less frequent causes of hypoglycemic coma were insulin-secreting pancreatic adenomas, retroperitoneal sarcomas, and hemochromatosis with liver disease. In patients taking either insulin or oral hypoglycemics, the addition of fluoroquinolones, mostly gatifloxacin or ciprofloxacin, may induce severe hypoglycemia[150] (gatifloxacin can also cause hyperglycemia[151]). The intake of alcohol and perhaps psychoactive drugs in insulin-treated diabetics with severe hypoglycemia is relatively common. In fact, alcohol alone is responsible for a significant percentage of patients with severe hypoglycemia.[152] It is therefore important to check blood glucose even in patients in whom cognitive impairment can be attributed to alcohol ingestion. Fortunately, in most emergency departments, a blood glucose from a fingerstick is done as a matter of course in any patient with altered mental status.

Pathologically, hypoglycemia directs its main damage at the cerebral hemispheres, producing laminar or pseudolaminar necrosis in fatal cases, but largely sparing the brainstem. Clinically, the picture of acute metabolic encephalopathy caused by hypoglycemia usually presents in one of four forms: (1) As a delirium manifested primarily by mental changes with either quiet and sleepy confusion or wild mania. (2) As coma accompanied by signs of multifocal brainstem dysfunction, including neurogenic hyperventilation and decerebrate spasms. In this form, pupillary light reactions, as well as oculocephalic and oculovestibular responses, are usually preserved to suggest that the underlying disorder is metabolic. The patients sometimes have shiver-like diffuse muscle activity and many are hypothermic (33–35°C). (3) As a stroke-like illness characterized by focal neurologic signs with or without accompanying coma. In one series of patients requiring hospital admission, 5% suffered transient focal neurologic abnormalities.[149] In patients with focal motor signs, permanent motor paralysis is uncommon and the weakness tends to shift from side to side during different episodes of metabolic worsening. This kind of shifting deficit, as well as the fact that focal neurologic signs also occur in children in coma with severe hypoglycemia, stands against explaining the localized neurologic deficits as being caused by cerebral vascular disease. And (4), as an epileptic attack with single or multiple generalized convulsions and postictal coma. In one series, 20% of hypoglycemic patients had generalized seizures.[149] Many hypoglycemic patients convulse as the blood sugar level drops, and some have seizures as their only manifestation of hypoglycemia, leading to an erroneous diagnosis of epilepsy. The varying clinical picture of hypoglycemia often leads to mistaken clinical diagnoses, particularly when, in a given patient, the clinical picture varies from episode to episode, as in Patient Vignette 5.7.

Patient Vignette 5.7

A 45-year-old woman was hospitalized for treatment of a large pelvic sarcoma. She had liver metastases and was malnourished. On morning rounds she was found to be unresponsive. Her eyes were open, but she did not respond to questioning, although she moved all four extremities in response to noxious stimuli. She was sweating profusely. The blood glucose was 40 mg/dL. Her symptoms cleared immediately after an intravenous glucose infusion. The next day her roommate called for help when the patient did not respond to her questions. This time she was awake and alert but globally aphasic with a right hemiparesis. Again she was hypoglycemic, and the symptoms resolved after the infusion of glucose.

Comment

The variability and neurologic findings from episode to episode make hypoglycemia a great imitator, particularly of structural disease of the nervous system, raising the question of whether prehospital blood glucose measurement should be done in all patients suspected by emergency medical services of having had a stroke. In one such series of 185 patients suspected of "cerebral vascular accident," five were found to be hypoglycemic and all were medication-controlled diabetics. All of these patients improved after receiving glucose.[153]

Neither the history nor the physical examination reliably distinguishes hypoglycemia from other causes of metabolic coma, although (as is true in hepatic coma) an important clinical point is that the pupillary and vestibulo-ocular reflex pathways are almost always spared. The great danger of delayed diagnosis is that the longer hypoglycemia lasts, the more likely it is to produce irreversible neuronal loss. This may be the reason that more diabetics treated with insulin have EEG abnormalities than those treated with diet alone.[154] Insidious and progressive dementia is not rare among zealously controlled diabetics who often suffer recurrent minor hypoglycemia. Hypoglycemic seizures cause permanent cognitive deficits in children with diabetes,[155] but even repetitive episodes of hypoglycemia without seizures can lead to cognitive dysfunction.[156] Patients with severe hypoglycemia often have changes on MRI suggesting cerebral infarction (hyperintensity on diffusion-weighted images).[157] These abnormalities may reverse after treatment with glucose and thus do not imply permanent damage.[158] Subtle hypoglycemia can go unrecognized, as Patient Vignette 5.8 illustrates.

Patient Vignette 5.8

A 77-year-old man with unresectable mesothelioma who had lost his appetite and was losing weight awoke one morning feeling "unusually good" and, for the first time in weeks, having an appetite. He got dressed and while descending the stairs from his bedroom slipped and fell but did not injure himself. He seated himself at the breakfast table, but despite indicating an appetite did not attempt to eat. His wife noticed that his speech was slurred, his balance was poor, and he did not respond appropriately to questions. She finally coaxed him to eat, and, after breakfast, he returned entirely to normal. The following morning the same thing happened, and his wife brought him to the emergency department, where his blood sugar was determined to be 40 mg/dL. He responded immediately to glucose.

Comment

What appeared to be hunger should have been a clue that he was hypoglycemic, but because the patient was not a diabetic, neither he nor his family had any suspicion of the nature of the problem. His wife dismissed the first episode because he recovered after breakfast. Alert emergency department physicians recognized the nature of the second episode and treated him appropriately.

Once recognized, the treatment is simple. Ten percent glucose given intravenously in 50-mL (5 g) aliquots to restore blood glucose to normal levels prevents the possible deleterious overshoot of giving 50% glucose.[159] Restoring blood glucose will almost always return neurologic function to normal, although sometimes not immediately. However, prolonged coma and irreversible diffuse cortical injury can occasionally result from severe hypoglycemia. Relapses, particularly in patients taking sulfonylureas, are common. The sulfonylurea agents cause hypoglycemia by binding to a receptor on pancreatic beta cells, with the inactive ATP-dependent potassium channels causing depolarization of the beta cell and opening voltage-gated calcium channels to release insulin. Octreotide binds to a second receptor of the pancreatic beta cell and inhibits calcium influx, reducing the secretion of insulin after depolarization. This drug has been used to treat those patients with sulfonylurea overdose who are resistant to intravenous glucose.[160]

Cofactor Deficiency

Energy metabolism requires a number of enzymatic cofactors, and when these are deficient, the damage can resemble that seen with hypoxia. Deficiency of one or more of the B vitamins, for example, can cause delirium, stupor, and, ultimately, dementia, but only thiamine deficiency seriously contends for a place in the differential diagnosis of coma.[161–163]

Thiamine deficiency produces Wernicke's encephalopathy, a symptom complex caused by neuronal dysfunction that, if not reversed, promptly leads to damage of the gray matter and blood vessels surrounding the third ventricle, cerebral aqueduct, and fourth ventricle.[162] Why the lesions have such a focal distribution is not altogether understood since, when thiamine is not ingested, it disappears from all brain areas at about the same rate. One investigator has proposed that with severe thiamine deficiency, glutamate and glutamic acid decarboxylase accumulate in peripheral tissues. The elevated levels of glutamate in the blood pass through circumventricular organs (brain areas without a blood–brain barrier) into the cerebral ventricles and contiguous brain, finally diffusing into the extracellular space of diencephalic and brainstem tissues. The damage to cells in this area is then produced by glutamate excitotoxicity.[164] Because alpha-ketoglutarate dehydrogenase is thiamine-dependent and rate-limiting in the tricarboxylic acid cycle, focal lactic acidosis, decreases in cerebral energy, and resultant depolarization have also been postulated as causes of the focal defect.[165] In addition, a thiamine-dependent enzyme, transketolase, loses its activity in the pontine tegmentum more rapidly than in other areas, and it is presumed that a focal effect such as this is related to the restricted pathologic changes. Thiamine reverses at least some of the neurologic defects in Wernicke's encephalopathy so rapidly that for years physicians have speculated that the vitamin is involved in synaptic transmission. Thiamine-deficient animals have a marked impairment of serotonergic neurotransmitter pathways in the cerebellum, diencephalon, and brainstem.[166]

The areas of diencephalic and brainstem involvement in animals correspond closely to the known distribution of pathologic lesions in humans with Wernicke's encephalopathy.

Thiamine affects active ion transport at nerve terminals and is necessary for regeneration and maintenance of the membrane potential.[167]

The ultimate cause of thiamine deficiency is absence of the vitamin from the diet, and the most frequent reason is that patients have substituted alcohol for vitamin-containing foods. A danger is that the disease can be precipitated by giving vitamin-free glucose infusions to chronically malnourished subjects. A significant number of elderly hospitalized patients have evidence of moderate to severe thiamine deficiency. Before it was routine to add thiamine to intravenous infusions in hospitalized patients, we encountered on the wards in a cancer hospital one or two very sick patients per year who were not eating and developed Wernicke's disease when being nourished by intravenous infusions[168] without vitamins. We still encounter occasional such patients on the wards in a general hospital. In some cases that we have seen, thiamine had been prescribed orally. However, its absorption orally is unreliable, particularly in patients who are malnourished; hence, it must be supplied by intravenous or intramuscular injection for at least the first few days in any patient with suspected Wernicke's encephalopathy. Prompt diagnosis and treatment is crucial in order to minimize lasting deficits.[169]

As would be expected with lesions involving the diencephalic and periaqueductal structures, patients are initially obtunded and confused and often have striking memory failure. Deep stupor or coma is unusual, dangerous, and often a preterminal development. However, such behavioral symptoms are common to many disorders. They can be attributed to Wernicke's disease only when accompanied by nystagmus, oculomotor paralysis, and impaired vestibulo-ocular responses that are subsequently reversed by thiamine treatment. In advanced cases, involvement of oculomotor muscles may be sufficient to cause complete external ophthalmoplegia; fixed, dilated pupils are a rarity. Most patients also suffer from ataxia, dysarthria, and a mild peripheral neuropathy in addition to the eye signs. Many affected patients show a curious indifference to noxious stimulation, and some are hypothermic and hypophagic. Autonomic insufficiency is so common that orthostatic hypotension and shock are constant threats. The hypotension of Wernicke's disease appears to result from a combination of neural lesions and depleted blood volume and is probably the most common cause of death.

The MRI is characteristic. T2 and FLAIR images are symmetrically hyperintense in the mammillary bodies, dorsal medial thalami, periventricular areas of the hypothalamus, periaqueductal gray matter, and tectum of the midbrain. On rare occasions, hemorrhage can be demonstrated in the mammillary bodies by hyperintensity on T1-weighted image. Lesions do not usually contrast enhance.[163,170] Diffusion-weighted images may show restricted diffusion within the areas, a finding that may be more sensitive than standard sequences.[170,171] Restricted diffusion has also been reported in the splenium of the corpus callosum in acute Wernicke's encephalopathy.[171] Corpus callosum atrophy has been demonstrated in patients with Wernicke's disease related to alcohol, but not in those with Wernicke's disease related to intestinal surgery, anorexia, or hyperemeses gravidarum.[172]

Mitochondrial Disorders

Mitochondria provide the energy for the molecular operations of all eukaryotic cells, including neurons, and anything that interrupts the flow of electrons in the mitochondrial transport chain will prevent the formation of ATP on which neurons are so dependent. Cyanide, for example, inhibits cytochrome c oxidase, which is required for electron transport, and rapidly causes cell death due to collapse of energy reserves. While cyanide poisoning caused death quickly, mutations of DNA for mitochondrial proteins can cause a slower process, which can have acute exacerbations. For example, in Leigh disease, one of a number of mutations in DNA encoding mitochondrial proteins results in disruption of the electron transport chain.[173] These can be inherited in a variety of different ways, as some of the genes for mitochondrial proteins are found in somatic nuclear chromosomes, others in the X chromosome, and still others in the DNA that is intrinsic to the mitochondria themselves. The result is injury to the brain that is reminiscent of that seen in Wernicke disease: along the walls of the third ventricle and periaqueductal gray matter, but also in the basal ganglia and cerebellum.

Leigh disease typically presents in infancy, so is rarely a problem in the differential diagnosis of coma in adults, although minor forms may make some patients more susceptible to environmental insults, such as thiamine deficiency or hypoglycemia. Patients with some mutations, however, can present in adulthood with metabolic encephalopathy or even coma, focal signs including ophthalmoparesis reminiscent of Wernicke encephalopathy, and seizures.[174,175]

PART 4: DISORDERS OF THE INTERNAL MILIEU: IONIC AND OSMOTIC ENVIRONMENT

Acid-base status, CO_2 tension, and osmolarity are pathophysiologically closely intertwined and, in the following sections, somewhat artificially discussed as separate entities. Here the focus will be on elucidating the impact of changes in these measures and other ionic and osmotic alterations on consciousness. Sodium is the most abundant serum cation, and, for practical purposes, systemic alterations of osmolarity are related to changes in serum sodium or glucose. As sodium is functionally an impermeable solute hypo- and hypernatremia will at least transiently cause movement of water across the vascular membrane. Intra- and extracellular changes in sodium and water concentration together account for much of the encountered clinical symptoms in these disorders.

Hyponatremia

Systemic hypo-osmolarity occurs predominantly in hyponatremic states. On the other hand, not all hyponatremic states are necessarily hypo-osmolar. For example, hyponatremia may be hyperosmolar, as with severe hyperglycemia, or iso-osmolar, as, for example, during transurethral prostatic resection when large volumes of sodium-free irrigants are systemically absorbed.

Hyponatremia or *"water intoxication"* can cause delirium, obtundation, and coma, examples being encountered annually in almost all large hospitals. Symptoms result from water excess in the brain; hence the name "water intoxication"

(Figure 5.5A). The pathogenesis of the symptoms caused by hyponatremia is probably multifactorial.[176,177] Water entering both neurons and glia causes brain edema and thus increased ICP. Brain herniation is probably the event leading to death. In an attempt to compensate, sodium and potassium are excreted from cells via a sodium-potassium ATPase pump, altering membrane excitability[178] and perhaps causing the seizures that are common in severe hyponatremia. Seizures may lead to hypoxia, but whether hypoxia plays a significant role in the development of the clinical symptoms is unclear.[176]

The differential for underlying causes of hyponatremia is broad and includes large surface burns, diarrhea, diuretics, heart failure, kidney disease, liver cirrhosis, syndrome of inappropriate antidiuretic hormone secretion (SIADH),[179] cerebral salt wasting (CSW),[180] sweating, and vomiting. In the ICU hyponatremia (less than 130 mEqu/L) is encountered in up to 15–20% of acutely brain-injured patients, particularly in those with SAH.[181,182] Speed of repletion of sodium deficits depends on the presumed acuity of developing hyponatremia. In cases of chronic or subacute development of hyponatremia, sodium correction should not exceed 0.5 mmol/h (or more than 12 mmol/d)[183] as central pontine and extrapontine myelinolysis may develop.[184] Acute hyponatremia can be much more rapidly corrected.

For the management of hyponatremic patients with brain injury, for practical purposes, CSW needs to be differentiated from SIADH as both cause hyponatremia, but management is fundamentally different. In acute brain injury, CSW predominates, while SIADH is frequent in subacute and chronic presentations.[181,185–187] Differentiation of CSW and SIADH is at times challenging in the acute state as patients frequently get actively repleted with intravenous fluids and receive diuretics at the same time. The fundamental difference is that patients with CSW have extracellular volume depletion while patients with SIADH are in a euvolemic or mildly hypervolemic state.[188,189]

Although acute hyponatremia can be fatal, chronic hyponatremia is usually only mildly symptomatic. The reason appears to be that the brain adapts to the hyponatremia by decreasing organic osmols within the cell, especially amino acids.[178,190] Acute hyponatremia

is rarely a cause of emergency department visits. In a total of 44,826 emergency department visits, only 2.9% were hyponatremic, and of those, only 11 (0.8%) of the hyponatremic patients presented with acute neurologic symptoms. The cause of the symptomatic hyponatremia was variable, but included increased water intake either from polydipsia or the use of herbal teas for weight reduction, drug abuse with MDMA, and use of diuretic agents. Women appear more susceptible than men. Of the 11 patients in this series, 9 were women.[191] In Shapiro's syndrome, paroxysmal hypothermia and sometimes hyponatremia are seen in association with agenesis of the corpus callosum.[192]

The entry of water into the brain is promoted by aquaporin, a water channel protein present in both brain and choroid plexus.[193] In experimental animals, hyponatremia increases aquaporin-1 expression in the choroid plexus, allowing more water to enter the CSF and leading to apoptosis of cells surrounding the ventricular system.[193] There is also increased immunoreactivity of aquaporin-4, a channel that allows entry of water into glia.[194]

Most patients with slowly developing or only moderately severe hyponatremia are confused or delirious. With more severe or more rapidly developing hyponatremia, asterixis and multifocal myoclonus often appear. Coma is a late and life-threatening phase of water-intoxication, and both coma and convulsions are more common with acute than chronic hyponatremia. Neurologic symptoms are rare with serum sodium above 120 mg/L, and convulsions or coma generally do not occur until the serum sodium values reach 95–110 mEq/L (again, the more rapidly the serum sodium falls, the more likely the symptoms are to occur at a higher level). Permanent brain damage may follow hyponatremic convulsions, and treatment with antiepileptic drugs is generally useless. In a series of 136 patients with hyponatremic encephalopathy, premenopausal women developed severe symptoms at higher sodium levels than either postmenopausal women or men.[176]

The primary treatment of hyponatremia must be directed at treating the underlying cause and reversing the hyponatremia. In general hyponatremia can be restored either by administering sodium (i.e., by NaCl tablets, hypernatremic fluids) or in euvolemic patients by administration of vasopressin receptor antagonists (VAPs).[195] These inhibit the antidiuretic effect of vasopressin by binding to renal vasopressin receptors inducing aquaresis. As mentioned earlier, the acuity of development of hyponatremia dictates the speed of correcting sodium deficits. Hyponatremia is often corrected with hypertonic fluids, while SIADH is primarily managed with fluid restriction.[196] However, in the acute setting and given the challenges of differentiating SIADH from CSW and the fact that fluid restriction may cause additional injury (i.e., development of strokes in patients with SAH)[197,198] repletion with hypertonic fluids is often practiced. Interestingly, rapid increases of serum sodium in acute hyponatremia and rapid increases of sodium from a normo- to hypernatremic state in patients receiving hypertonic saline for ICP elevations are typically tolerated extremely well.[199]

Hypernatremia

Serum sodium elevations above normal are labeled hypernatremia and may be seen in patients with and without brain injury or occur iatrogenic. As sodium is functionally an impermeable solute, it will at least transiently cause dehydration of the extravascular environment such as surrounding cells. In the ICU setting, particularly for patients with neurological diseases, hypernatremia is frequent and associated with worse outcomes.[200] Physicians sometimes induce transient hyperosmolality by therapeutically using hypertonic solutions containing sodium chloride or mannitol to treat cerebral edema and ICP elevation. Thresholds for abnormality differ between studies, but these iatrogenic, rapid increases in serum sodium are typically well-tolerated unless exceeding 155–160 mEq/L, beyond which impaired consciousness and seizures may develop.

Severe water depletion producing acute hypernatremia occurs in children with intense diarrhea and, occasionally, in adults with diabetes insipidus during circumstances that impair their thirst or access to adequate water replacement. Acute hypernatremia also occurs in obtunded patients receiving excessively concentrated solutions by tube feeding. As with other hyperosmolar states, blood volumes tend

to be low because of excess free water losses (solute diuresis). Elevated levels of urea nitrogen, and sometimes glucose, contribute to the hyperosmolality. Symptoms of encephalopathy usually accompany serum sodium levels in excess of about 160 mEq/L or total osmolalities of 340 mOsm/kg or more, the earliest symptoms being delirium or a confusional state.[201] Hypernatremic osmolality also should be considered when patients in coma receiving tube feedings show unexplained signs of worsening, especially if their treatment has included oral or systemic dehydrating agents. In the hypernatremic patient, sodium enters muscle cells, displacing potassium, causing hypokalemia and a hypopolarized muscle cell that can be electrically inexcitable. Rhabdomyolysis may be the eventual result. Clinically, patients have weak, flaccid muscles and absent deep tendon reflexes, and the muscles are electrically inexcitable.[202]

In the neurologically ill critical care population, central diabetes insipidus as a cause for hypernatremia is most frequently seen in pituitary apoplexy and brain death, occasionally with brain tumors and TBI. Otherwise it is uncommon when compared to iatrogenic causes such as diuretic use, hypertonic fluid administration, and treatments given for ICP management.[203,204] Potential mechanisms of action for hypertonic saline are debated and include osmotic, vasoregulatory, hemodynamic, and immunomodulatory.[205–208] In patients with ICP elevation and hypernatremia, tromethamine (THAM) may offer an alternative.[209,210] In hospitalized patients, hypernatremia is clearly associated with increased mortality. Likewise, a number of studies have found hypernatremia in the critically ill population, including those with brain injury, to be associated with poor outcomes but this has been challenged in TBI.[211] In SAH patients, hypernatremia predicts mortality[212,213] but likely leads more indirectly to worse outcomes, for example, via its relationship to acute kidney failure.[214]

Mild chronic hypernatremia occasionally occurs in chronic untreated diabetes insipidus caused by uncompensated water loss, but severe chronic hypernatremia with serum sodium levels in excess of 155–160 mEq/L is practically confined to the syndrome of essential hypernatremia. Essential hypernatremia usually is caused by a diencephalic abnormality and is characterized by a lack of thirst and a failure of ADH secretion to respond to osmoreceptor stimulation. In essential hypernatremia, serum sodium concentrations sometimes rise in excess of 170 mEq/L.[215] This disorder is mainly seen in patients with lesions of the preoptic area along the lamina terminalis, but patients have been reported without macroscopic lesions. Most patients with significant hypernatremia complain of fatigue and weakness. They usually become lethargic when sodium levels exceed 160 mEq/L; with elevations above 180 mEq/L, most become confused or stuporous, and some die. A danger is that too rapid rehydration of such chronically hypernatremic subjects can produce symptoms of water intoxication in the presence of serum sodium levels as high as 155 mEq/L (i.e., about 25–30 mEq below the level at which hydrating efforts began). The problem is especially frequent in children.[44,216]

Rapid correction of hypernatremia is often asked for by renal specialists but should be done with extreme caution, particularly in acutely brain-injured patients, as cerebral swelling and subsequent herniation may result. The reason for this is that, in hypernatremic states, the brain as a compensatory response to restore brain volume will, after a few hours, generate idiogenic osmoles or organic brain osmoles.[217] Rapid correction of hyperosmolar states will then lead to brain swelling because the brain is unable to eliminate these osmols rapidly enough. Assessment of the hypernatremic patient should include an assessment of the volume status (examination, urine sodium concentration, and fractional excretion of sodium <1%) and exclusion of diabetes insipidus.

Hypercalcemia

An elevated serum calcium level may be due to the effects of primary hyperparathyroidism, immobilization, or cancer. Hypercalcemia is a common and important complication of cancer, resulting from either metastatic lesions that demineralize the bones or as a remote effect of parathyroid hormone-secreting tumors. Hyperparathyroidism due to a benign parathyroid adenoma is also a common cause.[218] The systemic clinical symptoms of hypercalcemia include anorexia, nausea and frequently vomiting, intense thirst, polyuria, and polydipsia. Muscle weakness can be prominent, and neurogenic atrophy has been reported. Some patients with hypercalcemia have as their first symptom a mild diffuse encephalopathy with headache. Delusions and changes in affect can be prominent, so that many such patients have been initially treated for a psychiatric disorder until the blood calcium level was measured. With severe hypercalcemia (typically if the serum calcium level is greater than 14 mg/dL [3.5 mmol/L]), stupor and finally coma occur,[218] which may be more common in the elderly.[219] Generalized or focal seizures are rare. The posterior leukoencephalopathy syndrome (see page 205) has been reported in association with severe hypercalcemia.[220,221]

Hypercalcemia should be suspected in a delirious patient who has a history of renal calculi, recent immobilization, cancer, or evidence of any other systemic disease known to cause the condition.[222] A serum calcium determination is therefore a routine part of the evaluation in patients with unexplained delirium or confusional states.

Hypocalcemia

Hypocalcemia is usually caused by hypoparathyroidism (often occurring late and unsuspected after thyroidectomy), pancreatitis, or, rarely, an idiopathic disorder of calcium metabolism. The cardinal peripheral manifestations of hypocalcemia are neuromuscular irritability and tetany, but these may be absent when hypocalcemia develops insidiously. Accordingly, patients with hypoparathyroid hypocalcemia can sometimes present with a mild diffuse encephalopathy as their only symptom. Seizures, either focal or generalized, are common, especially in children, and may occur even late after thyroid surgery.[223] With more severe cases, excitement, delirium, hallucinations, and stupor have been reported. Coma is, however, primarily seen in the setting of seizures. Papilledema has been reported, associated with an increased ICP. This hypocalcemic pseudotumor cerebri[224] apparently is a direct effect of the metabolic abnormality, but the precise mechanism remains unexplained.[225]

Hypocalcemia is commonly misdiagnosed as mental retardation, dementia, or epilepsy, and occasionally a brain tumor is suspected. Hypocalcemia should be suspected if the patient has cataracts, and the correct diagnosis sometimes can be inferred from observing calcification in the basal ganglia on CT scan. Normally, serum calcium levels run from 8.5 to 10.5 mg/dL. About half of this is bound to albumin and half represents free ions. For each 1.0 g/dL drop in serum albumin below about 5, the serum calcium falls by about 0.8 mg/dL. Thus, with an albumin of 2.0 g/dL, a normal serum calcium may be as low as 7.0 mg/dL. To avoid making this extrapolation, if there is any question about the calcium level, the free serum calcium should be measured. A free calcium level below 4.0 mg/dL is diagnostic of hypocalcemia.

Chronic hypocalcemia may cause chorea and parkinsonism, along with calcifications in the basal ganglia. Tetany caused by spontaneous, irregular, repetitive nerve action potentials is a common complication of hypocalcemia, as Patient Vignette 5.9 demonstrates.

Patient Vignette 5.9

An 18-year-old woman had been treated for an osteogenic sarcoma. Surgery was followed by cisplatin-based chemotherapy. Five years later, following reconstructive surgery on her leg, she complained of numbness and tingling of both hands and arms spreading into the face and followed by spasms of her arms, which lasted several hours. A diagnosis of panic attack was made, and, after sedation, the symptoms cleared. Other attacks followed but were milder, but eventually while the patient was in bed with a viral illness, the symptoms were so severe that she was taken to an emergency department where sedation was again applied. She was referred for evaluation of anxiety and panic attacks. The general neurologic examination was entirely normal. However, a Trousseau's sign elicited by raising the pressure in a blood pressure cuff above systolic pressure for 3 minutes demonstrated carpal spasms bilaterally. Voluntary hyperventilation for 2 minutes reproduced the carpal spasms and paresthesias in both hands. Chvostek's sign elicited by tapping over the facial nerve in front of the ear also elicited contraction of the facial muscles, particularly the orbicularis oculi. Serum calcium was 7.5 mEq/L (normal = 8.5–10.5); serum albumin was normal, but ionized calcium was 3.8 mEq/L (normal = 4.8–5.3). Serum magnesium and potassium were also low. The patient responded to electrolyte replacement.

Comment

Cisplatin and ifosfamide are drugs that can cause calcium- and magnesium-losing nephropathy. Both low magnesium (see later discussion) and low ionized calcium that result from a magnesium loss can cause hyperventilation that further lowers ionized calcium, presumably by increasing the binding of calcium to albumin, thus causing tetany. The patient's two severe attacks probably resulted from anxiety-induced hyperventilation.

Metabolic Acidosis (Disorders of Systemic Acid–Base Balance)

Systemic acidosis and alkalosis accompany several diseases that cause metabolic coma, and the attendant respiratory and acid–base changes can give important clues about the cause of coma. However, of the four disorders of systemic acid–base balance (respiratory and metabolic acidosis and respiratory and metabolic alkalosis), respiratory acidosis is the most commonly associated with stupor and coma.[226] Even then, the associated hypoxia or hypercapnia may be as important as the acidosis in producing the neurologic abnormality. Acidosis is frequently encountered in critically ill unconscious patients and associated with poor outcomes.[227] Metabolic acidosis, the most immediately medically dangerous of the acid–base disorders, by itself only rarely produces coma. Usually, metabolic acidosis is associated with alternating states of unconsciousness and agitation (also known as delirium) or, at most, confused obtundation. The impact of acidosis on brain physiology and consciousness depends on multiple factors, including the etiology of acidosis (respiratory vs. metabolic), the degree of acidosis (reflected in the pH and bicarbonate), and the acuity of its development (which dictates whether or not compensatory or adaptive mechanisms play a role).

Systemic measurements of acidosis and pH are not necessarily reflective of brain pH. Direct measurements of intracranial pH are possible in critically ill brain injured patients using intracranial tonometers[228] or microdialysis techniques,[229–231] the former primarily reflecting gray and the latter white matter pH. Following acute brain injury, brain metabolism may shift to an anaerobic state with associated lactic acidosis, fall in brain pH, and resultant changes in brain perfusion.[228,232–234] In patients with TBI, direct cerebral measurements of pH values below 7.2 were found to be associated with worse outcomes.[228]

In brain-injured patients, metabolic (hyperchloremic) acidosis may not only be seen as a consequence of injury but also result from therapeutic interventions such as hypertonic saline administration given for the treatment of ICP elevations in unconscious patients.[235,236] Interestingly, preliminary data show that administration of sodium bicarbonate results in reduction of brain water content in animal experiments[237] and an increase in CBF in humans.[238,239]

Respiratory alkalosis under most circumstances causes no more than light-headedness and confusion, which is believed to be due to decreased CBF in the face of low PCO_2. However, when respiratory alkalosis[240] is caused by overcorrection of chronic pulmonary failure, the resulting large drop in PCO_2, while serum bicarbonate corrects more slowly, can cause stupor or coma associated with multifocal myoclonus due to cerebral ischemia resulting from the large decrease of CBF.[241]

Severe metabolic alkalosis has occasionally been reported to cause encephalopathy and, rarely, seizures. Tetany may occur, probably related to decreased ionized calcium.[242] Compensation for metabolic alkalosis with hypoventilation and a rising PCO_2 may play a role in decreasing consciousness, and, in adult patients with cystic fibrosis, it may contribute to respiratory failure.[243] If patients with acid–base disorders other than respiratory acidosis or severe and protracted metabolic acidosis are in stupor or coma, it is unlikely that the acid–base disturbance by itself is responsible. Instead, it is more likely that the metabolic defect responsible for the acid–base disturbance (e.g., uremia, hepatic encephalopathy, or circulatory depression leading to lactic acidosis) also is directly interfering with brain function.

A useful clinical clue to the presence and possible cause of metabolic acidosis or certain other electrolyte disorders comes from estimating the anion gap from the measured blood electrolytes. The calculation is based on the known electroneutrality of the serum, which requires the presence of an equal number of anions (negative charges) and cations (positive charges). For practical purposes, sodium and potassium (or sodium alone) represent 95% of the cations, whereas the most abundant and conveniently measured anions, chloride and bicarbonate, add up to only 85% of the normal total. The result is an anion gap in unmeasured electrolytes that amounts normally to about 12 ± 4 mEq/L:

$$(Na^+ + K^+) - (Cl^- + HCO_{3^-}) = 8 \text{ to } 16 \text{ meq/L}$$

An increase in the anion gap ordinarily implies the presence of an undetected electrolyte (either an endogenous or exogenous toxin) causing a metabolic acidosis and should prompt an immediate search by deduction and specific testing for the "missing anion."

Hyperglycemic Hyperosmolar State

Brain damage from chronic hyperglycemia (i.e., either type 1 or type 2 diabetes) is well established.[244] Sustained hyperglycemia causes hyperosmolality, which in turn induces compensatory vasopressin secretion. Although adaptive in the short term, in the long term sustained hyperglycemia damages vasopressin-secreting neurons in the supraoptic and paraventricular nuclei of the hypothalmus. In addition, some evidence suggests that sustained hyperglycemia damages hippocampal neurons as well,[245] leading to cognitive defects in both humans[246] and experimental animals. These effects appear to be independent of diabetes-induced damage to brain vasculature leading to stroke, a common complication of chronic poorly controlled diabetes.[247,248]

Acute, hyperosmolar hyperglycemic states are life-threatening emergencies that most frequently are encountered in but not limited to elderly patients with type 2 diabetes. Clinically these patients present with elevated serum glucose levels, with or without ketoacidosis, and dehydration. Neurological symptoms range from cognitive impairment to unconsciousness.

The effect of acute hyperglycemia on patients with damaged brains is less clear-cut, but hyperglycemia is frequently seen in the immediate post brain injury period.[249] Clinical evidence demonstrates that patients who are hyperglycemic after brain injury, either due to global or focal ischemia,[250,251] intracranial hemorrhage,[252] or to brain trauma, do less well than patients who are euglycemic. The same may well be true for critically ill patients, even those without direct brain damage.[253,254] These findings have led investigators to recommend careful control of blood glucose in critically ill patients and those with brain injury of various types.[255] Clinical trials have shown mixed results,[253,254,256] which may be due to logistical reasons and the ability to safely control blood glucose without the risk of hypoglycemia or that patients with acute brain injury may need different glucose targets than patients without acute brain injury.[257] Invasive brain monitoring using microdialysis suggests that intracranial hypoglycemia may be seen in patients managed with tight targets for systemic glucose.[258,259] Preliminary work suggests that abrupt changes in serum glucose[260] and increased glucose variability[261] may be particularly harmful. If available, guidelines suggest targeting interstitial glucose levels instead of systemic values.[262,263] Furthermore, the impact of timing, amount, and content of nutritional input in acutely brain-injured patients is largely not understood but clearly affects glucose levels. Insulin administration by itself may lead to brain hypoglycemia independently of the effect on serum glucose in metabolically distressed brain[264] following brain injury.

The mechanism by which hyperglycemia worsens the prognosis in such patients is not clear. Some believe that the increased production of lactate and lowering of the pH leads to the cellular damage.[265] However, lactate is probably a good substrate for neurons,[35] and the increased blood glucose should be protective. In patients with acute brain injury, a study using ^{13}C-labled acetate and lactate and nuclear magnetic resonance (NMR) analysis of microdialysis fluid demonstrated that the brain is able to utilize lactate instead of glucose.[266] In fact, in experimental animals, a glucose load given 2–3 hours before an ischemic insult is protective, but the same glucose load administered 15–60 minutes before ischemia aggravates the ischemic outcome,[267] although these findings have been challenged.[268] Another possible mechanism by which hyperglycemia

may damage the brain is that a glucose load leads to release of glucocorticoids that in turn can cause cellular damage.[245,269,270] Whatever the mechanism, careful control of blood glucose allowing neither cerebral hyper- nor hypoglycemia appears essential for the best care of critically ill and brain-injured patients.

PART 5: DISORDERS OF THE INTERNAL MILIEU: HORMONAL AND TEMPERATURE

Hypothyroidism

Both hyperthyroidism and hypothyroidism interfere with normal cerebral function, but exactly how the symptoms are produced is unclear.[271] Thyroid hormone (or more strictly triiodothyronine) binds to nuclear receptors that function as ligand-dependent transcription factors. The hormone is absolutely essential for development of the brain, such that in infantile hypothyroidism the neurologic abnormality (cretinism) is rarely reversed unless the defect is almost immediately recognized and corrected.[272] One reason may be that thyroid hormone regulates hippocampal neurogenesis in both the juvenile and adult brain.[273] Thyroid hormone also has effects on cerebral metabolism[274]; hypothyroidism causes a generalized decrease in regional CBF by more than 20% and a 12% decrease in cerebral glucose metabolism without specific regional changes. On the other hand, hyperthyroidism appears to have little effect on cerebral metabolism.

MYXEDEMA

Severe, decompensated hypothyroidism may be associated with life-threatening unconsciousness in a syndrome called *myxedema crisis* or *myxedema coma*.[275,276] Coma is a rare complication of myxedema,[277–279] but one that is often associated with a fatal outcome. Mortality is high, with approximately every second to fourth patient with myxedema coma not surviving hospitalization.[279–283] In a series of 11 patients either stuporous or comatose from hypothyroidism, three of four patients who were in a coma on admission died, whereas only one of seven patients with less severe changes of consciousness died.[279] Many authors have commented on the appearance of "suspended animation" in these profoundly hypometabolic patients. Characteristically, the patients are hypothermic with body temperatures between 87°F and 91°F. They appear to hypoventilate and, indeed, usually have elevated blood PCO_2 values and mild hypoxia. The EEG shows nonspecific changes, with diffuse background slowing and triphasic waves, but the voltage may be either depressed or increased.[284,285] Decreases in CBF and glucose metabolism may be seen in patients with hypothyroidism,[274,286] but it is unclear if this is even more exacerbated in the unconscious hypothyroid patient. It is unclear if this pathological mechanism plays a role for alterations of consciousness in patients with myxedema coma.

The onset of myxedema coma is usually acute or subacute and precipitated by stressors such as infection, congestive heart failure, trauma, exposure to cold, or sedative or anesthetic drug administration in an untreated hypothyroid patient. Occasionally, discontinuation of thyroid supplementation in a patient with diagnosed hypothyroidism is the trigger. The diagnosis of myxedema in a patient in coma is suggested by the systemic stigmata of hypothyroidism, plus a low body temperature and the finding of pseudomyotonic stretch reflexes (i.e., normal jerk, but slow relaxation phase). The diagnosis is also often suggested by the presence of elevated muscle enzyme levels in the serum but can be confirmed definitively only by thyroid function tests. As myxedema coma frequently results in death, however, treatment with intravenous administration of triiodothyronine or thyroxine, as well as treatment of the precipitating cause, should begin once the clinical diagnosis has been made and blood for laboratory tests has been drawn; treatment should not be delayed while awaiting laboratory confirmation.

The greatest diagnostic challenge in myxedema coma is to regard one or more of its complications as the whole cause of the encephalopathy. CO_2 narcosis may be suspected if hypoventilation and CO_2 retention are present, but $PaCO_2$ values are rarely above 50–55 mm Hg in hypothyroidism, and hypothermia is not part of CO_2 narcosis.[287] Some authors have attributed the cause of coma and profound hypothyroidism to respiratory failure with CO_2 retention, but this is unlikely as not all patients with myxedema hypoventilate. Hyponatremia

is often present in severe myxedema, probably the result of inappropriate antidiuretic hormone (ADH) secretion,[288] and sometimes is severe enough to cause seizures. Gastrointestinal bleeding and shock also can complicate severe myxedema and divert attention from hypothyroidism as a cause of coma. Hypothermia, which is probably the most dramatic sign, should always suggest hypothyroidism, but may also occur in other metabolic encephalopathies, especially hypoglycemia, depressant drug poisoning, primary hypothermia due to exposure, and brainstem infarcts. Critical care management focuses on emergent administration of thyroid hormone replacement (bolus T4 300–500 µg parenteral, continue T4 at 50–100 µg daily) in addition to supportive measures, fluid and vasopressor administration, and aggressive management of precipitating factors (consider steroid supplementation if required).[276] When managing hypothermia in these patients using external warming devices, hypotension due to accompanying vasodilatation should be expected and appropriately managed.

Hypothyroidism is especially challenging to diagnose in patients with Parkinson's disease, whose main manifestation may be worsening of their parkinsonian symptoms.

STEROID-RESPONSIVE ENCEPHALOPATHY AND ASSOCIATED AUTOIMMUNE THYROIDITIS

Steroid-responsive encephalopathy and associated autoimmune thyroiditis (SREAT), also known as Hashimoto's encephalopathy, is an encephalopathy associated with autoimmune thyroiditis characterized by high titers of antithyroid antibodies in the serum.[289–291] Patients may be hypothyroid, but also may be euthyroid or even hyperthyroid. The disorder is a relapsing and remitting encephalopathy and may be characterized by seizures, either focal or generalized (seen in approximately 60%); myoclonus (65% of cases); confusion; and, in some instances, stupor and coma.[292] There may be associated pyramidal tract and cerebellar signs (tremor in 80%, gait ataxia 65%). Transient aphasia (in 80%) and sleep abnormalities (in 55%) have been reported.[289]

MRI and cerebral angiography are generally uninformative; in the few cases that have come to autopsy,[289] there is no evidence of vasculitis.[293] The EEG shows generalized slowing with frontal intermittent rhythmic delta activity and often triphasic waves.[294] Only a quarter of patients will have an inflammatory CSF picture.[289] Antithyroid antibodies are found in serum and spinal fluid, and antineuronal antibodies have also been reported in some cases, although the pathophysiologic significance of either type of antibody for the encephalopathy is not clear.[293] Histopathology may be normal or show patchy myelin pallor, scant perivascular chronic inflammation, mild gliosis, and microglial activation.[289]

The importance of the syndrome is that it is steroid-responsive and should be suspected when a hypothyroid patient does not show an improved level of consciousness in response to thyroxin. The diagnosis is established by elevated anti-thyroid antibodies and responsiveness to steroids. Alternative treatments include intravenous immunoglobulin and plasmapheresis.[292]

Hyperthyroidism

Thyrotoxicosis usually presents with signs of increased CNS activity (i.e., anxiety, tremor, or hyperkinetic behavior).[278] Subtle changes in cognitive function accompany the more obvious emotional disturbances. Rarely, in "thyroid storm," these symptoms can progress to confusion, stupor, or coma.[278] Thyroid storm usually develops in a patient with preexisting thyrotoxicosis, often partially treated, who encounters precipitating factors such as an infection or a surgical procedure, although in some patients no trigger can be identified.[295] Patients with Graves's disease are at particularly high risk, but the life-threatening condition may also develop in patients with a toxic multinodular goiter or a TSH-secreting pituitary adenoma.[296] Only 1–2% of hospital admissions for thyrotoxicosis fulfill criteria of thyroid storm.[295]

The early clinical picture is dominated by signs of hypermetabolism. Fever is invariably present, profuse sweating occurs, there is marked tachycardia, and there may be signs of pulmonary edema and congestive heart failure. A more difficult problem is so-called *apathetic* thyrotoxicosis.[297,298] Such patients are usually elderly and present with neurologic signs of depression and apathy. If untreated, the clinical symptoms progress to delirium and finally to stupor and coma. Nothing distinctive marks the neurologic picture, but seizures may occur.[299] Hypermetabolism is not clinically prominent, nor can one observe the eye signs generally associated with thyrotoxicosis. However, almost all patients show evidence of severe weight loss and have cardiovascular symptoms, particularly atrial fibrillation and congestive heart failure. Many have signs of a moderately severe proximal myopathy.

The diagnosis is established by obtaining tests that reflect thyroid hyperfunction, and the neurologic signs are reversed by antithyroid treatment. Management aims at inhibiting synthesis (e.g., by giving propylthiouracil or methimazole) and release of thyroid hormone (e.g., by giving sodium iodine or lithium). Additionally, treatment attempts to block the peripheral effects (e.g., by giving beta blockers) and to increase the clearance of thyroid hormone (e.g., by giving cholestyramine or starting plasma exchange). Supportive measures focus on treating fever and hypovolemia and may include stress dose steroids for hypoadrenal states.[296]

Adrenal Gland

Both hyper- and hypoadrenal corticosteroid states are occasional causes of altered consciousness,[300] but the exact mechanisms responsible for those alterations are not fully understood. Adrenal corticosteroids have profound effects on the brain, influencing genes that control enzymes and receptors for biogenic amines and neuropeptides, growth factors, and cell adhesion factors.[300] Adrenal insufficiency may occur due to destruction of the adrenal gland (i.e., autoimmune etiology; this type of adrenal insufficiency is also known as primary adrenal insufficiency), hypopituitarism from pituitary apoplexy (secondary adrenal insufficiency), or possibly most commonly from medication-induced adrenal insufficiency (withdrawal from chronic glucocorticoid therapy). In situations of stress (e.g., surgery), life-threatening Addisonian crisis or coma may develop. Primary adrenal insufficiency is associated with both glucocorticoid and mineralocorticoid deficiency, while secondary adrenal insufficiency only manifests as a glucocorticoid deficiency state as the secretion of mineralocorticoid under control of the renin-angiotensin system is preserved. Despite standard of care management, patients with primary adrenal insufficiency experience an average of 8.3 adrenal crises per 100 patient-years, and those with secondary adrenal insufficiency have 0.5 adrenal crisis-related deaths per 100 patient-years.[301] Adrenal crisis may be part of the initial presentation in almost half of patients with adrenal insufficiency.

ADRENAL INSUFFICIENCY: ADDISON'S DISEASE

The pathogenesis of the encephalopathy of adrenal cortical failure in Addison's disease probably involves several factors in addition to the removal of the effect of cortisol on brain tissue.[302,303] The untreated disease also produces hypoglycemia as well as hyponatremia and hyperkalemia due to hypoaldosteronism. Hypotension is the rule, and, if severe, this alone can cause cerebral symptoms from orthostatic hypotension. Symptoms do not entirely clear until both mineralocorticosteroids and glucocorticosteroid are replaced. Some untreated and undertreated patients with Addison's disease are mildly delirious. In a series of 86 patients with adrenal insufficiency associated with the antiphospholipid syndrome, altered mental status was present in only 16 (19%). The major symptoms were abdominal pain (55%), hypotension (54%), and nausea or vomiting (31%). Weakness, fatigue, malaise, or asthenia was present in 31%.[304] Stupor and coma usually appear, if at all, only during addisonian crises. Changes in consciousness, respiration, pupils, and ocular movements are not different from those of other types of metabolic coma. The presence of certain motor signs, however, may be helpful in suggesting the diagnosis. Patients in addisonian crises have flaccid weakness and either hypoactive or absent deep tendon reflexes, probably resulting from hyperkalemia; a few suffer from generalized convulsions, which have been attributed to hyponatremia and water intoxication.[305] Papilledema is occasionally present and presumably results from brain swelling caused by fluid shifts perhaps exacerbated by increased capillary permeability, which is normally limited by corticosteroids. The EEG is diffusely slow and not different from the pattern in other causes of metabolic encephalopathy.[306]

The neurologic signs of addisonian coma are only rarely sufficiently distinctive to be diagnostic, although the combination of metabolic coma, absence of deep tendon reflexes, and papilledema may suggest adrenal insufficiency. Hyperpigmented skin (due to elevated secretion of ACTH by pituitary corticotrophs) and hypotension are helpful supplementary signs and, when combined with low serum sodium and a high serum potassium levels, strongly suggest the diagnosis. The definitive diagnosis of adrenal insufficiency is made by the direct measurement of low blood or urine cortisol levels. Life-threatening hypotension may develop and requires emergent attention.[307,308]

Surgical procedures and other acute illnesses put severe stress on the adrenal glands. A patient whose adrenal function has been marginal prior to an acute illness or surgical procedure may suddenly develop adrenal failure with its attendant delirium. The symptoms may be attributed inappropriately to the acute illness or to a "postoperative delirium" unless adrenal function studies are carried out. Some patients without known preexisting adrenal insufficiency develop acute adrenal failure following surgical procedures, particularly cardiac surgery or during sepsis (Waterhouse-Friderichsen syndrome). Acute pituitary failure, as in pituitary apoplexy, may also cause an addisonian state.

The main error in differential diagnosis of Addison's disease is with regard to the hyponatremia, hyperkalemia, or hypoglycemia as the primary cause of the metabolic coma, rather than recognizing the combination as caused by underlying adrenal insufficiency. This error can be avoided only by considering Addison's disease as a potential cause of metabolic coma and by heeding the other general physical signs and laboratory values. Hypotension and hyperkalemia, for example, rarely combine together in other diseases causing hyponatremia or hypoglycemia. Patients with Addison's disease are exceedingly sensitive to sedative drugs, including barbiturates and narcotics; ingestion of standard doses of these drugs may produce coma.

Treatment with fluid resuscitation and steroid replacement should be initiated immediately if addisonian insufficiency is suspected in a comatose patient. Electrolytes need to be monitored and replaced carefully.

Hypothermia

Body core temperature (Tc) is typically held within a very narrow range in mammals, across the day, across the entire lifetime, and even across species. In a typical human, Tc is held at 37°C plus or minus 1° for the entire lifetime when the individual is healthy. There are daily circadian fluctuations, so that the Tc is usually 0.5–1.0°C cooler during sleep. Some have attributed this to the overall lack of motor activity that generates heat during sleep, but the fall in Tc begins before sleep itself, and calorimetric measurements indicate that the lack of movement cannot account for the tightly regulated fall in Tc. Women also undergo a similar range of fluctuation in daily temperature over their menstrual cycle, with a fall in Tc signaling ovulation and the most fertile period of the cycle.

Deviation of Tc by even 0.1°C causes brisk activation of either heat conservation mechanisms (if the Tc falls) or heat dissipating mechanisms (if it rises). In fact, raising or lowering the ambient temperature has surprisingly little effect on Tc, because the changes in ambient temperature are picked up by skin thermoreceptors, and counter-regulatory mechanisms are activated before Tc even changes. The neurons and pathways that regulate Tc have recently received considerable attention, and we know that skin thermoreceptors innervate neurons in the spinal dorsal horn that send this information on to the lateral parabrachial nucleus in the pons.[309] The parabrachial neurons then relay both cold and warm sensation to the preoptic area, where mechanisms for maintaining thermoregulation are integrated with control of body fluids and electrolytes, as well as the wake–sleep cycle. Preoptic neurons generally drive the inhibition of heat-producing pathways, including the dorsal hypothalamic area (which responds to both metabolic and stress inputs by raising body temperature) and its target in the medulla, the raphe pallidus.[310] The raphe pallidus is a midline cell group just above and between the pyramidal tracts, which drives both vasomotor pathways necessary to conserve heat (cutaneous vasoconstriction) and production of heat by brown adipose tissue (BAT). Although BAT was thought at one time to be present primarily in small mammals, such as rodents, that depend upon heat generation to avoid hypothermia, fluoro-deoxyglucose

PET studies have identified BAT deposits along the paraspinal regions in humans as well.

In addition to the autonomic mechanisms for producing heat or for dissipating it (cutaneous vasodilation, sweating), humans have a wide range of behavioral methods (ranging from putting additional layers of clothing on or taking them off, to moving to a different environment, to changing the temperature of their ambient environment) that allow them to control the ambient temperature and adjust it to keep Tc in a narrow range. If Tc falls despite these adjustments, shivering is recruited to increase generation of heat from the muscles.

The tight regulation of Tc within such a narrow range is required because it provides the optimum environment for a wide range of biochemical processes that sustain life in mammals. For example, at temperatures a few degrees out of the normal range for Tc, ion channels and ion pumps that are necessary to maintain a normal resting membrane potential and to generate synaptic potentials and action potentials become unable to maintain their normal function. Thus, at temperatures below about 34°C, there is often generalized cognitive impairment, with stupor and then coma intervening as Tc reaches 30–31°C. At temperatures reached during the deep hypothermia required for cardiac procedures that include any period of cardiac arrest, Tc of 19°C permits complete cessation of flow of blood and oxygen to the brain for periods of up to 20 minutes without injury. Some animals use this slowing of metabolism to survive periods of lack of food. Many mammals have regulated periods of *torpor* when the temperature is cold and sufficient food is not available to maintain a normal Tc.[311] The temperature of these animals will drop into the range of 20–30°C, associated with profound slowing of heart rate and metabolism and deep unresponsiveness. Periodically, the animals rewarm spontaneously, search for food, and, in its absence, go back into *torpor*.

Because it slows metabolism, humans may also survive surprisingly long periods of deep hypothermia. Typically this occurs due to exposure, often in homeless individuals, especially if they have been imbibing ethanol which causes vasodilation and loss of judgment. A common story is that the person felt warm, despite cold temperatures and inadequate clothing, but was tired and lay down to rest on a snowbank. The heart rate in such individuals may become so slow that emergency medical crews may declare the person to be dead. Such individuals wake up in the morgue and often recover full consciousness with little cognitive impairment (although they usually lose some fingers and toes to frostbite due to a combination of peripheral vasoconstriction and tissue freezing).

It is important to rewarm a patient who has suffered from hypothermia relatively slowly, so that the body has a chance to readjust. Rapid rewarming may result in cardiac arrhythmias.

A variant of hypothermia due to exposure is often seen in the ICU setting, where the temperature is generally set around 20°C so that staff who are wearing gowns during procedures are comfortable, but bare cutaneous areas are often exposed to the air (particularly in burn units). In addition, certain drugs that may impair thermoregulation, such as dopaminergic or serotonergic or noradrenergic inhibitors, may contribute to hypothermia.

Paroxysmal hypothermia is a mysterious condition that occurs in patients who have had damage to the preoptic area, usually during development or in childhood. It is also seen in patients with agenesis of the corpus callosum (Shapiro's syndrome),[192] which is associated with malformation of the preoptic area. (During development, both the corpus callosum and the preoptic area develop along the lamina terminalis, the rostral wall of the third ventricle.) Such individuals typically have mild to moderate cognitive disability, although some are cognitively normal, but intermittently, usually once or more per year, they will undergo a period of 3–10 days in which their Tc will drop to the range of 30–34°C. During the time when their Tc is falling, the patients may feel hot, seek to lower the temperature in the room, and drink ice water, as if they were too warm, leading to the implication that the fall in Tc is regulated by the CNS, similar to the process in torpor. At Tc of less than 34°C, there is generally cognitive impairment. Attempts to warm the patient are generally rebuffed if the patient is awake and fruitless if the patient is not. At the end of the period, the patient spontaneously rewarms and resumes his or her normal life.

The mechanism of paroxysmal hypothermia is not understood. Some have proposed that it may be due to hypothalamic seizures, but attempts to treat it with antiepileptic drugs have met with uniform failure. Perhaps a clue may be found in the conditions under which the preoptic area normally causes hypothermia. One of these conditions is torpor, as noted earlier, but there is no obvious trigger for this. On the other hand (see later discussion), fever responses include competing, regulated hyperthermic and hypothermic mechanisms, both controlled by the preoptic area.[312] In healthy young adults, immune stimuli produce predominantly an elevation of Tc (fever) although this alternates with periods of normothermia (thus giving rise to "fever spikes"). However, in older adults and in neonates, immune stimuli can cause unalloyed hypothermia (and even in healthy young adults, overwhelming sepsis can induce hypothermia). Because the time course of paroxysmal hypothermia in those who are disposed resembles that of a typical viral febrile illness, and such individuals seem rarely to experience hyperthermic fevers, we have treated these events with inhibitors of prostaglandin synthesis (acetaminophen and nonsteroidal anti-inflammatory drugs) with modest success.

Hyperthermia

FEVER

Elevation of Tc is a common experience during a febrile illness. Fever is a regulated increase in Tc, usually by about 2–3°C, that is thought to be adaptive because the cells of the immune system (lymphocytes, macrophages) are more active at that temperature, while the metabolism of most organisms that are adapted to the carefully maintained milieu of 37° C in homeothermic mammals is impaired at higher temperatures.[313] The immune system maintains receptors (the native immune system) that recognize common invaders by molecular patterns typically expressed on their surface (pathogen-associated molecular pattern [PAMPs]). This sets off a cascade of events, including secretion of lipid molecules, such as prostaglandins, as well as protein hormones called cytokines, that signal the presence of the organism and prepare the immune response.[314] Other inflammatory diseases or cancers presumably can also set off fever by activating portions of the immune cascade in the absence of an extrinsic organism.

The actual increase in Tc in the case of a bacterial infection appears to be due to the generation of prostaglandin E2 by cells along the blood vessels, including those in the preoptic area.[315,316] Genetic deletion or pharmacological inhibition of the enzymes that produce PGE2 in this region prevents fever to systemic lipopolysaccharide (a bacterial cell wall component). Prostaglandin E2 can enter the brain directly, bypassing the blood–brain barrier because it is a lipid, and it acts on type 3 E prostaglandin (EP3) receptors located on neurons in the preoptic area. Genetic deletion of these receptors in just the preoptic area also prevents fever responses to circulating lipopolysaccharide.[317]

Dissection of the fever response in animals lacking different EP receptors has been informative.[312] In the absence of the EP3 receptors, the predominant response to circulating lipopolysaccharide is hypothermia, not hyperthermia. The hypothermic response appears to be due to EP1 and -4 receptors, also in the preoptic area. Thus, during a normal response to a bacterial invader, the PGE2 system normally sets up competing hyperthermic and hypothermic responses. Presumably the result (fever in a healthy young adult; hypothermia in an elderly person or a neonate) is due to the predominance of these receptor systems at different stages of life or to the dose of the immune stimulus, as profound septicemia can cause hypothermia even in a young adult and in healthy adult animals.

Although cognitive function is typically impaired to some extent during a fever, and there is often a degree of sleepiness,[314] the patient generally remains responsive. The extent to which the cognitive involvement is due to the change in Tc is difficult to judge, as the cytokine storm induced by the systemic infectious or inflammatory illness may potentially act on the brain independently.

Fever due to an infection or inflammatory disease of the brain itself may have additional mechanisms of action because once the blood–brain barrier is breached by an organism there is a flux of cytokines and inflammatory cells into the brain that are not be seen in the brain during a systemic illness and which may have direct effects ranging from causing local vasoconstriction to necrosis of neural tissue. Much of the brain injury during a brain infection may, in fact, be due to the immune response, rather than the organism itself. Thus, while the brain is designed to produce an elevation of Tc during an infectious process and to return to normal after weathering the infection, the set of responses and the recovery of the brain are much less predictable during a brain infection.

Although the concept of "central fever" is sometimes used to explain fever in someone who has no known infectious or inflammatory disease, this is almost always erroneous. Fever is always of central origin, but even that produced by brain injury or subarachnoid blood is nearly always due to the inflammatory reaction to the injury. Only under rare circumstances, such as pontine hemorrhage, is the hyperthermia produced by damage to the thermoregulatory pathways themselves. On the other hand, in the setting of acute brain injuries, the "fever burden" (cumulative time spent above the normal range for Tc) has been associated with poor outcomes for a number of brain injuries such as subarachnoid hemorrhage[318] and traumatic brain injury[319] (please refer to Chapter 8 for details).

FEBRILE SEIZURES

During any febrile illness, when there is an increase in Tc, there is an increased probability of a seizure in those who are predisposed (e.g., have epilepsy or a previous brain injury). This reduction in seizure threshold is sufficiently predictable for many physicians to treat fever aggressively in patients with unstable seizure disorders.[320]

On the other hand, seizures during febrile illnesses are particularly common in children under the age of 3 or 4. Most of these children will not go on to develop further seizures, even during febrile illnesses in later years. Thus many clinicians do not treat simple febrile seizures in this age group.

HYPERTHERMIA DUE TO EXPOSURE: HEAT STROKE

During very hot weather, the body typically maintains its normal temperature by peripheral vasodilatation and sweating. The thin coating of moisture on the skin, which is constantly evaporating, cools the body. To keep up with the demand for this cooling action, it is necessary to greatly increase the intake of fluids. Some people, particularly elderly individuals who live alone in facilities without air conditioning, may find it difficult to keep up with fluid intake and thus experience a rise in Tc into, and then above the usual febrile range. Alternatively, when the ambient temperature rises above 37°C, vasodilation no longer cools the blood, particularly if sweating also fails. Another group at risk for hyperthermia are those who take drugs, including some of the older drugs for mental illness with antimuscarinic activity. Patients with mental illness who may live in buildings without air conditioning and with little supervision, are at particular risk during summer hot spells.

Patients brought to the emergency department with heat stroke typically have a Tc above 40°C, and in some cases it may go above 42°C.[321] This is important because at 42°C the effects on potassium channels become sufficiently potent that patients may slip into ventricular tachycardia or fibrillation. Thus, the first thing to do in assessing a patient with impaired consciousness due to hyperthermia is to record an electrocardiogram (EKG). The second order of business is to put in at least two large-bore intravenous lines and begin fluid resuscitation. Although the patient may be hypertonic and hypernatremic, it is important to give isotonic fluids to avoid too rapid a drop in serum sodium. Ideally these interventions are accomplished in parallel and not sequentially. The third approach is rapid cooling. In the past, this was done by packing the patient in ice or putting the patient in a pool of ice-water. However, that stimulus may actually increase serum catecholamines and cause peripheral vasoconstriction, making the heart less stable and impairing passive heat exchange. Modern less extreme cooling equipment and if needed intravascular cooling that allows a gradual more controlled temperature modulation may be preferable.

Although most patients who survive the initial hyperthermia rapidly regain cognitive function, sustained temperatures of 42°C or above may cause permanent brain injury.

PART 6: DISORDERS OF THE INTERNAL MILIEU: ELECTRICAL ENVIRONMENT

Seizure Disorders

Seizures represent excessive, synchronized firing of a population of neurons. In general, most seizures take origin in cerebral cortical structures (including the hippocampus and amygdala) which are composed of large numbers of glutamatergic neurons with extensive cortico-cortical network connections. These networks include positive feedback loops, which are typically held in check by inhibitory interneurons. When the balance of excitatory and inhibitory connections is disturbed, however, this excitatory pattern of recurrent excitation can underlie excessive firing, or seizures.

Several but by no means all types of seizures are associated with impairment of consciousness. Partial seizures can cause mainly motor or sensory phenomena, without impairing consciousness. However, impairment of consciousness is a hallmark of seizures that involve most of the cortex (e.g., in generalized tonic-clonic seizures or convulsive SE), or if they primarily involve structures that maintain awareness of one's self and one's environment (as in absence, complex partial seizures, or nonconvulsive SE).[322] SE consists of prolonged or repeated seizure activity without regaining baseline neurological function, including consciousness. Continual partial seizures are generally called *epilepsy partialis continua*, and as they generally do not impair consciousness will not be discussed further here. While patient profiles, EEG and MRI features, and management of these conditions differ, seizures with impairment of consciousness all converge on a set of common anatomical structures. Functional imaging and EEG studies have implicated frontoparietal association cortex, thalamus, and upper brainstem in seizures associated with impairment of consciousness. These resemble anatomical structures implicated in other disorders of consciousness (see Chapter 1).

In this chapter, seizures are discussed in the context of a differential diagnosis for patients with more prolonged states of unconsciousness. The child with absence seizure presents with brief staring episodes and behavioral arrest or ongoing repetitive behavioral tasks with rapid return to preictal function. Patients with complex partial seizures typically exhibit staring and stereotyped motor movements, but again, these are generally self-limited in time (unless the patient develops partial complex SE). Neither condition would be on the likely differential for the patient with unexplained unconsciousness and will not be discussed here further. Similarly, most generalized tonic-clonic seizures are self-limited in time, and the postictal state, which may include confusion or a postictal deficit (Todd's paralysis) of the cortical area in which the seizure was most intense, is also usually transient. Even if the initial seizure is not observed, there is often evidence on exam (tongue bite, incontinence, unexplained upgoing toe or toes) to suggest a seizure as the cause. Instead, we will focus on patients with generalized convulsive or nonconvulsive SE. See Patient Vignette 5.10.

Patient Vignette 5.10

An 83-year-old woman who lived with her daughter's family was found on the living room sofa, slumping toward the right and unable to speak. She was brought to the hospital emergency department, where she was found to be globally aphasic with a left gaze preference and to have a right hemiparesis with a right Babinski sign. She was thought to have had a left middle cerebral artery embolus, but computed tomography (CT) and magnetic resonance angiography (MRA) failed to disclose a source, and there was no infarct on diffusion weighted MR imaging (MRI). She cleared over the next 24 hours and was discharged in her baseline condition, with the diagnosis of a transient ischemic attack (TIA). This occurred twice more over the next 6 months, and, on the third admission, when her aphasia and hemiparesis had cleared, she was witnessed to have a seizure with right focal motor onset (arm jerking, head to right, eyes to right with right-beating nystagmus) and rapid generalization. Postictally, she had reinstatement of her aphasia and hemiparesis, which cleared again over the next day. She was started on antiepileptic drugs and did not have any more seizures or episodes of aphasia or hemiparesis.

Comment

This patient was worked up three times for TIA before the source of her transient episodes of aphasia and hemiparesis was discovered. In retrospect, the aphasia probably prevented the examiners from detecting a typical postictal confused state, and the right upgoing toe seemed to be part of the right hemiparesis, thus muddying the clues which might otherwise have led to an earlier diagnosis of a postictal state. However, patients with unexplained impairment of consciousness and transient confusion are common, and the examiner must have a high index of suspicion for (missed) seizure in such cases.

GENERALIZED CONVULSIVE STATUS EPILEPTICUS

Convulsive seizures show initially widespread low-voltage, fast, or polyspike activity (tonic muscle contraction) followed by polyspike wave discharges (clonic motor movements), and ultimately generalized attenuation and slowing (postictal lethargy).[322] The untreated patient with convulsive seizures may transition from tonic to clonic movements (duration typically about 2 minutes) to an ultimately motionless comatose state with characteristic accompanying EEG stages: discrete seizures with interictal slowing, waxing and waning of ictal discharges, continuous ictal discharges, continuous ictal discharges punctuated by flat periods, and ultimately to slow periodic epileptiform discharges on a flat background. The sustained depolarizations which characterize SE alter the extracellular milieu, most importantly by excitatory amino acid–mediated opening of ion channels causing elevation of intracellular free calcium, free oxygen radicals and nitric oxide, and phosphorylating enzyme and receptor systems; increasing intracellular osmolality; and activating of autolytic enzyme systems. Repetitive seizures, as seen in SE, result in a progressive, abnormal increase in the permeability of the blood–brain barrier.[64] Breakdown of mechanisms to stop seizures, which allows ongoing SE, include reduced surface expression and sensitivity of $GABA_A$ receptors (which also reduces sensitivity to antiepileptic drugs that act to potentiate $GABA_A$ transmission, such as barbiturates and benzodiazepines), upregulation of N-methyl-D-aspartate (NMDA) receptors, and overexpression of drug efflux transporters.[323–325]

The intense, repetitive neuronal discharges of seizures are followed by postictal metabolic cerebral depression of varying degrees and duration.

In general, the metabolic demand of seizures is created by that massive firing of re-entrant neuronal circuits that mainly occurs in the structures of the cortical mantle. In experimental animals, major seizures produce a 200–300% increase in cerebral metabolic demand, a substantial degree of systemic hypertension, and an enormously increased CBF.[63] The massive metabolic demand of seizures has been demonstrated using intrinsic optical imaging and direct intracranial brain monitoring, both in animals[326–328] and humans.[329–332] These studies revealed deoxygenation (drop in partial brain tissue oxygenation), hypermetabolism (increase of cerebral metabolic rate of oxygen, lactate, glutamate, aspartate, GABA), and increased in regional CBF. The degree of oxygen and blood flow changes has been linked tightly to spike density.[328]

If substrate depletion or a relative decline in blood flow occurs during seizures, the brain maintains its metabolism by the consumption of endogenous substrates. Sustained SE in animals results in progressive hypoxic-ischemic structural neuronal damage. Similar, but necessarily less comprehensive analyses, indicate that seizures cause comparable changes in the human brain. Life-threatening systemic changes accompany the effects on the brain, including elevation of systemic and pulmonary arterial pressures, fever, tachycardia, hyperglycemia, hypercarbia and hypoxia, and lactic acidosis. A combined respiratory and metabolic acidosis is seen, associated with hyperkalemia and later rhabdomyolysis.

Consciousness is probably impaired during seizures by either the excessive firing in structures implicated supporting consciousness (Chapter 1) or by cortical spreading depression due to release of intracellular potassium stores during the excessive firing. This has been suggested by ictal single-photon emission computed tomography (SPECT) scans showing bilateral increases of blood flow in the lateral frontal and parietal, medial parietal, thalamus, and upper brainstem[333,334] during seizures. During the postictal lethargy that is associated with EEG slowing and attenuation, frontoparietal structures show hypoperfusion.[335,336]

NONCONVULSIVE STATUS EPILEPTICUS

Approximately 20% of patients with convulsive status will transition to nonconvulsive SE despite adequate treatment.[337] In addition, nonconvulsive seizures and nonconvulsive SE are frequently seen among unconscious patients with acute brain injury.[338] In these patients, coma may be secondary, both to the seizures as well as to the underlying acute brain injury that also may be the cause for the seizure. Therefore, recovery of consciousness with adequate treatment of seizures may or may not be seen. Many underlying destructive and metabolic cerebral disorders produce both seizures and coma and must be differentiated by other signs, symptoms, and laboratory studies. Nonconvulsive SE is seen in up to 10% of unconscious patients in a general medical or surgical ICU,[339–341] even after excluding all patients with any evidence of brain injury. The prevalence of nonconvulsive seizures and nonconvulsive SE are not known because clinical symptoms are nonspecific, and EEG is required for making the diagnosis. A population-based study of nonconvulsive SE reports an incidence of 1.5 per 100,000/year.[342] Nonconvulsive seizures and SE are most prevalent in patients admitted for CNS infections (i.e., encephalitis, meningitis, brain abscesses), slightly less often in hemorrhages (i.e., subarachnoid, intracerebral, and subdural hemorrhage), TBI, and least often seen in ischemic strokes.

The diagnosis can be suspected if the patient has a history of risk factors such as noncompliance with anticonvulsant drugs[343] or a careful neurologic examination reveals particular abnormalities such as subtle motor activity (particularly twitching of the face and distal extremities)[343] or intermittent bouts of nystagmoid eye movements. If the EEG identifies unequivocal continuous epileptic activity,[344] the diagnosis is established. Unfortunately, an electrographic diagnosis is often difficult. Patients may have electrographic activity that suggests seizures but may simply represent diffuse brain damage, or the seizure activity may occur in a part of the brain, such as the medial temporal or orbitofrontal cortex, from which it may be difficult to record electrographic seizure activity. When the diagnosis is suspected, a trial of an intravenous anticonvulsant (usually a benzodiazepine) may be warranted. Improvement in both the EEG and the patient's clinical state confirms the diagnosis.

In acute brain injury, seizures may cause more damage than in the healthy brain. In patients with acute brain injury, orderly progression of seizures may be disrupted and focal seizures may be an indicator of disrupted neuronal circuitry.[70] Epileptic activity in patients with acute brain injury, such as TBI and intracerebral or subarachnoid hemorrhage, is associated with elevation of serum neuron-specific enolase,[345,346] cerebral interstitial glutamate,[347] midline shift and brain edema,[348,349] and hippocampal atrophy.[350] All taken together, this suggests additional injury encountered from the abnormal nonconvulsive electrical activity. The burden of nonconvulsive seizure activity is associated with worse functional and cognitive outcomes, both in children[351] and adults[352] with acute brain injury.

Invasive brain monitoring has revealed that—just as in animal models—patients with acute brain injury have increased metabolic demand (suggested by a brief drop in jugular bulb oxygenation), hypoxia (supported by a drop in brain oxygenation), raised ICP, and metabolic crisis (indicated by an elevation of the interstitial lactate pyruvate ratio and drop in cerebral glucose as measured by microdialysis) associated with nonconvulsive seizures.[70,353,354] Furthermore, in brain-injured patients, the mechanisms for compensating for increased metabolic demand (e.g., via increased blood flow) may be impaired. For example, impaired vasoreactivity[70,353] may explain the association of seizures with poor outcomes in these patients.[70] Brain tissue hypoxia may develop in patients not only with nonconvulsive seizures and SE, but also with higher frequency periodic epileptiform discharges.[355]

It is an axiom of treatment that convulsions and electrographic seizures should be stopped as promptly as possible, as both the seizures themselves and the accompanying tissue hypoxemia are sources of potentially serious brain damage. Aggressiveness for treatment of these patients is controversial,[356,357] but clearly, patients may have a good functional outcome,[358] which depends on age, seizure history and type, underlying etiology, and extent of consciousness impairment.[359]

Cortical Spreading Depression

Intracortical EEG recording via subdural strips or depth electrodes may allow detection of cortical spreading depression (CSD).[360,361] This phenomenon, first described by Leao in cats, is triggered by excess potassium on cortical neurons. As all neurons achieve their negative membrane potential by maintaining a gradient of potassium across their membrane (high on the inside, low outside), the sudden increase in external potassium reduces the normal polarization of the membrane potential. This causes the neurons to open their potassium channels further to attempt to reestablish their membrane potential, which causes further increase in external potassium. Without sufficient repolarization between action potentials, neurons can no longer fire new action potentials and enter a state of depolarization block. The state of sustained depolarization during CSD leads to neuronal swelling and distortion of dendritic spines.[362] Eventually, the activation of ATP-dependent sodium-potassium pumps restore the ionic gradient, usually after 15–20 minutes in healthy tissue.[53,363] Experimentally, CSD can be triggered by a number of pathophysiological conditions that result in loss of membrane polarization such as manipulation of the ionic environment (i.e., potassium administration, inhibition of the sodium-potassium pump), neurotransmitter release (i.e., glutamate), and alterations of the electrical environment (i.e., SE) or neuronal substrates (i.e., hypoxia, ischemia, and hypoglycemia).

CSDs may originate in healthy brain and are thought to be the basis for migrainous auras.[364] CSDs may also invade healthy brain tissue from their origins in nearby injured brain tissue—spread occurs across a sheet of cortical neurons at an approximate rate of 2–6 mm per minute. In healthy brain, hyperperfusion may be observed as part of the transient physiological hemodynamic response mediated via dilation of resistance vessels. This perfusion change allows the brain to match increased metabolic demand.

In patients with ischemia following SAH, intracerebral hemorrhage, TBI, and large hemispheric infarction, CSDs are frequent. Patients with acute brain injury and CSD are typically unconscious.[365,366] The role CSD plays in relation to consciousness is not well understood, but, based on migraine auras, it is likely that the cortex that is depolarized is incapacitated. Thus, widespread, repeated waves of CSDs could presumably act like a massive, but potentially reversible, cortical lesion. In acute brain injury, neurovascular coupling is impaired and increased metabolic demands cannot be adequately met. This mismatch potentially leads to further exacerbation of brain dysfunction and ultimately to damage.[52] Impaired relaxation of resistance vessels seen in injured brain is part of an inverse hemodynamic response leading to severe hypoperfusion and additional brain injury. In patients with brain hemorrhage, erythrocyte products trigger impaired vasodilation, microcirculatory vasospasm, and additional CSDs. A prospective, observational, multicenter study associated CSD following TBI with poor outcomes after controlling for established predictors.[366] CSD or the associated pathologic hemodynamic response may represent potential targets in the management of acutely brain-injured patients. Ketamine has been shown to inhibit CSD, but the impact on outcomes is unclear.[367] A major challenge for interventional trials, however, is the limited ability of surface EEG recordings to reliably identify CSD.[368]

PART 7: DISORDERS OF THE INTERNAL MILIEU: ABNORMAL CSF PRESSURE OR CONSTITUENTS

Intracranial Hypertension

The role of acute increases in ICP are discussed in Chapter 3. The brain can withstand fairly high ICPs as long as they are applied slowly and the pressure is evenly distributed among the intracerebral compartments. In Chapter 3, we dealt mainly with the consequences of unequal distribution of pressure, such as caused by an expansile mass, and how this leads to brain herniation syndromes. Here we will consider the problem caused by a rapid and diffuse increase in ICP, such as caused by an SAH, acute ventricular obstruction, or cerebral edema.

Perfusion pressure of the brain is typically mean arterial pressure measured at the brachial artery (100 mm Hg = 1,360 mm H_2O), minus the distance from the brachial fossa to the base of the brain (approximately 400 mm H_2O), or about 960 mm H_2O, minus the ICP (which is typically less than 160 mm H_2O), so about 800 mm H_2O. During benign intracranial

hypertension, the ICP can be increased by 400 mm H_2O further, reducing perfusion pressure of the brain to 400 mm H_2O (30 mm Hg). At this point, cerebral perfusion pressure is barely adequate to maintain normal brain function, and even minimal changes in brain perfusion pressure (such as suddenly standing up) can result in failure of brain function. One of the first signs of imminent brain failure in patients with very high ICP is "visual obscuration," the sudden loss of vision when changing position.

One consequence of the drop in cerebral perfusion pressure with elevated ICP is that the medullary cerebral pressor reflex is activated. This is a reflex increase in peripheral resistance that increases BP. Typically there is not an increase in heart rate, such as is seen during the carotid baroreceptor reflex, particularly in children. The lack of increase in heart rate during the cerebral pressor reflex may reflect the fact that the carotid sinus nerve sees an increase in blood pressure, and the carotid sinus reflex actually tries to slow the heart rate.

If the cause of the sudden increase in ICP is SAH, however, the increased systemic blood pressure may actually pump more blood into the intracranial compartment under higher pressure, thus further raising ICP. This vicious cycle rapidly leads to death, which may be why so many patients with SAH do not live long enough to make it to the hospital. See Patient Vignette 5.11.

Patient Vignette 5.11

A 63-year-old man noticed problems with his vision, and his ophthalmologist found bitemporal field deficits. A magnetic resonance imaging (MRI) scan of the brain revealed a pituitary adenoma with suprasellar extension. He was referred to a neurosurgeon, who decided to remove the tumor via a transsphenoidal approach. While working on the pituitary gland, an intracranial artery feeding the tumor tore, resulting in a rapid increase in intracranial pressure (ICP). The anesthesiology record showed a rapid rise in arterial blood pressure even while there was a fall in heart rate as the cerebral pressor response tried to keep cerebral perfusion pressure above ICP. After a few minutes, the blood pressure began to fall off, eventually reaching a level of 70 mm Hg mean arterial pressure. Examination off anesthesia was compatible with brain death.

Comment

The anesthesia records from this unfortunate incident demonstrated the cerebral pressor reflex, as well as the fact that the ICP was inexorably rising due to the subarachnoid ejection of blood to equal the arterial pressure. This rapid upward spiral in blood pressure resulted in inadequate cerebral perfusion pressure to maintain the brain, at which point brain death ensued, and the blood pressure fell to the levels of spinal shock (i.e., those maintained by the heart in the absence of neural input).

Another cause of sudden increase in intracranial pressure is acute ventricular obstruction causing hydrocephalus. The exit from the foramen of Monro into the third ventricle may be blocked by a colloid cyst of the third ventricle. Depending on head position, the cyst may act like a ball valve, causing acute hydrocephalus of the lateral ventricles. This probably impairs consciousness mainly due to the sudden increase in the contents of the lateral ventricles forcing the forebrain downward and compressing the junction of the diencephalon and mesencephalon (central herniation). The subsequent rostrocaudal deterioration of the brainstem can be prevented by acute decompression of the lateral ventricles via an extraventricular drain.

Cerebral edema, following either trauma or cerebral infarction, may be either focal or diffuse. When the edema is asymmetric, involving predominantly one hemisphere or the posterior fossa, the local pressure can reduce perfusion of adjacent tissue whose perfusion may already be compromised (ischemic penumbra), resulting in gradual extension of the edema and involvement of even more tissue. There is also the danger of herniation of tissue from one intracranial compartment into the adjacent compartments if their tissue pressure is lower. When damage is confined to or worse in one hemisphere, it may be possible to reduce the local pressure by hemicraniectomy. In the posterior fossa, if the edema is due to infarction or trauma to the cerebellum, it may be necessary

to remove the damaged cerebellar tissue if the patient is to survive.

Diffuse increase in cerebral edema can occur with certain metabolic insults, such as in severe liver failure. The cerebral edema is thought to be due to toxicity of the elevated ammonia in such patients causing astrocytic swelling,[369] but the exact mechanism is not known. Nevertheless, the increased ICP often is sufficient to deprive the brain of adequate perfusion pressure and is a frequent cause of death in such patients.

Intracranial Hypotension

Clinicians are probably most familiar with intracranial hypotension as a complication of lumbar puncture. The continued leak of CSF from a tear in the dura results in pooling of CSF outside the spinal canal and low CSF pressure within the CSF. Because the brain is normally suspended in a pool of CSF that provides buoyancy, the low pressure causes the brain to sag through the tentorial opening, and the resulting tension on the meninges causes a severe headache. Lying flat brings the head down to the level of the lumbar spine, thus reducing CSF pressure and the volume of the leak. This positional head pain is the hallmark of the post-lumbar puncture headache. Typically this can be eliminated by using a blood patch. Some of the patient's own blood is drawn, and a needle is reintroduced at the same interspace as the original lumbar puncture. However, the needle is not advanced far enough to result in return of CSF, and instead the patient's blood is injected at that site. This tends to coat the epidural space in blood and seals the hole.

Patients with post-lumbar puncture headache sometimes also experience traction on their cranial nerves that run from the posterior to the middle fossa. The most common deficit is a sixth-nerve palsy, which can be on one or both sides. However, impairments of CN III and IV have been reported as well during post-lumbar puncture headache.

A similar condition can occur spontaneously. This spontaneous intracranial hypotension is generally due to a tear in a dural sleeve diverticulum that accompanies a spinal root. Sometimes pooling of CSF can be visualized adjacent to the root. The symptoms and appearance of brain sagging on the MRI scan are essentially identical to post-lumbar puncture headache. However, on rare occasions, the tension at the midbrain–diencephalic junction may result in stupor or even coma in patients with spontaneous intracranial hypotension.[370,371]

Subarachnoid Hemorrhage

Up to half of patients with SAH suffer from unconsciousness. The underlying causes for this are many and differ depending on the timing of unconsciousness in relation to the timing of the bleed. Consciousness is lost at the time of the bleed in approximately 40% of SAH patients,[372–374] and they may or may not recover rapidly. This initial loss of consciousness is primarily thought to be related to an acute, massive reduction of cerebral perfusion pressure due to an increase in ICP with resultant transient cessation of CBF. This pathophysiologic explanation is based on experimental studies and incidental observations in patients who sustained aneurysmal rupture while undergoing transcranial Doppler ultrasonography or digital subtraction angiography studies.[375–377] The mechanism of loss of consciousness is similar to that responsible for unconsciousness in other hypotensive syncopal events.

Additional reasons for unconsciousness by the time of hospital admission include seizures, brain hypoperfusion in the setting of stunned myocardium or frank cardiac arrest, and hypoxia from respiratory failure. Occasionally patients with SAH present with trauma due to falling at the time of loss of consciousness, but the pattern of intracranial blood on CT suggests an underlying aneurysmal etiology (i.e., predominantly blood in the cerebral cisterns surrounding the circle of Willis, but very little blood over the hemispheres or deep in cortical sulci). In these cases, differentiating the "chicken from the egg"—or, in other words, the trauma causing SAH from aneurysmal rupture causing loss of consciousness and trauma—can be challenging. Digital angiography is highly recommended in all of these cases to identify a potentially treatable underlying aneurysm as the cause for the SAH.

Patients with loss of consciousness at presentation more frequently have larger amounts of subarachnoid and intraventricular blood, a higher frequency of diffuse brain swelling known as global cerebral edema, prehospital

tonic-clonic seizures, and cardiopulmonary arrest when compared to SAH patients without loss of consciousness.[373,378,379] Earlier studies also had associated early loss of consciousness with rebleeding and delayed cerebral ischemia.[380,381] Unconsciousness at presentation has been consistently linked to severe long-term disability and higher rates of mortality after SAH.[213,373] Even in patients with lower grade SAH, in whom overall mortality is low, loss of consciousness at the time of bleeding remains associated with poor functional outcomes.[382]

Consciousness may be lost secondarily following SAH with a whole host of etiologies, mostly related to the presence of blood contents in the subarachnoid and ventricular spaces. Within the first hours, patients with SAH may develop hydrocephalus from mechanical obstruction of the arachnoid granulations and flow obstruction within the ventricular system if intraventricular hemorrhage is prominent. Some patients may develop hydrocephalus insidiously, several months or years after SAH, often with opening pressures in the range of 160–180 mm H_2O; although this may cause dementia, especially with poor judgment and memory, it is typically not associated with prominent impairment of consciousness. Elevated ICP without hydrocephalus may be seen particularly in those with poor-grade SAH, including patients with global cerebral edema. Underlying mechanisms causing diffuse brain swelling are not completely clear but are thought to include rebound hyperemia with disruption of the blood–brain barrier with impaired vasoreactivity following the initial arrest of CBF[379] (similar to reperfusion injury after reopening a major cerebral artery in occlusive stroke).

Blood contents in the subarachnoid space cause a prominent inflammatory response,[383] which potentially may directly or indirectly impair consciousness via delayed cerebral ischemia,[384] seizures,[385] and fever, including dysautonomia or autonomic storm. Seizures may occur within the first 2 weeks following SAH, possibly linked to underlying metabolic and electrolyte disturbances, infections, and medications. A vicious cycle between SAH-triggered inflammation and seizures has been identified, and this may cause secondary fluctuation in states of unconsciousness.[385] These delayed seizures are often nonconvulsive and only accurately diagnosable using EEG. Other concerns in SAH patients with secondary unconsciousness include possible ventriculitis in those with external ventricular drainage catheters, postoperative CNS infections, rebleeding, hypoxia (which may be due to neurogenic pulmonary edema), and other medical complications.

Even patients who do well initially may be subject to delayed vasospasm, usually from 3–14 days after SAH. Vasospasm is thought to be due to the breakdown products of hemoglobin activating microglia and causing release of vasoactive substances that result in arterial spasm, but the exact underlying mechanisms are not fully understood.[386] The likelihood of spasm increases with the amount of intracisternal blood, and blood vessels most likely to go into spasm are those surrounded by the most blood.[387] Spasm may cause dysfunction or infarction in the tissue that is not adequately perfused. Clinical symptoms vary depending on the insufficiently perfused brain tissue.[388] However, the substances released in the inflammatory response that causes the spasm may by themselves contribute to impairment of consciousness.

In addition to these many potential causes of unconsciousness in patients with SAH, the hemorrhage may have caused injury to components of the ascending arousal system. Preliminary evidence suggests that this damage can be visualized with diffusion tensor MRI sequences.[389] Conflicting evidence exists regarding the association between perfusion deficits and impairment of consciousness.[390,391] Please refer to Chapter 8 for details on the prevalence, clinical features, and management of delayed cerebral ischemia from vasospasm.

Clinical recovery of patients with SAH may be delayed, and prediction remains challenging,[392] although models have been proposed for predicting functional, cognitive, and quality-of-life outcomes.[393] Overall recovery is tightly linked to initial loss and eventual recovery of consciousness, but understanding the causes of the impaired consciousness and trying to treat them remains challenging.[394] Fortunately, accumulating evidence supports using functional neurophysiologic and neuroimaging studies[395,396] both to monitor the many potential causes, to manage the treatment, and to predict the outcome. Recovery of consciousness even with delayed onset of recovery beyond 6 months after SAH has been described,[394] and therefore overly pessimistic early withdrawal should be cautioned against.

Acute Bacterial Meningitis

Infections of the subarachnoid space are among the most common and most deadly causes of stupor or coma. Because the doubling time of many bacteria is less than an hour, in a few hours time an infection can go from being inapparent to being life-threatening. Hence it is important for the clinician seeing a patient with sudden onset of stupor or coma to consider and rule out this entity as quickly as possible. Prior to the advent of CT scanning, it was common to do a lumbar puncture routinely on any patient with unexplained loss of consciousness. This practice saved many lives, but did result in rare complications, such as when a brain abscess or subdural empyema caused herniation. Currently, where access to CT scanning is ubiquitous, a patient with impairment of consciousness and signs of bacterial infection (fever, elevated white blood count, stiff neck) would receive a dose of broad-spectrum antibiotics before being sent for a CT scan and then a lumbar puncture (please refer to Chapters 7 and 8 for details on diagnosis and management of acute bacterial meningitis).

CNS infections in immunocompromised patients, including infants and elderly adults, are particularly difficult to diagnose and treat for two reasons: (1) symptoms and signs, save for delirium or stupor, may be absent and the patient may have other reasons for being encephalopathic. Furthermore, the immunosuppression may prevent the patient from mounting an inflammatory response and thus the spinal fluid may not suggest infection. In addition, imaging may either be normal or nonspecific. (2) The organisms infecting the CNS in an immunocompromised patient are different from those encountered in the general population. However, being aware of the nature of the immunocompromise, and the variety of organisms that tend to affect such patients, can often lead to an effective early diagnosis and treatment.[397,398] In one series of 696 episodes of community-acquired acute bacterial meningitis, 69% of patients had some alteration of consciousness and 14% were comatose.

Seizures had occurred in 5%.[399] In a review of 317 patients with CNS *Listeria*, 59 (19%) were stuporous and 76 (24%) were comatose.[400] Leptomeningeal infections produce stupor and coma in one of several ways, as detailed next.

TOXIC ENCEPHALOPATHY

Both the bacterial invaders and the inflammatory response to them can have profound effects on cerebral metabolism, causing neuronal injury or death. The injury is mediated by a release of reactive oxygen species, proteases, cytokines, and excitatory amino acids. Both apoptosis and necrosis can occur.[401]

BACTERIAL ENCEPHALITIS AND VASCULITIS

The bacteria that cause acute leptomeningitis often invade the cerebrum, penetrating via the Virchow-Robin perivascular spaces and causing inflammation of both penetrating meningeal vessels and the brain itself.[402] The effects on the brain are both vascular and metabolic. Vasculitis induces diffuse or focal ischemia of the underlying brain and can lead to focal areas of necrosis. Diffuse necrosis of the subcortical white matter has also been reported as a complication of such bacterial vasculitis. Cerebral veins may be occluded, as well as arteries.[402]

INAPPROPRIATE THERAPY

The fluid therapy employed for patients with acute leptomeningitis carries a potential risk of inducing acute water intoxication unless carefully regulated. Many patients with bacterial meningitis suffer from inappropriate ADH secretion, which leads to hyponatremia and cerebral edema when excessive amounts of water are infused.

CEREBRAL HERNIATION

As a result of the preceding mechanisms, severe leptomeningeal infection is often accompanied by considerable cerebral edema, especially in young persons. Cerebral edema is an almost invariable finding in fatal leptomeningitis, and the degree may be so great that it causes both transtentorial and cerebellar tonsillar herniation. In a series of 87 adults with pneumococcal meningitis, diffuse brain edema was

encountered in 29%.[402] In addition, leptomeningeal infections occlude CSF absorptive pathways and, depending on the site of occlusion, cause either communicating or noncommunicating hydrocephalus in about 15% of patients.[402] Shunting of the ventricles may be required to relieve the pressure. The enlargement of the ventricles by nonreabsorbed CSF adds to increased ICP and increases the risk of cerebral herniation.

All of these mechanisms lead to a form of stupor and coma that closely resembles that produced by other metabolic diseases, leading us to include acute leptomeningitis in this section. However, it is important not to lose sight of the possibility that, as the patient's condition worsens, a structural component may also supervene.

The meningeal infections that produce coma are principally those caused by acute bacterial organisms. The major causes of community-acquired bacterial meningitis include *Streptococcus pneumoniae* (51%) and *Neisseria meningitis* (37%).[399] In immunocompromised patients, *Listeria monocytogenes* meningitis accounts for about 4% of cases.[400,403,404] *Listeria* meningitis may be noticeably slower in its course, but it has a tendency to cause brainstem abscesses. *Staphylococcus aureus* and, since a vaccine became available, *Haemophilus influenzae* are uncommon causes of community-acquired meningitis.[399]

The *clinical appearance* of acute meningitis is one of an acute metabolic encephalopathy with drowsiness or stupor accompanied by the toxic symptoms of chills, fever, tachycardia, and tachypnea. Most patients have either a headache or a history of it. However, the classic triad of fever, nuchal rigidity, and alteration of mental status was present in only 44% of patients in a large series of community-acquired meningitis.[399] Focal neurologic signs were present in one-third and included cranial nerve palsies, aphasia, and hemiparesis; papilledema was found in only 3%. CT or MRI may show enhancement in cerebral sulci (Figure 5.6).

Meningitis, particularly in children, can cause acute brain edema with transtentorial herniation as the initial sign. Clinically, such children rapidly lose consciousness and develop hyperpnea disproportionate to the degree of fever. The pupils dilate, at first moderately and then widely, then fix, and the child

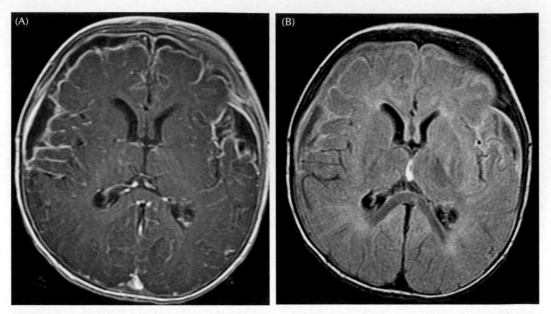

Figure 5.6 (A) A contrast-enhanced T1 image of a patient with acute bacterial meningitis. There is marked enhancement in several of the cerebral sulci. The cortex and the underlying brain appear normal. Hyperintensity in cerebral sulci is apparent on the FLAIR (B) image.
Magnetic resonance image courtesy Dr. Linda Hier.

develops decerebrate motor signs. Urea, mannitol, or other hyperosmotic agents, if used properly, can prevent or reverse the full development of the ominous changes that are otherwise rapidly fatal. In this situation, some believe that a diagnostic lumbar puncture may lead to transtentorial herniation and death. On the other hand, delaying lumbar puncture to procure a CT scan places the patient at major risk, and if the edema is diffuse, the scan does not indicate the risk of herniation.[405–407] Hence, it is now standard practice to draw blood cultures, start steroids and empiric antibiotic therapy, procure a CT scan, and then do a lumbar puncture if there does not appear to be evidence of marked cerebral edema or shift.[408]

In elderly patients, bacterial meningitis sometimes presents as insidiously developing stupor or coma in which there may be focal neurologic signs but little evidence of severe systemic illness or stiff neck. In older patients, a stiff neck may result from cervical osteoarthritis. However, the neck is usually also stiff in the lateral direction as well as in the anterior-posterior direction, a finding not present in meningitis. Furthermore, a positive Kernig

sign (resistance to extension of the knee when the hip is flexed) or Brudzinski sign (flexion of the hips when the neck is flexed) is pathognomonic of meningeal irritation.

In one series, 50% of patients with meningitis were admitted to the hospital with an incorrect diagnosis.[406,407] Such patients can be regarded incorrectly as having suffered a stroke, but this error is readily avoided by accurate spinal fluid examinations. Another pitfall is the difficulty of assessing the CSF when blood due to a traumatic lumbar puncture obscures the elevated spinal fluid white cell count. With acute subarachnoid bleeding, there is approximately 1 white cell to each 1,000 red cells in the CSF. When there are more than two or three white cells beyond this ratio, the patient should be treated as if there were meningitis until proven otherwise by a repeat tap or negative cultures.

Patients are occasionally observed who develop the encephalopathy of meningitis before white cells appear in the lumbar spinal fluid. The series of Carpenter and Petersdorf[409] includes several such cases, and Patient Vignette 5.12 is an example from our own series.

Patient Vignette 5.12

A 28-year-old man complained of mild diurnal temperature elevation for several days with intermittent sore throat, chills, and malaise. He had no muscle or joint complaints or cough, but his chest felt tight. He saw his physician, who found him to be warm and appearing acutely ill, but he lacked significant abnormalities on examination, except that his pharynx and ear canals were reddened. A diagnosis of influenza was made, but the next afternoon he had difficulty thinking clearly and was admitted to the hospital.

His blood pressure was 90/70 mm Hg, pulse 120 per minute, respirations 20 per minute, and body temperature 38.6°C. He was acutely ill, restless, and unable to sustain his attention to cooperate fully in the examination. No rash or petechiae were seen. There was slight nuchal rigidity and some mild spasm of the back and hamstring muscles. The remainder of the physical and the neurologic examination was normal. The white blood count was 18,000/mm^3 with a left shift. Urinalysis was normal. A lumbar puncture was performed with the patient in the lateral recumbent position; the opening pressure was 210 mm, the closing pressure was 170 mm, and the clear cerebrospinal fluid (CSF) contained one red cell and no white cells. The protein was reported as 80 mg/dL, the glucose content as 0.

The first evening at 9 P.M. his temperature had declined to 38°C and he was seemingly improved. Two hours later, he had a chill followed by severe headache and he became slightly irrational. The body temperature was 37.6°C. There was an increase in the nuchal rigidity with increased hamstring and back muscle spasm. The white blood count had increased to 23,000/mm^3. Shortly before 1:30 A.M., he became delirious and then comatose with irregular respiration. The pupils were equal and reactive, the optic fundi were normal, the deep tendon reflexes were equal and active throughout. The left plantar response was extensor, the right was equivocal. Because of the high white cell count, fever, and coma, administration of large doses of antibiotics was started, but the diagnosis was uncertain.

The next morning, the spinal fluid and throat cultures that had been obtained the evening before were found to contain *Neisseria meningitides* and a lumbar puncture now revealed purulent spinal fluid containing 6,000 white cells/mm^3 under a high pressure, with high protein and low glucose contents.

Comment

The error in diagnosis in this patient was in failing to ensure that a CSF Gram stain, protein, and glucose were done and checked immediately by the physicians, who were lured into a false sense of security by the absence of white blood cells in the CSF. In addition, if meningitis or other CNS infection is suspected, even if no cells are found in the initial examination, the lumbar puncture should be repeated in about 6 hours. Patients with overwhelming meningococcal septicemia and few or no polymorphonuclear leukocytes in their spinal fluid represent the worst prognostic group of patients with acute bacterial meningitis. Although a high concentration of polymorphonuclear leukocytes and a decreased spinal fluid glucose strongly suggest the diagnosis of bacterial meningitis, viral infections including mumps and herpes simplex can also occasionally cause hypoglycorrhachia.

Chronic Bacterial or Fungal Meningitis

Chronic meningitis, by its nature, rarely comes into the differential diagnosis of impairment of consciousness. Most of the bacterial causes of chronic meningitis, including syphilis, Lyme disease, nocardia, and actinomycosis, produce a classic meningitic pattern, with headache, stiff neck, and fever. Fungal causes such as cryptococcus, histoplasmosis, coccidiomycosis, or parasitic infections such as babesiosis or amoebiasis are similar. Eventually any of these causes of chronic meningitis may enter a vasculitic phase, where damage to penetrating blood vessels causes small infarcts, which may impair consciousness. However, only a few causes of chronic meningitis routinely cause disorders of consciousness.

TUBERCULOUS MENINGITIS

Although tuberculosis is usually considered a subacute or chronic disease, tuberculous meningoencephalitis may have a fulminant course. Fewer than 50% of adults with meningoencephalitis have a history of pulmonary tuberculosis.[410] On examination patients are lethargic, stuporous, or comatose with nuchal rigidity. The CSF is characterized by an elevated opening pressure with 1–500 white blood cells, which are mainly lymphocytes or monocytes, resembling more an aseptic than an infective meningitis. The protein concentration is elevated (above 100 mg/dL) and the glucose concentration is usually decreased but rarely below 20 mg/dL. Organisms are seen on smear in a minority of patients. Cultures of the CSF may be negative, but even if positive, take several weeks to develop. Polymerase chain reaction (PCR) techniques are rapid and specific; however, sensitivity has been reported to range from 25% to 80%.[410] Neuroimaging is nonspecific, demonstrating contrast enhancement of the meninges and often hydrocephalus.

Because the cell count in the spinal fluid is often low or even absent, the disorder may be confused with other causes of so-called aseptic meningitis including sarcoidosis, leptomeningeal metastases, Wegener's granulomatosis with polyangiitis, and Behçet's disease. The severity of the illness should lead one to suspect the possibility of tuberculosis. Untreated, patients usually die within a few weeks.

LISTERIA MENINGITIS

Listeria monocytogenes is an unusual bacterium in that it generally is found only in patients who are immune-compromised. In such patients, the organism can cause a chronic infection that can continue for several weeks without killing the host. It has an unusual predilection for causing cystic lesions or abscesses in the brainstem (see Fig. 4.12). These can cause cranial neuropathies, or rarely, impair consciousness.[411] It is important to consider Listeria in patients with meningitis because it responds to ampicillin, but not to many of the advanced widespectrum antibiotics currently used to treat bacterial meningitis. Thus, whenever Listeria is in the differential diagnosis, it is useful to include ampicillin in the antibiotic mix.

WHIPPLE'S DISEASE

Whipple's disease is a systemic inflammatory disorder caused by a bacterium, Trophermyma whippleii.[412] It most commonly affects middle-aged men. There may be systemic symptoms including weight loss, abdominal pain, diarrhea, arthralgias, and uveitis. However, in some cases, the symptoms are restricted to the CNS and often are characterized by encephalopathy or even coma.[413] Brainstem signs, especially ataxia and focal or generalized seizures, are common, as is dementia. The characteristic neurologic abnormality in these patients is oculomasticatory myorhythmia, a slow convergence nystagmus accompanied by synchronous contraction of the jaw. The myorhythmias are present in only about 20% of patients and are always associated with a supranuclear vertical gaze palsy. The spinal fluid may demonstrate a pleocytosis but may be entirely benign. MRI is nonspecific, showing hyperintense signal in the hypothalamus and brainstem sometimes with abnormal enhancement, but without mass effect.[414] Lesions are frequently multiple.

The diagnosis, if suspected, can often be made by intestinal biopsy or sometimes by PCR of the spinal fluid, but may require meningeal biopsy.[415] The disease is curable with antibiotics but lethal if not treated.

Viral Meningitis Versus Encephalitis

Viruses, bacteria, rickettsia, protozoa, and nematodes can all invade brain parenchyma. However, only viruses and bacteria (including the obligate intracellular rickettsial species causing Rocky Mountain spotted fever[416]) invade the brain acutely and diffusely enough to cause altered states of consciousness and to demand immediate attention in the diagnosis of stupor or coma. Bacterial encephalitis has been considered earlier as a part of meningitis. Viral encephalitis is discussed in this section.

Viral encephalitis can be divided into four pathologic syndromes. These syndromes are sometimes clinically distinct as well, but the clinical signs of the first three are often so similar as to preclude specific diagnosis without biopsy, CSF PCR,[417] or, sometimes, autopsy. (1) Acute viral encephalitis results from invasion of the brain by a virus that produces primarily or exclusively a CNS infection.[418] Delays in diagnosis of viral meningitis will lead to higher morbidity.[419] We will primarily discuss these in this section.

(2) *Parainfectious encephalomyelitis,* also called acute disseminated encephalomyelitis (ADEM), occurs during or after viral infections, particularly during childhood. Historically ADEM was most often associated with infections of measles, mumps, and varicella,[418] which are rarely seen anymore in developed countries due to vaccination programs. However, ADEM is seen in all age ranges and can follow any type of viral infection. Because ADEM can begin while the acute infection is still present, the two can be very difficult to distinguish in some cases. We will also consider it in detail later.

(3) *Progressive viral infections* are encephalitides caused by conventional viral agents but occurring in susceptible patients, usually those who are immunosuppressed or who develop the infection in utero or during early childhood. Such infections lead to slow or progressive destruction of the nervous system. During intrauterine development these disorders include cytomegalovirus, rubella, Zika, and herpes infections, although nonviral causes such as toxoplasma or syphilis can have a similar result. During childhood, progressive brain damage used to be seen with measles (subacute sclerosing panencephalitis) or rubella (progressive panencephalitis), but these are now rarely seen in vaccinated populations. In children as well as adults, progressive multifocal leukoencephalopathy, a slow infection with JC virus, may occur at any time of life in an immune-compromised host. These progressive viral infections are subacute or gradual in onset, producing stupor or coma in their terminal stages. Hence, they do not cause problems in the differential diagnosis of stupor or coma and are not dealt with here in detail. Progressive multifocal leukoencephalopathy is considered along with the primary neuronal and glial disorders of brain. *Prion infections,*[420,421] including Creutzfeldt-Jakob disease, Gerstmann-Sträussler disease, and fatal familial insomnia,[420] were at one time also thought to be "slow viral" illnesses, but they are now known to be due to a misfolded protein. With the occasional exception of Creutzfeldt-Jakob disease, these disorders likewise are gradual in onset; they do not represent problems in differential diagnosis of disorders of consciousness and are not discussed here.

(4) *Acute toxic encephalopathy* and its variant *Reye's syndrome* historically also occurred mainly in children, often during the course of a systemic infection with a common virus. Since the association of Reye's syndrome with aspirin treatment led to abandoning use of aspirin in those younger than 12 years of age, this consequence of viral infection has become rare. We will consider this category only briefly below.

In each of the pathologically defined viral encephalitides, the viruses produce neurologic signs in one of three ways: (1) they invade, reproduce in, and destroy neurons and glial cells (acute viral encephalitis). Cell dysfunction or death may occur even in the absence of any inflammatory or immune response. (2) They evoke an immune response that can cause hemorrhage, inflammation, and necrosis, or demyelination (parainfectious encephalomyelitis). (3) They provoke cerebral edema and sometimes vascular damage (the premed mechanism in toxic encephalopathy), both of which increase the ICP and, like a supratentorial mass lesion, lead to transtentorial herniation

Acute Viral Encephalitis

The clinical findings in each of the viral encephalitides are sometimes sufficiently different to allow clinical diagnosis even when the illness has progressed to the stage of stupor or coma. Furthermore, within each of these categories, specific viral illnesses may have individual clinical features that strongly suggest the diagnosis. Unfortunately, all too often, though, the specific virus cannot be distinguished on a clinical basis, and the generic term "acute encephalitis" must be used unless PCR, biopsy, or autopsy material establishes the exact pathologic cause. Despite these difficulties in diagnosis, an attempt should be made to separate the acute encephalitides into pathologic categories and to establish the causal agent since the treatment and prognosis are different in the different categories. Brain biopsy is only rarely necessary, as discussed in detail in Chapter 8.

Although a number of viruses cause human encephalitis, only two major types are both common and produce coma in the United States: arboviruses (Eastern equine, Western equine, and St. Louis encephalitis) and herpes viruses. Uncommon causes of stupor and coma include West Nile virus (especially between

August and October),[422,423] severe acute respiratory syndrome (SARS), and other emerging neurotropic viruses that may become more common causes of encephalitis-induced coma in the future.[424] (The varicella-zoster virus typically causes a focal encephalitis or myelitis, but can also infect cerebral blood vessels and cause brain injury or even coma via vascular occlusion and stroke). We will consider each of these here.

HERPES SIMPLEX ENCEPHALITIS

This disease is pathologically characterized by extensive neuronal damage in the cerebral hemispheres with a remarkable predilection by the virus for the gray matter of the medial temporal lobe as well as other limbic structures, especially the insula, cingulate gyrus, and medial frontal lobe (Figure 5.7). Neuronal destruction is accompanied by perivascular invasion with inflammatory cells and proliferation of microglia with frequent formation of glial nodules. The vascular endothelium often swells and proliferates. Areas of focal cortical necrosis are common. Local hemorrhage into brain tissue may occur. Cowdry type A inclusion bodies in neurons and glial cells are a distinctive feature.

Clinically, herpes simplex encephalitis begins with the acute onset of a confusional state, aphasia, or behavioral changes, often accompanied by headache, fever, and seizures. The illness progresses acutely or subacutely to produce stupor or coma. In one series of 45 patients, 28 had Glasgow Coma Score of less than 10, and 13 were deeply comatose.[425] This early stage may be fulminating and, in some instances, may transition from full health to stupor in only a few hours. Often, behavioral disturbances or agitated delirium, particularly with olfactory or gustatory hallucinations, precedes coma by hours or days, a pattern so characteristic as to suggest the diagnosis. Focal motor signs frequently accompany the onset of coma, and tremors of the extremities, face, and even trunk commonly complement the agitated delirium of herpes encephalitis. Occasionally the neurologic signs of herpes simplex encephalitis, either type 1[426] or type 2,[427] are limited to the brainstem, with cranial nerve palsies predominating.

The CSF pressure is usually increased (180–400 mm water) and the white cell count is usually elevated (10–1,000/mm^3, mostly mononuclear). Both may be normal, particularly early in the course of the illness. Up to 500 red cells/mm^3 are common, and the CSF protein

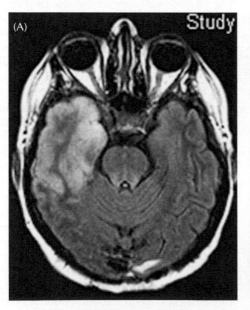
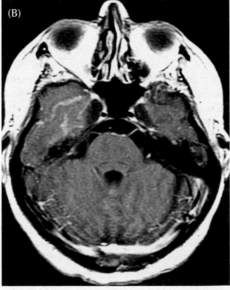

Figure 5.7 Magnetic resonance images of herpes simplex encephalitis. (A) and (B) are, respectively, the FLAIR and contrast-enhanced images of a patient with acute herpes simplex encephalitis. She also suffered from non-small cell lung cancer, and a left occipital metastasis had been previously resected (scar obvious on FLAIR image).

content usually is elevated (values up 870 mg/dL having been reported). The CSF sugar is usually normal but occasionally depressed. Identification of viral DNA by PCR establishes the diagnosis.[428,429] The EEG is always abnormal. Distinctive, periodic, high-voltage, 1-Hz sharp waves from one or both temporal lobes are highly characteristic of herpes simplex encephalitis and suggest a poor prognosis. Imaging with MRI typically identifies the lesions much earlier than CT. Abnormalities in the pattern of the medial temporal lobes, insula, and medial prefrontal cortex including the cingulate gyrus, strongly suggest the diagnosis. (While limbic encephalitis, an autoimmune disorder, can have a similar pattern of MRI abnormality, it generally has a much slower and more progressive onset.) Functional imaging identifies hyperperfusion in the temporal lobe.[428]

Early treatment of herpes simplex encephalitis is vital as treatment with acyclovir or an equivalent antiviral drug yields the best results when administered before patients become comatose. Most patients with suspected herpes encephalitis are now treated immediately, with the drug discontinued later if the diagnosis is not confirmed.

Sometimes, as in Patient Vignette 5.13 and Historical Patient Vignette 5.14, severe temporal lobe brain swelling produces transtentorial herniation and may lead to death.

Patient Vignette 5.13

A 71-year-old woman was brought into the emergency department for a headache and confusion. Her temperature was 98°F and she complained of a diffuse headache, but could not answer questions coherently. Neurologic examination showed a mild left hemiparesis and some left-sided inattention. A right hemisphere ischemic event was suspected, but the computed tomography (CT) did not disclose any abnormality. She was admitted to the stroke service. The following day, her temperature spiked to 102°F, and a lumbar puncture was done showing 7 white blood cells, 19 red blood cells, a protein of 48, and a glucose of 103 with a normal opening pressure. A magnetic resonance imaging (MRI) scan showed T2 signal involving the medial and lateral temporal lobe, as well as the insular and cingulate

cortex on the right, with less intense but similar involvement of the left cingulate cortex. By this time, she had lapsed into a stuporous state, with small but reactive pupils, full roving eye movements, and symmetric increase in motor tone. She was started on acyclovir. Despite treatment, she developed edema of the right temporal lobe with uncal herniation.

Comment

Because the initial presentation suggested a right hemisphere ischemic event, the patient was treated according to standard stroke protocols, which do not require lumbar puncture. By the time the MRI scan was done, revealing the typical pattern of herpes simplex encephalitis, the patient had progressed to a stuporous state and acyclovir was not able to prevent the swelling and herniation of her right temporal lobe.

Historical Patient Vignette 5.14

This case was seen in the era prior to computed tomography (CT) and antiviral therapy. It is presented because it illustrates the natural history of herpes encephalitis and included a pathologic examination.

A 32-year-old children's nurse was admitted to the hospital in coma. She had felt vaguely unwell 5 days before admission and then developed occipital headache and vomiting. Two days before admission, a physician carefully examined her but found only a temperature of 39°C and a normal blood count. She remained alone for the next 48 hours and was found unconscious in her room and brought to the emergency department.

Examination showed an unresponsive woman with her head and eyes deviated to the right. She had small ecchymoses over the left eye, left hip, and knee. Her neck was moderately stiff. The right pupil was slightly larger than the left, both reacted to light, and the oculocephalic reflex was intact. The corneal reflex was bilaterally sluggish, and the gag reflex was intact. Her extremities were flaccid, the stretch reflexes were 3+, and the plantar responses were flexor.

In the emergency department, she had a generalized convulsion associated with deviation of the head and the eyes to the left. The opening pressure on lumbar puncture was 130 mm of cerebrospinal fluid (CSF). There were 550 mononuclear cells and 643 red blood cells/mm³. The CSF glucose was 65, and the protein was 54 mg/dL. Skull x-ray findings were normal. A right carotid arteriogram showed marked elevation of the sylvian vessels with only minimal deviation of the midline structures, suggesting temporal lobe mass effect. Burr holes were placed; no subdural blood was found. A ventriculogram showed the third ventricle curved to the right. The electroencephalogram (EEG) contained 1- to 2-Hz high-amplitude slow waves appearing regularly every 3–5 seconds from a background of almost complete electrical silence. Low-amplitude 10- to 12-Hz sharp-wave bursts of gradually increasing voltage began over either frontal area and occurred every 1–2 minutes; they lasted 20–40 seconds and were associated with seizure activity.

Her seizures were partially controlled with anticonvulsants, and she received 20 million units of penicillin/day and chloramphenicol for possible bacterial meningitis. Her condition gradually deteriorated, and, on the eighth hospital day, she developed midposition fixed pupils with absence of oculovestibular responses and diabetes insipidus with a serum osmolality of 313 mOsm/L and urine specific gravity of 1.005. Eight days after admission, lumbar puncture yielded a serosanguineous fluid with 26,000 red blood cells and 2,200 mononuclear cells. The protein was 210 mg/dL. CSF antibody titers for herpes simplex virus were 1:4 at admission but 1:32 by day 8. She died 10 days after admission, having been maintained with artificial ventilation and pressor agents for 48 hours.

At autopsy, herpes simplex virus was cultured from the cerebral cortex. The leptomeninges were congested, and the brain was swollen and soft with bilateral deep tentorial grooving along the hippocampal gyrus. The diencephalon was displaced an estimated 8–10 mm caudally through the tentorial notch. On cut section, the medial and anterior temporal lobes as well as the insula were bilaterally necrotic, hemorrhagic, and soft. Linear and oval hemorrhages were found in the thalamus bilaterally and extended down the central portion of the brainstem as far as the pons.

Hemorrhages were also found in the cerebellum, and there was a small, intact arteriovenous malformation in the right sylvian fissure. There were meningeal infiltrations predominantly of lymphocytes, some plasma cells, and polymorphonuclear leukocytes. The perivascular spaces were also infiltrated, in places extending to the subcortical white matter. In some areas, the entire cortex was necrotic with shrunken and eosinophilic nerve cells. Numerous areas of extravasated red blood cells were present in the cortex, basal ganglia, and upper brainstem. Marked microglial proliferation and astrocytic hyperplasia were present. Cowdry type A intranuclear inclusion bodies were present primarily in the oligodendroglia, but were also seen in astroglia, small neurons, and occasional capillary endothelial cells.

Comment

This patient's history, findings, and course in the days before imaging, polymerase chain reaction, or antiviral agents were available were characteristic of herpes simplex encephalitis. The pathologic examination of the brain complements the imaging available in modern cases and was able to demonstrate the presence of viral inclusions.

ARBOVIRUS INFECTIONS

Arboviruses are so-named because they are transmitted by arthropod insects (ARthropod-BOrne virus). Arthropod vectors such as mosquitos, tics, and sandflies typically infect animals, including humans, when they consume their blood. Arboviruses typically infect the salivary glands of the arthropod, whose saliva contacts the blood of the host animal. Once the virus has replicated in the host and is plentiful in its bloodstream, later arthropods who feed on the same host become infected.

Some arboviruses cause mainly a systemic febrile illness with severe body aches, such as dengue, Zika, or chikungunya, all of which have found a wider distribution in the temperate parts of the Western hemisphere in recent years. Some can cause a hemorrhagic fever. Still others are neurotropic and cause encephalitis, including Japanese encephalitis, Eastern equine encephalitis, St. Louis encephalitis, and West Nile fever (among others). Because these infections depend on the life cycle of arthropods, they typically occur from late spring through early fall, but are rare during the winter.

These infections begin as a febrile illness with lethargy and body aches, but progress rapidly to stupor and coma. Examination of the patient in West Nile virus infection often shows evidence of a polioencephalopathy, a lower motor neuron type weakness and loss of muscle stretch reflexes reminiscent of polio virus. There is usually nuchal rigidity, and lumbar puncture shows CSF with mild elevation of white blood cells (usually less than 100) and protein (less than 100), but normal glucose. MRI scan may show a pattern of T2 hyperintensity in the basal ganglia and thalamus.

Many noninfectious illnesses may mimic infections. Some present as acute meningeal reactions, others as more chronic reactions. Table 5.1 lists some of these.

PARAINFECTIOUS ENCEPHALITIS (ACUTE DISSEMINATED ENCEPHALOMYELITIS)

ADEM is an autoimmune disorder that typically follows a viral illness, although it can also be triggered by vaccination and rarely by bacterial or parasitic infection.[430,431] In some cases, the initiating infection may be so mild that it is not remembered. In other cases, where ADEM occurs during the course of viral encephalitis, it may be difficult to distinguish where one problem ends and the other begins. ADEM has been described by different terms in the literature depending on the circumstances of its appearance (e.g., as parainfectious disseminated encephalomyelitis and as acute hemorrhagic leukoencephalopathy). Two pathogenetic mechanisms have been advanced. In the first, the invading organism or vaccine is molecularly similar to a brain protein (molecular mimicry), but sufficiently different for the immune system to recognize it as nonself and mount an immune attack against the brain or spinal cord. In the second, the virus invades the brain, causing tissue damage and leakage of antigens into the systemic circulation. Because the brain is a relatively immune-privileged site, the immune system may not have been exposed to the brain protein before and it mounts an immune attack.[430] Similar clinical and pathologic disorders can be produced in experimental animals by the injection of brain extracts of myelin basic protein mixed with appropriate adjuvants (experimental allergic encephalomyelitis [EAE]) and by Theiler virus.[430] Hemorrhagic changes appear to signify a hyperacute form of allergic encephalomyelitis. The disorder largely affects children, but adults and even the elderly are sometimes affected. The estimated incidence is 0.8 per 100,000 population per year.[430] Fifty percent to 75% of patients have a febrile illness within the 30 days preceding the onset of neurologic symptomatology.

Table 5.1 Disorders that Imitate Central Nervous System Infections and the Types of Infection that they Most Commonly Mimic

Acute meningitis	Chronic meningitis	Encephalitis/Meningoencephalitis
Behçet's disease	Chemical meningitis	Acute disseminated encephalomyelitis
Chemical meningitis	Granulomatous angiitis	Acute hemorrhagic leukoencephalitis
Cyst rupture	Lymphomatoid granulomatosis	Acute toxic encephalopathy
Drug-induced meningitis	Meningeal malignancy	Behçet's disease
Parameningeal infection	Sjögren syndrome	Serum sickness
Systemic lupus erythematosus	Systemic lupus erythematosus	Systemic lupus erythematosus
Vogt-Koyanagi-Harada syndrome	Sarcoidosis	Vogt-Koyanagi-Harada syndrome

Modified from Wasay et al.,[432] with permission.

In ADEM, the brain and spinal cord contain multiple perivascular zones of demyelination in which axons may be relatively spared, resembling acute multiple sclerosis. There is usually striking perivascular cuffing by inflammatory cells. Clinically, the illness occasionally arises spontaneously, but usually it follows by several days a known or presumed viral infection, frequently an exanthem (e.g., rubella, varicella), but occasionally a banal upper respiratory infection or another common viral infection (e.g., mumps or herpes). The onset is usually rapid, with headache and a return of fever. In most cases, there is early evidence of behavioral impairment, and, as the disorder progresses, the patient may lapse into delirium, stupor, or coma. In one series of 26 patients, 5 (19%) were comatose.[433] Nuchal rigidity may be present. Both focal and generalized convulsions are common, as are focal motor signs such as hemiplegia or paraplegia, or even extrapyramidal movement disorders.

Careful examination often discloses evidence for disseminated focal CNS dysfunction in the form of optic neuritis, conjugate and dysconjugate eye movement abnormalities, and sensory losses or motor impairment. In 80% of cases, the CSF white cell count is elevated, usually to less than 500 lymphocytes/mm^3, but in the remainder there may be no elevation of CSF white blood count. The CSF protein may be slightly increased, but the glucose is normal. Oligoclonal bands may be present but are commonly absent. Even in patients in whom the CSF is normal, MRI scanning usually discloses multiple white matter lesions that are bright on T2 and FLAIR imaging and which may show contrast enhancement. Sometimes gray matter is involved as well as white matter, which may explain the tendency for seizures to occur. However, early in the course of the illness, the MRI scan may be normal. We observed one patient who became comatose during the first few days of a severe attack, but whose MRI scan was normal for another week, at which time it progressed rapidly to diffuse T2 signal throughout the white matter of the brain (see Patient Vignette 4.4). The diagnosis of ADEM should be suspected when a patient becomes neurologically ill following a systemic viral infection or vaccination. Evidence of widespread or multifocal nervous system involvement and of mild lymphocytic meningitis supports the diagnosis. An MRI strongly supports the diagnosis when it is consistent with multifocal areas of demyelination.

Acute hemorrhagic leukoencephalopathy is usually considered to be an especially severe variant of ADEM.[434] However, a recent report suggests that organisms may be found in the brains of patients who die of the disorder. The organisms, measured by PCR, include herpes simplex virus, herpes zoster virus, and HHV-6. Whether the virus itself or an immune reaction to it was causal was unclear.[435] This disorder is marked pathologically by inflammation and demyelination similar to ADEM, plus widespread hemorrhagic lesions in the cerebral white matter. The hemorrhagic lesions vary in diameter from microscopic to several centimeters and are accompanied by focal necrosis and edema. The perivascular infiltrates frequently contain many neutrophils, and there is often perivascular fibrinous material. The clinical course is as violent as the pathologic response. The illness begins abruptly with headache, fever, nausea, and vomiting. Affected patients rapidly lapse into coma with high fever but little or no nuchal rigidity. Convulsions and focal neurologic signs, especially hemiparesis, are common. Focal cerebral hemorrhages and edema may produce both the clinical and radiographic signs of a supratentorial mass lesion. The CSF is usually under increased pressure and contains from 10 to 500 mononuclear cells and up to 1,000 red blood cells/mm^3. The CSF protein may be elevated to 100–300 mg/dL or more.

As a rule, the problem in the differential diagnosis of coma presented by disseminated and hemorrhagic encephalomyelitis is to distinguish it from viral encephalitis and acute toxic encephalopathy. At times a distinction may be impossible, either clinically or virologically. As a general rule, patients with viral encephalitis tend to be more severely ill and have higher fevers for longer periods of time than patients with disseminated encephalomyelitis, with the exception of the hemorrhagic variety. Acute toxic encephalopathy usually is more acute in onset and is associated with higher ICP and with fewer focal neurologic signs, either clinically or radiographically.

ACUTE TOXIC ENCEPHALOPATHY DURING VIRAL ENCEPHALITIS

Acute toxic encephalopathy is the term applied to a nervous system disorder, seen predominantly in children under the age of 5, which usually occurs during or after a systemic viral infection and is characterized clinically by the acute onset of increased ICP, with or without focal neurologic signs, and without CSF pleocytosis. The disorder is distinguished pathologically from acute viral encephalitis by the absence of inflammatory change or other pathologic abnormalities of acute viral encephalitis, save for cerebral edema and its consequences. The cause of acute toxic encephalopathy is unknown and may represent several different illnesses. The best characterized of these was Reye's syndrome (see later discussion), which rarely is seen after the use of aspirin was abandoned in children with febrile illnesses. It often accompanies viral infection, particularly influenza,[436] but also the common exanthems such as measles and mumps; it also appears without evidence of preceding systemic viral infection. In some instances, viruses have been identified in the brain at autopsy. There may be accompanying evidence of an acute systemic illness, such as liver and kidney damage in Reye's syndrome, or the patient may be free of symptoms other than those of CNS dysfunction. Death is caused by cerebral edema with transtentorial herniation. At autopsy neither inflammation nor demyelination are encountered in the brain, only evidence of severe and widespread cerebral edema.

Clinically, the disease is characterized by an acute or subacute febrile onset associated with headache, sometimes nausea and vomiting, and often delirium or drowsiness followed by stupor or coma. Focal neurologic signs usually are absent but may be prominent and include hemiparesis or hemiplegia, aphasia, or visual field defects. In its most fulminant form, the untreated illness progresses rapidly, with signs of transtentorial herniation leading to coma with impaired ocular movements, abnormal pupillary reflexes, abnormal posturing, and, eventually, respiratory failure and death. SE marks the early course of a small proportion of the patients. Patient Vignette 5.15 illustrates such a case.

Historical Patient Vignette 5.15

A 46-year-old man was in hospital 10 days following a negative inguinal lymph node dissection for the treatment of urethral cancer.

He was well and ready for discharge when he complained of a sudden left temporal headache and was noted by his roommate to be confused. Neurologic examination revealed a modest temperature elevation to 38.1°C in an awake but confused individual who was disoriented to time and had difficulty carrying out three-step commands. The neurologic examination was entirely intact, and laboratory evaluation for infection or metabolic abnormalities was entirely normal. The electroencephalogram (EEG) was bilaterally slow, more so on the right side than the left. The lumbar puncture pressure was 160 mm cerebrospinal fluid (CSF). There were two red cells, one white cell, and a protein of 41 mg/dL. The glucose was 75 mg/dL. Within 48 hours, he became agitated and mildly aphasic, with a right homonymous visual field defect. He then had a generalized convulsion. The day following the seizure, the lumbar puncture pressure was 230 mm CSF; there was one white cell, a protein of 90 mg/dL, and glucose of 85 mg/dL. A computed tomography (CT) scan was normal, as were bilateral carotid arteriograms. Cultures of blood and CSF for bacteria, viruses, and viral titers were all negative, as was a coagulation profile. Within 48 hours after the convulsion, the patient lapsed into coma with evidence of transtentorial herniation leading to respiratory arrest and death despite treatment with mannitol and steroids. At autopsy, the general examination was normal except for evidence of his previous surgery. There was no evidence of residual cancer. The brain weighed 1,500 g and was grossly swollen, with evidence of both temporal lobe and tonsillar herniation and a Duret hemorrhage in the pons. Microscopic examination was consistent with severe cerebral edema and herniation, but there was no inflammation, nor were there inclusion bodies.

Comment

Except for his age and a somewhat protracted course, this patient is typical of patients with acute toxic encephalopathy.

A clinical distinction between acute, sporadic viral encephalitis and acute, toxic encephalopathy often cannot be made. Certain clues, when present, help to differentiate the two entities: acute encephalopathy appears with or shortly after a banal viral infection, usually occurs in children under 5 years of age, may be associated with hypoglycemia and liver function abnormalities, and usually produces only a modest degree of fever. Rapidly developing increased ICP in the absence of focal signs or neck stiffness also suggests acute toxic encephalopathy. Conversely, prominent focal signs, particularly those of temporal lobe dysfunction accompanied by an abnormal CT or MRI, indicate an acute viral encephalitis such as herpes simplex. The presence of pleocytosis (with or without additional red cells) in the CSF suggests acute viral encephalitis, whereas a spinal fluid under very high pressure but with a normal cellular content suggests acute toxic encephalopathy. In many instances, however, neither a clinical nor laboratory diagnosis can be made immediately.

Reye's syndrome is a variant of acute toxic encephalopathy. This disorder seemed to appear out of nowhere in the 1950s and then, except for rare reports, disappeared in North America and Europe before 1990. In children, it was believed to be precipitated by the use of aspirin to treat viral infections, and the disappearance coincided with the recommendation that aspirin not be given to children for febrile illnesses.[437] It is still seen, however, in countries in which administration of aspirin to children is practiced.[438] Reye's syndrome, like other acute toxic encephalopathies, was characterized by progressive encephalopathy with persistent vomiting often following a viral illness (particularly influenza B and varicella). It differs from other forms of acute toxic encephalopathy in that it occurred in epidemics, and there was usually evidence of hepatic dysfunction and often hypoglycemia. The illness was pathologically characterized by fatty degeneration of the viscera, particularly the liver but also the kidney, heart, lungs, pancreas, and skeletal muscle.

CEREBRAL BIOPSY FOR DIAGNOSIS OF ENCEPHALITIS

When faced with a delirious or stuporous patient suspected of suffering acute encephalitis, the physician is often perplexed about how best to proceed. The clinical pictures of the various forms of encephalitis are often so similar that only cerebral biopsy will distinguish them, but the treatment of the various forms differs. Of the acute viral encephalitides, herpes simplex can be effectively treated by antiviral agents, and it is likely that in some immune-suppressed patients other viral infections such as varicella-zoster and cytomegalovirus also respond to antiviral treatment. Acute parainfectious encephalomyelitis is not reported to respond to either antiviral treatment or control of ICP, but often does respond to steroids or immunosuppressive agents.

Weighing the pros and cons, when noninvasive imaging (MRI, magnetic resonance spectroscopy [MRS], PET) and other tests (CSF PCR for organisms, cytology, oligoclonal bands, and immune globulins) are unrevealing, the risk of biopsy is often small compared to the risk of missing treatment for a specific diagnosis. If there is a focal lesion, a stereotactic needle biopsy will often suffice.[439,440] If there is no focal lesion, an open biopsy, ensuring that one procures leptomeninges and gray and white matter,[441] is required. The biopsy should be taken either from the edge of an involved area (as necrotic tissue from the center of a lesion may be nondiagnostic) or, if the illness is diffuse, from the right frontal or temporal lobe. Complications of either stereotactic or open biopsy are uncommon. However, nondiagnostic biopsies are common. In one series of 90 brain biopsies for evaluation of dementia, only 57% were diagnostic.[441] However, in this and other studies, the biopsy sometimes identified treatable illnesses such as multiple sclerosis, Whipple's disease, cerebral vasculitis, or paraneoplastic encephalopathy.[441,442]

Carcinomatous Meningitis

Diffuse encephalopathy leading to delirium, stupor, or coma is frequently seen in patients with disseminated cancer.[432] About 20% of the neurologic consultations in a cancer hospital are requested for the evaluation of confused or stuporous patients.[443] The causes of the mental changes are many (Table 5.2) and may include all those discussed in this book.[444] In a series of 140 patients with encephalopathy and cancer, two-thirds had multiple causes of their encephalopathy. However, when a single cause was identified, multiple brain metastases were the most common. In some cases, the metastases are leptomeningeal and may be discovered only by lumbar puncture. Other single causes included drugs, sepsis, multiorgan failure, and hypoxia.[444] As with other patients suffering from metabolic encephalopathy, the cancer patient can often be restored to a fully sentient state if the underlying metabolic cause is corrected (Table 5.2).

The key feature of carcinomatous meningitis is multilevel dysfunction (cognitive, cranial nerves, spinal nerves) of the nervous system. This is sometimes, but not always associated meningismus. MRI scanning may show evidence of deposits of tumor along the meninges, particularly thickening of the spinal roots or cranial nerves. CSF may show elevated white blood cells or protein or low glucose, but is seldom entirely normal. The diagnosis is made by finding tumor cells in the CSF via cytology. However, this requires that a fresh specimen of

Table 5.2 Some Neurologic Complications of Cancer Causing Stupor or Coma

Lesion	Example
Primary brain tumor	Hypothalamic glioma
	Gliomatosis cerebri
Brain metastasis	Carcinomatous encephalitis
Leptomeningeal	
metastasis	Hydrocephalus
Vascular disease,	Nonbacterial
Large stroke	thromboendocarditis
	Cerebral venous occlusion
Multiple small	Disseminating intravascular
strokes	coagulation
	Intravascular lymphoma
Infections	
Viral	PML
	Herpes simplex/zoster
Fungi	*Aspergillus*
Bacteria	*Listeria*
Side effects of therapy	
Radiation	Radiation necrosis
Chemotherapy	Methotrexate
	leukoencephalopathy
Metabolic	Hypoglycemia
	Liver, renal failure
Nutritional	Wernicke's encephalopathy
	Pellagra
	B_{12} deficiency
	encephalopathy

CSF be prepared with an appropriate preservative almost immediately after lumbar puncture. The longer the delay before the spinal fluid is fixed properly, the lower the yield of the cytological examination. Even under ideal circumstances in patients with pathological proven carcinomatous meningitis, it is possible to have multiple false-negative lumbar punctures, so if the index of suspicion is high, repeated attempts are warranted. See Patient Vignette 5.16.

Patient Vignette 5.16

A 42-year-old woman with breast cancer known to be metastatic to bone was admitted to the hospital because of stupor. When stimulated vigorously she would answer with her name, but could not answer other questions or follow commands. On examination there was bilateral papilledema. Pupils were 2 mm bilaterally, with roving eye movements and full responses to oculocephalic maneuvers. There were diminished tendon reflexes in the left triceps and right knee jerk. Toes were upgoing. A computed tomography (CT) scan with contrast disclosed several small enhancing lesions along the surface of the cerebral cortex. Lumbar puncture showed increased opening pressure of 300 mm cerebrospinal fluid (CSF), protein of 228, 14 WBCs, no RBCs, and multiple large atypical cells, which, on cytologic examination, were similar to the adenocarcinoma cells of her breast cancer. She was treated with dexamethasone and whole-brain radiation therapy, resulting in rapid clearing of her cognitive function. Intraventricular chemotherapy with methotrexate and cytosine arabinoside was initiated. When she died of a pulmonary embolus 18 months later, autopsy revealed no evidence of residual cancer in the brain.

Comment

Leptomeningeal metastasis from cancer generally presents with multilevel dysfunction of the central nervous system, spinal cord, and spinal nerve roots. The loss of several tendon reflexes in this setting is a critical clue to the diagnosis. Radiologic evaluation may show nothing, or it may reveal superficial tumor implants along the surface of the brain, the meninges, or the spinal roots. Although often a sign of far advanced cancer, in occasional patients, particularly with breast cancer or lymphoma, vigorous treatment may clear the tumor cells and dramatically improve and extend the patient's life.

On the other hand, even in patients who have a well-established diagnosis of cancer, it is sometimes necessary to look elsewhere for the origin of impaired consciousness. See Patient Vignette 5.17.

Patient Vignette 5.17

A 60-year-old man with multiple myeloma became obtunded while in the hospital. Treatment with chemotherapy had produced a severe pancytopenia, which had led to pneumonia. In addition, he suffered from renal failure and required intermittent hemodialysis. At 6:50 A.M., he was given 4 mg of levorphanol because of low back pain. Early in the afternoon he began hemodialysis, but he became hypotensive and hemodialysis was stopped. He was noted early in the evening to be markedly obtunded, with the right eye slightly deviated outward and upward. His respirations "appeared agonal." On neurologic examination, the patient was stuporous. With vigorous stimuli, however, he could be aroused to say his name and to identify Memorial Hospital. No other verbal responses could be secured. His pupils were 1.5 mm and reactive. In the resting position, the left eye was straight ahead and the right eye was slightly externally and superiorly deviated. Ice water caloric testing yielded a few beats of nystagmus in the appropriate direction. His respirations were 8 per minute, irregular, and shallow. Bilateral asterixis and extensor plantar responses were present. Laboratory abnormalities that morning had included a white blood cell count of 1,100/mm^3, a hemoglobin of 9.3 g/dL, and platelets of 21,000/mm^3, and D-dimer concentrations (fibrin degradation products suggesting mild disseminated intravascular coagulation) were elevated. The serum sodium was 130 mEq/L, blood urea nitrogen 82 mg/dL, creatinine 5.7 mg/dL, total protein 8.1 g/L, albumin 3.0 g, and alkaline phosphatase 106. Because of

the small pupils and slow and shallow respiration, the patient was given 0.4 mg of naloxone intravenously. The pupils dilated to 6 mm, respirations went from 8 to 24 per minute, and he became awake and alert, complaining of the low back pain for which he had been given the drug that morning. The following morning, he again became obtunded but less severely than the evening before. Pupils were 3 mm, and respirations were 20 and relatively deep. Another 0.4 mg of naloxone was given, the pupils dilated to 7 mm, respirations accelerated to 30 and deeper, and again he became alert and oriented.

Comment

The clues to opioid overdosage in this patient were the small pupils and the shallow, irregular respirations despite pneumonia. The patient's other metabolic defects made him particularly sensitive to small doses of opioids, as did the fact that he had not received the drug in the past for pain and thus had not developed tolerance to it. Furthermore, the long action of levorphanol compared to that of naloxone resulted in a relapse the next morning after the effects of the naloxone had worn off.

PART 8: DISORDERS OF ENDOGENOUS TOXINS

Hypercarbia

During hypoventilation or complete ventilatory failure (which may be due to asphyxia or neuromuscular failure), there is a combination of hypoxia and hypercarbia, which can lead to encephalopathy.[445] It is often difficult in such circumstances to dissect the effects of hypercarbia from hypoxia. On the other hand, in patients with chronic obstructive lung disease, it is not uncommon for the patient to live most of his or her life with both pO_2 and PCO_2 in the 50–60 torr range. At low levels of ventilatory insufficiency, the main drive to breathe is typically the elevated pCO_2. However, CO_2 causes ventilatory drive by combining with water to form hydrogen and bicarbonate ion. It is the hydrogen, as measured by a falling pH, that is monitored by the brain and which causes increased ventilation.

In patients with chronic elevation of pCO_2, there is reduced renal excretion of the bicarbonate ion, which rises to the point where it largely buffers the hydrogen ion, and the pH becomes only slightly acidic (compensated respiratory alkalosis). As a result, ventilatory drive decreases, and the high buffering capacity means that the patient becomes desensitized to further changes in pCO_2 driving ventilatory responses. On the other hand, the hypoxic drive to breathe is increased in the presence of chronically elevated pCO_2.

When such a patient is then given oxygen to breathe, often a well-meaning act for a hypoxic patient in the hospital setting, this blunts the hypoxic drive to breathe, and, as the patient breathes less deeply, the pCO_2 becomes even more elevated. It is in this situation when the sudden increase in pCO_2 causes hypercarbic encephalopathy. The patient becomes progressively more obtunded, despite being at a higher level of pO_2 than they are usually accustomed.

Such patients may be erroneously suspected of having sedative poisoning or other causes of coma, but, as Patient Vignette 5.18, blood gas measurements make the diagnosis.

Patient Vignette 5.18

A 60-year-old woman with severe chronic pulmonary disease went to a physician complaining of nervousness and insomnia. An examination disclosed no change in her pulmonary function, and she was given a sedative to help her sleep. Her daughter found her unconscious the following morning and brought her to the hospital. She was comatose but withdrew appropriately from noxious stimuli. She was cyanotic, and her respirations were labored at 40 per minute. Her pupils were 3 mm in diameter and reacted to light. There was a full range of extraocular movements on passive head turning. No evidence of asterixis or multifocal myoclonus was encountered, and her extremities were flaccid with slightly depressed tendon reflexes and bilateral extensor plantar responses. The arterial blood pH was 7.17, the $PaCO_2$ was 70 mm Hg, the serum bicarbonate was 25 mEq/L, and the PaO_2 was 40 mm Hg.

She was intubated and received artificial ventilation with a respirator for several days before she awakened and was able by her own efforts to maintain her arterial $PaCO_2$ at its normal level of 45 mm Hg.

Comment

This is not an unusual history. It is possible that the increased nervousness and insomnia were symptoms of increasing respiratory difficulty. The sedative hastened the impending decompensation and induced severe respiratory insufficiency as sleep stilled voluntary respiratory efforts. The rapidity with which her $PaCO_2$ rose from 45 to 70 mm Hg is indicated by her normal serum bicarbonate, there having been no time for the development of the renal compensation that usually accompanies respiratory acidosis.

When CO_2 accumulates slowly, the complaints of insidiously appearing headache, somnolence, and confusion may occasionally attract more attention than the more direct signs of respiratory failure. The headache, like other headaches associated with increased ICP, may be maximal when the patient first awakens from sleep and disappears when activity increases respiration, lowering the PCO_2 and, thus, the ICP.

In its most severe form, pulmonary encephalopathy may cause increased ICP, papilledema,[446] and bilateral extensor plantar responses, symptoms that may at first raise the question of a brain tumor or some other expanding mass. The important differential features are that in CO_2 retention focal signs are rare, blood gases are always abnormal, and the encephalopathy usually improves promptly if artificial ventilation is effectively administered.

Two associated conditions are closely related to CO_2 narcosis and often accentuate its neurologic effects. One is hypoxemia and the other is metabolic alkalosis, which often emerges as the result of treatment. Hypoxia accompanying CO_2 retention must be treated because lack of oxygen is immediately dangerous both to the heart and brain. Traditional teaching has been that oxygen therapy for hypercapnic patients with an acute exacerbation of chronic obstructive pulmonary disease may be dangerous, as it may reduce respiratory drive and further worsen hypercapnia. Even careful oxygen replacement that is titrated to what is required to restore pO_2 to greater than 50 torr can cause respiratory arrest,[447] so oxygen replacement in patients with chronic lung disease and associated hypercarbia should be done in a facility where emergency intubation is available.

Renal bicarbonate excretion is a relatively slow process. As a result, correction of CO_2 narcosis by artificial respiration sometimes induces severe metabolic alkalosis if the CO_2 tension is returned quickly to normal in the face of a high serum bicarbonate level. Although metabolic alkalosis is usually asymptomatic, Rotheram and colleagues[448] reported five patients with pulmonary emphysema treated vigorously by artificial ventilation in whom metabolic alkalosis was associated with serious neurologic symptoms. These patients, after initially recovering from CO_2 narcosis, developed severe alkalosis with arterial blood pH values above 7.55–7.60 and again became obtunded. They developed multifocal myoclonus, had severe convulsions, and three died. Two patients regained consciousness after blood CO_2 levels were raised again by deliberately reducing the level of ventilation. We have observed a similar sequence of events in deeply comatose patients treated vigorously with artificial ventilation, but have found it difficult to conclude that alkalosis and not hypoxia, possibly from hypotension,[241] was at fault. What seems likely is that too sudden hypocapnia induces cerebral vasoconstriction, which more than counterbalances the beneficial effects to the brain of raising the blood oxygen tension. Rotheram and his colleagues recommended that the PCO_2 should be lowered gradually during treatment of respiratory acidosis to allow renal compensation to take place and prevent severe metabolic alkalosis. This is a reasonable approach so long as hypoxemia is prevented.

Hepatic Encephalopathy

Hepatic insufficiency can present in a wide range of ways, from slow insidious and fluctuating onset in a patient with cryptogenic liver disease, to coma in a patient with hepatic failure waiting for a liver transplant.[449,450]

Neurological morbidity in acute liver failure is associated with cerebral edema and intracranial hypertension,[451] though other complications such as seizures and ischemic and hemorrhagic strokes may contribute to the poor outcome.[449] The major site of pathology in hepatic encephalopathy appears to reside in astrocytes. In chronic liver disease, morphologic changes include an increase in large Alzheimer type-2 astrocytes.[452] The astrocytes exhibit an alteration in the expression of benzodiazepine receptors, glutamate transporters, and glial acidic fibrillary protein. In the more acute encephalopathy, or with deterioration of chronic encephalopathy, permeability of the blood–brain barrier increases without loss of tight junctions. The resultant cerebral edema, along with an increase in CBF, leads to intracranial hypertension.[453] All these pathologic processes are believed to be initiated by an interaction between gut-derived neurotoxins like ammonia, abnormal neurotransmission due to excess glutamine and GABA, and the inflammatory cascade.[454] The ammonia is metabolized by astrocytes to glutamine. The glutamine may be retained within the cell, leading to swelling. There is no consistent correlation between the level of ammonia and the patient's clinical symptoms, suggesting that there are other factors, including intercurrent infectious processes.[455] This hypothesis is further supported by studies showing improvement in transplant-free survival in acute liver failure patients by ameliorating the IL-17 production using N-acetylcysteine.[456] Oxidative stress may also contribute to worsening of hepatic encephalopathy.[452]

The clinical picture of hepatic encephalopathy is fairly consistent, but its onset often is difficult to define.[449] Mild hepatic encephalopathy may fluctuate markedly in severity,[457] and it is sometimes confused with psychiatric disturbances or acute alcoholism. Comatose patients in whom hepatic coma has developed rapidly often have motor signs (but not neuro-ophthalmologic changes) that may suggest structural disease of the brainstem. They are sometimes mistakenly believed to have subdural hematoma or basilar artery thrombosis. In anything short of preterminal hepatic coma, however, pupillary and caloric responses are normal, patients hyperventilate, and signs of rostral-caudal deterioration are absent, all of which are often abnormal in patients with subdural hematoma. Normal pupillary and caloric responses as well as fluctuating and inconstant quality motor signs are atypical for subtentorial structural disease.

The incipient mental symptoms usually consist of a quiet, apathetic delirium, which either persists for several days or rapidly evolves into profound coma. Less often, in perhaps 10–20% of cases, the earliest symptoms are of a boisterous delirium verging on mania, an onset suggesting rapidly progressive liver disease. The degree of impairment may fluctuate substantially from day to day, perhaps as a result of changes in diet, especially the amount of protein intake. One of our patients with chronic cirrhosis suffered two episodes of hepatic coma spaced 2 weeks apart. The first began with an agitated delirium, the second, with quiet obtundation. It was impossible to distinguish between the two attacks by biochemical changes or rate of evolution.

Respiratory changes are a hallmark of severe liver disease. Hyperventilation, as judged by low arterial PCO_2 and high pH levels, occurs at all depths of coma and usually becomes clinically obvious as patients become deeply comatose. This almost invariable hyperventilation is well-confirmed by our own series of 83 patients; all had plasma alkalosis and all but three had low PCO_2 values. These three exceptions had concomitant metabolic alkalosis of other causes, correction of which was followed by hyperventilation and respiratory alkalosis. Although some authors have reported instances of metabolic acidosis, particularly in terminal patients, in our experience it is likely that encephalopathy unaccompanied by either respiratory or metabolic alkalosis is not hepatic.

Moderately obtunded patients with hepatic encephalopathy typically have roving eye movements with easily elicited brisk and conjugate oculocephalic and oculovestibular responses; these findings are generally so striking that in an unresponsive patient they should suggest hepatic encephalopathy. If the patient is more awake, there may sometimes be nystagmus on lateral gaze. Tonic conjugate downward or downward and lateral ocular deviation has marked the onset of coma in several of our patients; we have once observed reversible, vertical skew deviation during an episode of hepatic coma. Focal neurologic signs are not rare. In one series of 34 cirrhotic patients with 38 episodes of hepatic encephalopathy, 8 demonstrated focal signs: 2 hemiplegia and 4 hemiparesis, 2 had agnosia, and 1 developed a lower limb monoplegia.[458] Other signs that have been described include disconjugate eye movements[459] and ocular bobbing.[460] Only one of our patients convulsed. Others have reported the seizure incidence to be between 2% and 33%. When seizures occur they may be related to alcohol withdrawal, cerebral edema, or hypoglycemia accompanying the liver failure.[461] Peripheral oculomotor paralyses are rare in hepatic coma unless patients have concomitant Wernicke's disease or cerebral edema has caused transtentorial herniation. The pupils are usually small but react to light. Asterixis[14] or mini-asterixis[462] (see page 192) is characteristic and frequently involves the muscles of the feet, tongue, and jaw, as well as the hands. Patients with mild to moderate encephalopathy are usually found to have bilateral *gegenhalten*. Decorticate and decerebrate posturing responses, muscle spasticity, and bilateral extensor plantar responses frequently accompany deeper coma. See Patient Vignette 5.19.

Patient Vignette 5.19

A 76-year-old woman was found in her apartment in a shelter for homeless women, smeared with feces and unable to answer questions coherently. She was brought to a local hospital emergency department, where she was assumed to be indigent and demented and was treated with intravenous fluids for dehydration. Shortly after arrival she had a tonic-clonic grand mal seizure, and neurology was called to consult.

On examination, she was able to give her name but not the date, and she did not know where she was. She was confused and perseverated in her answers. She was unable to follow directions to test eye movements, but had brisk oculocephalic responses. She had atrophy of the right side of her tongue as well as in the muscles of her right upper extremity. There was generally increased muscle tone, and her toes were upgoing. Computed tomography (CT) and later magnetic resonance imaging (MRI) scan of the brain were unrevealing.

When her medical records were accessed, it was found that she was living in the shelter for homeless women because she had been its executive director and generally had a high level of cognitive function in the past. She had a history of poliomyelitis as a child causing her right tongue and upper extremity muscle atrophy, and a long-standing tonic-clonic seizure disorder which was being treated with valproic acid, as documented in the notes by her neurologist. While her hepatic function had been documented as normal in the past, her aspartate amino-transferase (AST) and alanine amino-transferase (ALT) on admission were now elevated to several times the normal range. Valproic acid was replaced with levetiracetam, and the liver function returned to the normal range, as did her cognitive function.

Comment

Valproic acid is known to cause hepatotoxicity in elderly individuals. However, she had been on it for many years, with no previous problems. The onset of the encephalopathy was sufficiently insidious that the patient's co-workers at the shelter for homeless women were unaware of a problem until she did not show up for work, which was very unusual for her, at which point they called the police to enter her apartment.

Acute liver failure causes brain edema with resultant intracranial hypertension.[463] About 30% of patients with acute liver failure succumb when ICPs increase to levels that impair CBF, causing brain infarction, increased edema, and eventual transtentorial herniation. Chronic liver failure, usually from cirrhosis or after portocaval shunting, is characterized only by defects in memory and attention with increased reaction time and poor concentration. One striking and frustrating problem in liver failure is that the encephalopathy may fluctuate widely without obvious cause. More severe forms can lead to delirium, stupor, and coma. The most severe forms often occur in a cirrhotic patient with mild, chronic hepatic encephalopathy who develops an infection, has gastrointestinal bleeding, or takes in an excessive amount of protein (so-called *meat intoxication*).[464] Cerebral dysfunction occurs either when liver function fails or when the liver is bypassed so that the portal circulation shunts intestinal venous drainage directly into the systemic circulation.

Hepatic coma is rarely a difficult diagnosis to make in patients who suffer from severe chronic liver disease and gradually lose consciousness displaying the obvious stigmata of jaundice, spider angiomata, fetor hepaticus, and enlarged livers and spleens. The diagnosis can be more difficult in patients whose coma is precipitated by an exogenous factor and who have either mild unsuspected liver disease or portal-systemic shunts. In this situation, hepatic coma can be suspected by finding clinical evidence of metabolic encephalopathy combined with respiratory alkalosis and brisk oculocephalic reflexes. The diagnosis is strengthened by identifying a portal-systemic shunt, plus an elevated serum ammonia level. The blood sugar should be measured in patients with severe liver disease since diminished liver glycogen stores may induce hypoglycemia and complicate hepatic coma. When the diagnosis remains doubtful, analysis of spinal fluid may reveal markedly elevated levels of either glutamine or alpha-ketoglutaramate (α-KGM). Of the two, α-KGM levels give almost no false positives as well as the strongest discrimination between patients with and without brain involvement.[465] The spinal fluid in hepatic encephalopathy is usually clear and free of cells and has a normal protein content. In severe cases, the opening pressure may be elevated, sometimes to very high levels. It is rare to detect bilirubin in the CSF unless patients have serum bilirubin levels of at least 4–6 mg/dL and chronic parenchymal liver failure as well. The EEG undergoes progressive slowing in hepatic coma, with slow activity beginning symmetrically in the frontal leads and spreading posteriorly as unconsciousness deepens. The changes are characteristic but not specific; they thus help in identifying a diffuse abnormality but do not necessarily diagnose hepatic failure. Nonspecific EEG findings correlate with clinical grading in adults[466] and spectral power changes with in outcomes in pediatric patients with acute liver failure.[467]

CT or MRI is usually only helpful in ruling out structural disease such as cerebral hematomas, although in advanced stages there may be substantial cerebral edema. In cases of severely elevated ICP, compromise of CBF may even result in global cerebral infarction. MRS identifies a lowered myoinositol and choline with increased glutamine levels in the basal ganglia of patients in early stages of hepatic encephalopathy when compared with cirrhotic controls[468] (Figure 5.8). The basal ganglia may be hyperintense on the T1-weighted image, believed to be a result of manganese deposits. Mild cerebral atrophy is frequently present. PET scanning demonstrates hypometabolism in frontal and parietal lobes, sometimes with increased uptake in the infra- and medial temporal regions, cerebellum, and posterior thalamus.[464] Fluorodeoxyglucose PET studies of the brain in cirrhotic patients shows a relative decrease of glucose utilization in the cingulate gyrus, the medial and lateral frontal regions, and the parieto-occipital cortex, with a relative increase in the basal ganglia, hippocampus, and cerebellum.[469]

Renal Failure

Renal failure causes uremic encephalopathy. The treatment of uremia, in turn, potentially causes two additional disorders of cerebral function: the dialysis dysequilibrium syndrome and cognitive issues that may accompany renal transplantation. Confusion, delirium, stupor, and sometimes coma can occur with each of these conditions.

UREMIC ENCEPHALOPATHY

Before the widespread use of dialysis and renal transplantation, the uremic syndrome was common in North America and Western Europe.[470] Today, the early correction of biochemical abnormalities in patients with known acute or chronic renal disease often prevents the development of cerebral symptoms. As a result, the physician more often encounters uremic encephalopathy as a problem of differential diagnosis in patients with a systemic disease causing multiorgan failure such as a collagen vascular disorder, malignant hypertension, the ingestion of a toxin, bacteremia, or disseminated anoxia-ischemia. Most of these primary disorders themselves produce abnormalities of brain function, adding to the complexities of diagnosis.

Despite extensive investigations, the precise cause of the brain dysfunction in uremia eludes identification. However, certain notable associations exist. Once azotemia develops, the uremic syndrome correlates only in a general way with biochemical changes in the blood. As with other metabolic encephalopathies, the more rapid the development of the toxic state, the less disturbed is the systemic chemical equilibrium. The level of BUN associated with uremic encephalopathy can vary widely. Urea itself cannot be the toxin, as urea infusions do not reproduce uremic symptoms and hemodialysis reverses the syndrome even when urea is added to the dialyzing bath so as not to lower the blood level. Although it is rare to see uremic encephalopathy with a creatine lower than 7.0, levels of creatinine and other serum biochemical or electrolyte abnormalities do not correlate with the neurologic state. Serum sodium or potassium levels can be abnormally low or high in uremia, depending on its duration and treatment, but symptoms associated with these electrolyte changes are distinct from the typical panorama of uremic encephalopathy. Systemic acidosis is not the cause; the systemic acidosis does not involve the CNS, and treatment of the reduced blood pH has no effect on uremic cerebral symptoms.

Morphologically, the brains of patients dying of uremia show no consistent abnormality. Uremia uncomplicated by hypertensive encephalopathy does not cause cerebral edema. The cerebral oxygen consumption declines in uremic stupor, just as it does in most other metabolic encephalopathies, although perhaps not as much as might be expected from the degree of impaired alertness. Levels of cerebral high-energy phosphates remain high during experimental uremia, while rates of glycolysis and energy utilization are reduced below normal. Uremic brains show a decrease in sodium and potassium flux along with depressed sodium-stimulated, potassium-dependent ATPase activity. However, all the preceding changes appear to be effects rather than causes of the disorder.

Calcium concentration in the brain is elevated in uremia,[471] and in humans with uremia both cognitive function and the EEG may be improved by parathyroidectomy,[472] suggesting that calcium plays a role in the encephalopathy. In addition, 1-guanidino compounds are elevated in uremia, and this may affect the release of GABA.[473] In uremic experimental animals, tryptophan is diminished both in plasma and brain, but levels of its metabolic product, 3-hydroxykinurine, a known

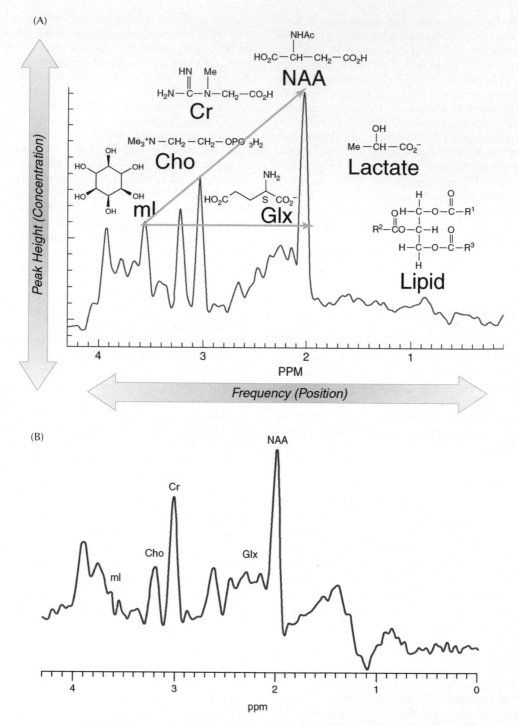

Figure 5.8 (A) Representative magnetic resonance spectrum of the human brain in vivo. Each peek is labeled with the molecule and its structure. The absorption spectra of lipid and lactate are not observed in a normal brain. The diagonal arrow represents Hunter's angle, which is drawn starting from myoinositol to *N*-acetylaspartate. In a normal spectrum, Hunter's angle is 45 degrees and is formed by the peaks of myoinositol, creatinine, choline, and *N*-acetylaspartate. (B) Magnetic resonance spectroscopy in a patient with chronic hepatic encephalopathy, demonstrating the three changes characteristic of hepatic encephalopathy: decreased myoinositol, increased glutamate-glutamine, and decreased choline. After transplant and metabolic changes, the patient returned to normal.

From Lin et al.,[474] with permission.

neurotoxin, are elevated in the brain, particularly in the striatum and the medulla.[475] Also in uremic animals, upregulation of the superoxide-producing enzyme nicotinamide adenine dinucleotide phosphate oxidase and downregulation of supraoxide dismutase cause oxidative stress in the brain via the nitration of brain proteins and the oxidation of myelin. Oxidative stress is also caused during dialysis treatment by interaction of the patient's blood with both the dialysis membrane and dialysate impurities.[476] Turnover of dopamine in the striatum, mesencephalon, and hypothalamus is decreased in uremic animals, whereas turnover of norepinephrine and 5-hydroxytriptomine is unchanged. Whether suppression of central dopamine turnover contributes to motor impairment in uremic animals is not clear.[477]

The clinical picture of uremic encephalopathy is nonspecific in most instances, although the characteristic combination of dulled consciousness, hyperpnea, and motor hyperactivity should immediately give high suspicion to the diagnosis. Untreated patients with uremic encephalopathy have metabolic acidosis, generally with respiratory compensation. Like many other metabolic encephalopathies, uremia, particularly when it develops rapidly, can produce a florid delirium marked by noisy agitation, delusions, and hallucinations. More often, however, progressive apathetic, dull, quiet confusion with inappropriate behavior blends slowly into stupor or coma accompanied by characteristic respiratory changes, focal neurologic signs, tremor, asterixis, muscle paratonia, and convulsions or, more rarely, nonconvulsive SE.[478] In uremic patients, both generalized convulsions and nonconvulsive SE may be caused by antibiotics, particularly cephalosporins.[479] Untreated patients with uremic encephalopathy all have serum acidosis. Pupillary and oculomotor functions are seldom disturbed in uremia, certainly not in any diagnostic way. On the other hand, motor changes are rarely absent. Patients with chronic renal disease are weak and unsteady in their movements. As uremia evolves, many of them develop diffuse tremulousness, intense asterixis, and, often, so much multifocal myoclonus that the muscles can appear to fasciculate. Action myoclonus has also been reported.[480,481] Tetany is frequent. Stretch reflex asymmetries are common, as are focal neurologic weaknesses; 10 of our 45 patients

with uremia had a hemiparesis that cleared rapidly after hemodialysis or shifted from side to side during the course of the illness.

Laboratory determinations tell one only that patients have uremia, but do not delineate this as the cause of coma. Renal failure is accompanied by complex biochemical, osmotic, and vascular abnormalities, and the degree of azotemia varies widely in patients with equally serious symptoms. One of our patients, a child with nephritis, had severe delirium proceeding to stupor despite a BUN of only 48 mg/dL. Other patients were free of cerebral symptoms with BUN values higher than 200 mg/dL. Uremia also causes aseptic meningitis accompanied by stiff neck, with as many as 250 lymphocytes and polymorphonuclear leukocytes/mm^3 in the CSF. The spinal fluid protein often rises as high as 100 mg/dL, and the CSF pressure can be abnormally elevated to more than 160–180 mm in some patients. EEG slowing correlates with increasing degrees of azotemia, but many patients with slow recordings have little or no accompanying mental changes.[482] The electrophysiologic changes are nonspecific and of no help in establishing the diagnosis.

In differential diagnosis, uremia must be distinguished from other causes of acute metabolic acidosis, from acute water intoxication, and from hypertensive encephalopathy. Penicillin and its analogs can be a diagnostic problem when given to uremic patients as these drugs can cause delirium, asterixis, myoclonus, convulsions, and nonconvulsive SE.[479] Laboratory studies distinguish uremia from other causes of metabolic acidosis causing the triad of clouded consciousness, hyperpnea, and a low serum bicarbonate (uremia, diabetes, lactic acidosis, ingestion of exogenous poisons), but only uremia is likely to cause multifocal myoclonus, tetany, and generalized convulsions, and the others do not cause azotemia during their early stages.

Hyponatremia is common in uremia and can be difficult to dissociate from the underlying uremia as a cause of symptoms. Patients with azotemia are nearly always thirsty, and they have multiple electrolyte abnormalities. Excessive water ingestion, inappropriate fluid therapy, and hemodialysis all potentially reduce the serum osmolarity in uremia and thereby risk inducing or accentuating delirium and convulsions. The presence of water intoxication is confirmed by measuring a low serum osmolarity (less than 260 mOsm/L), but the disorder can be suspected when the serum sodium concentration falls below 120 mEq/L. Interestingly, rapid correction of hyponatremia does not seem to be associated with pontine myelinolysis when it occurs in uremic patients. The osmotic pressure of urea in the brain that is eliminated more slowly than in the blood appears to protect the brain against the sudden shifts in brain osmolality, although such shifts may emerge during treatment unless special precautions are taken (see later discussion).[483] Patients with uremia are often deficient in thiamine, which may cause neurologic manifestations that mimic uremia.[484]

It may be difficult to separate the symptoms of uremia from those of hypertensive encephalopathy if both azotemia and advanced hypertension plague the same patient. Each condition can cause seizures, focal neurologic signs, increased ICP, and delirium or stupor. The MRI of typical posterior leukoencephalopathy establishes the diagnosis of hypertensive encephalopathy.

The treatment of uremia by hemodialysis sometimes adds to the neurologic complexity of the syndrome. Neurologic recovery does not always immediately follow effective dialysis, and patients often continue temporarily in coma or stupor. One of our own patients remained comatose for 5 days after his blood nitrogen and electrolytes returned to normal. Such a delayed recovery did not imply permanent brain damage, as this man, like others with similar but less protracted delays, enjoyed normal neurologic function on chronic hemodialysis.

DIALYSIS DYSEQUILIBRIUM SYNDROME

Some patients undergoing dialysis, particularly during the first treatment, develop headache, nausea, muscle weakness, cramps, and fatigue. At one time, occasional patients had more serious symptoms caused by a sudden osmolar gradient shifting of water into the brain, including asterixis, myoclonus, delirium, convulsions, stupor, coma, and very rarely death,[485] but these are now prevented by slower dialysis and the addition of osmotically active solutes such as urea, glycerol, mannitol, or sodium to the dialysate.[473]

An occasional patient will develop a subdural hematoma, probably resulting from a combination of anticoagulants used for dialysis and the coagulopathy that often accompanies uremia. Wernicke's encephalopathy with its attendant confusional state (see page 211) has developed in patients receiving chronic dialysis who were not being given vitamin supplements.[484] At one time, patients undergoing long-term renal dialysis were found to experience *dialysis dementia*. This was found to be due to elevated levels of aluminum in the dialysate, and when this was reduced, it largely disappeared.[486]

All agree on the general mechanism of the dialysis dysequilibrium syndrome, although not on the details.[487] The blood–brain barrier is only slowly permeable to urea as well as to a number of other biologic molecules, including electrolytes and idiogenic osmols[488] (molecules, e.g., organic acids, amino acids, that form during pathologic processes and increase tissue osmolality) that are found in the brain during serum hyperosmolarity. The brain and blood are in osmotic equilibrium in steady states such as uremia; electrolytes and other osmols are adjusted so that brain concentrations of many biologically active substances (e.g., H^+, Na^+, Cl^-) remain more normal than those in blood. A rapid lowering of the blood urea by hemodialysis is not paralleled by equally rapid reductions in brain osmols. As a result, during dialysis, the brain becomes hyperosmolar relative to blood and probably loses sodium, the result being that water shifts from plasma to brain, potentially resulting in water intoxication. Concurrently, rapid correction of blood metabolic acidosis can induce brain tissue acidosis because the increased PCO_2 in the blood rapidly diffuses into the brain, whereas the bicarbonate moves much more slowly into the brain. Symptoms of water intoxication can be prevented by slower dialysis and by adding agents to maintain blood osmolarity.

In a small study of patients with ICP monitoring who underwent hemodialysis, an increase in ICP was seen several hours after the start of dialysis.[489] It is not clear whether, for patients at risk early after brain injury, continuous veno-venous hemofiltration (CVVH) is advantageous over regular hemodialysis.[490,491]

RENAL TRANSPLANTATION

Immunosuppression accompanying renal transplant can lead to a variety of neurologic disorders.[482,492] Cyclosporin and taxolimus can cause posterior leukoencephalopathy and the anti-CD3 murine monoclonal antibody, muromonab-CD3, can be neurotoxic, causing aseptic meningitis with headache and blurred vision and sometimes encephalopathy and seizures.[492,493] MRI shows patchy enhancement in the corticomedullary junction, indicating blood–brain barrier dysfunction. The pathogenesis of the encephalopathy is believed to be cerebral edema from a capillary leak syndrome.[494]

Renal transplant patients also are at risk for a variety of opportunistic infections and tumors similar to other immune-suppressed patients, such as those with HIV infection. These include lymphomas, which may occur primarily in the CNS, and lead to stupor or coma. Opportunistic infections include fungi, such as *Aspergillus*, *Cryptococcus*, or *Candida*, and viruses, including cytomegalovirus, varicella-zoster, papova virus (JC virus), or progressive multifocal leukoencephalopathy. On rare occasions, the transplanted kidney carries a virus and may cause encephalitis within a few days of the transplant.[192]

Pancreatic Encephalopathy

Failure of either the exocrine or endocrine pancreas can cause stupor or coma. Failure of the endocrine pancreas (diabetes) is discussed in the section on disorders of the internal milieu: hyperglycemia and hyperosmolar states. Failure of the exocrine pancreas causes pancreatic encephalopathy, a rare complication of acute or chronic pancreatitis. Chronic relapsing pancreatitis may cause episodic stupor or coma.[495] Estrada and associates reported that 6 of 17 non-alcoholic patients with acute pancreatitis, whom they followed prospectively, developed encephalopathy.[496] The pathogenesis of pancreatic encephalopathy is not known. Postmortem evidence of patchy demyelination of white matter in the brain has led to the suggestion that enzymes liberated from the damaged pancreas are responsible for the encephalopathy.[496] Other hypotheses include

coexistent viral pancreatitis and encephalitis, disseminated intravascular coagulation complicating pancreatitis, and fat embolism. In one patient with relapsing pancreatitis and episodic coma, there were marked increases in CSF and plasma citrulline and arginine levels, and moderate increases of other amino acids.[495] Pathologically, autopsies have revealed cerebral edema, patchy demyelination, occasional perivascular hemorrhages, and, at times, plugging of small vessels with fat or fibrin thrombi.[497] Biochemical complications of acute pancreatitis also may cause encephalopathy. These include cerebral ischemia secondary to hypotension, hyperosmolality, hypocalcemia,[498] and diabetic acidosis.

Pancreatic encephalopathy usually begins between the second and fifth day after the onset of pancreatitis. The clinical features include an acute agitated delirium with hallucinations, focal or generalized convulsions, and often signs of bilateral corticospinal tract dysfunction. The mental status may wax and wane, and patients often become stuporous or comatose. The CSF is usually normal or occasionally has a slightly elevated protein concentration. The CSF lipase level is elevated.[496] The EEG is always abnormal with diffuse or multifocal slow activity. The diagnosis usually suggests itself when, after several days of abdominal pain, the patient develops acute encephalopathy. The MRI may be normal[499] or show diffuse white matter lesions.[497] The differential diagnosis should include other factors complicating pancreatitis listed above, including, of course, mumps that can cause both pancreatitis and encephalopathy. CSF lipase is elevated in pancreatic encephalopathy. See Patient Vignette 5.17.

Patient Vignette 5.20

A 72-year-old man with no significant past medical history presented to the hospital with abdominal pain and was diagnosed with acute pancreatitis. The next day the patient was noted to be confused with waxing and waning mental status changes, which became an acute agitated delirium on the fifth day requiring four-point restraints. Electroencephalogram (EEG) done at the time showed a diffuse theta rhythm. Initial computed tomography (CT) and magnetic resonance imaging (MRI) studies were unrevealing, and the patient remained mute in an awake state for several days, following which he recovered to a confused state with occasional lucid periods. Neurologic examination was notable for preserved arousal and confabulation, decreased spontaneous movements of the lower extremities, and increased muscle tone. Diffuse hyperreflexia and bilateral extensor plantar response were noted. Repeat MRI revealed diffuse white matter abnormalities consistent with demyelination.

Systemic Septic Encephalopathy

During inflammatory illness, there are a number of adaptive responses involving the CNS, such as fever, which increased body temperature a few degrees in response to a prostaglandin E2 (PGE2) stimulus from inflammatory cells. PGE2 crosses the blood–brain barrier into the hypothalamus, where it acts on preoptic neurons that increase body temperature. At the same time, there are changes in behavior which have been termed the "sickness syndrome."[314] Animals show lower pain thresholds and become sleepy and anorexic. The syndrome is in part due to the effects of prostaglandins, but may also involve other mediators, including lipid inflammatory mediators and cytokines, acting on the CNS.

Underlying pathomechanisms that are invoked include changes in blood–brain barrier permeability,[500] altered cerebral microcirculation,[501] mitochondrial and vascular endothelial dysfunction,[502] endotoxins and oxidative stress,[503] direct neuronal damage, increased level of cytokines and proinflammatory factors,[504] and neurotransmitter disturbances, and changes in amino acid levels.[505]

During more severe infectious illness, many patients show even more severe lethargy and may even become stuporous or comatose. Of course, infectious illnesses can affect the brain in many ways, including directly via meningitis or encephalitis; by causing failure of other organ systems such as the lungs, kidneys, or liver (see preceding discussion); or, in the case of bacteremia, by causing septic shock, in which blood pressure may fall below the threshold needed to maintain normal cerebral function.

In addition, such patients often have other reasons for delirium, including medications, sleep deprivation, and living in a hospital environment with few if any circadian clues. Under such circumstances, in a patient who is severely ill with an infectious process, it may be difficult to sort out whether elements of the cognitive impairment are due to a direct effect on the brain, septic shock, or many other potential complications of the infection.

In favor of the concept of the sickness syndrome due to systemic inflammation causing cerebral impairment is the common presentation to neurologists of patients who are much less severely ill, often with infection confined to a limited area of the body, normal blood pressure, are not taking drugs that could affect the sensorium, do not have seizure activity on EEG, and who nevertheless show lethargy, stupor, or coma. One feature of this group is that they frequently have hyperventilation with a respiratory alkalosis.[506] While they rarely have other motor phenomena (such as asterixis or motor restlessness), they do generally have diffuse increase in muscle tone (*gegenhalten*).

In our experience, in a patient who has hyperventilation and impaired consciousness with no other obvious metabolic cause, it is worthwhile to mount a search for an infectious process. Often when an innocuous appearing urinary tract infection or leg ulcer is treated, the patient also wakes up.

Autoimmune Disorders: Specific Antibodies

The phenomenon of experimental allergic encephalomyelitis, caused by inoculating an animal with CNS myelin, has long led to the suspicion that other central demyelinating disorders, such as acute disseminated encephalomyelitis or multiple sclerosis have an autoimmune origin. Surprisingly, however, to this day no specific causative autoantibody has been demonstrated in either of these disorders.

By contrast, specific autoantibodies have been discovered in a variety of paraneoplastic neurological disorders. For example, patients with myasthenia gravis have been found to have antibodies against acetylcholine nicotinic receptors in many cases; others have additional antibodies against other muscle components, such as muscle-specific kinase (MuSK).[507] Posner and colleagues identified a series of autoantibodies (anti-Hu, anti-Yo, etc.), which were named for the immunohistochemical and Western blot staining pattern of the serum of the index patient (whose initials were used to name the antibody pattern) when used to stain human brain tissue. The first of these, anti-Hu, was found associated with a sensory neuronopathy in patients with small-cell cancer of the lung. The antibody was found to stain the nuclei of neurons and was found within the nuclei of neurons of dorsal root ganglia in a postmortem analysis of one case. The antibody stained a protein band of 35-38 kD molecular weight in Western blots from both normal brain and the patient's tumor.[508] Anti-Yo antibodies were found in the sera of patients with paraneoplastic cerebellar degeneration, and stained Purkinje cells as well as 34 and 62 kD Purkinje cell proteins.[509]

Later it was recognized that specific antibody types could be elicited from a variety of tumors (e.g., both lung and breast tumors may have associated cerebellar degeneration), and that the clinical phenotypes of the patients with specific paraneoplastic antibodies could vary considerably (e.g., anti-Hu was associated with both sensory neuronopathy and with a much more aggressive generalized encephalomyelitis). To better understand this diversity, Darnell and colleagues used the high-affinity antibodies from some patients with these syndromes to clone and characterize a series of onconeural antigens (i.e., antigens shared between neurons and tumors that the paraneoplastic antibodies bound).[510] They found that the anti-Hu antibodies bound to neuron-specific ribonuclear proteins and that Nova antibodies, which cause paraneoplastic opsoclonus myoclonus, bind to other neuronal ribonuclear proteins. By contrast, anti-Yo antibodies bound to three cerebellar degeneration–related (cdr) proteins, of which cdr2 turned out to be the protein also made in tumors of patients with cerebellar degeneration. Interfering with the role of cdr2, or of recoverin, the target of the paraneoplastic antibody in cancer-associated retinopathy, can lead to apoptosis.

Other anti-tumor antibodies have turned out to target the receptors and ion channels that neurons use to generate their membrane potentials and to communicate. "Limbic encephalitis" was first described by Brierley and colleagues in 1960 as an encephalitis with elevated CSF white blood cells and protein in patients with a memory disorder and postmortem evidence of encephalitis with a predilection for the medial temporal lobes.[511] The disorder was distinguished from herpes simplex encephalitis in that it occurred over several months and there was no pathological evidence of viral inclusions.[512] Others found a variety of behavioral disorders, including seizures, especially of the medial temporal lobe type.[513] Over the years, limbic encephalitis has been associated with antibodies against various molecules involved in neural transmission, including glutamate alpha-amino-3-hydroxy-5-methyl-4-isoxazolepropionic acid (AMPA) or NMDA receptors, voltage-gated potassium channels (including antibodies against LGI1 and Caspr2), and glutamic acid decarboxylase 65.[514–516] Depending on the antibody involved, limbic encephalitis may not be associated with an underlying cancer, and the phenotype can involve other features ranging from peripheral nerve hypersensitivity to dysautonomia. Recently a number of autoimmune encephalitides have been identified and better characterized, both based on the associated antibody pattern as well as the clinical spectrum.[517]

Among the neuronal autoantibody disorders, the ones most likely to come into the differential diagnosis in a patient with an acute or subacute disorder of consciousness would be limbic encephalitis or the more diffuse paraneoplastic encephalitis. Limbic encephalitis is now most often considered in patients who have behavioral disturbances, with or without seizures, and MRI evidence of high T2 signal in the medial temporal lobe. If the onset is rapid, the main concern is usually for herpes simplex encephalitis. As the CSF picture does not distinguish the two entities, such patients are usually treated with acyclovir until the CSF PCR result is available. If the result is negative, the patient is usually taken off acyclovir, although there is a low but real percentage of false-negative herpes simplex PCR (<5%), so that, if the clinical suspicion for herpes is high (e.g., rapid onset and fever), the patient should be given the complete course of acyclovir.

The treatment of an autoantibody encephalitis is usually two-fold. First, it is necessary to reduce the level of autoantibody, either by intravenous immune globulin infusion or by plasmapheresis. Patients in whom the syndrome relapses later may benefit from longer term treatment with monoclonal antibodies against B lymphocytes, such as rituximab. Second, it is usually necessary to mount a search for a potential underlying cancer. The cancer may be occult, as the antibodies may be holding the tumor in check. However, if the antibodies are against an antigen made by the tumor, long-term relief is available only if the tumor can be extirpated. On the other hand, in patients with anti-tumor antibodies, removing the tumor may not improve the condition of the patient if the neurological deficits are due to CNS cellular death that precedes the treatment.

PART 9: DISORDERS OF EXOGENOUS TOXINS

Neurons in the brain communicate via neurotransmitters. Not surprisingly, most of the psychotropic drugs that people have discovered over the millennia, both for recreation and for treating pain, seizures, stress, anxiety, sleeplessness, depression, psychosis, and other common human ills that originate in the brain, are based on enhancing or inhibiting the actions of various neurotransmitters.

Many drugs in common use can cause delirium, stupor, or coma when taken in large amounts (Box 5.3).

A few drugs, such as salicylates and acetaminophen, can be tested at the bedside.[518] Combined high-performance liquid chromatography (HPLC)-immunoenzymatic screening is available in some emergency departments to detect amphetamines, barbiturates, benzodiazepines, cocaine, opioids, and phencyclidine and other drugs in 20–45 minutes.[519] Others can be inferred from the physical examination (e.g., pupil size and response to antidotes) or rapidly procured laboratory tests. Examples include an anion gap, unidentifiable osmoles, or an oxygen saturation gap[520] (Table 5.3). Measurement of the anion gap helps in establishing a diagnosis. An increased anion gap is found in toxic ingestion of drugs such as ethylene glycol, propylene glycol, methanol, paraldehyde, and salicylates. A decreased anion gap may be found after ingestion of lithium, bromides, or iodides.[520] An increased osmol gap can be found with ethanol and ethylene ingestion. The so-called oxygen saturation gap exists when there is more than a 5% difference between calculated saturation, as measured from arterial blood and that measured by an oximeter. If the oximeter reading is too high after carbon monoxide intoxication, there may be severe methemoglobinemia. In addition, if the venous blood has a high oxygen content with the appearance of arterial blood, one should consider cyanide or hydrogen sulfide poisoning.[520]

However, in many instances, an accurate immediate diagnosis leans heavily on the physical findings and clinical deduction (Box 5.4). Laboratory confirmation of the clinical diagnosis is desirable, but the delay in conducting the tests often means that the information becomes available too late to be useful in guiding treatment. Furthermore, blood levels of sedatives or alcohol sometimes provide a poor guide to the depth or anticipated duration of coma. Several reasons account for the potential discrepancy. Persons who chronically take these drugs develop a tolerance to their effects and require larger doses with resulting higher blood levels to produce coma. Pharmacologic interaction between drug mixtures and the inability to anticipate the effects of still unabsorbed material in the gut further interfere with making a correlation (Box 5.4).

Sedatives such as benzodiazepines, neuroleptics, antihistamines, alcohol, and sedating antidepressants, as well as older drugs such as meprobamate and bromides, can all produce coma if enough is taken. The mechanism of action of each drug depends partly on its structure and partly on the dose. Many of the sedative drugs cause delirium or coma by increasing GABAergic input to the ascending arousal system, thus extinguishing wakefulness.[520,521] Antidepressant drugs interfere with the reuptake of neurotransmitters, including serotonin and norepinephrine, and neuroleptics block dopamine receptors, but the more sedating ones also have antihistamine and anticholinergic effects. These effects may produce autonomic dysfunction, and, in fact, the most dangerous effect of overdose with tricyclic antidepressants is their cardiotoxicity.

Box 5.3 Drugs Commonly Causing Delirium, Stupor, or Coma

Medicinal agents
  Antihistamines
  Anticholinergics (muscarinic)
Psychotropic agents
  Tricyclic antidepressants
  Selective serotonin or norepinephrine reuptake inhibitors
  Lithium
  Phenothiazines
Atypical antipsychotics
Sedative/hypnotic drugs
  Benzodiazepines
  "Nonbenzodiazepines"
  Barbiturates
Chloral hydrate
  Trazadone
Analgesics
Opioids
  Acetaminophen
Aspirin
Anticonvulsants
Phenytoin
Barbiturates
Valproic acid
Carbamazepine/oxcarbazepine
Levetiracctam

Nonmedicinal agents

Alcohols
  Alcohol
  Ethylene glycol/propylene glycol
  Methanol
Illicit drugs
  Cocaine
  Methamphetamine
  Gamma-hydroxybutyrate
  Methylenedioxymethamphetamine (MDMA)
  Phencyclidine
  Ketamine
  Flunitrazepam (Rohypnol)

The list of such drugs is legion; also, the agents favored by drug abusers change from time to time and differ in different geographic areas. Agents causing delirium or coma may include (1) medicinal agents prescribed but taken in overdose; (2) medicinal agents procured illicitly (e.g., opioids); (3) agents substituted for alcohol, such as ethylene glycol and methanol; and (4) illicit drugs (e.g., "party" or "club" drugs).[522] If it is known what agents the patient has taken, there is not much of a diagnostic problem. However, patients who are stuporous but arousable may deny drug ingestion, and, if comatose, no history may be available at all.

Table 5.3 Clues to Specific Drugs Frequently Causing Delirium, Stupor, or Coma

Drug	Chemical diagnosis	Behavior	Physical signs
Amphetamine	Blood or urine	Hypertension; aggressive, sometimes paranoid, repetitive behavior progressing into agitated paranoid delirium; auditory and visual hallucinations	Hyperthermia, hypertension, tachycardia, arrhythmia; pupils dilated; tremor, dystonia, occasionally convulsions
Cocaine	None available	Similar to above but more euphoric, less paranoid	Variable
Club drugs such as Methylenedioxy-methamphetamine (MDMA), phencyclidine	Blood or urine	Confused, disoriented, perceptual distortions, distractible, withdrawn or eruptive; can lead to accidents or violence	See text
Atropine-scopolamine	None available	Delirium; often agitated; responding to visual hallucinations; drowsiness; rarely coma	Fever, flushed face; dilated pupils; sinus or supraventricular tachycardia; hot dry skin
Tricyclic antidepressants	Blood or urine	Drowsiness; delirium; agitation; rarely coma	Fever; supraventricular tachycardia; conduction defects; ventricular tachycardia or fibrillation; hypotension; dystonia
Phenothiazines	Blood	Somnolence; coma rare	Arrhythmias, hypotension, dystonia
Lithium	Blood	Lethargic confusion, mute state, eventually coma. Multifocal seizures can occur. Onset can be delayed by hours or days after overdose	Appearance of distraction; roving conjugate eye movement; pupils intact; paratonic resistance; tremors, akathisia
Benzodiazepines	Blood or urine	Stupor, rarely unarousable	Minimal cardiovascular or respiratory depression
Methaqualone *(no longer available in US)*	Blood or urine	Hallucinations and agitation blend into depressant drug coma	Mild: resembles barbiturate intoxication. Severe: increased tendon reflexes, myoclonus, dystonia, convulsions. Tachycardia and heart failure
Barbiturates	Blood or urine	Stupor or coma	Hypothermia; skin cool and dry; pupils reactive; doll's eyes absent; hyporeflexia; flaccid hypotension; apnea
Alcohol	Blood or breath	Dysarthria, ataxia, stupor. Rapidly changing level of alertness with stimulation	With stupor: hypothermia, skin cold and moist; pupils reactive, midposition to wide; tachycardia
Opioids/opiates	Blood or urine	Stupor or coma	Hypothermia; skin cool and moist; pupils symmetrically pinpoint reactive; bradycardia, hypotension; hypoventilation; pulmonary edema

Box 5.4 Laboratory Clues to Specific Toxins

Anion gap
  Increased
    Ethylene glycol
    Methanol
    Paraldehyde
    Salicylate
    Acetaminophen
    Cocaine
  Decreased
    Bromides
    Lithium
    Iodide
Osmolal gap
  Increased
    Ethanol
    Ethylene glycol
    Propylene glycol
O_2 saturated gap
  Increased
    Carbon monoxide
    Methemoglobin
    Cyanide
    Hydrogen sulfate

Modified from Fabbri et al.[519] and Mokhlesi and or-bridge,[520] with permission.

Sedative/Hypnotic Drugs and Anesthetics (GABA$_A$ Receptor Enhancers)

The range of drugs that rely on enhancing transmission of GABA$_A$ receptors is very large. In part, this reflects the ubiquity of the GABA$_A$ receptor as an inhibitory receptor found on almost all neurons, and, in part, the biochemistry of the receptor itself. GABA$_A$ receptors are composed of five subunits that form a ligand-gated chloride channel in their center. There are generally two alpha (α) subunits, drawn from six different possibilities (α1 through α6), two beta (β) subunits drawn from among three types (β1 to β3), and a fifth subunit which may be a gamma (γ; from γ1 to γ3) or a delta (δ), or one of several other alternatives.[523] Altogether, there are at least

17 possible subunits that can participate in a GABA$_A$ receptor, and the properties of the ion channel, its disposition on the cell surface, and what drugs affect the channel vary with the subunit composition.

GABA$_A$–enhancing drugs are among the oldest known, as ethanol, prized since antiquity for both its euphoric and medicinal sedative (and antiseptic) qualities acts mainly by this mechanism. So, too, do older sedative drugs such as chloral hydrate and barbiturates. More recently developed sedative-hypnotic drugs such as benzodiazepines and nonbenzodiazepines (drugs that affect the same site on the GABA$_A$ receptor as benzodiazepines, but do not have the same structure, such as eszopiclone and zolpidem) have in general eclipsed use of the older drugs but share a similar mechanism (and side effects such as ataxia and respiratory depression). In addition, many anesthetics, including gas anesthetics such as ether, but also including isoflurane and halothane, as well as intravenous compounds such as propofol, all act via GABA$_A$ receptors.

At dosages of GABA$_A$ enhancers used in social settings, such as ethanol consumed with a dinner, they cause muscle relaxation and are anxiolytic. At higher doses used in social settings, however, they can produce cognitive impairment and ataxia, as well as loss of judgment. Slightly higher dosages, commonly used to promote onset of sleep, appear to engage the normal wake–sleep systems in the brain.[524] The ventrolateral preoptic nucleus, which inhibits the key elements of the arousal system at the onset of sleep, relies on GABA as a neurotransmitter, and so potentiating its effect reduces the level of arousal (and results in increased activity of the ventrolateral preoptic sleep-promoting neurons because they are inhibited by the arousal systems).[525] At this level of administration, the subject may be sleepy but arousable, although cognitively impaired and ataxic, which can provide problems if the sleeper is aroused by an emergency during the night or must negotiate the way to the bathroom in a darkened house.

At higher dosages, such as those used for conscious sedation or in a drunken stupor, the GABA$_A$ enhancers begin to potentiate GABAergic transmission throughout the brain nondiscriminantly. This causes hypotonia, and it is difficult if not impossible to fully waken the individual in case of danger. There is suppression of response to pain, which makes these drugs useful for minor procedures, such as endoscopy, and these drugs provided the only known source of anesthesia for surgical procedures prior to the twentieth century. Doses of GABA-enhancers at this level suppress respiration and can cause respiratory arrest. Even higher doses, such as those used to produce a surgical plane of anesthesia, require intubation to be administered safely.

The EEG during low-dose administration of GABA$_A$ enhancers is typical of a sleepy state, with increased delta activity. At doses used for conscious sedation, the EEG is in a high-voltage, continuous delta state. At a surgical plane of anesthesia, though, the EEG changes to burst-suppression, and at the very high doses used to treat SE, the EEG may become isoelectric.

Some of the GABA$_A$ enhancers wear off very quickly after administration. Gas anesthetics and propofol, for example last only about 10 minutes. The half-lives of most modern benzodiazepines (lorazepam, oxazepam, triazolam) or nonbenzodiazepines (eszopiclone) used clinically to induce sleep is in the range of 4–8 hours, although some are even shorter (e.g., zolpidem is 1.5 hours). On the other hand, some of the older benzodiazepines (e.g., flurazepam, diazepam, chlorazepam, clonazepam) have half-lives of 12–24 hours or longer. This long half-life leads to two issues that clinicians need to be aware of: first, repeated dosing of these drugs in a patient who is having trouble sleeping (or who is being treated for alcohol withdrawal) can build up a very high level, sufficient to cause respiratory arrest. Second, when treating patients who have taken these drugs with a specific antidote, such as flumazenil, it may be necessary to keep up treatment for 2–3 days to wait for the drug to be metabolized.

Clinically, overdoses with most depressant drugs produce fairly consistent findings; individual drugs usually cause relatively minor clinical differences. Almost all of these agents depress vestibular and cerebellar function as readily as cerebral cortical function so that nystagmus, ataxia, and dysarthria accompany or even precede the first signs of impaired consciousness. Larger amounts of drug produce coma, and, at this quantity, all the agents depress brainstem autonomic responses. Respiration tends to be depressed at least as much as and sometimes more than somatic motor function. The pupils are usually small and reactive and ciliospinal reflexes are preserved. The oculocephalic responses are depressed or absent, and the oculovestibular responses to cold caloric testing are depressed and may be lost altogether in deep coma. Patients with depressant drug poisoning are usually flaccid, with stretch reflexes that are diminished or absent. This typical picture is not always immediately seen, especially if coma develops rapidly after the ingestion of a fast-acting sedative. In such cases, respiratory depression may ensue almost as rapidly as does unconsciousness; signs in the motor system may initially evolve as if function was being depressed in a rostral-caudal fashion, with a brief appearance of hyperreflexia and even clonus and extensor plantar responses.

Failure to recognize this short-lived phase (it rarely lasts more than 30–45 minutes) as being due to depressant drugs can be fatal if one leaves the patient temporarily unattended or delays needed ventilatory assistance. The identifying clue to the toxic-metabolic basis of the changes in such cases is that the pupillary reflexes are preserved and the motor signs are symmetric.

Treatment of sedative-hypnotic drugs largely involves meticulous supportive care. This includes prevention of further absorption of the poison, elimination of the toxin that has already been absorbed, and support of respiration, blood pressure, and cardiac rhythm. While at one time it was common to lavage the stomach of a patient who had taken an overdose of sedative medication, it is important to avoid this in the sleepy patient who may then aspirate the stomach contents resulting in pneumonia that is more dangerous than the overdose. In general, it is better to wait until the patient is intubated before beginning gastric lavage. It may also be possible to remove some toxins from the GI tract with adsorptive substances such as charcoal or from the blood via dialysis. Some toxins, such as use of flumazenil for benzodiazepine overdoses or naloxone for opiate overdoses, have specific antidotes.[520]

The neurologic examination itself cannot categorically separate drug poisoning from other causes of metabolic brain disease. The most common diagnostic error is to mistake deep coma from sedative poisoning for the coma of brainstem infarction. The initial distinction between these two conditions may be difficult, but small, reactive pupils, absence of caloric responses, failure to respond to noxious stimuli, absence of stretch reflexes, and muscular flaccidity suggest a profound metabolic disorder. Persistent extensor responses, hyperactive stretch reflexes, spasticity, dysconjugate eye movements to caloric tests, and unreactive pupils more likely occur with brainstem destruction. If both the pupillary light reflexes and ciliospinal responses are present, deep coma is metabolic in origin. However, even if both the pupillary reactions and the ciliospinal reflexes are lost, deep coma can still be due to severe sedative intoxication. Thus, demonstration of brain death requires eliminating the possibility of a sedative overdose. See Historical Patient Vignette 5.21.

Historical Patient Vignette 5.21

A 48-year-old woman ingested 50 g of chloral hydrate, 1.5 g of chlordiazepoxide (150 tablets of Librium), and 2.4 g of flurazepam (80 capsules of Dalmane) in a suicide attempt. Shortly afterward, her family found her in a lethargic condition, and, by the time they brought her to the emergency department, she was deeply comatose, hypotensive, and apneic. Examination following endotracheal intubation and the initiation of artificial ventilation showed a blood pressure of 60/40 mm Hg, pupils that were 2 mm in diameter and light fixed, absent corneal and oculovestibular responses, and total muscle flaccidity accompanied by areflexia. Arterial and Schwann-Ganz catheters were placed to assist in physiologic monitoring in view of the overwhelmingly large depressant drug dose. There was already evidence of aspiration pneumonia by the time she reached the hospital. A broad-spectrum antibiotic was given, and a dopamine infusion was started, which initially succeeded in raising the blood pressure to 80/60 mm Hg. By 12 hours following admission, progressively increasing amounts of dopamine to a level of 40 pg/kg/minute were unable to keep the blood pressure above 60/40 mm Hg and urine flow ceased. Treatment with L-norepinephrine was initiated at an intravenous dose that reached 12 pg/minute. This induced a prompt rise in blood pressure to 80/40 mm Hg accompanied by a brisk urine flow. Toxicologic analysis of an admission blood sample showed the qualitative presence of chloral hydrate (quantitative assay was not available). The chlordiazepoxide level was 59.4 µg/mL and flurazepam was 6.6 µg/mL.

Early management was complicated by the effects of radiographically demonstrated aspiration pneumonia and by pulmonary edema, as well as by atrial, junctional, and ventricular premature cardiac contractions. Hypotension hovering between 80/60 and 60/40 mm Hg was a serious problem for the first 48 hours, and declines in blood pressure were repeatedly accompanied by a marginal urinary flow. The woman remained unresponsive, but by day 4 it was possible to maintain mean blood pressures above 80/60 mm Hg using dopamine; the L-norepinephrine was discontinued.

Isosthenuria and polyuria developed, reflecting the probable complication of renal tubular necrosis, but meticulous attention to electrolyte balance, pulmonary toilet, and the avoidance of overhydration managed to prevent the various complications from worsening. Ice water caloric stimulation first elicited a reaction of ocular movement on day 4 and the pupillary light reflexes reappeared on the same day. On day 8, spontaneous breathing began and one could detect stretch reflexes in the extremities. She first responded to noxious stimuli by opening her eyes and withdrawing her limbs on day 10, and she mumbled words 1 day later. Not until day 13 did she fully awaken to follow commands and answer questions. The quick phase of nystagmus to caloric stimulation did not return until day 15. She subsequently made a complete physical and intellectual recovery and received psychiatric treatment.

Comment

This woman's course emphasizes the maxim that if patients with depressant drug poisoning survive to reach the hospital, they are potentially salvageable no matter what the blood levels of the ingested agent. The toxicologic analyses in this instance showed an amount of drug in the body that is generally regarded as a fatal dose. Whether hemodialysis would have shortened this patient's course can be questioned, since none of the ingested agents was dialyzable. Generally speaking, among younger patients seen with drug intoxication, only those who have ingested large amounts of barbiturates have periods of unconsciousness that approach the length of this woman's coma. However, patients put into pentobarbital coma therapeutically to treat status epilepticus may have a very similar course, and prolonged drug-induced coma does not appear to injure the brain. Her case illustrates that any sedative taken in sufficiently large amounts is capable of producing many days of coma that require meticulous systemic care to accomplish survival. Her outcome further emphasizes that even very long periods of unresponsive coma need not produce any measure of brain injury so long as blood gases and arterial perfusion pressures are maintained at levels close to the physiologic norm.

Table 5.4 Severity of Depressant Drug Coma*

Grade:

0- Asleep but arousable
1- Unarousable to talk but withdraws appropriately
2- Comatose; most reflexes intact; no cardiorespiratory depression
3- Comatose; no tendon reflexes; no cardiorespiratory depression
4- Respiratory failure, hypotension, pulmonary edema or arrhythmia present. Comatose for more than 36 hours

*Adapted from Reed et al.[526]

In diagnosing coma caused by depressant drug poisoning, one must not only identify the cause, but also judge the depth of coma because the latter influences the choice of treatment. Several years ago, Reed and colleagues[526] suggested a grading scheme for patients with depressant drug poisoning, as outlined in Table 5.4. The practical aspect of the classification is that only patients with grade 3 or 4 depression are at risk of losing their lives. By the same token, comparisons of the potential value of one treatment over another can only be judged by comparing them on patients in grade 3 or 4 coma, where essentially all deaths occur.

Benzodiazepines and nonbenzodiazepine agonists of the same receptors (e.g., drugs like zolpidem and eszopiclone) have replaced barbiturates as hypnotic agents. They cause much less respiratory depression, but at very high dosages may still cause respiratory arrest, particularly if the patient has underlying chronic pulmonary disease or has been taking other drugs, such as ethanol or opiates, at the same time. An overdose can be reversed by the specific antagonist flumazenil.[527] Flumazenil is useful in assessing multiagent poisoning because it reverses the side effects of the benzodiazepine; however, in some circumstances, it may cause acute withdrawal seizures.[528] Flumazenil does not affect coma due to alcohol, barbiturates, tricyclic antidepressants, or opioids (Table 5.4).

Intoxication with "Endogenously Produced" Benzodiazepines

Over the years there have been scattered case reports of patients with recurrent episodes of stupor resembling drug overdose,[529] but no drug ingestion could be identified. Lugaresi and colleagues suggested the possibility that such attacks might be due to elevated levels of an endogenous benzodiazepine-like agent which they called 'endozepine'.[530,531] Patients clinically resemble those who have taken benzodiazepines in overdose, and, in fact, some have called into question whether the disorder is really due to surreptitious ingestion of benzodiazepines[532]; at least one of Lugaresi's cases turned out to be due to surreptitious loraz-epam ingestion.[533] Stupor in such patients may last hours or days; it has an unpredictable onset and frequency. Patients are entirely normal between attacks. Like patients with benzodi-azepine intoxication, these patients respond to flumazenil, which both wakes the patient and normalizes the EEG. Measures of endogenous benzodiazepine-like levels are increased during the stupor. Patients can be treated with oral flumazenil to reduce the frequency of attacks. Recent reports with more sensitive methods of drug detection have found that all or nearly all of these cases are due to surreptitious self-administration of benzodiazepines. However, recently Rye and colleagues have proposed that many patients with chronic excessive daytime sleepiness have evidence of a $GABA_A$ receptor enhancer that is similar to benzodiazepines and which is blocked by flumazenil or by administering clarithromycin.[534] The nature of this benzodiazepine-like agent, however, re-mains elusive.

Ethanol Intoxication and Ethanol Withdrawal

A secure diagnosis of alcoholic intoxica-tion and its severity requires blood level determinations. Measurement of breath eth-anol is not as accurate as measurement of blood ethanol and often underestimates the degree of toxicity.[535] However, in a stuporous or comatose patient with a breath ethanol level of less than 50 mg/dL, alcohol intoxication is probably not the culprit and other causes need to be searched for.

Alcohol levels also interact with measurements of osmolality.[520] Alcohol adds osmols to blood in a degree proportional to its blood level. Each 50 mg/dL of ethanol will add about 10 mOsm/L to blood osmolality.

Because alcohol is uniformly distributed in body water, the hyperosmolality does not lead to fluid shifts out of the brain, and thus the hyperosmolality produced by alcohol is not in itself a cause of symptoms. Although ethanol is one of the $GABA_A$ enhancers, it also affects other neurotransmitters, including causing increases in dopaminergic transmission, which is a critical component of the reward system to the brain. It also promotes the release of noradrenaline, blocks the NMDA glutamate receptor, and stimulates the serotonin ($5HT_3$) receptor.[536]

Alcohol deserves special attention among $GABA_A$ enhancers for three reasons. First, it has pride of place as the only sedative-hypnotic substance that is officially sanctioned for sale to any adult, hence it is ubiquitous in our society. For this reason, it is the most common party drug, and one that is found in many types of food and even medications. This makes alco-holic intoxication difficult to diagnoses because so many patients who are unconscious for other reasons (e.g., head trauma or drug ingestion) will have the odor of "alcohol" (actually caused by impurities in the liquor) on their breath.

The patient in an alcoholic stupor (blood level 250–300 mg/dL, although highly tolerant alcoholics may be awake at these levels) usu-ally has a flushed face, a rapid pulse, low blood pressure, and mild hypothermia, all resulting from the vasodilatory effects of alcohol. As the coma deepens (blood levels of 300–400 mg/dL), such patients become pale and quiet, and the pupils may dilate and become sluggishly re-active. With deeper depression respiration fails. The depth of alcoholic stupor or coma may be deceptive when judged clinically. Repetitive stimulation during medical examinations often arouses such patients to the point where they awaken and require little further stimulation to remain awake, only to lapse into a deep coma with respiratory failure when left alone in bed. Alcohol is frequently taken in conjunction with psychotropic or sedative drugs in suicide attempts. Because ethanol is also a $GABA_A$ ag-onist, it synergizes with the other depressant drugs. Under such circumstances of double in-gestion, blood levels are no longer reliable in predicting the course, and sudden episodes of respiratory failure or cardiac arrhythmias are more frequent than in patients who have taken only a sedative.

Large doses of alcohol produce a coma that, at greater than 400 mg/dL, can be fatal primarily due to respiratory depression. A major problem with alcohol ingestion is that the ensuing uninhibited behavior leads to the impulsive ingestion of other sedative, hypnotic, or antidepressant drugs or to careless, headstrong, and uncoordinated activity (e.g., fighting, driving while intoxicated) that invites head trauma. As a result, the major diagnostic problem in altered states of consciousness associated with acute alcoholic intoxication lies in separating the potentially benign and spontaneously reversible signs of alcoholic depression from evidence of more serious injury from other drugs or head trauma.

As noted earlier, in pure alcohol intoxication, blood levels correlate fairly well with clinical signs of intoxication. Dose levels correlate less well because the rate of absorption from the stomach and intestine depends heavily on the presence or absence of other stomach contents. Chronic ingestion induces moderate tolerance, but, in general, the associations in Table 5.5 represent dependable guidelines. When estimating dosage, the physician should recall that, in the United States, the alcoholic content of distilled spirits equals 50% of the stated proof on the label.

Clinical signs of acute drunkenness can closely resemble those caused by several other

metabolic encephalopathies, especially including other depressant drug intoxication, diabetic ketoacidosis, and hypoglycemia. Innate psychologic traits influence the behavior of many drunks, adding to the complexities of diagnosis. As mentioned above, the odor of the breath depends on impurities and is an unreliable sign. Patients with alcohol intoxication are ataxic, clumsy, and dysarthric. They are easily confused, are often uninhibited and boisterous (or, more severely, stuporous), and commonly vomit. The conjunctivae are often hyperemic, and with severe poisoning, the pupils react sluggishly to light. Severe intoxication or stupor produces a remarkable degree of analgesia ("feeling no pain") to noxious stimuli such that, prior to the discovery of modern anesthetics, alcohol was often used for this purpose (Table 5.5).

A second reason that ethanol deserves a special discussion is because many individuals who are addicted to alcohol will look for a substitute when none is available. This may lead them to ingest methanol (wood alcohol) or ethylene glycol (found in radiator antifreeze solutions). Both of these will cause intoxication similar to ethanol, but later lead to damage to other organ systems. Because these compounds cause systemic acidosis, which is often the most striking laboratory finding early on in an intoxicated patient, they are discussed later under that topic.

The third reason for separating ethanol from the other GABA-enhancers is that withdrawal from imbibing alcohol is also a common cause of impaired consciousness.[537] In some cases this is due to the occurrence of seizures. Both ethanol intoxication and withdrawal from ethanol can lower the seizure threshold. The seizures are usually generalized tonic-clonic seizures, but if the individual is not accompanied at the time, he or she may be found afterward in a sleepy and confused postictal state. Because such patients often fall and may hit their heads as well, it is often difficult to sort out what component of the exam is due to the head trauma, what to the ethanol, and what to the seizure.

Other patients during ethanol withdrawal experience *delirium tremens*. Although it is caused by withdrawal of alcohol and generally follows complete cessation of drinking, usually by 3–4 days, it may occur in a patient still drinking a diminished amount of ethanol. Similar clinical findings may follow benzodiazepine, barbiturate, or other sedative drug

Table 5.5 Clinical Effects and Blood Levels in Acute Alcoholism

Symptoms	Blood level (mg/dL)
Euphoria, giddiness, verbosity	25–100
Long reaction time, impaired mental status examination	
Mild incoordination, nystagmus	
Hypalgesia to noxious stimuli	
Boisterousness, withdrawal, easily confused	100–200
Conjunctival hyperemia	
Ataxia, nystagmus, dysarthria	
Pronounced hypalgesia	
Nausea, vomiting, drowsiness	200–300
Diplopia, wide sluggish pupils	
Marked ataxia and clumsiness	
Hypothermia, cold sweat, amnesic stupor	>300
Severe dysarthria or anarthria	
Anesthesia	
Stertor, hypoventilation	
Coma	

withdrawal.[538] Particularly perplexing to the physician are those patients not known to be alcoholics or chronic sedative drug users who enter the hospital for elective surgery and, during the course of workup or shortly following the operation, become acutely delirious. The disease generally runs its course in less than a week. If treated with sedative drugs and good supportive therapy, most patients recover fully, although a mortality ranging from 2% to 15% has been reported from various sources. Much of this mortality is probably due to other complications of alcoholism, such as liver failure, or to sympathetic activation that commonly accompanies the disorder. The pathogenesis of drug withdrawal syndromes may depend on their effect on receptors, particularly NMDA and $GABA_A$ receptors. NMDA receptors are up-regulated during chronic alcohol exposure and because it is a $GABA_A$ potentiator, $GABA_A$ receptors may be down-regulated. Hence, abrupt cessation increases brain excitability leading to clinically evident anxiety, irritability, agitation, and tremor.[539]

Finally, both alcohol intoxication as well as recovering from alcohol intoxication lower the seizure threshold.[537] In addition, many chronic alcoholics have histories of repeated head trauma or may have other reasons (e.g., brain injuries or malformations that produce poor societal adjustment resulting in drinking behavior) for a lower seizure threshold. Alcoholic seizures may, therefore, occur at any time from ingestion out to about a week later. As the initial seizure may be missed, particularly if the patient is "found down" and unable to give a history, it is always important to consider a seizure as the cause of impaired consciousness in a patient who has been drinking. In addition, it is important to perform an lumbar puncture to check for possible infection if the patient is not known to have seizures in the past.

There are two schools of thought concerning treatment of alcoholic seizures or withdrawal seizures. Some clinicians treat with another $GABA_A$ enhancer, usually either phenobarbital or a benzodiazepine, which will both prevent further seizures and forestall alcohol withdrawal symptoms, especially during an acute hospitalization.[540] Others, particularly if the seizures are recurrent and if the alcoholism is chronic and unlikely to abate, prefer to treat with an antiepileptic drug that uses a different mechanism of action, so that the patients are protected from seizures during future cycles of intoxication and withdrawal.

Many other drugs of abuse are proconvulsive and may produce seizures, as indicated in Table 5.6.

Ketamine, Phencyclidine (NMDA Receptor Antagonist Drugs)

This class of drugs acts by antagonizing NMDA-class glutamate receptors involved in excitatory transmission, rather than enhancing inhibition in the brain. At moderate dosages, they produce a peculiar dissociative state in which the individual is not truly unconscious, but may have hallucinations. Because there is very little respiratory depression, they were used as anesthetics, but occasional patients would wake up after surgery and complain that they had been awake the entire time and could repeat conversations the surgeons had had in the operating room. And yet, while they could feel the actual surgery, they did not care, and could not do anything about it. As a result neither drug is in common use for human anesthesia, but both are used widely as veterinary anesthetics. Ketamine was recently introduced for use at low dosages to treat severe depression.[541,542] However, ketamine is still available as a Class III drug in the United States and used as an additive drug in anesthesia in combination with GABAA acting drugs such as Propofol[543] or in combination with benzodiazepines in the management of refractory status epilepticus.[544]

A key feature of drugs in this class is that they cause little cardiovascular and respiratory depression and, in fact, may increase blood pressure or heart rate. Overdosage with phencyclidine, also known as "angel dust,[545] can result in bizarre behavior and agitation and, at higher doses, can produce delirium and coma. Both vertical and horizontal nystagmus are common. Seizures and dystonic reactions are less common. Many patients have pinpoint pupils when they are awake and agitated, and this can be a clue to the diagnosis. Patients may develop hypertensive encephalopathy; intracerebral and subarchnoid hemorrahges have been reported. Ketamine[546] is also abused as a club drug, and it can either be ingested or smoked. It causes delirium, often with hallucinations. Side effects may include

Table 5.6 Proconvulsant Agents: Classification by Source and Use

Pharmaceuticals		Nonpharmaceuticals	
Class	Example(s)	Class	Example(s)
Analgesics	Meperidine/normeperidine, propoxyphene, pentazocine, salicylate, tramadol	Alcohols	Methanol, ethanol (withdrawal)
Anesthetics	Local anesthetics (lidocaine, benzocaine)	Antiseptics/preservatives	Ethylene oxide, phenol
Anticonvulsants	Carbamazepine	Biologic toxins	
Antidepressants	Tricyclics (amitriptyline/nortriptyline), amoxapine, bupropion, selective serotonin reuptake inhibitors (citalopram), venlafaxine	Marine animals	Domoic acid (shellfish [blue mussels])
		Mushrooms	Monomethylhydrazine (*Gyromitra* spp.)
		Plants	Conine (poison hemlock) Water hemlock Camphor
Antihistamines	Diphenhydramine, doxylamine, tripelennamine	Gases (naturally and/or anthropogenically occurring)	Carbon monoxide, hydrogen sulfide, hydrogen cyanide
Antimicrobials		Metals/organometallics	Alkyl mercurials (dimethylmercury), arsenic, lead, thallium, tetraethyl lead, organotins (trimethyl ...)
Antineoplastics	Alkylating agents (chlorambucil, busulfan)	Metal hydrides	Pentaborane, phosphine
Antipsychotics	Clozapine, loxapine	Pesticides	
Asthma medications		Fungicides/herbicides	Dinitrophenol, diquat, glufosinate
Cardiovascular drugs	Propranolol, quinidine	Insecticides	Organochlorines (lindane, DDT), organophosphates (parathion), pyrethroids (type II), sulfuryl fluoride, alkyl halides (methyl bromide)
Cholinergics	Pilocarpine, bethanechol	Molluscacides	Metaldehyde
Muscle relaxants	Baclofen, orphenadrine	Rodenticides	Strychnine, zinc or aluminum phosphide
Nonsteroidal anti-inflammatory drugs	Mefenamic acid, phenylbutazone		
Psychostimulants/anorectics	Amphetamine, caffeine, cocaine, methamphetamine, methylenedioxymethamphetamine (MDMA)		
Vitamins/supplements	Vitamin A, iron salts (ferrous sulfate)		

hypothermia and respiratory depression.[547] With either drug, a benzodiazepine may help control violent behavior.[548] Treatment is largely supportive.

Antidepressants

The antidepressant class of drugs was discovered accidentally in the 1950s, when isoniazid was tested as a treatment for tuberculosis. The patients felt better more quickly than their disease improved, and other drugs with antidepressant properties, such as monoamine oxidase inhibitors, including deprenyl, were soon developed. Meanwhile, a tricyclic antihistamine derivative with antidepressant properties, imipramine, was identified, and, over the years, a large number of tricyclic antidepressant drugs with similar effects on serotonin and norepinephrine reuptake were developed. Although the early tricyclic antidepressants were antihistaminergic and anticholinergic, therefore causing a dry mouth and sleepiness as side effects, these properties were reduced in later generations. The development of selective serotonin or norepinephrine reuptake inhibitors, with minimal side effects, has made the medications more tolerable, as well as reducing the chances of coma or cardiovascular arrhythmias or hypotension in case of an overdose.

Nevertheless, tricyclic antidepressants such as amitriptyline and desipramine are still used, and it is useful to be able to recognize the effect of overdoses, which can cause stupor or coma. The major toxicity of the tricyclic antidepressants is on the cardiovascular system, causing cardiac arrhythmias and hypotension. The CNS is affected by the change in blood pressure as well as by the anticholinergic effects of the drugs that can lead to anhydrosis, fever, and multifocal myoclonus.[548] In some cases, patients with tricyclic overdoses can lose some or all of their eye movements, even with oculocephalic maneuvers or cold water caloric stimulation.

Selective serotonin reuptake inhibitors (SSRIs) and monoamine oxidase (MAO) inhibitors taken alone generally are not neurotoxic. When taken together, however, they may result in the serotonin syndrome characterized by delirium, myoclonus, hyperreflexia, diaphoresis, flushing, fever, nausea, and diarrhea.

Disseminated intravascular coagulation may be a side effect and add to the CNS difficulties. Methysergide and cyproheptadine have been reported to be effective in reversing this disorder.[548]

Lithium is used to treat bipolar disorder. Intoxication is characterized by tremor, ataxia and nystagmus, choreoathetosis, photophobia, and lethargy. A key finding in many cases is nephrogenic diabetes insipidus, resulting in volume depletion and hyperosmolarity. Delirium, seizures, coma, and cardiovascular instability may occur with severe intoxication.[549] Cerebellar toxicity occurs at levels higher than 3.5 mEq/L and may be nonreversible.[550] With a decreased serum anion gap, hemodialysis may be required for severe intoxication.[549]

Neuroleptics

The first neuroleptic drug, chlorpromazine, was synthesized in 1950 from synthetic antihistamines. Like most of the early antipsychotic drugs, it retained its anticholinergic and antihistaminergic effects and was heavily sedating. Other drugs with similar properties were soon developed, but nearly all of the drugs in this group also were dopamine antagonists, which caused slowing and stiffness of movement (i.e., parkinsonism). These properties were noticed by psychiatrists, who tested the drugs on agitated psychotic patients. The neuroleptic drugs made it practical to treat these patients, who were often delusional and agitated, with less use of restraints and less danger to themselves and to the hospital staff. Like the antidepressants, later neuroleptic drugs have had less anticholinergic and antihistaminergic effects, which improves patient compliance. However, only two drugs in this class have minimal anti-dopaminergic effects, clozapine and quetiapine, and hence do not cause or worsen parkinsonism.

The effect of overdosage with a neuroleptic depends on the specific pharmacological properties of that agent. For example, the older neuroleptic drugs, which have anticholinergic effects, are similar to the tricyclic antidepressants in causing cardiovascular side effects. All drugs in this class cause sedation, which can reach the level of stupor or coma. However, the neuroleptics with dopamine antagonist properties also produce a parkinsonian state in which the patient may be unable to swallow adequately to protect the airway and may be quite stiff and rigid.

A particularly dangerous effect is the *neuroleptic malignant syndrome*.[551] Although this may occur with overdosage of any of the neuroleptics with dopaminergic antagonist properties, it may also be seen occasionally in patients on clozapine or quetiapine, or in patients with Parkinson's disease in whom levodopa has suddenly been reduced.[552,553] There is generally a high fever, with intense muscular rigidity associated with tachycardia and hypertension, which may result in cardiovascular collapse, with rhabdomyolysis, renal failure, or seizures. Treatment includes stopping the neuroleptic (or restarting dopamine in a Parkinson patient), cooling, and supportive care. Some have suggested using dantrolene (to break muscular rigidity), bromocriptine (as a dopamine agonist), or sedation with a benzodiazepine. However, once the body temperature is under control, supportive measures may be sufficient.

Opiates

Although opiates are one of the oldest classes of drugs that are still in common medical use, their mechanism of action only became clear in the late 1970s, when it was discovered that they interact with a series of endogenous receptors which respond to endogenous opioid peptides.[554] It is now recognized that there are five classes of opioid receptors (delta, kappa, mu, sigma [δ, κ, μ, σ], and the nociceptin receptor) and that the first four recognize peptides with the consensus opioid sequence of YGGFL or YGGFM (Leucine- or Methionine-encephalin). These sequences are found on the N-terminal of the various other opioid peptides, which include the enkephalins, endorphins, dynorphins, and nociceptin. Endomorphins have a different N-terminal (YPWF or YPFF) but also act on the μ receptor.

Alkaloids derived from the poppy plant, known as opiates, have been known since antiquity to cause analgesia and sedation. It has also been known for many centuries that overdosage of these drugs can cause coma and respiratory depression or even arrest and also that they are among the most highly addictive drugs known. The indispensable nature of opiates for

pain control has thus resulted in their widespread use and abuse. In recent years, with the availability of high-potency synthetic opiates such as fentanyl, this has led to an epidemic of deaths due to addicts taking unintended overdoses.

These drugs can be taken either by injection, nasally, orally, or by smoking or sniffing the fumes ("chasing the dragon"). Overdosage with narcotics may occur from suicide attempts or, more commonly, when an addict or neophyte misjudges the amount or the quality of the opiate that he or she is injecting or sniffing. Characteristic signs of opioid coma include pinpoint pupils that generally constrict to a bright light and dilate rapidly if a narcotic antagonist is given. Respiratory slowing, irregularity, and cessation are prominent features and result either from direct narcotic depression of the brainstem or from pulmonary edema, which is a frequent complication of heroin overdosage,[555] although the pathogenesis is not understood. Opiates can cause hypothermia, but by the time such patients reach the hospital, they frequently have pneumonitis due to aspiration, so that body temperatures may be normal or elevated. Some opioids such as propoxyphene and meperidine can cause seizures. Intravenous naloxone at an initial dose of 0.2–0.4 mg usually reverses the effects of opioids. In patients who are physically dependent, the drug may also cause acute withdrawal. Repeated boluses at intervals of 1–2 hours may be needed, as naloxone is a short-acting agent and the patient may have taken a long-acting opioid.[548]

Individuals who had respiratory insufficiency during an overdosage may also suffer from *posthypoxic leukoencephalopathy*. This begins about a week after the hypoxic episode, with gradual onset of cognitive impairment, and frequently blindness or a dyskinetic movement disorder, and it may progress to impaired consciousness or even an unresponsive state. This is associated with diffuse symmetric increased T2 signal in the white matter of the cerebral hemispheres, gray matter, or both. A similar picture has been reported in patients who were "chasing the dragon."[559] It is not clear if this is due to a period of respiratory depression or to some impurity in the heroin that was inhaled along with the vapors of the opiate drug, but the MRS in "chasing the dragon" cases has been reported to show increased lactic acid and myo-inositol, decrease *N*-acetyl-aspartate and creatine, with normal[557] or slightly increased choline and normal lipid peaks. These findings are similar to MRS in posthypoxic encephalopathy,[558] lending credence to speculation that the two phenomena may be related.

Intoxication with Antipyretic/ Analgesic Medications

Acetaminophen overdose is the most common poisoning reported to poison information centers. The drug's metabolite (NAPQI)[559] can cause acute liver necrosis, and doses above 5 g can lead to liver failure and hepatic coma. Alkalosis and grossly elevated liver function studies are a clue to its presence; prompt treatment with *N*-acetylcysteine may prevent fatality.[549]

Salicylate intoxication is less common with the advances in other nonsteroidal anti-inflammatory drugs that have less gastric toxicity and do not cause long-term antiplatelet effects. However, some patients still do still take aspirin for various pain syndromes, and there are topical salicylates (usually for musculoskeletal aches) which may be absorbed through the skin and add to systemic salicylate levels. Salicylate toxicity may appear in two principal forms. Relatively younger persons sometimes take aspirin or similar agents in suicide attempts. Although many become severely ill and a few die with terminal coma or convulsions, most of these younger patients lack prominent neurologic complaints except for tinnitus and dyspnea. Older persons, by contrast, often ingest salicylates in excessive amounts more or less accidentally in proprietary analgesics; in these patients, neurologic symptoms can dominate the early illness, producing an encephalopathy that initially obscures the etiologic diagnosis. Salicylates act as a "metabolic uncoupler" in oxidative phosphorylation and stimulate net organic acid production. Aspirin (acetylsalicylic acid) also contains 1.7 mEq of acid per 300-mg tablet. In experimental animals, death from salicylate poisoning comes from convulsions and relates directly to the concentration of the drug in the brain; clinical evidence suggests that similar principles apply in humans.

Salicylates in adults stimulate respiration neurogenically to a degree that nearly always produces a respiratory alkalosis in the blood that overshadows its intrinsic tendency toward metabolic acidosis unless simultaneous ingestion of a sedative drug suppresses the respiratory response.[548] The metabolic acidosis of the tissues is reflected usually by a disproportionately lowered serum bicarbonate and always by an acid urine. Depending on age, associated illness, and the rapidity of accumulation, the first symptoms of salicylate intoxication usually appear at a blood level of about 40–50 mg/dL. Blood levels of more than 60 mg/dL usually produce symptoms of severe toxicity. Initial complaints are of tinnitus and, less often, deafness. As many as one-half of older persons with severe salicylate intoxication develop confusion, agitation, slurred speech, hallucinations, convulsions, stupor, or coma. Hyperpnea, intact pupillary responses, intact oculocephalic responses, diffuse paratonia, and, in many instances, extensor plantar responses are present. In a patient with metabolic encephalopathy, a respiratory alkalosis and mildly abnormal anion gap in the blood combined with aciduria are almost always diagnostic of salicylate toxicity and can be quickly confirmed by determination of salicylate blood levels. Salicylate intoxication may be complicated by gastrointestinal bleeding, pulmonary edema, and multiorgan failure. Hemodialysis may be necessary to treat the disorder. Patient Vignette 5.22 illustrates the problem.

Patient Vignette 5.22

A 74-year-old woman with osteoarthritis, self-treated with aspirin, developed peptic ulcer disease. She was admitted to the hospital, where she was noted to be lethargic and confused after she fell out of bed. With a dysarthric, deepened voice, she complained of a recent loss of hearing. The examination showed fluctuating lethargy, asterixis, and bilateral extensor plantar responses, but little else. A computed tomography (CT) scan was unremarkable, and the changes were at first ascribed to the nonfocal effects of trauma. The next day, however, she was barely arousable, severely dysarthric, and disoriented when she did respond. The pupils were 2 mm and reactive, the oculocephalic responses full and conjugate, and prominent bilateral asterixis involved the upper extremities. Both plantar responses were extensor, and the respiratory rate was 32 per minute. Arterial blood gases were pH 7.48, PCO_2 24 mm Hg, PO_2 81 mm Hg, and HCO_3 19 mEq/L. Serum sodium was 134, potassium 3.5, and chloride 96 mEq/L, giving an anion gap of approximately 19. Serum salicylate level was 54 mg/dL. She was treated cautiously with alkaline diuresis and became alert without abnormal neurologic symptoms or signs within 48 hours. Her aspirin was found in the bedside table.

Intoxication with Drugs of Abuse

Party or club drugs include GHB (sodium oxybate), ketamine, Rohypnol (flunitrazepam), methamphetamine, lysergic acid diethylamide (LSD), and 3,4-methylenedioxymethamphetamine (MDMA; Ecstasy).[560,522] Other drugs include cocaine, opioids (see preceding sections), and phencyclidine. These drugs may be taken alone or in combination and can cause critical illness.[548]

Cocaine may be taken nasally, orally, or intravenously. The drug inhibits neuronal uptake of catecholamines and causes CNS stimulation. Patients are often euphoric and may be anxious, agitated, and delirious, and sometimes have seizures. Agitation can be controlled with benzodiazepines. Some patients are febrile and require cooling. There is no specific antidote. Some patients develop CNS bleeds, presumably due to increased blood pressure due to drug ingestion; others develop later cerebral infarction.[560] This is currently one of the most common causes of stroke in young adults without the usual risk factors for atherosclerotic disease. GHB causes a state of deep sleep with high-voltage delta EEG. It has been released in the United States to treat narcolepsy, in which fragmented sleep at night contributes to daytime symptoms such as cataplexy. Because it induces such deep unresponsiveness, it has achieved a reputation as a date rape drug[350] and, at high doses, can cause coma and respiratory insufficiency. It has a rather short half-life, so that recovery usually

occurs within several hours. Some uncontrolled studies have suggested physostigmine as an antidote, but the evidence for this is poor and experimental studies have failed to find an effect.[561,562]

MDMA has its major effect on the serotonin system. It is an indirect serotonin agonist that inhibits tryptophan hydroxylase and thus decreases serotonin production. It also induces the release of serotonin and blocks serotonin reuptake. The drug also increases the release of dopamine and norepinephrine from presynaptic neurons and prevents their metabolism by inhibiting monamine oxydase. The usual adverse effects include anxiety, ataxia, and difficulty concentrating; seizures can occur and pupillary dilation is common. Hyperthermia may lead to death.[563] Agitation and seizures can be treated with benzodiazepines.

Flunitrazepam (Rohypnol) is a benzodiazepine and, like other drugs in this class, potentiates $GABA_A$ receptors. Its effects are similar to other drugs in this class, such as benzodiazepines or alcohol intoxication, except that it is more likely to produce respiratory depression, so that overdose can be life-threatening. Flumazenil, a benzodiazepine antagonist, can reverse the toxicity.[563]

Many poisons have specific antidotes, and some of the most common are indicated in Table 5.7.

Intoxication with Drugs Causing Metabolic Acidosis

This section considers specific exogenous poisons causing metabolic acidosis.[565] These include methyl alcohol, ethylene glycol, and paraldehyde. Salicylate poisoning, as noted earlier, also produces a metabolic acidosis in the tissues, but in adults this aspect of the disorder often is overshadowed in the blood by evidence of respiratory alkalosis.

The metabolic acidosis and neurotoxicity of methyl alcohol, ethylene glycol, and paraldehyde all result from their metabolic breakdown products rather than the original agent. Poisoning from all three drugs is most common in chronic alcoholics who ingest the agents either by mistake or in ignorance of their risks as a substitute for ethanol. All three agents initially cause symptoms of alcohol intoxication, progressing to confusion and stupor, by

Table 5.7 **Selected Drugs and Poisons with Specific Antidotes**

Drug/Poison	Antidotes
Acetaminophen	*N*-acetylcysteine
Anticholinergics	Physostigmine
Anticholinesterases	Atropine
Benzodiazepines	Flumazenil
Carbon monoxide	Oxygen
Cyanide	Amyl nitrite, sodium nitrite, sodium thiosulfate, hydroxocobalamin
Ethylene glycol	Ethanol/fomepizole, thiamine, and pyridoxine
Hypoglycemic agents	Dextrose, glucagon, octreotide
Methanol	Ethanol or fomepizole, folic acid
Methemoglobinemia	Methylene blue
Opioids	Naloxone
Organophosphate	Atropine, pralidoxime

Modified from Fabbri et al.,[519] with permission.

which point symptoms and signs of severe acidosis and systemic organ complications usually emerge as well.

Methanol is degraded by alcohol dehydrogenase into formic acid.[548] The presence of ethanol in the system slows its metabolic breakdown, thereby influencing the clinical course. The earliest and most frequent neurologic damage of methyl alcohol poisoning affects retinal ganglion cells. The symptoms of methanol poisoning can evolve over several days or appear abruptly. Stupor, coma, or seizures occur only in severely poisoned patients. Most subjects at first give the appearance of advanced inebriation and develop visual loss ("blind drunk"). Hyperpnea (respiratory compensation for metabolic acidosis) is the rule. Effective early intervention depends on recognizing the presence of an organic acidosis and treating it vigorously by using an inhibitor of alcohol dehydrogenase, such as fomepizole.[566] Because ethanol competes with methanol for alcohol dehydrogenase and thus slows its metabolism, it may be used to minimize the damage from methanol if a specific inhibitor is not readily available. If these drugs fail, hemodialysis may be indicated.[548] Patient Vignette 5.23 illustrates the point.

Patient Vignette 5.23

A 39-year-old man had been intermittently drinking denatured alcohol for 10 days. He was admitted complaining that for several hours his vision was blurred and he was short of breath. He was alert, oriented, and coherent, but restless. His blood pressure was 130/100 mm Hg, his pulse was 130 per minute, and his respirations were 40 per minute, regular and deep. The only other abnormal physical findings were 20/40 vision, engorged left retinal veins with pink optic disks, and sluggishly reactive pupils, 5 mm in diameter. His serum bicarbonate level was 5 mEq/L, and his arterial pH was 7.16. An intravenous infusion was begun immediately; 540 mEq of sodium bicarbonate was infused during the next 4 hours. By that time, his arterial pH had risen to 7.47 and his serum bicarbonate to 13.9 mEq/L. He was still hyperventilating but less restless. The infusion was continued at a slower rate for 20 hours to a total of 740 mEq of bicarbonate. He recovered completely.

Comment

Denatured alcohol, usually sold as a solvent, contains about 83% ethanol and 16% methanol. Hence, it is not unusual for alcoholics to ingest denatured alcohol despite the required warnings on the label, and this source should be sought in the emergency department when a patient who appears intoxicated with ethanol complains of visual symptoms and is hyperventilating. It is likely that the presence of ethanol sufficiently slowed the metabolism of methanol in this patient so that he was able to recover. This patient had profound acidosis, as was reflected by the requirement of 540 mEq of parenteral sodium bicarbonate to raise his serum bicarbonate from 5 to 13 mEq/L. However, it is not clear that bicarbonate therapy improves outcome.[565] Some patients suffer from hypercalcemia and hypoglycemia, and these need to be corrected. Patients may be chronically malnourished, and treatment with vitamins, particularly thiamine but also folate and pyridoxine, should be administered. These same general guidelines apply to ingestion of other alcohols as indicated in the text. The acidosis of methyl alcohol poisoning can be lethal with alarming rapidity. One of our patients walked into the hospital complaining of blurred vision. He admitted drinking "a lot" of methyl alcohol and was hyperventilating. During the 10 minutes that it took to transfer him to a treatment unit, he lost consciousness. By the time an intravenous infusion could be started, his breathing and heart had stopped and resuscitation was unsuccessful. No bicarbonate could be detected in a serum sample drawn simultaneously with death.

Paraldehyde is no longer available in the United States, as it has been replaced by other drugs for treating SE, although it may still be available in other countries.[567] It was used, mainly as a rectal gel, for acute suppression of seizures. Paraldehyde is metabolized to acetic acid, which may cause acidosis, but the degree of acidosis in these patients exceeds the amount of detectable acetic acid in the serum, implying the presence of other acid products as well. Distinctive clinical features, in addition to the manifestations of metabolic acidosis, include the odor of paraldehyde on the breath, abdominal pain, a marked leukocytosis, and obtunded, lethargic behavior. All patient overdoses reported to date have recovered.

Ethylene glycol (antifreeze) is metabolized by alcohol dehydrogenase, the end products being formic, glyoxylic, and oxalic acids.[548] A relatively severe metabolic acidosis occurs during the early hours of toxicity. The initial clinical signs are similar to alcohol intoxication but without ethanol's characteristic odor. Patients with severe poisoning go on to disorientation, stupor, coma, convulsions, and death. Neuro-ophthalmologic abnormalities including papilledema, nystagmus, and ocular bobbing can be prominent. Metabolic abnormalities, if uncorrected, can lead to cardiopulmonary failure. A late complication of ethylene glycol poisoning is renal damage caused by oxalate crystalluria. Diagnosis should be suspected by a history of ingestion of antifreeze in an alcoholic or after a suicide attempt, the identification of an anion gap metabolic acidosis, and the detection of characteristic oxalic acid crystals in the urine. The treatment is the same as that of methanol poisoning (see earlier discussion).[549]

Propylene glycol is a widely available organic solvent used in a variety of oral and injectable pharmaceutical agents, food preparations, and cosmetic materials. Because of its typically pharmacologically inert nature, propylene glycol overdose is not considered in the differential diagnosis of acute large anion gap acidosis and is not included in standard toxicologic studies (or may be used as an internal standard masking overdose). However, propylene glycol overdose may produce profound CNS compromise including stupor and coma, cardiovascular collapse, and marked hematologic changes including leukocytosis, thrombocytosis, microcytic anemia, and bone marrow abnormalities. Animal studies indicate reduction in arousal following repeated intoxication, suggesting that long-term CNS depression results from chronic propylene glycol exposure.[568] Commercial preparations of propylene glycol contain a racemic mixture and are metabolized in vivo to both D- an L-lactic acid isomers. Cats that developed CNS depression were noted to accumulate D-lactate on a dose-dependent basis that was positively correlated with an elevated anion gap. Preferential accumulation in the brain is thought to occur because of the low level of catabolizing enzyme in this site. D-lactic acidosis is known to produce a toxic encephalopathy in humans, usually in the setting of short bowel syndrome.[569]

Lactic acidosis presenting with a depressed level of consciousness is most often due to a postictal state (i.e., a missed generalized seizure, following which the patient was "found down"). Lactic acidosis may also appear in association with a number of other conditions that cause impairment of consciousness,[570] including anxiety, and other conditions that elevate blood epinephrine, in diabetic ketoacidosis, and in alcohol intoxication, but there is little evidence that the lactic acidosis itself actually alters consciousness. For example, more intense, but still systemically benign, lactic acidosis with arterial blood levels of 20 mEq/L or more and blood pH levels below 7.00 can follow vigorous muscular exercise without alteration of consciousness. Lactic acid crosses the blood–brain barrier via a carrier mechanism that saturates at about three to four times the normal plasma concentration of 1 mEq/L. Thus, although high concentrations of lactate in the brain are believed to be neurotoxic, possibly by promoting excitotoxicity,[571] these probably only occur when produced by local brain ischemia or in conditions in which systemic hypoxia, circulatory failure, or drug poisoning also affect directly the oxidative metabolism of the CNS. Finally, elevated CSF lactic acid is seen in mitochondrial encephalopathies. However, even though these may cause stroke-like events, as in mitochondrial encephalopathy, lactic acidosis, and stroke-like (MELAS) events, there is rarely an acute change in level of consciousness.

REFERENCES

1. Ely EW, Inouye SK, Bernard GR, et al. Delirium in mechanically ventilated patients: validity and reliability of the confusion assessment method for the intensive care unit (CAM-ICU). *JAMA* 2001;286:2703–2710.
2. Meah MS, Gardner WN. Post-hyperventilation apnoea in conscious humans. *J Physiol* 1994;477 (Pt 3): 527–538.
3. Jennett S, Ashbridge K, North JB. Post-hyperventilation apnoea in patients with brain damage. *J Neurol Neurosurg Psychiatry* 1974;37:288–296.
4. Flinta I, Ponikowski P. Relationship between central sleep apnea and Cheyne-Stokes respiration. *Int J Cardiol* 2016;206 Suppl:S8–S12.
5. Guyenet PG, Bayliss DA. Neural control of breathing and CO2 homeostasis. *Neuron* 2015;87.946–961.
6. Reeves AG, Posner JB. The ciliospinal response in man. *Neurology* 1969;19:1145–1152.
7. Simon RP. Forced downward ocular deviation. Occurrence during oculovestibular testing in sedative drug-induced coma. *Arch Neurol* 1978;35: 456–458.
8. Cadranel JF, Lebiez E, Di Martino V, et al. Focal neurological signs in hepatic encephalopathy in cirrhotic patients: an underestimated entity? *Am J Gastroenterol* 2001;96(2):515–518.
9. Liberman AL, Prabhakaran S. Stroke chameleons and stroke mimics in the emergency department. *Curr Neurol Neurosci Rep.* 2017;17(2):15.
10. Huff JS. Stroke mimics and chameleons. *Emerg Med Clin North Am.* 2002;20(3):583–595.
11. Adams RD, Foley JM. The neurological disorder associated with liver disease. *Res Publ Assoc Res Nerv Ment Dis* 1953;32:198–237.
12. Rio J, Montalban J, Pujadas F, Alvarezsabin J, Rovira A, Codina A. Asterixis associated with anatomic cerebral lesions: A study of 45 cases. *Acta Neurol Scand* 1995;91:377–381.
13. Apartis E, Vercueil L. To jerk or not to jerk: A clinical pathophysiology of myoclonus. *Rev Neurol (Paris).* 2016;172(8-9):465–476.
14. Young RR, Shahani BT. Asterixis: one type of negative myoclonus. *Adv Neurol* 1986;43:137–156.
15. Leavitt S, Tyler HR. Studies in asterixis. I. *Arch Neurol* 1964;10:360–368.
16. Noda S, Ito H, Umezaki H, Minato S. Hip flexion-abduction to elicit asterixis in unresponsive patients. *Ann Neurol* 1985;18:96–97.
17. Leavitt S, Tyler HR. Studies in asterixis. I. *Arch Neurol* 1964;10:360–368.

18. Adams RD, Foley JM. The neurological disorder associated with liver disease. *Res Publ Assoc Res Nerv Ment Dis*. 1953;32:198–237.
19. van Zijl JC, Beudel M, vd Hoeven HJ, et al. Electroencephalographic findings in posthypoxic myoclonus. *J Intensive Care Med*. 2016;31(4):270–275.
20. Ishii K, Sasaki M, Kitagaki H, Sakamoto S, Yamaji S, Maeda K. Regional difference in cerebral blood flow and oxidative metabolism in human cortex. *J Nucl Med* 1996;37(7):1086–1088.
21. Nair DG. About being BOLD. *Brain Res Brain Res Rev* 2005;50:229–243.
22. Magistretti PJ, Pellerin L. Cellular mechanisms of brain energy metabolism and their relevance to functional brain imaging. *Phil Trans Royal Soc Lond B Biol Sci* 1999;354(1387):1155–1163.
23. Iadecola C. Neurovascular regulation in the normal brain and in Alzheimer's disease. *Nat Rev Neurosci* 2004;5:347–360.
24. Filosa JA, Morrison HW, Iddings JA, Du W, Kim KJ. Beyond neurovascular coupling, role of astrocytes in the regulation of vascular tone. *Neuroscience.* 2016;323:96–109.
25. Magistretti PJ, Pellerin L. Cellular mechanisms of brain energy metabolism and their relevance to functional brain imaging. *Phil Trans Royal Soc Lond B Biol Sci* 1999;354:1155–1163.
26. Pellerin L, Magistretti PJ. Glutamate uptake stimulates Na+,K+-ATPase activity in astrocytes via activation of a distinct subunit highly sensitive to ouabain. *J Neurochem* 1997;69:2132–2137.
27. Pellerin L, Magistretti PJ. Glutamate uptake into astrocytes stimulates aerobic glycolysis: a mechanism coupling neuronal activity to glucose utilization. *Proc Nat Acad Sci USA* 1994;91:10625–10629.
28. Uhlirova H, Kilic K, Tian P, et al. Cell type specificity of neurovascular coupling in cerebral cortex. *eLife* 2016;5.
29. Jones TH, Morawetz RB, Crowell RM, et al. Thresholds of focal cerebral ischemia in awake monkeys. *J Neurosurg* 1981;54:773–782.
30. Kraig RP, Petito CK, Plum F, Pulsinelli WA. Hydrogen ions kill brain at concentrations reached in ischemia. *J Cereb Blood Flow Metab* 1987;7:379–386.
31. Clausen T, Khaldi A, Zauner A, et al. Cerebral acid-base homeostasis after severe traumatic brain injury. *J Neurosurg* 2005;103:597–607.
32. Zauner A, Daugherty WP, Bullock MR, Warner DS. Brain oxygenation and energy metabolism: part I-biological function and pathophysiology. *Neurosurgery* 2002;51:289–301; discussion 302.
33. Buonocore G, Perrone S, Tataranno ML. Oxygen toxicity: chemistry and biology of reactive oxygen species. *Semin Fetal Neonatal Med* 2010;15:186–190.
34. Pellerin L. How astrocytes feed hungry neurons. *Mol Neurobiol* 2005;32:59–72.
35. Gallagher CN, Carpenter KL, Grice P, et al. The human brain utilizes lactate via the tricarboxylic acid cycle: a 13C-labelled microdialysis and high-resolution nuclear magnetic resonance study. *Brain* 2009;132:2839–2849.
36. Gruetter R. Glycogen: the forgotten cerebral energy store. *J Neurosci Res* 2003;74:179–183.
37. Brown AM. Brain glycogen re-awakened. *J Neurochem* 2004;89:537–552.

38. Wu TW, Tamrazi B, Hsu KH, et al. Cerebral lactate concentration in neonatal hypoxic-ischemic encephalopathy: in relation to time, characteristic of injury, and serum lactate concentration. *Front Neurol* 2018;9:293.

39. Vujovic N, Gooley JJ, Jhou TC, Saper CB. Projections from the subparaventricular zone define four channels of output from the circadian timing system. *J Comp Neurol* 2015;523:2714–2737.

40. Hladky SB, Barrand MA. Mechanisms of fluid movement into, through and out of the brain: evaluation of the evidence. *Fluids Barriers CNS* 2014;11:26.

41. Chesler M. Regulation and modulation of pH in the brain. *Physiol Rev* 2003;83:1183–1221.

42. Posner JB, Swanson AG, Plum F. Acid-base balance in cerebrospinal fluid. *Arch Neurol* 1965;12:479–496.

43. Magnotta VA, Heo HY, Dlouhy BJ, et al. Detecting activity-evoked pH changes in human brain. *Proc Natl Acad Sci U S A* 2012;109:8270–8273.

44. Adrogue HJ, Madias NE. Hyponatremia. *N Engl J Med* 2000;342:1581–1589.

45. Lin M, Liu SJ, Lim IT. Disorders of water imbalance. *Emerg Med Clin North Am* 2005;23:749–770.

46. Videen JS, Michaelis T, Pinto P, Ross BD. Human cerebral osmolytes during chronic hyponatremia. A proton magnetic resonance spectroscopy study. *J Clin Invest* 1995;95:788–793.

47. Leao AAP. Spreading depression of activity in the cerebral cortex. *J Neurophysiol* 1944;7:359–390.

48. Strong AJ, Fabricius M, Boutelle MG, et al. Spreading and synchronous depressions of cortical activity in acutely injured human brain. *Stroke* 2002;33:2738–2743.

49. Fabricius M, Fuhr S, Bhatia R, et al. Cortical spreading depression and peri-infarct depolarization in acutely injured human cerebral cortex. *Brain* 2006;129:778–790.

50. Hadjikhani N, Sanchez Del Rio M, Wu O, et al. Mechanisms of migraine aura revealed by functional MRI in human visual cortex. *Proc Natl Acad Sci U S A* 2001;98:4687–4692.

51. Pietrobon D, Moskowitz MA. Pathophysiology of migraine. *Annu Rev Physiol* 2013;75:365–391.

52. Dreier JP. The role of spreading depression, spreading depolarization and spreading ischemia in neurological disease. *Nat Med* 2011;17:439–447.

53. Kraig RP, Nicholson C. Extracellular ionic variations during spreading depression. *Neuroscience* 1978;3:1045–1059.

54. Largo C, Cuevas P, Somjen GG, Martin del Rio R, Herreras O. The effect of depressing glial function in rat brain in situ on ion homeostasis, synaptic transmission, and neuron survival. *J Neurosci* 1996;16:1219–1229.

55. Lauritzen M. Pathophysiology of the migraine aura. The spreading depression theory. *Brain* 1994;117 (Pt 1):199–210.

56. Mutch WA, Hansen AJ. Extracellular pH changes during spreading depression and cerebral ischemia: mechanisms of brain pH regulation. *J Cereb Blood Flow Metab* 1984;4:17–27.

57. Saito R, Graf R, Hubel K, Fujita T, Rosner G, Heiss WD. Reduction of infarct volume by halothane: effect on cerebral blood flow or perifocal spreading depression-like depolarizations. *J Cereb Blood Flow Metab* 1997;17:857–864.

58. Cohen MX. Where does EEG come from and what does it mean? *Trends Neurosci* 2017;40:208–218.

59. Lopes da Silva F. EEG and MEG: relevance to neuroscience. *Neuron* 2013;80:1112–1128.

60. Siegel M, Donner TH, Engel AK. Spectral fingerprints of large-scale neuronal interactions. *Nat Rev Neurosci* 2012;13:121–134.

61. Weiss SA, McKhann G, Jr., Goodman R, et al. Field effects and ictal synchronization: insights from in homine observations. *Front Human Neurosci* 2013;7:828.

62. Smith EH, Liou JY, Davis TS, et al. The ictal wavefront is the spatiotemporal source of discharges during spontaneous human seizures. *Nat Commun* 2016;7:11098.

63. Ingvar M. Cerebral blood flow and metabolic rate during seizures. Relationship to epileptic brain damage. *Ann N Y Acad Sci* 1986;462:194–206.

64. Uzum G, Sarper Diler A, Bahcekapili N, Ziya Ziylan Y. Erythropoietin prevents the increase in blood-brain barrier permeability during pentylentetrazol induced seizures. *Life Sci* 2006;78:2571–2576.

65. Miyamoto O, Auer RN. Hypoxia, hyperoxia, ischemia, and brain necrosis. *Neurology* 2000;54:362–371.

66. Sharp FR, Ran R, Lu A, et al. Hypoxic preconditioning protects against ischemic brain injury. *NeuroRx* 2004;1:26–35.

67. Siggaard-Andersen O, Ulrich A, Gothgen IH. Classes of tissue hypoxia. *Acta Anaesthesiol Scand Suppl* 1995;107:137–142.

68. Dengler J, Frenzel C, Vajkoczy P, Wolf S, Horn P. Cerebral tissue oxygenation measured by two different probes: challenges and interpretation. *Intensive Care Med* 2011;37:1809–1815.

69. Oddo M, Bosel J. Monitoring of brain and systemic oxygenation in neurocritical care patients. *Neurocrit Care* 2014;21(Suppl 2):S103–S120.

70. Claassen J, Perotte A, Albers D, et al. Nonconvulsive seizures after subarachnoid hemorrhage: multimodal detection and outcomes. *Ann Neurol* 2013;74:53–64.

71. Menzel M, Doppenberg EM, Zauner A, Soukup J, Reinert MM, Bullock R. Increased inspired oxygen concentration as a factor in improved brain tissue oxygenation and tissue lactate levels after severe human head injury. *J Neurosurg* 1999;91:1–10.

72. Meixensberger J, Jaeger M, Vath A, Dings J, Kunze E, Roosen K. Brain tissue oxygen guided treatment supplementing ICP/CPP therapy after traumatic brain injury. *J Neurol Neurosurg Psychiatry* 2003;74:760–764.

73. Rosenthal G, Hemphill JC 3rd, Sorani M, et al. Brain tissue oxygen tension is more indicative of oxygen diffusion than oxygen delivery and metabolism in patients with traumatic brain injury. *Crit Care Med* 2008;36:1917–1924.

74. James PB, Calder IM. Anoxic asphyxia: a cause of industrial fatalities: a review. *J Royal Soc Med* 1991;84:493–495.

75. Hossmann KA. The hypoxic brain. Insights from ischemia research. *Adv Exp Med Biol* 1999;474:155–169.

76. Czosnyka M, Smielewski P, Piechnik S, et al. Continuous assessment of cerebral autoregulation: clinical verification of the method in head injured patients. *Acta Neurochir Suppl* 2000;76:483–484.

77. Rosenthal G, Sanchez-Mejia RO, Phan N, Hemphill JC 3rd, Martin C, Manley GT. Incorporating a parenchymal thermal diffusion cerebral blood flow probe in bedside assessment of cerebral autoregulation and

vasoreactivity in patients with severe traumatic brain injury. *J Neurosurg* 2011;114:62–70.

78. Jaeger M, Schuhmann MU, Soehle M, Meixensberger J. Continuous assessment of cerebrovascular autoregulation after traumatic brain injury using brain tissue oxygen pressure reactivity. *Crit Care Med* 2006;34:1783–1788.

79. Strandgaard S, Paulson OB. Cerebral autoregulation. *Stroke* 1984;15:413–416.

80. Fleidervish IA, Gebhardt C, Astman N, Gutnick MJ, Heinemann U. Enhanced spontaneous transmitter release is the earliest consequence of neocortical hypoxia that can explain the disruption of normal circuit function. *J Neurosci* 2001;21:4600–4608.

81. Kao LW, Nanagas KA. Carbon monoxide poisoning. *Med Clin North Am* 2005;89:1161–1194.

82. Ries NL, Dart RC. New developments in antidotes. *Med Clin North Am* 2005;89:1379–1397.

83. Kern KB. Cardiopulmonary resuscitation without ventilation. *Crit Care Med* 2000;28:N186–N189.

84. Ewy GA, Zuercher M, Hilwig RW, et al. Improved neurological outcome with continuous chest compressions compared with 30:2 compressions-to-ventilations cardiopulmonary resuscitation in a realistic swine model of out-of-hospital cardiac arrest. *Circulation* 2007;116:2525–2530.

85. group S-Ks. Cardiopulmonary resuscitation by bystanders with chest compression only (SOS-KANTO): an observational study. *Lancet* 2007;369:920–926.

86. Hallstrom A, Cobb L, Johnson E, Copass M. Cardiopulmonary resuscitation by chest compression alone or with mouth-to-mouth ventilation. *N Engl J Med* 2000;342:1546–1553.

87. Sharp FR, Ran R, Lu A, et al. Hypoxic preconditioning protects against ischemic brain injury. *NeuroRx* 2004;1:26–35.

88. Miller TH, Kruse JE. Evaluation of syncope. *Am Fam Physician* 2005;72:1492–1500.

89. Georgiou M, Papathanassoglou E, Xanthos T. Systematic review of the mechanisms driving effective blood flow during adult CPR. *Resuscitation* 2014;85:1586–1593.

90. Tobin JM, Mihm FG. A hemodynamic profile for consciousness during cardiopulmonary resuscitation. *Anesth Analg* 2009;109:1598–1599.

91. Olaussen A, Nehme Z, Shepherd M, et al. Consciousness induced during cardiopulmonary resuscitation: An observational study. *Resuscitation* 2017;113:44–50.

92. Munoz X, Marti S, Sumalla J, Bosch J, Sampol G. Acute delirium as a manifestation of obstructive sleep apnea syndrome. *Am J Respir Crit Care Med* 1998;158:1306–1307.

93. Basnyat B, Wu T, Gertsch JH. Neurological conditions at altitude that fall outside the usual definition of altitude sickness. *High Alt Med Biol* 2004;5:171–179.

94. Vaughan CJ, Delanty N. Hypertensive emergencies. *Lancet* 2000;356:411–417.

95. Schwartz RB. Hyperperfusion encephalopathies: hypertensive encephalopathy and related conditions. *Neurologist* 2002;8:22–34.

96. Hinchey J, Chaves C, Appignani B, et al. A reversible posterior leukoencephalopathy syndrome. *N Engl J Med* 1996;334:494–500.

97. Garg RK. Posterior leukoencephalopathy syndrome. *Postgrad Med J* 2001;77:24–28.

98. Stott VL, Hurrell MA, Anderson TJ. Reversible posterior leukoencephalopathy syndrome: a misnomer reviewed. *Intern Med J* 2005;35:83–90.

99. Fugate JE, Rabinstein AA. Posterior reversible encephalopathy syndrome: clinical and radiological manifestations, pathophysiology, and outstanding questions. *Lancet Neurol* 2015;14:914–925.

100. Quick AM, Cipolla MJ. Pregnancy-induced up-regulation of aquaporin-4 protein in brain and its role in eclampsia. *Faseb J* 2005;19:170–175.

101. Schiff D, Lopes M-B. Neuropathological correlates of reversible posterior leukoencephalopathy. *Neurocrit Care* 2005;2:303–305.

102. Lavigne CM, Shrier DA, Ketkar M, Powers JM. Tacrolimus leukoencephalopathy: a neuropathologic confirmation. *Neurology* 2004;63:1132–1133.

103. Mak W, Chan KH, Cheung RTF, Ho SL. Hypertensive encephalopathy: BP lowering complicated by posterior circulation ischemic stroke. *Neurology* 2004;63:1131–1132.

104. Duley L, Gulmezoglu AM, Henderson-Smart DJ, Chou D. Magnesium sulphate and other anticonvulsants for women with pre-eclampsia. *Cochrane Database Syst Rev* 2010:CD000025.

105. Chan PS, McNally B, Tang F, Kellermann A, Group CS. Recent trends in survival from out-of-hospital cardiac arrest in the United States. *Circulation* 2014;130:1876–1882.

106. Levy DE, Caronna JJ, Singer BH, Lapinski RH, Frydman H, Plum F. Predicting outcome from hypoxic-ischemic coma. *JAMA* 1985;253:1420–1426.

107. Levy DE, Bates D, Caronna JJ, et al. Prognosis in nontraumatic coma. *Ann Intern Med* 1981;94:293–301.

108. Bassetti C, Bomio F, Mathis J, Hess CW. Early prognosis in coma after cardiac arrest: a prospective clinical, electrophysiological, and biochemical study of 60 patients. *J Neurol Neurosurg Psychiatry* 1996;61:610–615.

109. Efthymiou E, Renzel R, Baumann CR, Poryazova R, Imbach LL. Predictive value of EEG in postanoxic encephalopathy: A quantitative model-based approach. *Resuscitation* 2017;119:27–32.

110. Chandrasekaran PN, Dezfulian C, Polderman KH. What is the right temperature to cool post-cardiac arrest patients? *Crit Care* 2015;19:406.

111. Reynolds AS, Guo X, Matthews E, et al. Post-anoxic quantitative MRI changes may predict emergence from coma and functional outcomes at discharge. *Resuscitation* 2017;117:87–90.

112. Forgacs PB, Fridman EA, Goldfine AM, Schiff ND. Isolation syndrome after cardiac arrest and therapeutic hypothermia. *Front Neurosci* 2016;10:259.

113. Choi IS. Delayed neurologic sequelae in carbon monoxide intoxication. *Arch Neurol* 1983;40:433–435.

114. Kwon OY, Chung SP, Ha YR, Yoo IS, Kim SW. Delayed postanoxic encephalopathy after carbon monoxide poisoning. *Emerg Med J* 2004;21:250–251.

115. Gilmer B, Kilkenny J, Tomaszewski C, Watts JA. Hyperbaric oxygen does not prevent neurologic sequelae after carbon monoxide poisoning. *Acad Emerg Med* 2002;9:1–8.

116. Kim HY, Kim BJ, Moon SY, et al. Serial diffusion-weighted MR Imaging in delayed postanoxic encephalopathy. A case study. *J Neuroradiol* 2002;29:211–215.

117. Plum F, Posner JB, Hain RF. Delayed neurological deterioration after anoxia. *Arch Intern Med* 1962;110:18–25.

118. Takahashi W, Ohnuki Y, Takizawa S, et al. Neuroimaging on delayed postanoxic encephalopathy with lesions localized in basal ganglia. *Clin Imaging* 1998;22:188–191.

119. Weinberger LM, Schmidley JW, Schafer IA, Raghavan S. Delayed postanoxic demyelination and arylsulfatase-A pseudodeficiency. *Neurology* 1994;44:152–154.

120. Wijdicks EF, Parisi JE, Sharbrough FW. Prognostic value of myoclonus status in comatose survivors of cardiac arrest. *Ann Neurol* 1994;35:239–243.

121. Custodio CM, Basford JR. Delayed postanoxic encephalopathy: a case report and literature review. *Arch Phys Med Rehabil* 2004;85:502–505.

122. Elmer J, Rittenberger JC, Faro J, et al. Clinically distinct electroencephalographic phenotypes of early myoclonus after cardiac arrest. *Ann Neurol* 2016;80:175–184.

123. Seder DB, Sunde K, Rubertsson S, et al. Neurologic outcomes and postresuscitation care of patients with myoclonus following cardiac arrest. *Crit Care Med* 2015;43:965–972.

124. Reynolds AS, Rohaut B, Holmes MG, et al. Early myoclonus following anoxic brain injury. *Neurol Clin Pract* 2018;8:249–256.

125. Reynolds AS, Holmes MG, Agarwal S, Claassen J. Phenotypes of early myoclonus do not predict outcome. *Ann Neurol* 2017;81:475–476.

126. Wijdicks EFM, Hijdra A, Young GB, Bassetti CL, Wiebe S, Quality Standards Subcommittee of the American Academy of N. Practice parameter: prediction of outcome in comatose survivors after cardiopulmonary resuscitation (an evidence-based review): report of the Quality Standards Subcommittee of the American Academy of Neurology. *Neurology* 2006;67:203–210.

127. Thomke F, Marx JJ, Sauer O, et al. Observations on comatose survivors of cardiopulmonary resuscitation with generalized myoclonus. *BMC Neurol* 2005;5:14.

128. Rossetti AO, Oddo M, Logroscino G, Kaplan PW. Prognostication after cardiac arrest and hypothermia: a prospective study. *Ann Neurol* 2010;67:301–307.

129. Lucas JM, Cocchi MN, Salciccioli J, et al. Neurologic recovery after therapeutic hypothermia in patients with post-cardiac arrest myoclonus. *Resuscitation* 2012;83:265–269.

130. Bouwes A, van Poppelen D, Koelman JHTM, et al. Acute posthypoxic myoclonus after cardiopulmonary resuscitation. *BMC Neurol* 2012;12:63.

131. Elmer J, Torres C, Aufderheide TP, et al. Association of early withdrawal of life-sustaining therapy for perceived neurological prognosis with mortality after cardiac arrest. *Resuscitation* 2016;102:127–135.

132. Levy A, Chen R. Myoclonus: pathophysiology and treatment options. *Curr Treat Options Neurol* 2016;18:21.

133. Wijdicks EF, Young GB. Myoclonus status in comatose patients after cardiac arrest. *Lancet* 1994;343:1642–1643.

134. Werhahn KJ, Brown P, Thompson PD, Marsden CD. The clinical features and prognosis of chronic posthypoxic myoclonus. *Mov Disord* 1997;12:216–220.

135. Galldiks N, Timmermann L, Fink GR, Burghaus L. Posthypoxic myoclonus (Lance-Adams syndrome) treated with lacosamide. *Clin Neuropharmacol* 2010;33:216–217.

136. Buonocore G, Perrone S, Tataranno ML. Oxygen toxicity: chemistry and biology of reactive oxygen species. *Semin Fetal Neonatal Med* 2010;15:186–190.

137. Rincon F, Kang J, Maltenfort M, et al. Association between hyperoxia and mortality after stroke: a multicenter cohort study. *Crit Care Med* 2014;42:387–396.

138. Kilgannon JH, Jones AE, Shapiro NI, et al. Association between arterial hyperoxia following resuscitation from cardiac arrest and in-hospital mortality. *JAMA* 2010;303:2165–2171.

139. Beynon C, Kiening KL, Orakcioglu B, Unterberg AW, Sakowitz OW. Brain tissue oxygen monitoring and hyperoxic treatment in patients with traumatic brain injury. *J Neurotrauma* 2012;29:2109–2123.

140. Brenner M, Stein D, Hu P, Kufera J, Wooford M, Scalea T. Association between early hyperoxia and worse outcomes after traumatic brain injury. *Arch Surg* 2012;147:1042–1046.

141. Raj R, Bendel S, Reinikainen M, et al. Hyperoxemia and long-term outcome after traumatic brain injury. *Crit Care* 2013;17:R177.

142. Nortje J, Coles JP, Timofeev I, et al. Effect of hyperoxia on regional oxygenation and metabolism after severe traumatic brain injury: preliminary findings. *Crit Care Med* 2008;36:273–281.

143. Tisdall MM, Tachtsidis I, Leung TS, Elwell CE, Smith M. Increase in cerebral aerobic metabolism by normobaric hyperoxia after traumatic brain injury. *J Neurosurg* 2008;109:424–432.

144. Rockswold SB, Rockswold GL, Zaun DA, Liu J. A prospective, randomized Phase II clinical trial to evaluate the effect of combined hyperbaric and normobaric hyperoxia on cerebral metabolism, intracranial pressure, oxygen toxicity, and clinical outcome in severe traumatic brain injury. *J Neurosurg* 2013;118:1317–1328.

145. Becker LB. New concepts in reactive oxygen species and cardiovascular reperfusion physiology. *Cardiovasc Res* 2004;61:461–470.

146. Floyd TF, Clark JM, Gelfand R, et al. Independent cerebral vasoconstrictive effects of hyperoxia and accompanying arterial hypocapnia at 1 ATA. *J Appl Physiol* (1985) 2003;95:2453–2461.

147. Bitterman H. Bench-to-bedside review: oxygen as a drug. *Crit Care* 2009;13:205.

148. Gabriely I, Shamoon H. Hypoglycemia in diabetes: common, often unrecognized. *Cleve Clin J Med* 2004;71:335–342.

149. Hart SP, Frier BM. Causes, management and morbidity of acute hypoglycaemia in adults requiring hospital admission. *QJM* 1998;91:505–510.

150. Bhasin R, Arce FC, Pasmantier R. Hypoglycemia associated with the use of gatifloxacin. *Am J Med Sci* 2005;330:250–253.

151. Park-Wyllie LY, Juurlink DN, Kopp A, et al. Outpatient gatifloxacin therapy and dysglycemia in older adults. *N Engl J Med* 2006;354:1352–1361.

152. Pedersen-Bjergaard U, Reubsaet JL, Nielsen SL, et al. Psychoactive drugs, alcohol, and severe hypoglycemia in insulin-treated diabetes: analysis of 141 cases. *Am J Med* 2005;118:307–310.

153. Abarbanell NR. Is prehospital blood glucose measurement necessary in suspected cerebrovascular accident patients? *Am J Emerg Med* 2005;23:823–827.

154. Izzo JL, Schuster DB, Engel GL. The electroencephalogram of patients with diabetes mellitus. *Diabetes* 1953;2:93–99.

155. Kaufman FR, Epport K, Engilman R, Halvorson M. Neurocognitive functioning in children diagnosed with diabetes before age 10 years. *J Diabetes Complications* 1999;13:31–38.

156. Frier BM. Morbidity of hypoglycemia in type 1 diabetes. *Diabetes Res Clin Pract* 2004;65(Suppl 1):S47–S52.

157. Jung SL, Kim BS, Lee KS, Yoon KH, Byun JY. Magnetic resonance imaging and diffusion-weighted imaging changes after hypoglycemic coma. *J Neuroimaging* 2005;15:193–196.

158. Aoki T, Sato T, Hasegawa K, Ishizaki R, Saiki M. Reversible hyperintensity lesion on diffusion-weighted MRI in hypoglycemic coma. *Neurology* 2004;63:392–393.

159. Moore C, Woollard M. Dextrose 10% or 50% in the treatment of hypoglycaemia out of hospital? A randomised controlled trial. *Emerg Med J* 2005;22:512–515.

160. Ries NL, Dart RC. New developments in antidotes. *Med Clin North Am* 2005;89:1379–1397.

161. Wallis WE, Willoughby E, Baker P. Coma in the Wernicke-Korsakoff syndrome. *Lancet* 1978;2:400–401.

162. Victor M, Adams RD, Collins GH. The Wernicke-Korsakoff syndrome. A clinical and pathological study of 245 patients, 82 with post-mortem examinations. *Contemp Neurol Ser* 1971;7:1–206.

163. Koguchi K, Nakatsuji Y, Abe K, Sakoda S. Wernicke's encephalopathy after glucose infusion. *Neurology* 2004;62:512.

164. McEntee WJ. Wernicke's encephalopathy: an excitotoxicity hypothesis. *Metab Brain Dis* 1997;12:183–192.

165. Hazell AS, Todd KG, Butterworth RF. Mechanisms of neuronal cell death in Wernicke's encephalopathy. *Metab Brain Dis* 1998;13:97–122.

166. Mousseau DD, Rao VL, Butterworth RF. Alterations in serotonin parameters in brain of thiamine-deficient rats are evident prior to the appearance of neurological symptoms. *J Neurochem* 1996;67:1113–1123.

167. Waldenlind L. Studies on thiamine and neuromuscular transmission. *Acta Physiol Scand Suppl* 1978;459:1–35.

168. Pepersack T, Garbusinski J, Robberecht J, Beyer I, Willems D, Fuss M. Clinical relevance of thiamine status amongst hospitalized elderly patients. *Gerontology* 1999;45:96–101.

169. Sechi G, Serra A. Wernicke's encephalopathy: new clinical settings and recent advances in diagnosis and management. *Lancet Neurol* 2007;6:442–455.

170. Halavaara J, Brander A, Lyytinen J, Setala K, Kallela M. Wernicke's encephalopathy: is diffusion-weighted MRI useful? *Neuroradiology* 2003;45:519–523.

171. Loh Y, Watson WD, Verma A, Krapiva P. Restricted diffusion of the splenium in acute Wernicke's encephalopathy. *J Neuroimaging* 2005;15:373–375.

172. Lee ST, Jung YM, Na DL, Park SH, Kim M. Corpus callosum atrophy in Wernicke's encephalopathy. *J Neuroimaging* 2005;15:367–372.

173. Gerards M, Sallevelt SC, Smeets HJ. Leigh syndrome: resolving the clinical and genetic heterogeneity paves the way for treatment options. *Mol Genet Metab* 2016;117:300–312.

174. Denier C, Balu L, Husson B, et al. Familial acute necrotizing encephalopathy due to mutation in the RANBP2 gene. *J Neurol Sci* 2014;345:236–238.

175. Fulham M, Lawrence C, Harper C. Diagnostic clues in an adult case of Leigh's disease. *Med J Aust* 1988;149:320–322.

176. Fraser CL, Arieff AI. Epidemiology, pathophysiology, and management of hyponatremic encephalopathy. *Am J Med* 1997;102:67–77.

177. Moritz ML, Ayus JC. The pathophysiology and treatment of hyponatraemic encephalopathy: an update. *Nephrol Dial Transplant* 2003;18:2486–2491.

178. Pasantes-Morales H, Franco R, Ordaz B, Ochoa LD. Mechanisms counteracting swelling in brain cells during hyponatremia. *Arch Med Res* 2002;33:237–244.

179. Schwartz WB, Bennett W, Curelop S, Bartter FC. A syndrome of renal sodium loss and hyponatremia probably resulting from inappropriate secretion of antidiuretic hormone. *Am J Med* 1957;23:529–542.

180. Peters JP, Welt LG, Sims EAH, Orloff J, Needham J. A salt-wasting syndrome associated with cerebral disease. *Trans Assoc Am Physicians* 1950;63:57–64.

181. Sherlock M, O'Sullivan E, Agha A, et al. Incidence and pathophysiology of severe hyponatraemia in neurosurgical patients. *Postgrad Med J* 2009;85:171–175.

182. Cuesta M, Hannon MJ, Thompson CJ. Diagnosis and treatment of hyponatraemia in neurosurgical patients. *Endocrinol Nutr* 2016;63:230–238.

183. Sterns RH, Hix JK, Silver SM. Management of hyponatremia in the ICU. *Chest* 2013;144:672–679.

184. Sterns RH, Riggs JE, Schochet SS, Jr. Osmotic demyelination syndrome following correction of hyponatremia. *N Engl J Med* 1986;314:1535–1542.

185. Cort JH. Cerebral salt wasting. *Lancet* 1954;266:752–754.

186. Mapa B, Taylor BES, Appelboom G, Bruce EM, Claassen J, Connolly ES, Jr. Impact of hyponatremia on morbidity, mortality, and complications after aneurysmal subarachnoid hemorrhage: a systematic review. *World Neurosurg* 2016;85:305–314.

187. Kalita J, Singh RK, Misra UK. Cerebral salt wasting is the most common cause of hyponatremia in stroke. *J Stroke Cerebrovasc Dis* 2017;26:1026–1032.

188. Chung HM, Kluge R, Schrier RW, Anderson RJ. Clinical assessment of extracellular fluid volume in hyponatremia. *Am J Med* 1987;83:905–908.

189. Sterns RH, Silver SM. Cerebral salt wasting versus SIADH: what difference? *J Am Soc Nephrol* 2008;19:194–196.

190. Massieu L, Montiel T, Robles G, Quesada O. Brain amino acids during hyponatremia in vivo: clinical observations and experimental studies. *Neurochem Res* 2004;29:73–81.

191. Hsu Y-J, Chiu J-S, Lu K-C, Chau T, Lin S-H. Biochemical and etiological characteristics of acute hyponatremia in the emergency department. *J Emerg Med* 2005;29:369–374.

192. Mooradian AD, Morley GK, McGeachie R, Lundgren S, Morley JE. Spontaneous periodic hypothermia. *Neurology* 1984;34:79–82.

193. Moon Y, Hong SJ, Shin D, Jung Y. Increased aquaporin-1 expression in choroid plexus

epithelium after systemic hyponatremia. *Neurosci Lett* 2006;395:1–6.

194. Vajda Z, Promeneur D, Doczi T, et al. Increased aquaporin-4 immunoreactivity in rat brain in response to systemic hyponatremia. *Biochem Biophys Res Commun* 2000;270:495–503.

195. Lee JJY, Kilonzo K, Nistico A, Yeates K. Management of hyponatremia. *Can Med Assoc J* 2014;186:E281–E286.

196. Jeon S-B, Choi HA, Lesch C, et al. Use of oral vasopressin V2 receptor antagonist for hyponatremia in acute brain injury. *Eur Neurol* 2013;70:142–148.

197. Wijdicks EF, Vermeulen M, Hijdra A, van Gijn J. Hyponatremia and cerebral infarction in patients with ruptured intracranial aneurysms: is fluid restriction harmful? *Ann Neurol* 1985;17:137–140.

198. Rosenwasser RH, Delgado TE, Buchheit WA, Freed MH. Control of hypertension and prophylaxis against vasospasm in cases of subarachnoid hemorrhage: a preliminary report. *Neurosurgery* 1983;12:658–661.

199. Froelich M, Ni Q, Wess C, Ougorets I, Hartl R. Continuous hypertonic saline therapy and the occurrence of complications in neurocritically ill patients. *Crit Care Med* 2009;37:1433–1441.

200. Aiyagari V, Deibert E, Diringer MN. Hypernatremia in the neurologic intensive care unit: how high is too high? *J Crit Care* 2006;21:163–172.

201. Lin M, Liu SJ, Lim IT. Disorders of water imbalance. *Emerg Med Clin North Am* 2005;23:749–770, ix.

202. Torchinsky MY, Deputy S, Rambeau F, Chalew SA. Hypokalemia and alkalosis in adipsic hypernatremia are not associated with hyperaldosteronism. *Horm Res* 2004;62:187–190.

203. Doyle JA, Davis DP, Hoyt DB. The use of hypertonic saline in the treatment of traumatic brain injury. *J Trauma* 2001;50:367–383.

204. Spatenkova V, Bradac O, Kazda A, Suchomel P. Central diabetes insipidus is not a common and prognostically worse type of hypernatremia in neurointensive care. *Neuro Endocrinol Lett* 2011;32:879–884.

205. Weed LH, McKibben PS. Pressure changes in the cerebro-spinal fluid following intravenous injection of solutions of various concentrations. *Am J Physiol* 1919;48:512–530.

206. Huang L, Cao W, Deng Y, Zhu G, Han Y, Zeng H. Hypertonic saline alleviates experimentally induced cerebral oedema through suppression of vascular endothelial growth factor and its receptor VEGFR2 expression in astrocytes. *BMC Neurosci* 2016;17:64.

207. Huang LQ, Zhu GF, Deng YY, et al. Hypertonic saline alleviates cerebral edema by inhibiting microglia-derived TNF-alpha and IL-1beta-induced Na-K-Cl Cotransporter up-regulation. *J Neuroinflammation* 2014;11:102.

208. Nakayama S, Migliati E, Amiry-Moghaddam M, Ottersen OP, Bhardwaj A. Osmotherapy with hypertonic saline attenuates global cerebral edema following experimental cardiac arrest via perivascular pool of Aquaporin-4. *Crit Care Med* 2016;44:e702–e710.

209. Wolf AL, Levi L, Marmarou A, et al. Effect of THAM upon outcome in severe head injury: a randomized prospective clinical trial. *J Neurosurg* 1993;78:54–59.

210. Zeiler FA, Teitelbaum J, Gillman LM, West M. THAM for control of ICP. *Neurocrit Care* 2014;21:332–344.

211. Tan SK, Kolmodin L, Sekhon MS, et al. The effect of continuous hypertonic saline infusion and hypernatremia on mortality in patients with severe traumatic brain injury: a retrospective cohort study. *Can J Anaesth* 2016;63:664–673.

212. Wartenberg KE, Schmidt JM, Claassen J, et al. Impact of medical complications on outcome after subarachnoid hemorrhage. *Crit Care Med* 2006;34:617–623; quiz 24.

213. Lantigua H, Ortega-Gutierrez S, Schmidt JM, et al. Subarachnoid hemorrhage: who dies, and why? *Crit Care* 2015;19:309.

214. Kumar AB, Shi Y, Shotwell MS, Richards J, Ehrenfeld JM. Hypernatremia is a significant risk factor for acute kidney injury after subarachnoid hemorrhage: a retrospective analysis. *Neurocrit Care* 2015;22:184–191.

215. Torchinsky MY, Deputy S, Rambeau F, Chalew SA. Hypokalemia and alkalosis in adipsic hypernatremia are not associated with hyperaldosteronism. *Hormone research* 2004;62:187–190.

216. Kang S-K, Kim W, Oh MS. Pathogenesis and treatment of hypernatremia. *Nephron* 2002;92(Suppl 1):14–17.

217. Lien YH, Shapiro JI, Chan L. Effects of hypernatremia on organic brain osmoles. *J Clin Invest* 1990;85:1427–1435.

218. Patten BM, Pages M. Severe neurological disease associated with hyperparathyroidism. *Ann Neurol* 1984;15:453–456.

219. Ohrvall U, Akerstrom G, Ljunghall S, Lundgren E, Juhlin C, Rastad J. Surgery for sporadic primary hyperparathyroidism in the elderly. *World J Surg* 1994;18:612–618.

220. Nakajima N, Ueda M, Nagayama H, Yamazaki M, Katayama Y. Posterior reversible encephalopathy syndrome due to hypercalcemia associated with parathyroid hormone-related peptide: a case report and review of the literature. *Intern Med* 2013;52:2465–2468.

221. Kastrup O, Maschke M, Wanke I, Diener HC. Posterior reversible encephalopathy syndrome due to severe hypercalcemia. *J Neurol* 2002;249:1563–1566.

222. Clines GA, Guise TA. Hypercalcaemia of malignancy and basic research on mechanisms responsible for osteolytic and osteoblastic metastasis to bone. *Endocr Relat Cancer* 2005;12:549–583.

223. Mrowka M, Knake S, Klinge H, Odin P, Rosenow F. Hypocalcemic generalised seizures as a manifestation of iatrogenic hypoparathyroidism months to years after thyroid surgery. *Epileptic Disord* 2004;6:85–87.

224. Sheldon RS, Becker WJ, Hanley DA, Culver RL. Hypoparathyroidism and pseudotumor cerebri: an infrequent clinical association. *Can J Neurol Sci* 1987;14:622–625.

225. Riggs JE. Neurologic manifestations of electrolyte disturbances. *Neurol Clin* 2002;20:227–239, vii.

226. Kirsch DB, Jozefowicz RF. Neurologic complications of respiratory disease. *Neurol Clin* 2002;20:247–264, viii.

227. Curley GF, Laffey JG. Acidosis in the critically ill—balancing risks and benefits to optimize outcome. *Crit Care* 2014;18:129.

228. Yokota H, Yamamoto Y, Naoe Y, et al. Measurements of cortical cellular pH by intracranial tonometer in severe head injury. *Crit Care Med* 2000;28:3275–3280.

229. Landolt H, Langemann H, Gratzl O. On-line monitoring of cerebral pH by microdialysis. *Neurosurgery* 1993;32:1000–1004; discussion 1004.

230. Langemann H, Mendelowitsch A, Landolt H, Alessandri B, Gratzl O. Experimental and clinical monitoring of glucose by microdialysis. *Clin Neurol Neurosurg* 1995;97:149–155.

231. Landolt H, Langemann H, Mendelowitsch A, Gratzl O. Neurochemical monitoring and on-line pH measurements using brain microdialysis in patients in intensive care. *Acta Neurochir Suppl (Wien)* 1994;60:475–478.

232. Baron JC, Rougemont D, Soussaline F, et al. Local interrelationships of cerebral oxygen consumption and glucose utilization in normal subjects and in ischemic stroke patients: a positron tomography study. *J Cereb Blood Flow Metab* 1984;4:140–149.

233. Marmarou A, Holdaway R, Ward JD, et al. Traumatic brain tissue acidosis: experimental and clinical studies. *Acta Neurochir Suppl (Wien)* 1993;57:160–164.

234. Rango M, Lenkinski RE, Alves WM, Cruz J, Gennarelli TA. Brain pH in acute head injury. *Minerva Anestesiol* 1993;59:835–836.

235. Qureshi AI, Suarez JI, Bhardwaj A, et al. Use of hypertonic (3%) saline/acetate infusion in the treatment of cerebral edema: effect on intracranial pressure and lateral displacement of the brain. *Crit Care Med* 1998;26:440–446.

236. Schwarz S, Georgiadis D, Aschoff A, Schwab S. Effects of hypertonic (10%) saline in patients with raised intracranial pressure after stroke. *Stroke* 2002;33:136–140.

237. Young RS, Yagel SK, Woods CL. The effects of sodium bicarbonate on brain blood flow, brain water content, and blood-brain barrier in the neonatal dog. *Acta Neuropathol* 1984;65:124–127.

238. Schieve JF, Wilson WP. The changes in cerebral vascular resistance of man in experimental alkalosis and acidosis. *J Clin Invest* 1953;32:33–38.

239. Nakashima K, Yamashita T, Kashiwagi S, Nakayama N, Kitahara T, Ito H. The effect of sodium bicarbonate on CBF and intracellular pH in man: stable Xe-CT and 31P-MRS. *Acta Neurol Scand Suppl* 1996;166:96–98.

240. Foster GT, Vaziri ND, Sassoon CS. Respiratory alkalosis. *Respir Care* 2001;46:384–391.

241. Faden A. Encephalopathy following treatment of chronic pulmonary failure. *Neurology* 1976;26:337–339.

242. Khanna A, Kurtzman NA. Metabolic alkalosis. *Respir Care* 2001;46:354–365.

243. Holland AE, Wilson JW, Kotsimbos TC, Naughton MT. Metabolic alkalosis contributes to acute hypercapnic respiratory failure in adult cystic fibrosis. *Chest* 2003;124:490–493.

244. Klein JP, Waxman SG. The brain in diabetes: molecular changes in neurons and their implications for end-organ damage. *Lancet Neurol* 2003;2:548–554.

245. Payne RS, Tseng MT, Schurr A. The glucose paradox of cerebral ischemia: evidence for corticosterone involvement. *Brain Res* 2003;971:9–17.

246. Cox DJ, Kovatchev BP, Gonder-Frederick LA, et al. Relationships between hyperglycemia and cognitive performance among adults with type 1 and type 2 diabetes. *Diabetes Care* 2005;28:71–77.

247. Aigner A, Grittner U, Rolfs A, Norrving B, Siegerink B, Busch MA. Contribution of established stroke risk factors to the burden of stroke in young adults. *Stroke* 2017;48:1744–1751.

248. O'Donnell MJ, Chin SL, Rangarajan S, et al. Global and regional effects of potentially modifiable risk factors associated with acute stroke in 32 countries (INTERSTROKE): a case-control study. *Lancet* 2016;388:761–775.

249. Rabinstein AA. Hyperglycemia in critical illness: lessons from NICE-SUGAR. *Neurocrit Care* 2009;11:131–132.

250. Baird TA, Parsons MW, Phan T, et al. Persistent poststroke hyperglycemia is independently associated with infarct expansion and worse clinical outcome. *Stroke* 2003;34:2208–2214.

251. Pulsinelli WA, Levy DE, Sigsbee B, Scherer P, Plum F. Increased damage after ischemic stroke in patients with hyperglycemia with or without established diabetes mellitus. *Am J Med* 1983;74:540–544.

252. Frontera JA, Fernandez A, Claassen J, et al. Hyperglycemia after SAH: predictors, associated complications, and impact on outcome. *Stroke* 2006;37:199–203.

253. van den Berghe G, Wouters P, Weekers F, et al. Intensive insulin therapy in critically ill patients. *N Engl J Med* 2001;345:1359–1367.

254. Van den Berghe G, Wilmer A, Hermans G, et al. Intensive insulin therapy in the medical ICU. *N Engl J Med* 2006;354:449–461.

255. Rady MY, Johnson DJ, Patel BM, Larson JS, Helmers RA. Influence of individual characteristics on outcome of glycemic control in intensive care unit patients with or without diabetes mellitus. *Mayo Clin Proc* 2005;80:1558–1567.

256. Investigators N-SS, Finfer S, Chittock DR, et al. Intensive versus conventional glucose control in critically ill patients. *N Engl J Med* 2009;360:1283–1297.

257. Australian N-SSIft, New Zealand Intensive Care Society Clinical Trials Group, the Canadian Critical Care Trials Group, et al. Intensive versus conventional glucose control in critically ill patients with traumatic brain injury: long-term follow-up of a subgroup of patients from the NICE-SUGAR study. *Intensive Care Med* 2015;41:1037–1047.

258. Oddo M, Schmidt JM, Carrera E, et al. Impact of tight glycemic control on cerebral glucose metabolism after severe brain injury: a microdialysis study. *Crit Care Med* 2008;36:3233–3238.

259. Vespa P, Boonyaputthikul R, McArthur DL, et al. Intensive insulin therapy reduces microdialysis glucose values without altering glucose utilization or improving the lactate/pyruvate ratio after traumatic brain injury. *Crit Care Med* 2006;34:850–856.

260. Helbok R, Schmidt JM, Kurtz P, et al. Systemic glucose and brain energy metabolism after subarachnoid hemorrhage. *Neurocrit Care* 2010;12:317–323.

261. Kurtz P, Claassen J, Helbok R, et al. Systemic glucose variability predicts cerebral metabolic distress and mortality after subarachnoid hemorrhage: a retrospective observational study. *Crit Care* 2014;18:R89.

262. Diringer MN, Bleck TP, Claude Hemphill J 3rd, et al. Critical care management of patients following aneurysmal subarachnoid hemorrhage: recommendations from the Neurocritical Care Society's Multidisciplinary Consensus Conference. *Neurocrit Care* 2011;15:211–240.

263. Schmutzhard E, Rabinstein AA; Participants in the International Multi-Disciplinary Consensus

Conference on the Critical Care Management of Subarachnoid Hemorrhage, et al. Spontaneous subarachnoid hemorrhage and glucose management. *Neurocrit Care* 2011;15:281–286.

264. Schmidt JM, Claassen J, Ko S-B, et al. Nutritional support and brain tissue glucose metabolism in poor-grade SAH: a retrospective observational study. *Crit Care* 2012;16:R15.

265. Rehncrona S. Brain acidosis. *Ann Emerg Med* 1985;14:770–776.

266. Gallagher CN, Carpenter KLH, Grice P, et al. The human brain utilizes lactate via the tricarboxylic acid cycle: a 13C-labelled microdialysis and high-resolution nuclear magnetic resonance study. *Brain* 2009;132:2839–2849.

267. Schurr A, Payne RS, Miller JJ, Tseng MT. Preischemic hyperglycemia-aggravated damage: evidence that lactate utilization is beneficial and glucose-induced corticosterone release is detrimental. *J Neurosci Res* 2001;66:782–789.

268. Li PA, He QP, Csiszar K, Siesjo BK. Does long-term glucose infusion reduce brain damage after transient cerebral ischemia? *Brain Res* 2001;912:203–205.

269. McKeown NJ, Tews MC, Gossain VV, Shah SM. Hyperthyroidism. *Emerg Med Clin N Am* 2005;23:669–685, viii.

270. Tews MC, Shah SM, Gossain VV. Hypothyroidism: mimicker of common complaints. *Emerg Med Clin N Am* 2005;23:649–667, vii.

271. Bauer M, Goetz T, Glenn T, Whybrow PC. The thyroid-brain interaction in thyroid disorders and mood disorders. *J Neuroendocrinol* 2008;20:1101–1114.

272. Konig S, Moura Neto V. Thyroid hormone actions on neural cells. *Cell Mol Neurobiol* 2002;22:517–544.

273. Desouza LA, Ladiwala U, Daniel SM, Agashe S, Vaidya RA, Vaidya VA. Thyroid hormone regulates hippocampal neurogenesis in the adult rat brain. *Mol Cell Neurosci* 2005;29:414–426.

274. Constant EL, de Volder AG, Ivanoiu A, et al. Cerebral blood flow and glucose metabolism in hypothyroidism: a positron emission tomography study. *J Clin Endocrinol Metab* 2001;86:3864–3870.

275. Kwaku MP, Burman KD. Myxedema coma. *J Intensive Care Med* 2007;22:224–231.

276. Mathew V, Misgar RA, Ghosh S, et al. Myxedema coma: a new look into an old crisis. *J Thyroid Res* 2011;2011:493462.

277. Pimentel L, Hansen KN. Thyroid disease in the emergency department: a clinical and laboratory review. *J Emerg Med* 2005;28:201–209.

278. Savage MW, Mah PM, Weetman AP, Newell-Price J. Endocrine emergencies. *Postgrad Med J* 2004;80:506–515.

279. Rodriguez I, Fluiters E, Perez-Mendez LF, Luna R, Paramo C, Garcia-Mayor RV. Factors associated with mortality of patients with myxoedema coma: prospective study in 11 cases treated in a single institution. *J Endocrinol* 2004;180:347–350.

280. Reinhardt W, Mann K. Haufigkeit, klinisches Bild und Behandlung des hypothyreoten Komas. Ergebnis einer Umfrage [Incidence, clinical picture and treatment of hypothyroid coma. Results of a survey]. *Med Klin (Munich)* 1997;92:521–524.

281. Dutta P, Bhansali A, Masoodi SR, Bhadada S, Sharma N, Rajput R. Predictors of outcome in myxoedema coma: a study from a tertiary care centre. *Crit Care* 2008;12:R1.

282. Wartofsky L. Myxedema coma. *Endocrinol Metab Clin North Am* 2006;35:687–698, vii-viii.

283. Yamamoto T, Fukuyama J, Fujiyoshi A. Factors associated with mortality of myxedema coma: report of eight cases and literature survey. *Thyroid* 1999;9:1167–1174.

284. River Y, Zelig O. Triphasic waves in myxedema coma. *Clin Electroencephalogr* 1993;24:146–150.

285. Pohunkova D, Sulc J, Vana S. Influence of thyroid hormone supply on EEG frequency spectrum. *Endocrinol Exp* 1989;23:251–258.

286. Bauer M, Silverman DHS, Schlagenhauf F, et al. Brain glucose metabolism in hypothyroidism: a positron emission tomography study before and after thyroid hormone replacement therapy. *J Clin Endocrinol Metab* 2009;94:2922–2929.

287. Massumi RA, Winnacker JL. Severe depression of the respiratory center in myxedema. *Am J Med* 1964;36:876–882.

288. Chen Y-C, Cadnapaphornchai MA, Yang J, et al. Nonosmotic release of vasopressin and renal aquaporins in impaired urinary dilution in hypothyroidism. *Am J Physiol Renal Physiol* 2005;289:F672–F678.

289. Castillo P, Woodruff B, Caselli R, et al. Steroid-responsive encephalopathy associated with autoimmune thyroiditis. *Arch Neurol* 2006;63:197–202.

290. Ferracci F, Bertiato G, Moretto G. Hashimoto's encephalopathy: epidemiologic data and pathogenetic considerations. *J Neurol Sci* 2004;217:165–168.

291. Chong JY, Rowland LP, Utiger RD. Hashimoto encephalopathy: syndrome or myth? *Arch Neurol* 2003;60:164–171.

292. Zhou JY, Xu B, Lopes J, Blamoun J, Li L. Hashimoto encephalopathy: literature review. *Acta Neurol Scand* 2017;135:285–290.

293. Oide T, Tokuda T, Yazaki M, et al. Anti-neuronal autoantibody in Hashimoto's encephalopathy: neuropathological, immunohistochemical, and biochemical analysis of two patients. *J Neurol Sci* 2004;217:7–12.

294. Schauble B, Castillo PR, Boeve BF, Westmoreland BF. EEG findings in steroid-responsive encephalopathy associated with autoimmune thyroiditis. *Clin Neurophysiol* 2003;114:32–37.

295. Chiha M, Samarasinghe S, Kabaker AS. Thyroid storm: an updated review. *J Intensive Care Med* 2015;30:131–140.

296. Ishii M. Endocrine emergencies with neurologic manifestations. *Continuum (Minneap Minn)* 2017;23:778–801.

297. Ghobrial MW, Ruby EB. Coma and thyroid storm in apathetic thyrotoxicosis. *South Med J* 2002;95:552–554.

298. Bailes BK. Hyperthyroidism in elderly patients. *AORN J* 1999;69:254–258.

299. Lee TG, Ha CK, Lim BH. Thyroid storm presenting as status epilepticus and stroke. *Postgrad Med J* 1997;73:61.

300. Torrey SP. Recognition and management of adrenal emergencies. *Emerg Med Clin North Am* 2005;23:687–702, viii.

301. Hahner S, Spinnler C, Fassnacht M, et al. High incidence of adrenal crisis in educated patients with chronic adrenal insufficiency: a prospective study. *J Clin Endocrinol Metab* 2015;100:407–416.

302. Arlt W, Allolio B. Adrenal insufficiency. *Lancet* 2003;361:1881–1893.

303. Ten S, New M, Maclaren N. Clinical review 130: Addison's disease 2001. *J Clin Endocrinol Metab* 2001;86:2909–2922.

304. Espinosa G, Santos E, Cervera R, et al. Adrenal involvement in the antiphospholipid syndrome: clinical and immunologic characteristics of 86 patients. *Medicine (Baltimore)* 2003;82:106–118.

305. Bertorini TE, Perez A. Neurologic complications of disorders of the adrenal glands. *Handb Clin Neurol* 2014;120:749–771.

306. Kaplan PW. The EEG in metabolic encephalopathy and coma. *J Clin Neurophysiol* 2004;21:307–318.

307. Bancos I, Hahner S, Tomlinson J, Arlt W. Diagnosis and management of adrenal insufficiency. *Lancet Diabetes Endocrinol* 2015;3:216–226.

308. Puar TH, Stikkelbroeck NM, Smans LC, Zelissen PM, Hermus AR. Adrenal crisis: still a deadly event in the 21st century. *Am J Med* 2016;129:339 e1–9.

309. Morrison SF, Nakamura K. Central mechanisms for thermoregulation. *Annu Rev Physiol* 2018.

310. Machado NLS, Abbott SBG, Resch JM, et al. A glutamatergic hypothalamomedullary circuit mediates thermogenesis, but not heat conservation, during stress-induced hyperthermia. *Curr Biol* 2018;28:2291–2301 e5.

311. Jastroch M, Giroud S, Barrett P, Geiser F, Heldmaier G, Herwig A. Seasonal control of mammalian energy balance: recent advances in the understanding of daily torpor and hibernation. *J Neuroendocrinol* 2016;28(11).

312. Oishi Y, Yoshida K, Scammell TE, Urade Y, Lazarus M, Saper CB. The roles of prostaglandin E2 and D2 in lipopolysaccharide-mediated changes in sleep. *Brain Behav Immun* 2015;47:172–177.

313. Kluger MJ, Kozak W, Conn CA, Leon LR, Soszynski D. The adaptive value of fever. *Infect Dis Clin North Am* 1996;10:1–20.

314. Saper CB, Romanovsky AA, Scammell TE. Neural circuitry engaged by prostaglandins during the sickness syndrome. *Nat Neurosci* 2012;15:1088–1095.

315. Elmquist JK, Scammell TE, Saper CB. Mechanisms of CNS response to systemic immune challenge: the febrile response. *Trends Neurosci* 1997;20:565–570.

316. Scammell TE, Griffin JD, Elmquist JK, Saper CB. Microinjection of a cyclooxygenase inhibitor into the anteroventral preoptic region attenuates LPS fever. *Am J Physiol* 1998;274:R783–R789.

317. Lazarus M, Yoshida K, Coppari R, et al. EP3 prostaglandin receptors in the median preoptic nucleus are critical for fever responses. *Nat Neurosci* 2007;10:1131–1133.

318. Fernandez A, Schmidt JM, Claassen J, et al. Fever after subarachnoid hemorrhage: risk factors and impact on outcome. *Neurology* 2007;68(13):1013–1019.

319. Bao L, Chen D, Ding L, Ling W, Xu F. Fever burden isan independent predictor for prognosis of traumatic brain injury. *PloS One* 2014;9(3):e90956.

320. Laino D, Mencaroni E, Esposito S. Management of pediatric febrile seizures. *Int J Environ Res Public Health* 2018;15(10):2232.

321. Hifumi T, Kondo Y, Shimizu K, Miyake Y. Heat stroke. *J Intensive Care* 2018;6:30.

322. Blumenfeld H. Impaired consciousness in epilepsy. *Lancet Neurol* 2012;11:814–826.

323. Mazarati AM, Baldwin RA, Sankar R, Wasterlain CG. Time-dependent decrease in the effectiveness of antiepileptic drugs during the course of self-sustaining status epilepticus. *Brain Res* 1998;814:179–185.

324. Kapur J, Macdonald RL. Rapid seizure-induced reduction of benzodiazepine and Zn2+ sensitivity of hippocampal dentate granule cell GABAA receptors. *J Neurosci* 1997;17:7532–7540.

325. Chen JW, Wasterlain CG. Status epilepticus: pathophysiology and management in adults. *Lancet Neurol* 2006;5:246–256.

326. Bahar S, Suh M, Zhao M, Schwartz TH. Intrinsic optical signal imaging of neocortical seizures: the 'epileptic dip'. *Neuroreport* 2006;17:499–503.

327. Zhao M, Nguyen J, Ma H, Nishimura N, Schaffer CB, Schwartz TH. Preictal and ictal neurovascular and metabolic coupling surrounding a seizure focus. *J Neurosci* 2011;31:13292–13300.

328. Geneslaw AS, Zhao M, Ma H, Schwartz TH. Tissue hypoxia correlates with intensity of interictal spikes. *J Cereb Blood Flow Metab* 2011;31:1394–402.

329. During MJ, Spencer DD. Extracellular hippocampal glutamate and spontaneous seizure in the conscious human brain. *Lancet* 1993;341:1607–1610.

330. Cavus I, Pan JW, Hetherington HP, et al. Decreased hippocampal volume on MRI is associated with increased extracellular glutamate in epilepsy patients. *Epilepsia* 2008;49:1358–1366.

331. Cavus I, Kasoff WS, Cassaday MP, et al. Extracellular metabolites in the cortex and hippocampus of epileptic patients. *Ann Neurol* 2005;57:226–235.

332. Zhao M, Suh M, Ma H, Perry C, Geneslaw A, Schwartz TH. Focal increases in perfusion and decreases in hemoglobin oxygenation precede seizure onset in spontaneous human epilepsy. *Epilepsia* 2007;48:2059–2067.

333. Enev M, McNally KA, Varghese G, Zubal IG, Ostroff RB, Blumenfeld H. Imaging onset and propagation of ECT-induced seizures. *Epilepsia* 2007;48:238–244.

334. Takano H, Motohashi N, Uema T, et al. Changes in regional cerebral blood flow during acute electroconvulsive therapy in patients with depression: positron emission tomographic study. *Br J Psychiatry* 2007;190:63–68.

335. Blumenfeld H, Varghese GI, Purcaro MJ, et al. Cortical and subcortical networks in human secondarily generalized tonic-clonic seizures. *Brain* 2009;132:999–1012.

336. Schridde U, Khubchandani M, Motelow JE, Sanganahalli BG, Hyder F, Blumenfeld H. Negative BOLD with large increases in neuronal activity. *Cereb Cortex* 2008;18:1814–1827.

337. DeLorenzo RJ, Waterhouse EJ, Towne AR, et al. Persistent nonconvulsive status epilepticus after the control of convulsive status epilepticus. *Epilepsia* 1998;39:833–840.

338. Claassen J, Mayer SA, Kowalski RG, Emerson RG, Hirsch LJ. Detection of electrographic seizures with

continuous EEG monitoring in critically ill patients. *Neurology* 2004;62:1743–1748.

339. Kurtz P, Gaspard N, Wahl AS, et al. Continuous electroencephalography in a surgical intensive care unit. *Intensive Care Med* 2014;40:228–234.

340. Oddo M, Carrera E, Claassen J, Mayer SA, Hirsch LJ. Continuous electroencephalography in the medical intensive care unit. *Crit Care Med* 2009;37:2051–2056.

341. Towne AR, Waterhouse EJ, Boggs JG, et al. Prevalence of nonconvulsive status epilepticus in comatose patients. *Neurology* 2000;54:340–345.

342. Tomson T, Lindbom U, Nilsson BY. Nonconvulsive status epilepticus in adults: thirty-two consecutive patients from a general hospital population. *Epilepsia* 1992;33:829–835.

343. Husain AM, Horn GJ, Jacobson MP. Non-convulsive status epilepticus: usefulness of clinical features in selecting patients for urgent EEG. *J Neurol Neurosurg Psychiatry* 2003;74:189–191.

344. Brenner RP. EEG in convulsive and nonconvulsive status epilepticus. *J Clin Neurophysiol* 2004;21:319–331.

345. Rabinowicz AL, Correale JD, Bracht KA, Smith TD, DeGiorgio CM. Neuron-specific enolase is increased after nonconvulsive status epilepticus. *Epilepsia* 1995;36:475–479.

346. DeGiorgio CM, Correale JD, Gott PS, et al. Serum neuron-specific enolase in human status epilepticus. *Neurology* 1995;45:1134–1137.

347. Vespa P, Prins M, Ronne-Engstrom E, et al. Increase in extracellular glutamate caused by reduced cerebral perfusion pressure and seizures after human traumatic brain injury: a microdialysis study. *J Neurosurg* 1998;89:971–982.

348. Claassen J, Jette N, Chum F, et al. Electrographic seizures and periodic discharges after intracerebral hemorrhage. *Neurology* 2007;69:1356–1365.

349. Vespa PM, O'Phelan K, Shah M, et al. Acute seizures after intracerebral hemorrhage: a factor in progressive midline shift and outcome. *Neurology* 2003;60:1441–1446.

350. Vespa PM, McArthur DL, Xu Y, et al. Nonconvulsive seizures after traumatic brain injury are associated with hippocampal atrophy. *Neurology* 2010;75:792–798.

351. Payne ET, Zhao XY, Frndova H, et al. Seizure burden is independently associated with short term outcome in critically ill children. *Brain* 2014;137:1429–1438.

352. De Marchis GM, Pugin D, Meyers E, et al. Seizure burden in subarachnoid hemorrhage associated with functional and cognitive outcome. *Neurology* 2016;86:253–260.

353. Vespa P, Tubi M, Claassen J, et al. Metabolic crisis occurs with seizures and periodic discharges after brain trauma. *Ann Neurol* 2016;79:579–590.

354. Vespa PM, Miller C, McArthur D, et al. Nonconvulsive electrographic seizures after traumatic brain injury result in a delayed, prolonged increase in intracranial pressure and metabolic crisis. *Crit Care Med* 2007;35:2830–2836.

355. Witsch J, Frey HP, Schmidt JM, et al. Electroencephalographic periodic discharges and frequency-dependent brain tissue hypoxia in acute brain injury. *JAMA Neurol* 2017;74:301–309.

356. Alvarez V, Lee JW, Westover MB, et al. Therapeutic coma for status epilepticus: Differing practices in a prospective multicenter study. *Neurology* 2016;87:1650–1659.

357. Fernandez A, Lantigua H, Lesch C, et al. High-dose midazolam infusion for refractory status epilepticus. *Neurology* 2014;82:359–365.

358. Claassen J, Lokin JK, Fitzsimmons BF, Mendelsohn FA, Mayer SA. Predictors of functional disability and mortality after status epilepticus. *Neurology* 2002;58:139–142.

359. Rossetti AO, Logroscino G, Milligan TA, Michaelides C, Ruffieux C, Bromfield EB. Status Epilepticus Severity Score (STESS): a tool to orient early treatment strategy. *J Neurol* 2008;255:1561–1566.

360. Dreier JP, Fabricius M, Ayata C, et al. Recording, analysis, and interpretation of spreading depolarizations in neurointensive care: Review and recommendations of the COSBID research group. *J Cereb Blood Flow Metab* 2017;37:1595–1625.

361. Leao AAP. Spreading depression of activity in the cerebral cortex. *Journal of Neurophysiology* 1944;7:359–390.

362. Takano T, Tian GF, Peng W, et al. Cortical spreading depression causes and coincides with tissue hypoxia. *Nat Neurosci* 2007;10:754–762.

363. Canals S, Makarova I, Lopez-Aguado L, Largo C, Ibarz JM, Herreras O. Longitudinal depolarization gradients along the somatodendritic axis of CA1 pyramidal cells: a novel feature of spreading depression. *J Neurophysiol* 2005;94:943–951.

364. Noseda R, Burstein R. Migraine pathophysiology: anatomy of the trigeminovascular pathway and associated neurological symptoms, CSD, sensitization and modulation of pain. *Pain* 2013;154 Suppl 1.

365. Dreier JP, Major S, Manning A, et al. Cortical spreading ischaemia is a novel process involved in ischaemic damage in patients with aneurysmal subarachnoid haemorrhage. *Brain* 2009;132:1866–1881.

366. Hartings JA, Bullock MR, Okonkwo DO, et al. Spreading depolarisations and outcome after traumatic brain injury: a prospective observational study. *Lancet Neurol* 2011;10:1058–1064.

367. Sakowitz OW, Kiening KL, Krajewski KL, et al. Preliminary evidence that ketamine inhibits spreading depolarizations in acute human brain injury. *Stroke* 2009;40:e519–e522.

368. Drenckhahn C, Winkler MK, Major S, et al. Correlates of spreading depolarization in human scalp electroencephalography. *Brain* 2012;135:853–868.

369. Dabrowska K, Skowronska K, Popek M, Obara-Michlewska M, Albrecht J, Zielinska M. Roles of glutamate and glutamine transport in ammonia neurotoxicity: state of the art and question marks. *Endocr Metab Immune Disord Drug Targets* 2018;18:306–315.

370. Collange O, Wolff V, Cebula H, et al. Spontaneous intracranial hypotension: an etiology for consciousness disorder and coma. *A Case Rep* 2016;7:207–211.

371. Davidson B, Nassiri F, Mansouri A, et al. Spontaneous intracranial hypotension: a review and introduction of an algorithm for management. *World Neurosurg* 2017;101:343–349.

372. Fontanarosa PB. Recognition of subarachnoid hemorrhage. *Ann Emerg Med* 1989;18:1199–1205.

373. Suwatcharangkoon S, Meyers E, Falo C, et al. Loss of consciousness at onset of subarachnoid hemorrhage as an important marker of early brain injury. *JAMA Neurol* 2016;73:28–35.

374. Linn FH, Rinkel GJ, Algra A, van Gijn J. Headache characteristics in subarachnoid haemorrhage and benign thunderclap headache. *J Neurol Neurosurg Psychiatry* 1998;65:791–793.

375. Grote E, Hassler W. The critical first minutes after subarachnoid hemorrhage. *Neurosurgery* 1988;22:654–661.

376. Asano T, Sano K. Pathogenetic role of no-reflow phenomenon in experimental subarachnoid hemorrhage in dogs. *J Neurosurg* 1977;46:454–466.

377. Hayashi T, Suzuki A, Hatazawa J, et al. Cerebral circulation and metabolism in the acute stage of subarachnoid hemorrhage. *J Neurosurg* 2000;93:1014–1018.

378. van Gijn J, Hijdra A, Wijdicks EF, Vermeulen M, van Crevel H. Acute hydrocephalus after aneurysmal subarachnoid hemorrhage. *J Neurosurg* 1985;63:355–362.

379. Claassen J, Carhuapoma JR, Kreiter KT, Du EY, Connolly ES, Mayer SA. Global cerebral edema after subarachnoid hemorrhage: frequency, predictors, and impact on outcome. *Stroke* 2002;33:1225–1232.

380. Hop JW, Rinkel GJ, Algra A, van Gijn J. Initial loss of consciousness and risk of delayed cerebral ischemia after aneurysmal subarachnoid hemorrhage. *Stroke* 1999;30:2268–2271.

381. Brouwers PJ, Dippel DW, Vermeulen M, Lindsay KW, Hasan D, van Gijn J. Amount of blood on computed tomography as an independent predictor after aneurysm rupture. *Stroke* 1993;24:809–814.

382. Wang J, Alotaibi NM, Akbar MA, et al. Loss of consciousness at onset of aneurysmal subarachnoid hemorrhage is associated with functional outcomes in good-grade patients. *World Neurosurg* 2017;98:308–313.

383. Provencio JJ, Vora N. Subarachnoid hemorrhage and inflammation: bench to bedside and back. *Semin Neurol* 2005;25:435–444.

384. Provencio JJ, Altay T, Smithason S, Moore SK, Ransohoff RM. Depletion of Ly6G/C(+) cells ameliorates delayed cerebral vasospasm in subarachnoid hemorrhage. *J Neuroimmunol* 2011;232:94–100.

385. Claassen J, Albers D, Schmidt JM, et al. Nonconvulsive seizures in subarachnoid hemorrhage link inflammation and outcome. *Ann Neurol* 2014;75:771–781.

386. Macdonald RL, Pluta RM, Zhang JH. Cerebral vasospasm after subarachnoid hemorrhage: the emerging revolution. *Nat Clin Pract Neurol* 2007;3:256–263.

387. Claassen J, Bernardini GL, Kreiter K, et al. Effect of cisternal and ventricular blood on risk of delayed cerebral ischemia after subarachnoid hemorrhage: the Fisher scale revisited. *Stroke* 2001;32:2012–2020.

388. Frontera JA, Fernandez A, Schmidt JM, et al. Defining vasospasm after subarachnoid hemorrhage: what is the most clinically relevant definition? *Stroke* 2009;40:1963–1968.

389. Jang SH, Kim HS. Aneurysmal subarachnoid hemorrhage causes injury of the ascending reticular activating system: relation to consciousness. *AJNR Am J Neuroradiol* 2015;36:667–671.

390. Nelson S, Edlow BL, Wu O, Rosenthal ES, Westover MB, Rordorf G. Default mode network perfusion in aneurysmal subarachnoid hemorrhage. *Neurocrit Care* 2016;25:237–242.

391. Hasan D, van Peski J, Loeve I, Krenning EP, Vermeulen M. Single photon emission computed tomography in patients with acute hydrocephalus or with cerebral ischaemia after subarachnoid haemorrhage. *J Neurol Neurosurg Psychiatry* 1991;54:490–493.

392. Jaja BN, Cusimano MD, Etminan N, et al. Clinical prediction models for aneurysmal subarachnoid hemorrhage: a systematic review. *Neurocrit Care* 2013;18:143–153.

393. Witsch J, Frey HP, Patel S, et al. Prognostication of long-term outcomes after subarachnoid hemorrhage: The FRESH score. *Ann Neurol* 2016;80:46–58.

394. Klein AM, Howell K, Straube A, Pfefferkorn T, Bender A. Rehabilitation outcome of patients with severe and prolonged disorders of consciousness after aneurysmal subarachnoid hemorrhage (aSAH). *Clin Neurol Neurosurg* 2013;115:2136–2141.

395. Claassen J, Velazquez A, Meyers E, et al. Bedside quantitative electroencephalography improves assessment of consciousness in comatose subarachnoid hemorrhage patients. *Ann Neurol* 2016;80:541–553.

396. Mikell CB, Banks GP, Frey HP, et al. Frontal networks associated with command following after hemorrhagic stroke. *Stroke* 2015;46:49–57.

397. Pruitt AA. Nervous system infections in patients with cancer. *Neurol Clin* 2003;21:193–219.

398. Cunha BA. Central nervous system infections in the compromised host: a diagnostic approach. *Infect Dis Clin North Am* 2001;15:567–590.

399. van de Beek D, de Gans J, Spanjaard L, Weisfelt M, Reitsma JB, Vermeulen M. Clinical features and prognostic factors in adults with bacterial meningitis. *N Engl J Med* 2004;351:1849–1859.

400. Mylonakis E, Hohmann EL, Calderwood SB. Central nervous system infection with Listeria monocytogenes. 33 years' experience at a general hospital and review of 776 episodes from the literature. *Medicine (Baltimore)* 1998;77:313–336.

401. Nau R, Bruck W. Neuronal injury in bacterial meningitis: mechanisms and implications for therapy. *Trends Neurosci* 2002;25:38–45.

402. Kastenbauer S, Pfister HW. Pneumococcal meningitis in adults: spectrum of complications and prognostic factors in a series of 87 cases. *Brain* 2003;126:1015–1025.

403. Gerner-Smidt P, Ethelberg S, Schiellerup P, et al. Invasive listeriosis in Denmark 1994-2003: a review of 299 cases with special emphasis on risk factors for mortality. *Clin Microbiol Infect* 2005;11:618–624.

404. Drevets DA, Leenen PJ, Greenfield RA. Invasion of the central nervous system by intracellular bacteria. *Clin Microbiol Rev* 2004;17:323–347.

405. van Crevel H, Hijdra A, de Gans J. Lumbar puncture and the risk of herniation: when should we first perform CT? *J Neurol* 2002;249:129–137.

406. Romer FK. Difficulties in the diagnosis of bacterial meningitis. Evaluation of antibiotic pretreatment and causes of admission to hospital. *Lancet* 1977;2:345–347.

407. Romer FK. Bacterial meningitis: A 15-year review of bacterial meningitis from departments of internal medicine. *Dan Med Bull* 1977;24:35–40.
408. Rennick G, Shann F, de Campo J. Cerebral herniation during bacterial meningitis in children. *BMJ* 1993;306:953–955.
409. Carpenter RR, Petersdorf RG. The clinical spectrum of bacterial meningitis. *Am J Med* 1962;33:262–275.
410. Roos KL. Mycobacterium tuberculosis meningitis and other etiologies of the aseptic meningitis syndrome. *Semin Neurol* 2000;20:329–335.
411. Ricard D, Sallansonnet-Froment M, Defuentes G, et al. Listeria monocytogenes abscess of the brain [in French]. *Rev Neurol (Paris)* 2008;164:388–393.
412. Ratnaike RN. Whipple's disease. *Postgrad Med J* 2000;76:760–766.
413. Mohm J, Naumann R, Schuler U, Ehninger G. Abdominal lymphomas, convulsive seizure and coma: a case of successfully treated, advanced Whipple's disease with cerebral involvement. *Eur J Gastroenterol Hepatol* 1998;10:893–895.
414. Compain C, Sacre K, Puechal X, et al. Central nervous system involvement in Whipple disease: clinical study of 18 patients and long-term follow-up. *Medicine (Baltimore)* 2013;92:324–330.
415. Mendel E, Khoo LT, Go JL, Hinton D, Zee CS, Apuzzo ML. Intracerebral Whipple's disease diagnosed by stereotactic biopsy: a case report and review of the literature. *Neurosurgery* 1999;44:203–209.
416. Bratton RL, Corey R. Tick-borne disease. *Am Fam Physician* 2005;71:2323–2330.
417. Davies NW, Brown LJ, Gonde J, et al. Factors influencing PCR detection of viruses in cerebrospinal fluid of patients with suspected CNS infections. *J Neurol Neurosurg Psychiatry* 2005;76:82–87.
418. Johnson RT. The pathogenesis of acute viral encephalitis and postinfectious encephalomyelitis. *J Infect Dis* 1987;155:359–364.
419. McGill F, Griffiths MJ, Bonnett LJ, et al. Incidence, aetiology, and sequelae of viral meningitis in UK adults: a multicentre prospective observational cohort study. *Lancet Infect Dis* 2018;18:992–1003.
420. Collinge J. Molecular neurology of prion disease. *J Neurol Neurosurg Psychiatry* 2005;76:906–919.
421. Johnson RT. Prion diseases. *Lancet Neurol* 2005;4:635–642.
422. Omalu BI, Shakir AA, Wang G, Lipkin WI, Wiley CA. Fatal fulminant pan-meningo-polioencephalitis due to West Nile virus. *Brain Pathol* 2003;13:465–472.
423. Sejvar JJ, Haddad MB, Tierney BC, et al. Neurologic manifestations and outcome of West Nile virus infection. *JAMA* 2003;290:511–515.
424. Olival KJ, Daszak P. The ecology of emerging neurotropic viruses. *J Neurovirol* 2005;11:441–446.
425. Kamei S, Sekizawa T, Shiota H, et al. Evaluation of combination therapy using aciclovir and corticosteroid in adult patients with herpes simplex virus encephalitis. *J Neurol Neurosurg Psychiatry* 2005;76:1544–1549.
426. Jereb M, Lainscak M, Marin J, Popovic M. Herpes simplex virus infection limited to the brainstem. *Wien Klin Wochenschr* 2005;117:495–499.
427. Chu K, Kang DW, Lee JJ, Yoon BW. Atypical brainstem encephalitis caused by herpes simplex virus 2. *Arch Neurol* 2002;59:460–463.
428. Chaudhuri A, Kennedy PG. Diagnosis and treatment of viral encephalitis. *Postgrad Med J* 2002;78:575–583.
429. Kennedy PG. Viral encephalitis: causes, differential diagnosis, and management. *J Neurol Neurosurg Psychiatry* 2004;75(Suppl 1):i10–i15.
430. Menge T, Hemmer B, Nessler S, et al. Acute disseminated encephalomyelitis: an update. *Arch Neurol* 2005;62:1673–1680.
431. Garg RK. Acute disseminated encephalomyelitis. *Postgrad Med J* 2003;79:11–17.
432. Wasay M, Mekan SF, Khelaeni B, et al. Extra temporal involvement in herpes simplex encephalitis. *Eur J Neurol* 2005;12:475–479.
433. Schwarz S, Mohr A, Knauth M, Wildemann B, Storch-Hagenlocher B. Acute disseminated encephalomyelitis: a follow-up study of 40 adult patients. *Neurology* 2001;56:1313–1318.
434. Gibbs WN, Kreidie MA, Kim RC, Hasso AN. Acute hemorrhagic leukoencephalitis: neuroimaging features and neuropathologic diagnosis. *J Comput Assist Tomogr* 2005;29:689–693.
435. An SF, Groves M, Martinian L, Kuo LT, Scaravilli F. Detection of infectious agents in brain of patients with acute hemorrhagic leukoencephalitis. *J Neurovirol* 2002;8:439–446.
436. Togashi T, Matsuzono Y, Narita M, Morishima T. Influenza-associated acute encephalopathy in Japanese children in 1994–2002. *Virus Res* 2004;103:75–78.
437. Orlowski JP, Hanhan UA, Fiallos MR. Is aspirin a cause of Reye's syndrome? A case against. *Drug Saf* 2002;25:225–231.
438. Lemberg A, Fernandez MA, Coll C, et al. Reyes's syndrome, encephalopathy, hyperammonemia and acetyl salicylic acid ingestion in a city hospital of Buenos Aires, Argentina. *Curr Drug Saf* 2009;4:17–21.
439. Whiting DM, Barnett GH, Estes ML, et al. Stereotactic biopsy of non-neoplastic lesions in adults. *Cleve Clin J Med* 1992;59:48–55.
440. Hornef MW, Iten A, Maeder P, Villemure JG, Regli L. Brain biopsy in patients with acquired immunodeficiency syndrome: diagnostic value, clinical performance, and survival time. *Arch Intern Med* 1999;159:2590–2596.
441. Warren JD, Schott JM, Fox NC, et al. Brain biopsy in dementia. *Brain* 2005;128:2016–2025.
442. Gray F, N'Guyen J P. Brain biopsy in systemic diseases [in French]. *Ann Pathol* 2002;22:194–205.
443. De Marcaida JA, Reik L Jr. Disorders that mimic central nervous system infections. *Neurol Clin* 1999;17:901–941.
444. Yao D, Kuwajima M, Kido H. Pathologic mechanisms of influenza encephalitis with an abnormal expression of inflammatory cytokines and accumulation of mini-plasmin. *J Med Invest* 2003;50:1–8.
445. Kirsch DB, Jozefowicz RF. Neurologic complications of respiratory disease. *Neurol Clin* 2002;20:247–264, viii.
446. Miller A, Bader RA, Bader ME. The neurologic syndrome due to marked hypercapnia, with papilledema. *Am J Med* 1962;33:309–318.
447. Gomersall CD, Joynt GM, Freebairn RC, Lai CK, Oh TE. Oxygen therapy for hypercapnic patients with chronic obstructive pulmonary disease and

acute respiratory failure: a randomized, controlled pilot study. *Crit Care Med* 2002;30:113–116.

448. Rotheram EB, Jr., Safar P, Robin E. CNS disorder during mechanical ventilation in chronic pulmonary disease. *JAMA* 1964;189:993–996.

449. Datar S, Wijdicks EF. Neurologic manifestations of acute liver failure. *Handb Clin Neurol* 2014;120:645–659.

450. Sarici KB, Karakas S, Otan E, et al. Can patients who develop cerebral death in fulminant liver failure despite liver transplantation be previously foreseen? *Transplant Proc* 2017;49:571–574.

451. Bernal W, Wendon J. Acute liver failure. *N Engl J Med* 2013;369:2525–2534.

452. Shawcross D, Jalan R. The pathophysiologic basis of hepatic encephalopathy: central role for ammonia and inflammation. *Cell Mol Life Sci* 2005;62:2295–2304.

453. Ott P, Larsen FS. Blood-brain barrier permeability to ammonia in liver failure: a critical reappraisal. *Neurochem Int* 2004;44:185–198.

454. Grover VP, Tognarelli JM, Massie N, Crossey MM, Cook NA, Taylor-Robinson SD. The why and wherefore of hepatic encephalopathy. *Int J Gen Med* 2015;8:381–390.

455. Miyake Y, Yasunaka T, Ikeda F, Takaki A, Nouso K, Yamamoto K. SIRS score reflects clinical features of non-acetaminophen-related acute liver failure with hepatic coma. *Intern Med* 2012;51:823–828.

456. Stravitz RT, Sanyal AJ, Reisch J, et al. Effects of N-acetylcysteine on cytokines in non-acetaminophen acute liver failure: potential mechanism of improvement in transplant-free survival. *Liver Int* 2013;33:1324–1331.

457. Weissenborn K, Ennen JC, Schomerus H, Ruckert N, Hecker H. Neuropsychological characterization of hepatic encephalopathy. *J Hepatol* 2001;34:768–773.

458. Cadranel JF, Lebiez E, Di Martino V, et al. Focal neurological signs in hepatic encephalopathy in cirrhotic patients: an underestimated entity? *Am J Gastroenterol* 2001;96:515–518.

459. Caplan LR, Scheiner D. Dysconjugate gaze in hepatic coma. *Ann Neurol* 1980;8:328–329.

460. Rai GS, Buxton-Thomas M, Scanlon M. Ocular bobbing in hepatic encephalopathy. *Br J Clin Pract* 1976;30:202–205.

461. Weissenborn K, Bokemeyer M, Krause J, Ennen J, Ahl B. Neurological and neuropsychiatric syndromes associated with liver disease. *AIDS* 2005;19 Suppl 3:S93–S98.

462. Timmermann L, Gross J, Kircheis G, Haussinger D, Schnitzler A. Cortical origin of mini-asterixis in hepatic encephalopathy. *Neurology* 2002;58:295–298.

463. Blei AT. The pathophysiology of brain edema in acute liver failure. *Neurochem Int* 2005;47:71–77.

464. Gerber T, Schomerus H. Hepatic encephalopathy in liver cirrhosis: pathogenesis, diagnosis and management. *Drugs* 2000;60:1353–1370.

465. Vergara F, Plum F, Duffy TE. Alpha-ketoglutaramate: increased concentrations in the cerebrospinal fluid of patients in hepatic coma. *Science* 1974;183:81–83.

466. Stewart J, Sarkela M, Koivusalo AM, et al. Frontal electroencephalogram variables are associated with the outcome and stage of hepatic encephalopathy in acute liver failure. *Liver Transpl* 2014;20:1256–1265.

467. Press CA, Morgan L, Mills M, et al. Spectral electroencephalogram analysis for the evaluation of encephalopathy grade in children with acute liver failure. *Pediatr Crit Care Med* 2017;18:64–72.

468. Tarasow E, Panasiuk A, Siergiejczyk L, et al. MR and 1H MR spectroscopy of the brain in patients with liver cirrhosis and early stages of hepatic encephalopathy. *Hepatogastroenterology* 2003;50:2149–2153.

469. Weissenborn K, Bokemeyer M, Ahl B, et al. Functional imaging of the brain in patients with liver cirrhosis. *Metab Brain Dis* 2004;19:269–280.

470. Tyler HR. Neurologic disorders seen in the uremic patient. *Arch Intern Med* 1970;126:781–786.

471. Arieff AI, Massry SG. Calcium metabolism of brain in acute renal failure. Effects of uremia, hemodialysis, and parathyroid hormone. *J Clin Invest* 1974;53:387–392.

472. Cogan MG, Covey CM, Arieff AI, et al. Central nervous system manifestations of hyperparathyroidism. *Am J Med* 1978;65:963–970.

473. Burn DJ, Bates D. Neurology and the kidney. *J Neurol Neurosurg Psychiatry* 1998;65:810–821.

474. Lin A, Ross BD, Harris K, Wong W. Efficacy of proton magnetic resonance spectroscopy in neurological diagnosis and neurotherapeutic decision making. *NeuroRx : The Journal of the American Society for Experimental NeuroTherapeutics* 2005;2:197–214.

475. Topczewska-Bruns J, Pawlak D, Chabielska E, Tankiewicz A, Buczko W. Increased levels of 3-hydroxykynurenine in different brain regions of rats with chronic renal insufficiency. *Brain Res Bull* 2002;58:423–428.

476. Vaziri ND. Oxidative stress in uremia: nature, mechanisms, and potential consequences. *Semin Nephrol* 2004;24:469–473.

477. Adachi N, Lei B, Deshpande G, et al. Uraemia suppresses central dopaminergic metabolism and impairs motor activity in rats. *Intensive Care Med* 2001;27:1655–1660.

478. Chow KM, Wang AY, Hui AC, Wong TY, Szeto CC, Li PK. Nonconvulsive status epilepticus in peritoneal dialysis patients. *Am J Kidney Dis* 2001;38:400–405.

479. Abanades S, Nolla J, Rodriguez-Campello A, Pedro C, Valls A, Farre M. Reversible coma secondary to cefepime neurotoxicity. *Ann Pharmacother* 2004;38:606–608.

480. Lance JW. Action myoclonus, Ramsay Hunt syndrome, and other cerebellar myoclonic syndromes. *Adv Neurol* 1986;43:33–55.

481. Chadwick D, French AT. Uraemic myoclonus: an example of reticular reflex myoclonus? *J Neurol Neurosurg Psychiatry* 1979;42:52–55.

482. Palmer CA. Neurologic manifestations of renal disease. *Neurol Clin* 2002;20:23–34, v.

483. Oo TN, Smith CL, Swan SK. Does uremia protect against the demyelination associated with correction of hyponatremia during hemodialysis? A case report and literature review. *Semin Dial* 2003;16:68–71.

484. Hung SC, Hung SH, Tarng DC, Yang WC, Chen TW, Huang TP. Thiamine deficiency and unexplained encephalopathy in hemodialysis and peritoneal dialysis patients. *Am J Kidney Dis* 2001;38:941–947.

485. Bagshaw SM, Peets AD, Hameed M, Boiteau PJ, Laupland KB, Doig CJ. Dialysis disequilibrium syndrome: brain death following hemodialysis for

metabolic acidosis and acute renal failure: a case report. *BMC Nephrol* 2004;5:9.

486. Mach JR Jr, Korchik WP, Mahowald MW. Dialysis dementia. *Clin Geriatr Med* 1988;4:853–867.

487. Silver SM, Sterns RH, Halperin ML. Brain swelling after dialysis: old urea or new osmoles? *Am J Kidney Dis* 1996;28:1–13.

488. Lien YH, Shapiro JI, Chan L. Study of brain electrolytes and organic osmolytes during correction of chronic hyponatremia. Implications for the pathogenesis of central pontine myelinolysis. *J Clin Invest* 1991;88:303–309.

489. Wu VC, Huang TM, Shiao CC, et al. The hemodynamic effects during sustained low-efficiency dialysis versus continuous veno-venous hemofiltration for uremic patients with brain hemorrhage: a crossover study. *J Neurosurg* 2013;119:1288–1295.

490. Fletcher JJ, Bergman K, Feucht EC, Blostein P. Continuous renal replacement therapy for refractory intracranial hypertension. *Neurocrit Care* 2009;11:101–105.

491. Tuchman S, Khademian ZP, Mistry K. Dialysis disequilibrium syndrome occurring during continuous renal replacement therapy. *Clin Kidney J* 2013;6:526–529.

492. Ponticelli C, Campise MR. Neurological complications in kidney transplant recipients. *J Nephrol* 2005;18:521–528.

493. Thaisetthawatkul P, Weinstock A, Kerr SL, Cohen ME. Muromonab-CD3-induced neurotoxicity: report of two siblings, one of whom had subsequent cyclosporin-induced neurotoxicity. *J Child Neurol* 2001;16:825–831.

494. Parizel PM, Snoeck HW, van den Hauwe L, et al. Cerebral complications of murine monoclonal CD3 antibody (OKT3): CT and MR findings. *AJNR Am J Neuroradiol* 1997;18:1935–1938.

495. Sjaastad O, Gjessing L, Ritland S, Blichfeldt P, Sandnes K. Chronic relapsing pancreatitis, encephalopathy with disturbances of consciousness and CSF amino acid aberration. *J Neurol* 1979;220:83–94.

496. Estrada RV, Moreno J, Martinez E, Hernandez MC, Gilsanz G, Gilsanz V. Pancreatic encephalopathy. *Acta Neurol Scand* 1979;59:135–139.

497. Ohkubo T, Shiojiri T, Matsunaga T. Severe diffuse white matter lesions in a patient with pancreatic encephalopathy. *J Neurol* 2004;251:476–478.

498. McMahon MJ, Woodhead JS, Hayward RD. The nature of hypocalcaemia in acute pancreatitis. *Br J Surg* 1978;65:216–218.

499. Ruggieri RM, Lupo I, Piccoli F. Pancreatic encephalopathy: a 7-year follow-up case report and review of the literature. *Neurol Sci* 2002;23:203–205.

500. Nico B, Ribatti D. Morphofunctional aspects of the blood-brain barrier. *Curr Drug Metab* 2012;13:50–60.

501. De Backer D. Hemodynamic management of septic shock. *Curr Infect Dis Rep* 2006;8:366–372.

502. Sharshar T, Polito A, Checinski A, Stevens RD. Septic-associated encephalopathy: everything starts at a microlevel. *Crit Care* 2010;14:199.

503. Berg RM, Moller K, Bailey DM. Neuro-oxidative-nitrosative stress in sepsis. *J Cereb Blood Flow Metab* 2011;31:1532–1544.

504. Jacob A, Brorson JR, Alexander JJ. Septic encephalopathy: inflammation in man and mouse. *Neurochem Int* 2011;58:472–476.

505. Basler T, Meier-Hellmann A, Bredle D, Reinhart K. Amino acid imbalance early in septic encephalopathy. *Intensive Care Med* 2002;28:293–298.

506. Chaudhry N, Duggal AK. Sepsis associated encephalopathy. *Adv Med* 2014;2014:762320.

507. Ghazanfari N, Trajanovska S, Morsch M, Liang SX, Reddel SW, Phillips WD. The mouse passive-transfer model of MuSK myasthenia gravis: disrupted MuSK signaling causes synapse failure. *Ann N Y Acad Sci* 2018;1412:54–61.

508. Graus F, Elkon KB, Cordon-Cardo C, Posner JB. Sensory neuronopathy and small cell lung cancer. Antineuronal antibody that also reacts with the tumor. *Am J Med* 1986;80:45–52.

509. Furneaux HM, Rosenblum MK, Dalmau J, et al. Selective expression of Purkinje-cell antigens in tumor tissue from patients with paraneoplastic cerebellar degeneration. *N Engl J Med* 1990;322:1844–1851.

510. Musunuru K, Darnell RB. Paraneoplastic neurologic disease antigens: RNA-binding proteins and signaling proteins in neuronal degeneration. *Annu Rev Neurosci* 2001;24:239–262.

511. Brierley J, Corsellis J, Hierons R, Nevin S. Subacute encephalitis of later adult life, mainle affecting the limbic areas. *Brain Behav Immun* 1960;83:357–368.

512. Corsellis JA, Goldberg GJ, Norton AR. "Limbic encephalitis" and its association with carcinoma. *Brain* 1968;91:481–496.

513. Serafini A, Lukas RV, VanHaerents S, et al. Paraneoplastic epilepsy. *Epilepsy Behav* 2016;61:51–58.

514. Arino H, Hoftberger R, Gresa-Arribas N, et al. Paraneoplastic neurological syndromes and glutamic acid decarboxylase antibodies. *JAMA Neurol* 2015;72:874–881.

515. Hoftberger R, van Sonderen A, Leypoldt F, et al. Encephalitis and AMPA receptor antibodies: novel findings in a case series of 22 patients. *Neurology* 2015;84:2403–2412.

516. Miya K, Takahashi Y, Mori H. Anti-NMDAR autoimmune encephalitis. *Brain Dev* 2014;36:645–652.

517. Graus F, Titulaer MJ, Balu R, Benseler S, Bien CG, Cellucci T, et al. A clinical approach to diagnosis of autoimmune encephalitis. *Lancet Neurol* 2016 Apr;15(4):391–404. doi:10.1016/S1474-4422(15)00401-9. Epub 2016 Feb 20. Review. PMID:26906964.

518. Dale C, Aulaqi AA, Baker J, et al. Assessment of a point-of-care test for paracetamol and salicylate in blood. *QJM* 2005;98:113–118.

519. Fabbri A, Ruggeri S, Marchesini G, Vandelli A. A combined HPLC-immunoenzymatic comprehensive screening for suspected drug poisoning in the emergency department. *Emerg Med J* 2004;21:317–322.

520. Mokhlesi B, Corbridge T. Toxicology in the critically ill patient. *Clin Chest Med* 2003;24:689–711.

521. Khom S, Baburin I, Timin EN, Hohaus A, Sieghart W, Hering S. Pharmacological properties of GABAA receptors containing gamma1 subunits. *Mol Pharmacol* 2006;69:640–649.

522. Maxwell JC. Party drugs: properties, prevalence, patterns, and problems. *Subst Use Misuse* 2005;40:1203–1240.

523. Antkowiak B, Rudolph U. New insights in the systemic and molecular underpinnings of general anesthetic actions mediated by gamma-aminobutyric acid A receptors. *Curr Opin Anaesthesiol* 2016;29:447–453.

524. Akeju O, Hamilos AE, Song AH, Pavone KJ, Purdon PL, Brown EN. GABAA circuit mechanisms are associated with ether anesthesia-induced unconsciousness. *Clin Neurophysiol* 2016;127:2472–2481.

525. Saper CB, Fuller PM, Pedersen NP, Lu J, Scammell TE. Sleep state switching. *Neuron* 2010;68:1023–1042.

526. Reed CE, Driggs MF, Foote CC. Acute barbiturate intoxication: a study of 300 cases based on a physiologic system of classification of the severity of the intoxication. *Ann Intern Med* 1952;37:290–303.

527. Young CC, Prielipp RC. Benzodiazepines in the intensive care unit. *Crit Care Clin* 2001;17:843–862.

528. Seger DL. Flumazenil—treatment or toxin. *J Toxicol Clin Toxicol* 2004;42:209–216.

529. Haimovic IC, Beresford HR. Transient unresponsiveness in the elderly. Report of five cases. *Arch Neurol* 1992;49:35–37.

530. Lugaresi E, Montagna P, Tinuper P, et al. Endozepine stupor. Recurring stupor linked to endozepine-4 accumulation. *Brain* 1998;121 (Pt 1):127–133.

531. Cortelli P, Avallone R, Baraldi M, et al. Endozepines in recurrent stupor. *Sleep Med Rev* 2005;9:477–487.

532. Granot R, Berkovic SF, Patterson S, Hopwood M, Mackenzie R. Idiopathic recurrent stupor: a warning. *J Neurol Neurosurg Psychiatry* 2004;75:368–369.

533. Lugaresi E, Montagna P, Tinuper P, Plazzi G, Gallassi R. Suspected covert lorazepam administration misdiagnosed as recurrent endozepine stupor. *Brain* 1998;121 (Pt 11):2201.

534. Trotti LM, Saini P, Koola C, LaBarbera V, Bliwise DL, Rye DB. Flumazenil for the treatment of refractory hypersomnolence: clinical experience with 153 patients. *J Clin Sleep Med* 2016;12:1389–1394.

535. Currier GW, Trenton AJ, Walsh PG. Innovations: Emergency psychiatry: relative accuracy of breath and serum alcohol readings in the psychiatric emergency service. *Psychiatr Serv* 2006;57:34–36.

536. McIntosh C, Chick J. Alcohol and the nervous system. *J Neurol Neurosurg Psychiatry* 2004;75(Suppl 3):iii16–iii21.

537. McKeon A, Frye MA, Delanty N. The alcohol withdrawal syndrome. *J Neurol Neurosurg Psychiatry* 2008;79:854–862.

538. Griffiths RR, Johnson MW. Relative abuse liability of hypnotic drugs: a conceptual framework and algorithm for differentiating among compounds. *J Clin Psychiatry* 2005;66(Suppl 9):31–41.

539. Bayard M, McIntyre J, Hill KR, Woodside J, Jr. Alcohol withdrawal syndrome. *Am Fam Physician* 2004;69:1443–1450.

540. Mo Y, Thomas MC, Karras GE, Jr. Barbiturates for the treatment of alcohol withdrawal syndrome: a systematic review of clinical trials. *J Crit Care* 2016;32:101–107.

541. McCloud TL, Caddy C, Jochim J, et al. Ketamine and other glutamate receptor modulators for depression in bipolar disorder in adults. *Cochrane Database Syst Rev* 2015:CD011611.

542. Andrade C. Ketamine for depression, 1: clinical summary of issues related to efficacy, adverse effects, and mechanism of action. *J Clin Psychiatry* 2017;78:e415–e419.

543. El Mourad MB, Elghamry MR, Mansour RF, Afandy ME. Comparison of Intravenous Dexmedetomidine-Propofol Versus Ketofol for Sedation During Awake Fiberoptic Intubation: A Prospective, Randomized Study. *Anesth Pain Med* 2019 Feb 26;9(1):e86442. doi:10.5812/aapm.86442. eCollection 2019 Feb. PMID:30881913.

544. Gaspard N, Foreman B, Judd LM, Brenton JN, Nathan BR, McCoy BM, et al. Intravenous ketamine for the treatment of refractory status epilepticus: a retrospective multicenter study. *Epilepsia* 2013 Aug;54(8):1498–1503. doi:10.1111/epi.12247. Epub 2013 Jun 12. PMID:23758557.

545. Siva A, Altintas A, Saip S. Behcet's syndrome and the nervous system. *Curr Opin Neurol* 2004;17:347–357.

546. Kidd D, Steuer A, Denman AM, Rudge P. Neurological complications in Behcet's syndrome. *Brain* 1999;122 (Pt 11):2183–2194.

547. Siva A, Kantarci OH, Saip S, et al. Behcet's disease: diagnostic and prognostic aspects of neurological involvement. *J Neurol* 2001;248:95–103.

548. Mokhlesi B, Leikin JB, Murray P, Corbridge TC. Adult toxicology in critical care: Part II: specific poisonings. *Chest* 2003;123:897–922.

549. Zimmerman JL. Poisonings and overdoses in the intensive care unit: general and specific management issues. *Crit Care Med* 2003;31:2794–2801.

550. Adityanjee, Munshi KR, Thampy A. The syndrome of irreversible lithium-effectuated neurotoxicity. *Clin Neuropharmacol* 2005;28:38–49.

551. Ware MR, Feller DB, Hall KL. Neuroleptic malignant syndrome: diagnosis and management. *Prim Care Companion CNS Disord* 2018;20(1).

552. Khaldi S, Kornreich C, Choubani Z, Gourevitch R. Neuroleptic malignant syndrome and atypical antipsychotics: a brief review [in French]. *Encephale* 2008;34:618–624.

553. Ikebe S, Harada T, Hashimoto T, et al. Prevention and treatment of malignant syndrome in Parkinson's disease: a consensus statement of the malignant syndrome research group. *Parkinsonism Relat Disord* 2003;9 Suppl 1:S47–S49.

554. Valentino RJ, Volkow ND. Untangling the complexity of opioid receptor function. *Neuropsychopharmacology* 2018;43:2514–2520.

555. Sterrett C, Brownfield J, Korn CS, Hollinger M, Henderson SO. Patterns of presentation in heroin overdose resulting in pulmonary edema. *Am J Emerg Med* 2003;21:32–34.

556. Kriegstein AR, Shungu DC, Millar WS, et al. Leukoencephalopathy and raised brain lactate from heroin vapor inhalation ("chasing the dragon"). *Neurology* 1999;53:1765–1773.

557. Bartlett E, Mikulis DJ. Chasing "chasing the dragon" with MRI: leukoencephalopathy in drug abuse. *Br J Radiol* 2005;78:997–1004.

558. Miura S, Ohyagi Y, Ohno M, et al. A patient with delayed posthypoxic demyelination: a case report of hyperbaric oxygen treatment. *Clin Neurol Neurosurg* 2002;104:311–314.

559. Rowden AK, Norvell J, Eldridge DL, Kirk MA. Updates on acetaminophen toxicity. *Med Clin North Am* 2005;89:1145–1159.

560. Toossi S, Hess CP, Hills NK, Josephson SA. Neurovascular complications of cocaine use at a tertiary stroke center. *J Stroke Cerebrovasc Dis* 2010;19:273–278.

561. Traub SJ, Nelson LS, Hoffman RS. Physostigmine as a treatment for gamma-hydroxybutyrate toxicity: a review. *J Toxicol Clin Toxicol* 2002;40:781–787.

562. Bania TC, Chu J. Physostigmine does not effect arousal but produces toxicity in an animal model of severe gamma-hydroxybutyrate intoxication. *Acad Emerg Med* 2005;12:185–189.

563. Britt GC, McCance-Katz EF. A brief overview of the clinical pharmacology of "club drugs". *Subst Use Misuse* 2005;40:1189–1201.

564. Mokhlesi B, Garimella PS, Joffe A, Velho V. Street drug abuse leading to critical illness. *Intensive Care Med* 2004;30:1526–1536.

565. Judge BS. Metabolic acidosis: differentiating the causes in the poisoned patient. *Med Clin North Am* 2005;89:1107–1124.

566. Megarbane B, Borron SW, Baud FJ. Current recommendations for treatment of severe toxic alcohol poisonings. *Intensive Care Med* 2005;31:189–195.

567. Perkin MR, Wey EQ. Emergency drug availability on general paediatric units. *Resuscitation* 2004;62:243–247.

568. Christopher MM, Eckfeldt JH, Eaton JW. Propylene glycol ingestion causes D-lactic acidosis. *Lab Invest* 1990;62:114–118.

569. Lalive PH, Hadengue A, Mensi N, Burkhard PR. Recurrent encephalopathy after small bowel resection. Implication of D-lactate [in French]. *Rev Neurol (Paris)* 2001;157:679–681.

570. Stacpoole PW, Wright EC, Baumgartner TG, et al. Natural history and course of acquired lactic acidosis in adults. DCA-Lactic Acidosis Study Group. *Am J Med* 1994;97:47–54.

571. Xiang Z, Yuan M, Hassen GW, Gampel M, Bergold PJ. Lactate induced excitotoxicity in hippocampal slice cultures. *Exp Neurol* 2004;186:70–77.

Chapter 6

Psychogenic Unresponsiveness

CONVERSION REACTIONS

CATATONIA

PSYCHOGENIC SEIZURES

CEREBELLAR COGNITIVE AFFECTIVE
   SYNDROME

"AMYTAL INTERVIEW"

Differentiating psychogenic neurologic symptoms from those caused by structural disease is often very difficult. The difficulty arises in part because some patients are very accurate in mimicking neurologic signs (actors are often used to train medical students in the diagnosis of neurologic illnesses) and, in part, because many patients with psychogenic neurologic disorders (conversion reactions) also have somatic disease, and the somatic illness may act as a stressor that causes psychologic problems. Examples abound: approximately one-half of patients with psychogenic seizures also have epilepsy.[1] Of those who do not have epilepsy, more than 20% show evidence of a brain disorder characterized either by epileptiform activity on electroencephalogram (EEG), magnetic resonance imaging (MRI) abnormalities, or neuropsychologic deficits.[2] Psychogenic neurologic symptoms sometimes complicate the course of multiple sclerosis.[3] Merskey and Buhrich studied 89 patients with classic motor conversion symptoms and found that 48% had a cerebral disorder.[4]

Of all the psychogenic illnesses that mimic structural disease, psychogenic unresponsiveness is among the most difficult to diagnose. With most psychogenic illnesses that mimic structural neurologic disease, the physician pursues a two-pronged diagnostic attack: a careful neurological examination to determine whether the patient's neurologic signs and symptoms are appropriate for the claimed disorder; and a probing history and mental status examination to determine whether the patient's psychologic problems can explain the discrepancy. In psychogenic unresponsiveness, the patient can neither give a history nor participate in a mental status examination. Hence, the physician is left with only the barest elements of a history that can be obtained from bystanders or family members (if present) and the neurological examination to discern whether, despite apparent unconsciousness, the patient is in fact physiologically awake. Testing, including MRI scan, EEG, or examination of the cerebrospinal fluid (CSF), can only provide "negative evidence" that may rule out some disorders, but cannot completely eliminate the presence of others.

Functional tests of the nervous system may, in fact, identify hypometabolism in the appropriate brain areas for the psychogenic deficits.[5] Vuilleumier and colleagues used single photon emission computed tomography (SPECT) to study seven patients with conversion symptoms mimicking motor or sensory dysfunction.[6] The scans revealed a consistent decrease of blood flow in the thalamus and basal ganglia contralateral to the deficit. These abnormalities resolved in those patients who recovered. Spence and colleagues studied two patients with psychogenic weakness affecting their left arms. They compared positron emission tomography (PET) scans of these patients with normal individuals and also with normal individuals who feigned paralysis of the left arm. The left dorsolateral prefrontal cortex was activated in the normal individuals and those feigning paralysis, but was hypofunctional in the patients with the conversion reaction. Interestingly, those feigning paralysis exhibited hypofunction of the right anterior prefrontal cortex when compared with controls.[7] A study of four patients with "hysterical anesthesia" using functional MRI revealed that stimuli to the anesthetic parts of the body did not activate areas in the thalamus, posterior region of the anterior cingulate cortex, or Brodmann's areas 44 and 45, which are typically activated in individuals who perceived the stimuli. A patient studied during catatonic stupor showed hypometabolism in a large area of the prefrontal cortex including anterior cingulate, medial prefrontal, and dorsolateral cortices when compared with controls.[5] The few other studies of functional imaging in patients with catatonia also showed hypometabolism in the frontal lobes, although frontal lobe hypometabolism is quite commonly seen in schizophrenic patients.[8–11] Although the catatonic subject was stuporous during the study, there is little evidence about potential alterations in brain metabolism during psychogenic coma. Thus, if after a meticulous examination of a patient with suspected psychogenic unresponsiveness any question remains about the diagnosis, a careful search for other causes of coma is obligatory.

Psychogenic unresponsiveness is uncommon; it was the final diagnosis in only 8 of the original 500 unresponsive patients collected by Plum and Posner in the first edition of this book (Table 1.1). In one study of conversion symptoms in 500 psychiatric outpatients, "unconsciousness" occurred in 17.[12] Two older series from London each report six patients with psychogenic unresponsiveness who were initially puzzling diagnostically.[13,14] However, it was not stated over how long a period of time these cases were collected or from how wide a patient population. Lempert and colleagues in 1990 found that 405 (9%) of 4,470 consecutive neurologic inpatients were found to have psychogenic rather than neurologic disorders (Table 6.1).[15] Among these only one was comatose. Another study conducted in a 566-bed tertiary care hospital identified a conversion disorder in 42 patients over 10 years.[16] In 17 patients, the presenting complaints were "seizure activity, syncope, or loss of consciousness." Patients admitted directly to the hospital without a definitive diagnosis were not included among the 42; how many this latter group included was not stated. A more recent study found that only 0.3% of 2,189 patients (i.e., 6 people) admitted to an ICU over an 8-year period were found to have psychogenic unresponsiveness.[17]

Because the diagnosis of psychogenic neurologic symptoms is often difficult, mistakes are sometimes made. Sometimes a structural disorder is initially diagnosed as psychogenic,[18,19] but other times the opposite occurs. The latter is typically true when psychogenic coma complicates a physical illness.[20,21] Although errors were common in the past, a systematic review of misdiagnosis of conversion symptoms suggests an error rate of only 4% since 1970.[22] Among the 390 patients with a diagnosis of nonepileptic seizures and/or loss of consciousness, only 9 were misdiagnosed.

Several psychiatric disorders can result in psychogenic unresponsiveness. These include (1) conversion reaction, which may in turn be secondary to a personality disorder, severe depression, anxiety, or an acute situational reaction[23]; (2) catatonic stupor, often a manifestation of schizophrenia; (3) a dissociative or "fugue" state; and (4) factitious disorder (Munchausen syndrome) or malingering. In the latter instance, the patient may actually take a drug or inject insulin to induce a real comatose state, which makes finding the correct diagnosis more complicated still. For example, in a patient with hypoglycemia suspected of Munchausen syndrome, measurement of blood insulin as well as C-peptide may be required to prove that the insulin that caused the coma was of exogenous origin.

Table 6.1 Signs and Symptoms (*N* = 717) of 405 Patients with Psychogenic Dysfunction of the Nervous System

Pain		*Vertigo/Dizziness*	
Trunk and extremities	89	Attacks of phobic postural vertigo	47
Headache	61	Continuous dizziness	38
Atypical facial pain	13	*Ocular symptoms*	
Motor symptoms		Amblyopia	10
Astasia/abasia	52	Amaurosis	6
Monoparesis	31	Visual field defects	6
Hemiparesis	20	Color blindness	2
Tetraparesis	18	Double vision	2
Paraparesis	10	Other visual phenomena	6
Paresis of both arms	2	Ptosis	1
Recurrent head drop	1	Convergence spasm	1
Tremor	11	Unilateral gaze paresis	1
Localized jerking	1	*Alimentary symptoms*	
Stereotyped motor behavior	1	Dysphagia	4
Hypokinesia	1	Vomiting	4
Akinesia	1	*Speech disturbances*	
Foot contracture	1	Dysarthria	9
Isolated ataxia of the upper extremities		Slow speech	1
		Aphonia	2
Sensory symptoms		Mutism	1
Hypesthesia/anesthesia	81		
Paresthesia/dysesthesia	63	*Neuropsychologic symptoms*	
Sensation of generalized vibration	1	Cognitive impairment	2
Sensation of fever	1	Amnestic aphasia	1
Pressure in the ears	1	Apathy	2
		Coma	**1**
Seizures			
With motor phenomena	47	*Other symptoms*	
Other (amnestic episodes, mental and emotional alterations)	34	Bladder dysfunction	11
		Stool incontinence	1
		Cough	1

From Lempert et al., with permission.[15]

The two most common categories of psychogenic unresponsiveness are those that result from a conversion disorder (often called *conversion hysteria*) and those that are part of the syndrome of catatonia (often thought to be a manifestation of schizophrenia). The two clinical pictures differ somewhat, but both may closely simulate delirium, stupor, or coma caused by structural or metabolic brain disease. The diagnosis of psychogenic unresponsiveness of either variety is made by demonstrating that both the cerebral hemispheres and the brainstem-activating pathways can be made to function in a physiologically normal way even though the patient will seemingly not respond to his or her environment.

The physician must recognize that, with the exception of factitious disorders and malingering, psychologically produced neurologic symptoms are not "imaginary."

The disorders are associated with measurable changes in brain function.

CONVERSION REACTIONS

A conversion reaction is the cause of most psychogenic comas. As used here, the term "conversion reaction" describes a psychogenic or nonphysiologic loss or disorder of neurologic function involving the special senses or the voluntary nervous system. Many physicians associate conversion reactions with a hysterical personality (conversion hysteria) but, in fact, conversion reactions may occur as a psychologic defense against a wide range of psychiatric syndromes, including depressive states and neuroses.[24] Furthermore, conversion symptoms, including psychogenic unresponsiveness, may be a reaction to organic disease and thus occur in a patient already seriously ill. We find it difficult to differentiate conversion reactions, presumably representing involuntary responses by patients to stress, from voluntary malingering except by the direct statement of the subject involved and perhaps by functional imaging.[7]

Patients suffering from psychogenic unresponsiveness, owing to either a conversion reaction or to malingering, usually lie with their eyes closed and do not attend to their surroundings. The respiratory rate and depth are usually normal, but in some instances the patient may be overbreathing as another manifestation of the psychologic dysfunction (hyperventilation syndrome). When one attempts to open the closed lids of a patient suffering from psychogenic unresponsiveness, the lids often resist actively and usually close rapidly when they are released. The slow, steady closure of passively opened eyelids that occurs in many comatose patients cannot be mimicked voluntarily.

When the eyelids are opened, the pupils may be slightly dilated, but are equal and reactive to light except in the instance of the individual who self-instills mydriatic agents. If this is done unilaterally, the combination of a "blown pupil" and impaired consciousness can cause the examiner to suspect temporal lobe herniation. Even full movement of the eye would not rule out an early uncal herniation syndrome or a ruptured posterior communicating artery aneurysm, and so an emergency computed tomography (CT) scan is often done. If this fails to disclose an anatomical cause, use of pharmacological agents, as discussed in Chapter 2, can demonstrate muscarinic blockade of the pupil.

Patients with psychogenic coma may show no eye movements at rest or even with oculocephalic maneuvers. Some examiners use a stimulus that is difficult to ignore to demonstrate following eye movements. These can range from an optokinetic strip or drum to a mirror to a $100 bill. Even if these tests fail, Henry and Woodruff described six patients with psychogenic unresponsiveness in whom the eyes deviated tonically toward the floor when the patient lay on his side.[13] The authors postulate that the deviation of the eyes was psychologically mediated as a way of avoiding eye contact with the examiner.

In some patients, the eyes deviate upward (Bell's phenomenon) when the eyelids are pried open against resistance. However, upward eye deviation also occurs during syncopal attacks.[25] On the other hand slow, roving eye movements cannot be mimicked voluntarily and so indicate an organic cause for the coma. Oculocephalic responses may or may not be present in psychogenic coma, but caloric testing invariably produces quick-phase nystagmus away from the cool water irrigation rather than the common results in structural coma (either tonic deviation of the eyes toward the irrigated ear or no response at all). *It is the presence of normal nystagmus in response to caloric testing that firmly indicates that the patient is physiologically awake and that the unresponsive state cannot be caused by structural or metabolic disease of the nervous system.* It is important to start with cool water, not ice water, if you suspect psychogenic coma, as this is usually sufficient to elicit the nystagmus, and ice water will make the patient very sick and may physically punish someone who is already tormented mentally. In the rare patient with preexisting vestibular dysfunction who may not respond to cool water but may have psychogenic unresponsiveness, you can always continue with ice water if there is no response. Similarly, other tests of noxious stimuli should be graded in approach, such as the "Harvey's second sign," in which application of a tuning fork (440–1,024 Hz) to the nasal mucosa on the inside of the nostril has been used to elicit response in functional coma.[26]

Patients suffering from psychogenic unresponsiveness as a conversion symptom usually offer no resistance to passive movements of the extremities although normal tone is present; if an extremity is moved suddenly, momentary resistance may be felt. The patient usually does not withdraw from noxious stimuli. Dropping the passively raised arm toward the face is a maneuver said to be positive when the patient's hand avoids hitting the face. However, the weight of the upper arm sometimes pulls the hand away from the face, giving the appearance of voluntary avoidance.[27] The deep tendon reflexes are usually normal, but they can be voluntarily suppressed in some subjects and thus may be absent or, rarely, asymmetric. The abdominal reflexes are usually present and plantar responses are invariably absent or flexor. The EEG is that of an awake patient, rather than one in coma.

Historical Patient Vignette 6.1

A 26-year-old nurse with a history of generalized convulsions was admitted to the hospital after a night of alcoholic drinking ostensibly followed by generalized convulsions. She had been given 50% glucose and 500 mg sodium amobarbital intravenously. Upon admission she was reportedly unresponsive to verbal command, but when noxious stimuli were administered she withdrew, repetitively thrust her extremities in both flexion and extension, and on one occasion spat at the examiner. Her respirations were normal. The remainder of the general physical and neurologic examination was normal. She was given 10 mg of diazepam intravenously and 500 mg of phenytoin intravenously in two doses 3 hours apart. Eight hours later, because she was still unresponsive, a neurologic consultation was requested. She lay quietly in bed, unresponsive to verbal commands and not withdrawing from noxious stimuli. Her respirations were normal; her eyelids resisted opening actively and, when they were opened, closed rapidly. The eyes did not move spontaneously, the doll's eye responses were absent, and the pupils were 3 mm and reactive. Her extremities were flaccid with normal deep tendon reflexes, normal superficial abdominal reflexes, and flexor plantar responses. When 20 mL of cold water was irrigated against the left tympanum, nystagmus with a quick component to the right was produced. The examiner indicated to a colleague that the production of nystagmus indicated that she was conscious and that an electroencephalogram (EEG) would establish that fact. She immediately "awoke." Her speech was dysarthric, and she was unsteady on her feet when she arose from bed. An EEG was marked by low- and medium-voltage fast activity in all leads with some 8-Hz alpha activity and intermittent 6- to 7-Hz activity, a recording suggesting sedation owing to drugs. She recovered full alertness later in the day and was discharged a day later with her neurologic examination having been entirely normal. An EEG done at a subsequent time showed background alpha activity of 8–10 Hz with a moderate amount of fast activity and little or no 5- to 7-Hz slow activity.

Comment

This patient illustrates a common problem in differentiating "organic" from psychogenic unresponsiveness. Patients with a history of a seizure disorder may have a psychogenic seizure and then be treated with medications for the presumed seizure. Note that phenytoin, which is used to treat seizures and status epilepticus, can also cause complete or partial loss of eye movements for several hours, which may complicate the diagnosis further. This patient had been sedated and had a mild metabolic encephalopathy due to these medications used to treat her seizures, but the preponderance of her signs represented psychogenic unresponsiveness. The presence of nystagmus on oculovestibular stimulation and an EEG that was only mildly slowed without other signs of neurologic abnormality effectively ruled out organic coma.

The converse of Historical Patient Vignette 6.1 is illustrated by Patient Vignette 5.2 (see page 190). In the latter, the initial examination suggested psychogenic unresponsiveness, but vestibular testing elicited tonic deviation of the eyes without nystagmus. The tonic eye deviation clearly indicated physiologic rather than psychologic unresponsiveness. A rare patient with psychogenic unresponsiveness is able to inhibit nystagmus induced by caloric testing (probably by intense visual fixation), but, in that instance, there is no tonic deviation of the eyes and the combination of other signs can establish the diagnosis.

When a patient with severe organic illness, whether systemic or neurologic, becomes unresponsive, the physician sometimes fails to entertain the possibility that the unresponsiveness is psychogenic and represents a conversion reaction to a difficult psychologic situation. Patient Vignette 6.2 illustrates this.

Patient Vignette 6.2

A 69-year-old woman was admitted to the coronary care unit complaining of chest pain.

On examination, she was diaphoretic and the electrocardiogram (EKG) showed changes suggestive of an acute anterior wall myocardial infarction. She was awake and alert at the time of admission and had a normal neurologic examination. The following morning, she was found to be unresponsive. On examination, her respiratory rate was 16 and regular, pulse 92, temperature 37.5, and blood pressure 120/80. The general physical examination was unremarkable, revealing no changes from the day before. On neurologic examination, she failed to respond to either verbal or noxious stimuli. She held her eyes in a tightly closed position and actively resisted passive eye opening; the lids, after being passively opened, sprung closed when released. Oculocephalic responses were absent. Cold caloric responses yielded normal, brisk nystagmus. Pupils were 4 mm and reactive. Tone in the extremities was normal. The deep tendon reflexes were equal throughout, and plantar responses were flexor. The neurologist who examined the patient suggested to the cardiologist that the unresponsiveness was psychogenic and that psychiatric consultation be secured. At the patient's bedside, the incredulous cardiologist began to discuss how the diagnosis of psychogenic unresponsiveness was made. When the decision was finally made to consult a psychiatrist, the patient, without opening her eyes, responded with the words, "No psychiatrist."

In this instance, the presence of severe heart disease led the patient's physicians to refuse initially to entertain a diagnosis of psychogenic unresponsiveness. In Historical Patient Vignette 6.3, the presence of severe organic neurologic disease masked the diagnosis for a considerable period.

Historical Patient Vignette 6.3

A 28-year-old man with hepatic carcinoma metastatic to the lungs was admitted to the hospital complaining of abdominal pain. His behavior was noted to be inappropriate a few days after admission, but this was believed secondary to the opioids given for pain. The inappropriate behavior progressed to lethargy and then stupor. When first examined by a neurologist,

he was unresponsive to verbal stimuli but grimaced when stimulated noxiously. He held his eyes open and blinked in response to a bright light. Nuchal rigidity and bilateral extensor plantar responses were present, but there were no other positive neurologic signs. A lumbar puncture revealed bloody cerebrospinal fluid (CSF) with xanthochromic supernatant fluid and a CSF glucose concentration of 15 mg/dL. The electroencephalogram (EEG) consisted of a mixture of theta and delta activity, which was bilaterally symmetric. Carotid arteriography failed to reveal the cause of his symptoms, which were believed to be caused by leptomeningeal metastases. For the next 2 weeks his state of consciousness waxed and waned. When awake, he continued to act oddly. Two weeks after the initial neurologic examination, he was noted to be lying in bed staring at the ceiling with no responses to verbal stimuli and with 6-mm pupils, which responded actively to light. Bilateral extensor plantar responses persisted. The EEG now was within normal limits, showing good alpha activity, which blocked with eye opening. Because of the confusion about the exact cause of his diminished state of consciousness, an "Amytal interview" was carried out (see page 302). After 300 mg of intravenous amobarbital was given slowly over several minutes, the patient awoke, was fully oriented, and was able to perform the serial sevens test without error. During the course of the discussion, when the problems of his cancer were broached, he broke into tears. Further history indicated that the patient's brother had a history of hospitalizations for both mania and depression. A diagnosis of psychogenic unresponsiveness superimposed on metastatic disease of the nervous system was made. The patient was started on psychotropic drugs, and he remained alert and responsive throughout the remainder of his hospital stay.

The two patients in the preceding vignettes illustrate the difficulties in making a diagnosis of psychogenic unresponsiveness in patients with organic disease. Merskey and Buhrich have stressed the frequency of conversion hysteria in patients suffering from structural disease.[4] Of 89 patients with hysterical conversion symptoms, 67% had some organic diagnosis; 48% of the group with organic diagnoses had either an organic cerebral disorder or a systemic illness affecting the brain. The authors believe that organic cerebral disease predisposes patients to the development of conversion reactions.

CATATONIA

The second major category of psychogenic unresponsiveness is catatonia. Catatonia is a symptom complex characterized by either stupor or excitement accompanied by behavioral disturbances that include, among others, mutism, posturing, rigidity, grimacing, waxy flexibility (a mild but steady resistance to passive motion, which gives the examiner the sensation that he is bending a wax rod), and catalepsy (the tonic maintenance for a long period of time of a limb in a potentially uncomfortable posture where it has been placed by an examiner). Some of these signs can be similar to those seen in patients with severe Parkinson's disease, and the use of neuroleptic drugs that can cause parkinsonism in many psychiatric patients adds to the confusion. There is a general impression among many psychiatrists that using "atypical" antipsychotic drugs reduces or eliminates the risk of parkinsonism. Nothing could be further from the truth. Except for quetiapine and clozapine, all of the other drugs in this class can and often do produce parkinsonism. Tables 6.2 and 6.3 list the signs of catatonia and some of its causes.

In a retrospective clinical study of patients admitted to a psychiatric unit with catatonic symptoms, only 4 of 55 were schizophrenic; 39 had affective disorders, 3 had reactive psychoses, and 9 suffered from organic brain diseases, which included toxic psychosis, encephalitis, alcoholic degeneration, and drug-induced psychosis.[28] Patients with catatonic stupor usually give the appearance of being obtunded or semi-stuporous rather than comatose. This state is compatible with normal pupillary and oculovestibular function even when the obtundation has a structural origin. In addition, catatonic stupor is accompanied by a variety of autonomic and endocrine abnormalities that give the patient a particularly strong appearance of organic neurologic disease. Catatonia may be

Table 6.2 **Signs of Catatonia**

Excitement	Nonpurposeful hyperactivity or motor unrest
Immobility	Extreme hypoactivity, reduced response to stimuli
Mutism	Reduced or absent speech
Stupor/coma	Unresponsive to all stimuli; eyes closed, flaccid, or rigid
Staring	Fixed, nonreactive gaze, reduced blinking
Posturing	Spontaneous maintenance of posture (the posture itself may or may not be abnormal) for longer than is usual
Grimacing	Maintenance of odd facial expressions
Echolalia	Mimicking of examiner's speech (may be delayed)
Echopraxia	Mimicking of examiner's movements (may be delayed)
Stereotypy	Repetitive, non-goal-directed movements
Mannerisms	Odd, purposeful voluntary movements
Verbigeration	Repetition of meaningless phrases or sentences
Rigidity	Maintenance of position despite efforts to be moved
Negativism	Apparently motiveless resistance to instructions or attempts to make contact
Waxy flexibility	During reposturing there is initial resistance, then the new posture is maintained
Withdrawal	Refusal to eat, drink, or make eye contact
Impulsivity	Sudden inappropriate behaviors with no explanation
Automatic	Exaggerated cooperation with request or continuation of obedience movement requested
Mitgehen	Raising of arm in response to light finger pressure (like an angle-poise lamp) despite instructions to the contrary
Gegenhalten	Resistance to passive movement in proportion to strength of stimulus
Ambitendency	Indecisive, hesitant movement
Grasp reflex	Reflex grasping movement of hand in response to stroking palm
Perseveration	Repeatedly returns to same topic or persists with movement
Combativeness	Usually undirected aggression or violent behavior

Modified from Bush et al.[29]

Table 6.3 **Some Reported Causes of Catatonia**

Category	Association
Idiopathic	Perhaps nearly 50% of patients
Psychiatric	Affective disorders, dissociative disorders, schizophrenia, drug-indued and other psychoses, obsessive compulsive disorder, personality disorder
Neurologic	Cerebral tumors, subarachnoid hemorrhage, subdural hemorrhage, hemorrhagic infarcts, closed head injury, multiple sclerosis, narcolepsy, tuberous sclerosis, epilepsy, Wernicke's encephalopathy, Parkinsonism, systemic lupus erythematosus
Metabolic	Addison's disease, Cushing's disease, diabetic ketoacidosis, hypercalcemia, acute intermittent porphyria, Wilson's disease
Drugs and toxins	Alcohol, anticonvulsants, disulfiram, neuroleptics, amphetamines, mescaline, phencyclidine, aspirin, L-dopa, steroids
Infections	Encephalitis (especially herpes), malaria, syphilis, tuberculosis, typhoid, acquired immunodeficiency mononucleosis, viral hepatitis

Modified from Philbrick and Rummans.[30]

seen in a number of critical care settings with and without previous psychiatric disease and should be considered as a cause of coma in the critically ill patient.[31]

The underlying pathophysiology is incompletely understood and a number of neurotransmitter systems have been implicated, including dopamine, glutamate, and gamma-aminobutyric acid (GABA).[32] A few studies using resting state MRI have identified reduced task activation in the primary and associative motor cortex areas.[33,34] Much of this research is performed in patients with schizophrenia, and alterations of the underlying psychiatric condition are difficult to distinguish from catatonia-related changes. Testing for catatonia can be approached with the trial use of GABAergic medications such as lorazepam or zolpidem.[35]

Catatonia occurs in two forms: retarded and excited. The patient in a catatonic stupor who presents a problem in the differential diagnosis of stupor or coma usually appears unresponsive to his or her environment. Severe and prolonged catatonic stupor, as described next, is uncommon since such patients are usually treated early with psychotropic medications before the full picture develops. The patient in catatonic stupor usually lies with the eyes open, apparently unseeing. The skin is pale and frequently marred by acne and has an oily or greasy appearance. The patient's pulse is rapid, usually between 90 and 120, and may be hypertensive. Respirations are normal or rapid. The body temperature is often elevated 1.0°–1.5°C above normal.

Such patients usually do not move spontaneously and appear to be unaware of their surroundings. If the febrile akinetic patient is taking a neuroleptic medication, the possibility of neuroleptic malignant syndrome must be entertained (see Chapter 5, p. 270). The patient may not blink to visual threat, although optokinetic responses are usually present. The pupils are often dilated and there is frequently alternating anisocoria; they are, however, reactive to light. Some patients hold their eyes tightly closed and will not permit passive eye opening. Oculocephalic eye movements are absent, and caloric testing with cool water produces normal ocular nystagmus rather than tonic deviation. At times there is increased salivation, the patient allowing the saliva either to drool from the mouth or to accumulate in the back of the pharynx without being swallowed. Such subjects may be incontinent of urine or feces or, on the contrary, may retain urine and require catheterization. The extremities may be relaxed, but more commonly are held in rigid positions and are resistant to passive motion. Many patients demonstrate waxy flexibility. Catalepsy is present in about 30% of retarded catatonics. Choreiform jerks of the extremities and grimaces are common. The deep tendon reflexes are usually present, and there are no pathologic reflexes.

Although appearing comatose, the patient is fully conscious. This normal level of consciousness is attested to both by a normal neurologic examination at the time the patient appears stuporous and by the fact that when he or she recovers, the patient is often (but not always) able to recall all the events that took place during the "stuporous" state (see Patient Vignette 6.4).

Patient Vignette 6.4

A 74-year-old woman with a history of hypertension and hypothyroidism, but otherwise in good health, was admitted to the hospital for replacement of her left hip. She had a previous replacement of the right hip several years before. She recovered well from the surgery, but 3 days later at 4:30 A.M., she was found unresponsive in bed. She lay quietly with eyes closed but did not respond to voice or noxious stimuli. She was seen by a neurologist at 7:30 A.M. She was unresponsive to voice, her eyes were open, and she would direct her eyes to sound and would blink to threat, but would not follow commands and did not respond to noxious stimuli. Tone was normal, as was the remainder of the neurologic exam. Ninety minutes later she "awoke" and responded entirely appropriately. She reported that, at 4:30 A.M., unable to sleep, she had the sudden feeling that she had died. Physicians whom she recognized entered the room, but she was unable to respond to them. She reported that the noxious stimuli were very painful, but she could not move, nor could she respond to questions. She continued to think that she was dead until somewhat later in the morning, when a nurse whom she knew well sat by the bedside and talked to her gently. Because the nurse was being so nice, she thought she had to respond and she began to talk. There had been no history of previous psychologic disorder nor was there any hint during the rest of her hospitalization of a psychologic abnormality.

Comment

It is hard to classify this patient with psychogenic coma, but the patient's mutism and inability or unwillingness to move suggest a *form fruste* of catatonia. That this disorder can be transient and occur in people without other underlying psychologic difficulty is well known and is illustrated by this patient.

While the patient with the retarded form of catatonia may be difficult to distinguish from a patient with stupor caused by structural disease, the patient with the excited type of catatonia may be difficult to distinguish from a patient with an acute delirium.[36] Both may be wildly agitated and combative, and such behavior may make it impossible to test for orientation and alertness. Hallucinatory activity can be caused by either organic or psychologic disease, although pure visual hallucinations are usually due to structural or metabolic disease and pure auditory hallucinations to psychologic disease. The segmental neurologic examination, insofar as it can be tested in a delirious or excited patient, may be normal with either structural or organic disease. Grimacing, stereotypic motor behavior, and posturing suggest catatonia rather than metabolic delirium.

Although the passage of time usually resolves the diagnostic problem, the only immediately distinguishing feature between psychogenic and organic delirious reactions is seen on the EEG. In patients with an acute toxic delirium caused by hepatic encephalopathy, encephalitis, alcohol, or other sedative drugs, slow EEG activity predominates. The EEG of the patient with the delirium of withdrawal from alcohol or barbiturates is dominated by low-voltage fast activity. The EEG is usually normal in patients with catatonia unless there is an underlying medical illness.[37,38] Thus, an entirely normal EEG with good background alpha activity that responds to eye opening and noise suggests that an either unresponsive or excessively excited patient is suffering from catatonia rather than structural or metabolic disease of the nervous system. If the EEG is dominated by high-voltage slow activity in the case of either a stuporous patient or an excited patient but not responsive patient, the likelihood is that the disorder is metabolic or structural rather than psychogenic.

PSYCHOGENIC SEIZURES

More difficult than identifying psychogenic coma is differentiating a psychogenic seizure from an epileptic seizure.[39] Psychogenic or non-epilpetic seizures are common; in one population study, psychogenic seizures affected 4% of the population.[1] The patient

Table 6.4 **Findings that can Help Distinguish Psychogenic from Epileptic Seizures**

	Psychogenic seizures	Epileptic seizures
History		
Started <10 years of life	Unusual	Common
Seizures in presence of doctors	Common	Unusual
Recurrent "status"	Common	Rare
Multiple unexplained physical symptoms	Common	Rare
Multiple operations/invasive tests	Common	Rare
Psychiatric treatment	Common	Rare
Sexual and physical abuse	Common	Rare
Observation		
Situational onset	Occasional	Rare
Gradual onset	Common	Rare
Precipitated by stimuli (noise, light)	Occasional	Rare
Purposeful movements	Occasional	Very rare
Opisthotonus, "arc de cercle"	Occasional	Very rare
Tongue biting (tip)	Occasional	Rare
Tongue biting (side)	Rare	Common
Prolonged ictal atonia	Occasional	Very rare
Vocalization during "tonic-clonic" phase	Occasional	Very rare
Reactivity during "unconsciousness"	Occasional	Very rare
Rapid postictal reorientation	Common	Unusual
Undulating motor activity	Common	Very rare
Asynchronous limb movements	Common	Rare
Rhythmic pelvic movements	Occasional	Rare
Side-to-side head shaking	Common	Rare
Ictal crying	Occasional	Very rare
Closed mouth in "tonic phase"	Occasional	Very rare
Closed eyelids	Very common	Rare
Convulsion >2 minutes	Common	Very rare
Resisted lid opening	Common	Very rare
Pupillary light reflex	Usually retained	Commonly absent
Lack of cyanosis	Common	Rare

Modified from Reuber and Elger.[40]

often presents in the emergency room having symptoms that may mimic a generalized tonic-clonic seizure or a complex partial seizure.[40] There is often no history available, and the patient may be unresponsive or appear to be stuporous or comatose. Because at least 50% of such patients also have epilepsy, differentiating a psychogenic from an epileptic seizure in a particular episode may be very difficult. Some clues both from the history and examination are given in Table 6.4. As indicated in the table, the physician should suspect a psychogenic seizure when the patient's motor movements are unusual (not rhythmic or repetitive), particularly when the seizure lasts a long time. An EEG may not be available unless the attack occurs on an inpatient unit during continuous EEG monitoring, but even

then may be marred by movement artifact. Furthermore, EEGs in patients with complex partial seizures may be normal. The physician should draw a prolactin level. An elevated prolactin level strongly suggests that a generalized tonic-clonic or complex partial seizure is epileptic.[41] A normal prolactin level does not rule out a nongeneralized seizure. Because the diagnosis is often uncertain and because, as indicated later, intravenous benzodiazepines treat psychogenic alterations of consciousness as well as epilepsy, one can often stop the episode with intravenous benzodiazepines. However, if there is a strong suspicion that the seizures are psychogenic, anticonvulsants should not be given. In most instances, a definitive diagnosis will require evaluation in an epilepsy unit with continuous video-EEG.

CEREBELLAR COGNITIVE AFFECTIVE SYNDROME

At times mistaken for catatonia, the cerebellar cognitive affective syndrome was originally described in children following surgery to the vermis of the cerebellum.[42] Because the children were awake but mute, the disorder was called the *cerebellar mutism syndrome*.[43] Cerebellar mutism also occurs in adults either after surgery involving the posterior fossa or as a result of lesions affecting the vermis and posterior lobes of the cerebellum. Such patients are awake, but may be somnolent. Whatever their level of alertness, they do not speak and often behave abnormally, either by not responding to the examiner or by behaving inappropriately. Patients may refuse to swallow food although they are not dysphagic. In children, the syndrome characteristically occurs after a period of normality in the postoperative period. The mutism begins hours to days after awakening from anesthesia. The syndrome is largely reversible, but neuropsychologic tests given long after apparent recovery demonstrate defects in executive function, affect, and language.[43] See Patient Vignette 6.5 and Figure 6.1.

Patient Vignette 6.5

A 32-year-old man with a cerebellar ependymoma complained of headache and mild imbalance. He had been operated on twice 2 years before with a vermis-splitting operation that removed most of the lesion, but left residual tumor in the lateral wall of the fourth ventricle. An operation was undertaken to remove the residual tumor. The surgeon did not invade the vermis but lifted the cerebellar tonsil to successfully resect the residual tumor. Neurologic consultation was sought in the immediate postoperative period when the patient appeared to be "unresponsive." He was lying in bed with his eyes open. He was still intubated, so that he could not speak, but he did not appear to respond to any verbal commands. He moved spontaneously and sometimes appeared to withdraw from noxious stimuli but never would look at the examiner or regard the examiner in any way. When

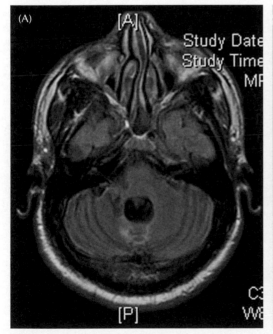 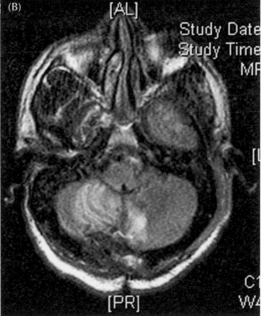

Figure 6.1 (A) A fluid-attenuated inversion recovery sequence from Patient Vignette 6.5 demonstrating hyperintensity in the vermis, a result of the first two operations, with residual tumor. (B) A 24-hour postoperative film done during the time when the patient was responding poorly. The hyperintensity in the vermis is more marked and there is new hyperintensity in the right posterior lobe of the cerebellum.

the patient was extubated he did not speak. Gradually, over the next 24–36 hours, the patient began to respond by closing his eyes to command but rarely looking at the examiner. He would carry out some commands, particularly grasping the examiner's hand. However, he had difficulty with commands involving the lips or tongue (oral buccal apraxia). Transiently, he demonstrated catalepsy. He would say his name, but to other questions he would only repeat his name. Later, when one of us asked him his name he responded "George Bush." It turned out that the nurse had asked him who the president was about 10 minutes before, and he had responded (at the time) appropriately.

Over time, he made a good recovery and was discharged from the hospital. However, even at discharge, his affect seemed flat and he himself reported that he was not the same as prior to surgery, although he could not describe what the changes were.

Comment

The cerebellar cognitive affective syndrome is rare in adults and can easily be mistaken for catatonia or psychogenic unresponsiveness. This patient had suffered modest damage to the vermis of the cerebellum from the first two operations (Figure 6.1A), and he suffered further transient damage to both the vermis and the right posterior lobe of the cerebellum as a result of the trauma of the third operation (Figure 6.1B). Interestingly, the surgeon noted that when she first interviewed him his affect seemed "flat." She referred him to a psychiatrist, who noted that his behavior had changed after the first operation in that he found himself "apathetic" and "not happy with the way I am." She found impaired memory and language "adequate, but not descriptive of his feelings and emotions." These changes were probably a result of the vermis damage from the first two operations.

"AMYTAL INTERVIEW"

In many instances, an immediate distinction between organic and psychologic delirium or stupor cannot be made on the basis of the neurologic examination or the EEG. In some of these instances, an Amytal interview has been used to successfully make the distinction immediately, although most psychiatrists these days recommend that if the examiner is fairly certain that the unresponsiveness is psychogenic, it is better to let a psychiatrist gradually break through to the patient, who may be using the unresponsiveness as a defense against severe psychiatric illness.

Although historically we have used amobarbital for this purpose, clinical evidence suggests that a benzodiazepine such as lorazepam works just as well and is more available.[44] We use the term *Amytal interview* loosely to describe the slow intravenous injection of an anxiolytic agent. The Amytal interview is conducted by injecting the drug intravenously at a slow rate while talking to the patient and doing repeated neurologic examinations. It is important that the discussion remains fairly neutral and not represent a direct challenge of the patient's veracity. Patients with structural or metabolic disease of the nervous system usually show immediately increasing neurologic dysfunction as the drug is injected. Neurologic signs not present prior to the injection of amobarbital (such as extensor plantar responses or hemiparesis) may appear after only a small dose has been introduced, and behavioral abnormalities, especially confusion and disorientation, grow worse. On the other hand, patients with psychogenic unresponsiveness or psychogenic excitement frequently require large doses of amobarbital before developing any change in their behavior, and the initial change is toward improvement in behavioral function rather than worsening of abnormal findings. Thus, a patient who is apparently stuporous may fully awaken after several hundred milligrams of amobarbital and carry out a rational conversation (see Historical Patient Vignette 6.3). A stuporous and withdrawn patient who is catatonic may become fully rational. An excited patient may calm down and demonstrate that he or she is alert, is oriented, and has normal cognitive functions. Patients in nonconvulsive status epilepticus may also awaken (see page 228). In some instances, Amytal interviews may provide a very useful method to disambiguate psychological reactions to new neurological disease by removing the symptoms of altered consciousness but preserving objective findings on the neurological examination.[45]

In a few instances, even the Amytal interview does not make a distinction between organic and psychologic delirium. In such instances, the patient must be hospitalized for observation while a meticulous search for a metabolic cause of the delirium is made. In one of our patients, a diagnosis of catatonic stupor, although strongly suspected, was confirmed after a thorough diagnostic evaluation had proved uninformative only when electroshock therapy was initiated and the patient fully awoke.[45] Once a psychogenic basis for unresponsiveness is established, a more extensive developmental and psychiatric history must be obtained to determine the type of psychiatric disturbance. The exact psychiatric diagnosis will determine the treatment. While the Amytal interview is a relatively safe procedure for diagnostic purposes, and is the first-line treatment for catatonia,[45] most psychiatrists do not recommend it for treatment if the patient relapses into psychogenic unresponsiveness after the diagnosis has been made. Intravenous sedatives given with the assumption that they will remove a symptom can be hazardous because the patient who has resolved his or her conflict by developing the conversion symptom may develop more serious psychologic disturbances should the symptom abruptly be removed.[46]

In summary, the diagnosis of psychogenic unresponsiveness requires exclusion of structural or metabolic causes of stupor and coma. The grave danger in making this diagnosis is that a treatable cause of the patient's condition will be missed. Hence, a complete workup for structural and metabolic causes of stupor and coma is necessary if the examiner has any doubt about the diagnosis.

REFERENCES

1. Sigurdardottir KR, Olafsson E. Incidence of psychogenic seizures in adults: a population-based study in Iceland. *Epilepsia* 1998;39:749–752.
2. Reuber M, Fernandez G, Helmstaedter C, Qurishi A, Elger CE. Evidence of brain abnormality in patients with psychogenic nonepileptic seizures. *Epilepsy Behav* 2002;3:249–254.
3. Caplan LR, Nadelson T. Multiple sclerosis and hysteria. Lessons learned from their association. *JAMA* 1980;243:2418–2421.
4. Merskey H, Buhrich NA. Hysteria and organic brain disease. *Br J Med Psychol* 1975;48:359–366.
5. De Tiege X, Bier JC, Massat I, et al. Regional cerebral glucose metabolism in akinetic catatonia and after remission. *J Neurol Neurosurg Psychiatry* 2003;74:1003–1004.
6. Vuilleumier P, Chicherio C, Assal F, Schwartz S, Slosman D, Landis T. Functional neuroanatomical correlates of hysterical sensorimotor loss. *Brain* 2001;124:1077–1090.
7. Spence SA, Crimlisk HL, Cope H, Ron MA, Grasby PM. Discrete neurophysiological correlates in prefrontal cortex during hysterical and feigned disorder of movement. *Lancet* 2000;355:1243–1244.
8. Manoach DS, Gollub RL, Benson ES, et al. Schizophrenic subjects show aberrant fMRI activation of dorsolateral prefrontal cortex and basal ganglia during working memory performance. *Biol Psychiatry* 2000;48:99–109.
9. Atre-Vaidya N. Significance of abnormal brain perfusion in catatonia: a case report. *Neuropsychiatry Neuropsychol Behav Neurol* 2000;13:136–139.
10. Lauer M, Schirrmeister H, Gerhard A, et al. Disturbed neural circuits in a subtype of chronic catatonic schizophrenia demonstrated by F-18-FDG-PET and F-18-DOPA-PET. *J Neural Transm (Vienna)* 2001;108:661–670.
11. Northoff G, Kotter R, Baumgart F, et al. Orbitofrontal cortical dysfunction in akinetic catatonia: a functional magnetic resonance imaging study during negative emotional stimulation. *Schizophr Bull* 2004;30:405-27.
12. Guze SB, Woodruff RA, Clayton PJ. A study of conversion symptoms in psychiatric outpatients. *Am J Psychiatry* 1971;128:643–646.
13. Henry JA, Woodruff GH. A diagnostic sign in states of apparent unconsciousness. *Lancet* 1978;2:920–921.
14. Hopkins A. Pretending to be unconscious. *Lancet* 1973;2:312–314.
15. Lempert T, Dieterich M, Huppert D, Brandt T. Psychogenic disorders in neurology: frequency and clinical spectrum. *Acta Neurol Scand* 1990;82:335–340.
16. Dula DJ, DeNaples L. Emergency department presentation of patients with conversion disorder. *Acad Emerg Med* 1995;2:120–123.
17. Weiss N, Regard L, Vidal C, et al. Causes of coma and their evolution in the medical intensive care unit. *J Neurol* 2012;259:1474–1477.
18. Slater E. Diagnosis of "hysteria". *Br Med J* 1965;1:1395–1399.
19. Shraberg D, D'Souza T. Coma vigil masquerading as psychiatric illness. *J Clin Psychiatry* 1982;43:375–376.
20. Meyers TJ, Jafek BW, Meyers AD. Recurrent psychogenic coma following tracheal stenosis repair. *Arch Otolaryngol Head Neck Surg* 1999;125:1267–1269.
21. Reuber M, Kral T, Kurthen M, Elger CE. New-onset psychogenic seizures after intracranial neurosurgery. *Acta Neurochir (Wien)* 2002;144:901–907; discussion 907.
22. Stone J, Smyth R, Carson A, et al. Systematic review of misdiagnosis of conversion symptoms and "hysteria." *BMJ* 2005;331:989.
23. Binzer M, Andersen PM, Kullgren G. Clinical characteristics of patients with motor disability due to conversion disorder: a prospective control group study. *J Neurol Neurosurg Psychiatry* 1997;63:83–88.
24. Hurwitz TA. Somatization and conversion disorder. *Can J Psychiatry* 2004;49:172–178.
25. Lempert T, von Brevern M. The eye movements of syncope. *Neurology* 1996;46:1086–1088.
26. Harvey P. Harvey's 1 and 2. *Pract Neurol* 2004;3:178–179.

27. Jackson AO. Faking unconsciousness. *Anaesthesia* 2000;55:409.
28. Gelenberg AJ. The catatonic syndrome. *Lancet* 1976;1:1339–1341.
29. Bush G, Fink M, Petrides G, Dowling F, Francis A. Catatonia. I. Rating scale and standardized examination. *Acta Psychiatr Scand* 1996;93:129–136.
30. Philbrick KL, Rummans TA. Malignant catatonia. *J Neuropsychiatry Clin Neurosci* 1994;6:1–13.
31. Saddawi-Konefka D, Berg SM, Nejad SH, Bittner EA. Catatonia in the ICU: an important and underdiagnosed cause of altered mental status. A case series and review of the literature. *Crit Care Med* 2014;42:e234–e241.
32. Walther S, Strik W. Motor symptoms and schizophrenia. *Neuropsychobiology* 2012;66:77–92.
33. Scheuerecker J, Ufer S, Kapernick M, et al. Cerebral network deficits in post-acute catatonic schizophrenic patients measured by fMRI. *J Psychiatr Res* 2009;43:607–614.
34. Payoux P, Boulanouar K, Sarramon C, et al. Cortical motor activation in akinetic schizophrenic patients: a pilot functional MRI study. *Mov Disord* 2004;19:83–90.
35. Sienaert P, Dhossche DM, Vancampfort D, De Hert M, Gazdag G. A clinical review of the treatment of catatonia. *Front Psychiatry* 2014;5:181.
36. Wilson JE, Carlson R, Duggan MC, et al. Delirium and catatonia in critically ill patients: the delirium and catatonia prospective cohort investigation. *Crit Care Med* 2017;45:1837–1844.
37. Louis ED, Pflaster NL. Catatonia mimicking nonconvulsive status epilepticus. *Epilepsia* 1995;36:943–945.
38. Carroll BT, Boutros NN. Clinical electroencephalograms in patients with catatonic disorders. *Clin Electroencephalogr* 1995;26:60–64.
39. Devinsky O, Thacker K. Nonepileptic seizures. *Neurol Clin* 1995;13:299–319.
40. Reuber M, Elger CE. Psychogenic nonepileptic seizures: review and update. *Epilepsy Behav* 2003;4:205–216.
41. Chen DK, So YT, Fisher RS. Use of serum prolactin in diagnosing epileptic seizures: report of the Therapeutics and Technology Assessment Subcommittee of the American Academy of Neurology. *Neurology* 2005;65:668–675.
42. Schmahmann JD, Sherman JC. The cerebellar cognitive affective syndrome. *Brain* 1998;121 (Pt 4):561–579.
43. Robertson PL, Muraszko KM, Holmes EJ, et al. Incidence and severity of postoperative cerebellar mutism syndrome in children with medulloblastoma: a prospective study by the Children's Oncology Group. *J Neurosurg* 2006;105:444–451.
44. Bush G, Fink M, Petrides G, Dowling F, Francis A. Catatonia. II. Treatment with lorazepam and electroconvulsive therapy. *Acta Psychiatr Scand* 1996;93:137–143.
45. Schiff ND, Moore DF, Winterkorn JM. Predominant downgaze ophthalmoparesis in anti-Hu encephalomyelitis. *J Neuroophthalmol* 1996;16:302–303.
46. Menza MA. A suicide attempt following removal of conversion paralysis with amobarbital. *General hospital psychiatry* 1989;11:137–138.

Chapter 7

Initial Management of Patients with Stupor and Coma

Of the acute problems in clinical medicine, none is more challenging than the prompt diagnosis and effective management of the patient in coma. The challenge exists in part because the causes of coma are so many and

the physician possesses only a limited time in which to make the appropriate diagnostic and therapeutic judgments. Coma caused by a subdural or epidural hematoma may be fully reversible when the patient is first seen, but if

305

treatment is not promptly undertaken, the brain injury may become either irreparable or fatal within a very short period of time. A comatose patient suffering from diabetic ketoacidosis or hypoglycemia may rapidly return to normal if appropriate treatment is begun immediately but may die or be rendered permanently brain damaged if treatment is delayed. In epidural hematoma, meticulous evaluation of acid–base balance and substrate availability may not only be useless, but it is also dangerous because precious time may be lost. In untreated diabetic coma, time spent performing imaging may interfere with life-saving treatment.

Outcomes of patients with severe acute brain injury in general and those with impaired consciousness in particular have improved significantly in the past decades, but what has become increasingly clear is that timeliness of interventions is crucial for patients with life-threatening neurological presentations. Millions of neurons, synapses, and myelinated fibers are lost every minute after onset of an ischemic stroke,[1] and seizures become increasingly difficult to control the later that treatment is initiated.[2] Time to deliver treatments is possibly the greatest variable to determine survival and functional outcome. This principle was put to the test in a number of clinical trials demonstrating the importance of early administration of intravenous thrombolytics[3] and endovascular clot removal[4] in patients with ischemic stroke, antiepileptic medications for patients with status epilepticus (SE),[5,6] and dexamethasone in adults with bacterial meningitis,[7] to highlight a few.

The physician evaluating a comatose patient requires a systematic approach that will allow directing the diagnostic and therapeutic endeavors along appropriate pathways. The preceding chapters of this text presented what may appear to be a bewildering variety of disease states that cause stupor or coma. However, these chapters have also indicated that for any disease or functional abnormality of the brain to cause unconsciousness, it must either (1) produce bilateral dysfunction of the cerebral hemispheres, (2) damage or depress the physiologic activating mechanisms in the upper brainstem and diencephalon, or (3) metabolically or physiologically damage or depress the brain globally. Conditions that can produce these effects can be divided into (1) supratentorial mass lesions that compress or displace the diencephalon and brainstem, (2) infratentorial destructive or expanding lesions that damage or compress the upper brainstem, or (3) metabolic, diffuse, or multifocal encephalopathies that affect the brain in a widespread or diffuse fashion. In addition, (4) the clinician must be alert to unresponsiveness of psychiatric causes. Examiners need to actively search for conditions without impairment of consciousness but limited ability to express consciousness, such as those associated with loss of motor response but intact cognition (e.g., brainstem infarction, degenerative loss of motor nerves, or acute peripheral neuropathy [Guillain-Barré syndrome] producing a locked-in state[8]).

These insights have led to efforts to streamline the initial management of patients with neurological emergencies, particularly those with impaired consciousness, and efforts to initiate targeted interventions in the emergency room or ideally prior to arrival to the hospital.[9] Using physiologic principles, one may considerably narrow the diagnostic possibilities and start specific treatment rapidly enough to make a difference in outcome. This chapter outlines a clinical approach that both stabilizes the patient to assure survival in most instances and allows the physician to assign the cause of unresponsiveness promptly into one of the preceding four main categories to start delivering targeted therapies to minimize irreversible damage to the patient's brain.

A CLINICAL REGIMEN FOR DIAGNOSIS AND MANAGEMENT

The initial objective of the first medical encounter with the comatose patient is to secure adequate vital body functions including airway, breathing, and circulation, which will be discussed in detail later. In addition to these measures focusing on cardiopulmonary resuscitation, a categorical clinical diagnosis for the underlying cause of coma should be made to guide the emergent management. The key to making a categorical clinical diagnosis of the patient in coma consists of two steps: first, the accurate interpretation of a limited number of physical signs that reflect the integrity or impairment of various levels of the brain; and, second, the determination of whether structural or metabolic dysfunction

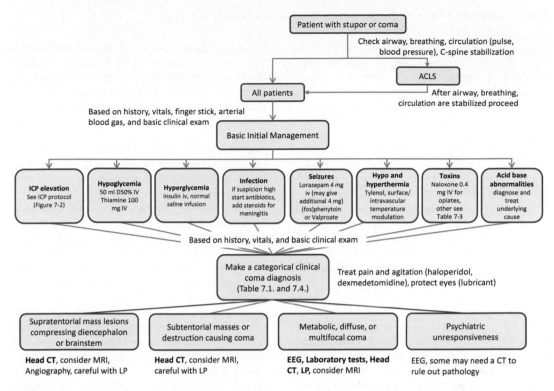

Figure 7.1 Flow diagram illustrating the initial management approach for the patient presenting with stupor or coma.

Table 7.1 **Differential Characteristics of States Causing Sustained Unresponsiveness**

I. *Supratentorial mass lesions compressing or displacing the diencephalon or brainstem*
 Signs of focal cerebral dysfunction present at onset
 Signs of dysfunction show a rostral-to-caudal progression through the brainstem
 Neurologic signs at any given time point to an anatomic level of progression (e.g., diencephalon, midbrain-pons, medulla)
 Motor signs often asymmetric

II. *Subtentorial masses or destruction causing coma*
 History of preceding brainstem dysfunction or sudden onset of coma
 Localizing brainstem signs precede or accompany onset of coma
 Pupillary and oculomotor abnormal findings usually present
 Abnormal respiratory patterns common and usually appear at onset

III. *Metabolic, diffuse, or multifocal coma*
 Confusion and stupor commonly precede motor signs
 Motor signs, if present, are usually symmetric
 Pupillary and oculomotor responses are usually preserved
 Asterixis, myoclonus, tremor, and seizures are common
 Acid-base imbalance with hyper- or hypoventilation is frequent

IV. *Psychiatric unresponsiveness*
 Lids close actively
 Pupils reactive or dilated (cycloplegics)
 Oculocephalic responses are unpredictable; oculovestibular responses physiologic for wakefulness (i.e., nystagmus is present)
 Motor tone is inconsistent or normal
 Eupnea or hyperventilation is usual
 No pathologic reflexes are present
 Electroencephalogram is normal

best explains the pattern and evolution of these signs (Figure 7.1). As Table 7.1 indicates, each of these pathophysiologic categories causes a characteristic group of symptoms and signs that usually evolve in a predictable manner. Once the patient's disease can be assigned to one of the three main categories, specific radiographic, electrophysiologic, or chemical laboratory studies can be employed to make disease-specific diagnoses or detect conditions that potentially complicate the patient's management. Once the diagnosis is made and treatment started, changes in these same clinical signs and laboratory tests can be used serially to extend or supplement treatment (medical or surgical), to judge its effect, and, as indicated in Chapter 9, to estimate recovery and prognosis.

Many efforts have been made to find an ideal clinical approach to the unconscious patient. Most such approaches repeat or even enlarge upon the complete neurologic examination, which makes them too time-consuming for practical daily use. A few are admirably brief and to the point (Chapter 2) (e.g., Glasgow Coma Scale) but have been designed for limited purposes, such as assessing patients with head injury; generally, they provide too little information to allow diagnosis or the monitoring of metabolic problems. The FOUR score scale (Chapter 2) gives more information, but is still limited.[10] The clinical profile described in Chapter 2, which has been employed extensively by ourselves and others, has advantages. The examination judges the normal and abnormal physiology of functions described earlier in Chapter 2: arousal, pupillary responses, eye movements, corneal responses, the breathing pattern, skeletal muscle motor function, and deep tendon reflexes. Most of these functions undergo predictable changes in association with localizable brain abnormalities that can locate the lesion or lesions. The constellation and evolution of these abnormal functions in a given patient can determine the cause of altered consciousness, whether supratentorial (focal findings start rostrally and evolve caudally), infratentorial (focal findings start in the brainstem), metabolic (lacks focal findings, but evidence of diffuse forebrain dysfunction), or psychiatric (lacks focal or diffuse signs of brain dysfunction). Of equal importance is that this examination is brief and does not delay implementation of effective treatment.

The need to initiate interventions as early as possible has generated interest in exploiting the out-of-hospital setting to start treatments. Success and challenges of initiating targeted therapy in the out-of-hospital setting are illustrated by randomized clinical trials for SE[5,6] and ischemic stroke.[11] Challenges of this setting include limited access to diagnostics such as imaging or EEG, limitations in medication choices such as those that need to be refrigerated, and, in most healthcare delivery systems, reliance upon nonphysician providers to assess and manage patients. Algorithms for out-of-hospital management of patients with decreased level of consciousness need to take these limitations into account while supporting optimally a relatively wide differential of underlying etiologies.

One problem that is frequently encountered is the tendency for paramedics in the field to intubate almost any patient with impaired consciousness "to protect the airway." Not all unconscious patients need to be intubated and, in fact, not infrequently unconscious patients can also be extubated. As long as patients have preservation of medullary reflexes that protect the airway and there is no concern for intracranial pressure (ICP) crises, many patients with coma caused by metabolic disarray, supratentorial mass lesion, and psychiatric conditions do not need to be intubated. Patients with impairment of the lower brainstem will require intubation. Because intubation usually involves giving patients sedative and paralytic drugs, the in-hospital evaluation of the patient requires either relying on the paramedic exam or stopping the drugs and waiting for them to clear. Initial assessment should therefore focus on determining if the out-of-hospital assessment/treatment was adequately provided so that this is not merely repeated, causing delay in more advanced treatment. In addition to stabilization of vital functions of the patient, diagnostic and interventional steps should be initiated as early as possible, taking the underlying cause of impaired consciousness into account.

ALGORITHM AND PRINCIPLES OF EMERGENCY MANAGEMENT

Support Vital Signs: Airway, Breathing, and Circulation

In patients with stupor or coma, vital cardiovascular and respiratory functions are frequently compromised and need to be supported. The primary injury linking consciousness and life-supporting vital body functions may either be directly in the cardiovascular or respiratory system (i.e., cardiac arrest leading to hypoxic brain injury; see Chapter 5), in the central nervous system (CNS) affecting both respiratory control pathways and pathways crucial to maintain consciousness (e.g., brainstem injury involving the respiratory centers in the ventrolateral medulla and that, at the same time, involve the ascending arousal system bilaterally such as seen with cerebellar hemorrhages with herniation causing mass effect on large areas of the brainstem; see Chapter 1, Figure 1.9 and Chapter 2, Figure 2.4), or conditions with effects both on cardiovascular and respiratory functions as well as brain areas crucial for supporting consciousness (e.g., tricyclic intoxication, see Chapter 5).

No matter what the diagnosis or the cause of coma, certain general principles of management apply to all patients with stupor or coma and should be prioritized as one pursues the examination and undertakes definitive therapy (Figure 7.1). All patients need to be screened and continuously monitored for development of cardiovascular and respiratory decompensation. In the out-of-hospital setting, diagnosis of cardiovascular and respiratory compromise typically consists of assessment of heart auscultation to determine rate and rhythm, blood pressure measurements, lung auscultation, observation of the breathing pattern, and oxygen saturation. In addition to the tests introduced in the out-of-hospital setting, laboratory tests, imaging, and ultrasound are readily available in most emergency room and intensive care unit settings. This allows rapid diagnosis, for example, of free fluid in the abdomen raising concerns for intra-abdominal bleeding in the trauma victim; pneumothorax for those with respiratory distress; or cardiac tamponade and function, as well as fluid status for those with hypotension. Initial evaluation of patients with impaired consciousness focuses on assessment and delivery of clinical interventions that are a fundamental part of the cardiopulmonary resuscitation protocol: airway, breathing, and circulation.

Ensure Oxygenation, Airway, and Ventilation

Stuporous or comatose patients with inadequate respirations will rapidly acquire

additional brain injury from lack of oxygen, have worsened impairment of consciousness from hypercarbia, and poor overall medical outcome from aspiration pneumonia. The initial focus needs to be an emergent assessment of the need for intubation, which can be categorized into a failure to oxygenate (assess skin color, check for cyanosis; if available and depending on the urgency of the respiratory decompensation, take into account pulse oximetry and arterial blood gas measurements), failure to ventilate (assess for excessive or inadequate work of breathing; if available and depending on the urgency, expiratory carbon dioxide and arterial blood gas measurements may be obtained), failure to protect the airway (to assess bulbar function, cough reflex and amount of secretions as well as presence of vomiting have to be weighed against each other), and anticipated neurological or cardiopulmonary decline. A protocol for assessment of the airway should take into account the risks and benefits to predict the level of airway difficulty as well as the ease of bag-mask ventilation.[12]

Providing an adequate airway includes basic maneuvers such as clearing mechanical obstructions and opening the airway using the jaw-thrust technique, as well as more advanced steps including the use of supraglottic devices (i.e., oropharyngeal or nasopharyngeal airways), tracheal intubation, and surgical approaches such as cricothyrotomy. Depending on the clinical scenario, level of expertise, and availability of the equipment, basic or more advanced airway support may be necessary and available. Breathing support includes application of artificial breaths via mouth-to-nose or mouth-to-mouth, and use of respiratory aids such as bag-valve-mask or ventilator-assisted respiratory support. Once the decision for endotracheal intubation has been made, the rapid sequence intubation is preferred to secure the airway, particularly of patients with suspected elevation of intracranial pressure.[13,14] This involves protection from the reflex sympathetic response induced by mechanical manipulation of the larynx during intubation resulting in tachycardia, hypertension, and ICP elevation. Steps include elevation of the head of the bed, intravenous access (allowing administration of pressors and fluids), preoxygenation for up to 5 minutes, and pretreatment with intravenous lidocaine (1.5 mg/kg 60–90 seconds before intubation;

this may also be given topically) to prevent the reflex sympathetic response, with fentanyl being an alternative.[15,16] Induction medications for patients with suspected elevation of ICP include the combination of etomidate and succinylcholine (2 mg/kg IV push), but alternative regimens including ketamine are available. For further details on intubation, please refer to published protocols.[15]

These primary resuscitation interventions are highly protocolized, but a few frequently encountered causes of unconsciousness require slight modification of these protocols. Stabilization of the cervical spine and replacing the head-tilt/chin-lift maneuver with the jaw-thrust technique is crucial for patients with any suspected trauma or any other cause for cervical spine instability as these interventions may otherwise further worsen the neurological injury. It is important to monitor all comatose patients carefully for hypotension as this may be a complication from medications given during intubation and worsen the outcome of all neurologically injured patients, particularly those with ischemia. Vagal discharge may occasionally lead to bradycardia or cardiac arrest, particularly in hypoxemic patients. As a general rule, keeping the mean arterial pressure between 70 and 90 mm Hg may serve as a guide to provide adequate cerebral perfusion.

Avoid hyperventilation in general but particularly if the underlying etiology is brain ischemia as this may cause cerebral vasoconstriction. If a patient shows signs of herniation, hyperventilation may be needed as an emergency temporizing measure. However, more definitive treatment of herniation and elevated ICP needs to be instituted as quickly as possible, as discussed later. Supraphysiologic oxygen levels are frequently provided to comatose or stuporous patients but have the potential to worsen outcome following traumatic brain injury[17] and cardiac arrest[18] due to formation of reactive oxygen species and impairment of mitochondrial function.[17]

Following intubation, appropriate placement of the endotracheal tube should be confirmed by checking for bilateral chest rise and lung sounds, lack of sounds on gastric auscultation, condensation in the endotracheal tube, and carbon dioxide measurements in the exhaled air (capnometer). Once confirmed, the patient should be connected to the ventilator (basic ventilator settings: volume-cycled ventilation at 8 cc/kg of ideal body weight and a respiratory rate of 12–14 per minute, unless the patient is herniating or medical conditions, such as adult respiratory distress syndrome, require adjustments), a pulse oximeter should be placed, an arterial blood gas sent, and a chest radiograph ordered. Patients comatose from drug overdose or who are hypothermic have depressed metabolism and require less ventilation than awake individuals. The comatose patient ideally should maintain a PaO_2 greater than 100 mm Hg and a $PaCO_2$ of between 35 and 45 mm Hg. All intubated patients should receive frequent chest physical therapy and suctioning of the airway, and many may need nebulizer treatments to loosen secretions. Sedation should be interrupted daily to assess spontaneous respiratory patterns and need for continued ventilation.[19] Caution is called for in any patients with suspected or confirmed elevation of ICP as mechanical manipulation may elevate the ICP. The optimal timing of tracheostomy in critically ill patients with neurological injury, such as those with stupor or coma, is controversial but many will discuss this option with families between the first and second week following the injury. Control of the airway and safety of regular feedings can be considered temporary measures that secure patient safety during a vulnerable period that can be re-evaluated over time.

Maintain the Circulation

Adequate blood supply to end organs including the brain is only achieved with an intact circulation. Emergent assessment of adequate circulation is crucial and involves checking the pulse, heart rate, cardiac rhythm, and blood pressure. When these are abnormal, additional diagnostic tools may be required to diagnose and treat the underlying problem, including electrocardiogram (EKG), arterial line placement, and emergency transthoracic echo.

Checking for a pulse should be the first diagnostic step. All pulseless patients are either already or will rapidly be comatose, and the primary treatment includes chest compressions (recommended ratio of 30:2 chest compressions to ventilations at 100 compressions/min).[20] The underlying cardiovascular abnormality needs to be identified rapidly and treatments initiated following the American Heart Association Advanced Cardiac Life Support (ACLS) protocol.[21] Treatments include defibrillations; cardiac medications such as epinephrine, atropine, adenosine, and others; intravenous fluids, and vasopressor support. Severe hypotension in patients with a pulse seen in all forms of shock needs to be addressed rapidly as additional brain injury will occur if untreated, and the cardiovascular condition may rapidly progress if untreated. Treatments include intravenous fluids, vasopressors, transfusion of red blood cells or other products, and stopping a bleeding source.

While treating the circulatory deficiency, the provider should focus actively on a search for the underlying cause as this may further guide the management. Hypotensive comatose patients with traumatic brain injury may also have a pelvic fracture resulting in hypovolemic shock from abdominal hemorrhage or have cardiac tamponade from chest trauma. However, damage to the brain above the level of the medulla does not cause systemic hypotension (see Chapter 2). The goal of maintaining an adequate blood pressure will depend on the underlying etiology, but, as an initial target, mean arterial pressure (MAP = 1/3 systolic + 2/3 diastolic) should be maintained between 70 and 90 mm Hg using hypertensive agents as necessary. In young, previously healthy patients, particularly those with depressant drug poisoning, a systolic blood pressure of 70–80 mm Hg is usually adequate.

In general, it is not necessary and may be dangerous to treat hypertension initially unless diastolic pressure exceeds 120 mm Hg or the patient is actively bleeding for example from a vascular cause. The elevation of blood pressure may be a reflex response to vascular occlusion (see Chapter 2), and, unless this is excluded, reducing blood pressure could worsen brain ischemia. In an older patient with known chronic hypertension, do not allow the blood pressure to fall below previously accustomed levels because the relative hypotension may cause cerebral hypoxia. However, if ICP is elevated, a higher MAP may be necessary to maintain cerebral perfusion pressure (e.g., MAP of 55–60 mm Hg above the ICP). When indicated, a number of intravenous agents are available to treat hypertensive emergencies, including labetalol (20–80 mg bolus over 10 minutes) and nicardipine (2–10 mg/hr).[22]

HISTORY, EXAM, AND BASIC DIAGNOSTICS

History and exam are crucial and also need to be assessed by first responders in the out-of-hospital setting as this information may be crucial to guide resuscitative efforts and be unobtainable at a later time point. Assessments should involve determination of the circumstances in which the patient is found (e.g., in an auto with the engine running, suggesting carbon monoxide poisoning), brief past medical history from bystanders or family (e.g., known polysubstance abuse may suggest overdose and prompt administration of naloxone), medication that the patient is taking (e.g., such as antiepileptic medication leading to administration of lorazepam or an antidepressant suggesting a suicide attempt), and a focused exam (e.g., may indicate herniation leading to administration of a hyperosmolar agent such as mannitol prior to obtaining imaging studies).

Emergency Neurological Examination of the Comatose or Stuporous Patient

Once the vital functions have been protected, proceed with the history and examination. The examination of the unconscious patient is covered in detail in Chapter 2, but a brief reprise is included here with emphasis on the elements that need to be covered quickly while initiating therapy in an emergency setting. Although the coma exam is, by necessity, relatively brief, the examiner has the luxury of time in doing the assessment when the patient has been under the continuous observation of other physicians on the ward or in an intensive care unit. In the emergency department, it is often necessary to weave obtaining the history and examination with urgent interventions. This goal of this emergency examination, together with the history and vital signs, is to allow the provider to categorize the etiology of unresponsiveness into one of four major categories (Table 7.1) that will guide emergent treatments.

The history should, to whatever extent possible, be obtained from relatives, friends, paramedics, bystanders, or sometimes even the

police. If it has not already been done, search
the patient's belongings and check for a medical alert bracelet. Implanted computer chips
that give full medical information are currently
available but are not yet in common use. The
history of onset is important. Coma of sudden
onset in a previously healthy patient usually
turns out to be self-induced drug poisoning,
subarachnoid hemorrhage, head trauma, or,
in older persons, brainstem hemorrhage or
infarction. Most examples of supratentorial
mass lesions produce a more gradual impairment of consciousness, as do the metabolic
encephalopathies.

In the general physical examination, after
assessing and dealing with abnormalities of
vital signs, look for evidence of trauma or signs
that might suggest an acute or chronic systemic medical illness or the ingestion of self-
administered drugs. Evaluate nuchal rigidity,
but take care first to ensure that the cervical
spine has not been injured.[23]

It is the neurologic examination that is
most helpful in assessing the nature of the
patient's unconsciousness. Table 7.2 outlines
the clinical neurologic functions that provide
the most useful information in making a categorical diagnosis. These clinical indices have
been extensively tested and applied to patients.
They have proved themselves to be easily and
quickly obtained and to have a high degree of
consistency from examiner to examiner.[10,24–26]
Furthermore, they give valuable information
upon which to base both diagnosis and prognosis. When serially recorded on a vital signs
sheet during each 24 hours, the result reflects
accurately the patient's clinical course. The following paragraphs give a detailed description
of each clinical sign.

Verbal Responses

Assessment of the verbal best response allows
assessment of orientation implying awareness of self and the environment. The patient
knows who he or she is, where he or she is,
why he or she is there, and the year, season,
and month. Confused conversation describes
conversational speech with syntactically correct phrases but with disorientation and confusion in the content. Inappropriate speech
means intelligible isolated words, which may

not be responsive or appropriate. The content
can include profanity but no sustained conversation. Incomprehensible speech refers to the
production of word-like mutterings or groans.
The worst verbal response, no speech, applies
to mutism.

Respiratory Pattern

The pattern is recorded as regular, periodic,
hyperpneic, ataxic, or a combination of these.
Respiratory rate is best determined in patients
not being mechanically ventilated.

Eye Opening

Patients with spontaneous eye opening
have some tone in the eyelids and generally
demonstrate spontaneous blinking, which
differentiates them from completely unresponsive patients whose eyes sometimes remain passively open. Though spontaneous eye
opening rules out coma by our definition, it
does not guarantee awareness. Some patients
remaining in a vegetative state, who by definition show eye opening, have been shown postmortem to have total loss of the cerebral cortex
(see Chapter 9). Eye opening in response
to verbal stimuli means that any verbal stimulus, whether an appropriate command or not,
produces eye opening. More severely brain-
injured patients demonstrate eye opening only
in response to a noxious stimulus applied to the
trunk or an extremity. The worst response, no
eye opening, applies to all remaining patients
except when local changes such as periorbital
edema preclude examination.

Pupillary Reactions

Pupillary reactions to an intense flashlight
beam are evaluated for both eyes, and the
better response is recorded; use a hand lens
or the plus 20 lens on the ophthalmoscope to
evaluate questionable responses. Record pupillary diameters and shape as well as if they
are ectopic (i.e., not centered).[27] Increasingly,
video-assisted quantification of pupillary reaction using pupillometer devices is used in clinical practice.[28,29]

Table 7.2 **A Score Sheet for Examination of the Comatose Patient**

Name of examiner

History (from relatives or friends)
Onset of coma (abrupt, gradual)
Recent complaints (headache, depression,
    focal weakness, vertigo)
Recent injury
Previous medical illnesses (diabetes, uremia,
    heart disease)
Previous psychiatric history
Access to drugs (sedatives, psychotropic
    drugs)
Occupation (pesticides, CO exposure)
Exposure to pathogens (ticks, mosquitoes)

General physical examination

Vital signs
Evidence of trauma
Evidence of acute or chronic
    systemic illness
Evidence of drug ingestion
    (needle marks, alcohol on breath)
Nuchal rigidity (examine with care)

Neurologic profile

Verbal responses
    Oriented speech
    Confused conversation
    Inappropriate speech
    Incomprehensible speech
    No speech
Respiratory pattern
    Regular
    Periodic (Cheyne-Stokes)
    Hyperpneic
    Ataxic
Eye opening
    Spontaneous
    Response to verbal stimuli
    Response to noxious stimuli
    None
Pupillary reactions
    Present and symmetric
    Asymmetric (describe)
    Absent

Date and time
    Eye positions at rest
    Conjugate or slight symmetric exo- or esodeviation
    Asymmetric deviation (describe)
    Spontaneous eye movements
    Orienting
    Roving conjugate
    Roving dysconjugate
    Abnormal movements (describe)
    None
Oculocephalic responses
    Normal awake
    Full comatose
    Abnormal (describe)
    Minimal
    None
*Oculovestibular responses (if oculocephalic responses
    are minimal or not obtainable)*
    Normal awake (nystagmus)
    Tonic conjugate
    Abnormal (describe)
    Minimal
    None
Corneal responses
    Present
    Asymmetric (describe)
    Absent
Motor responses
    Obeying commands
    Localizing (describe if asymmetric)
    Withdrawal
    Abnormal flexion posturing
    Abnormal extension posturing
    None
Deep tendon reflexes
    Normal
    Increased
    Asymmetric (describe)
    Absent
Skeletal muscle tone
    Normal
    Paratonic
    Flexor
    Extensor
    Flaccid
    Asymmetric (describe)

Eye Position at Rest

During sleep or metabolic coma, the eyes typically are slightly but symmetrically in exodeviation, although they may be conjugate or even have a slight symmetrical esodeviation. Any asymmetry in eye position should be noted, including exo-, eso-, superior or inferior deviation that is most marked in one eye, or skew deviation, when both eyes are out of the neutral position at rest. However, this must be interpreted in light of the baseline eye positions for that individual, as many people have congenital or acquired strabismus. Examining a photo ID or other photograph of the patient may be helpful.

Spontaneous Eye Movement

The best response is spontaneous, orienting eye movements in which the patient looks toward environmental stimuli. Record roving conjugate and roving dysconjugate eye movements when present, and reserve a miscellaneous movement category for patients without orienting eye movements who have spontaneous nystagmus, opsoclonus, ocular bobbing, or other abnormal eye movement. Absent spontaneous eye movements should be noted.

Oculocephalic Responses

These are evaluated in conjunction with passive, brisk, horizontal, and vertical head turning. Patients with normal waking responses retain orienting eye movements and do not have consistent oculocephalic responses. Full oculocephalic responses are brisk conjugate eye movements opposite to the direction of turning. Abnormal responses, which may include selective loss of horizontal or vertical movement of one or both eyes, should be described. Minimal responses are defined as conjugate movements of less than 30 degrees. Absence of response is the poorest level of function. *Remember, do not test oculocephalic reflexes in patients suspected of having sustained a neck injury.*

Caloric Vestibulo-Ocular Responses

In the absence of oculocephalic responses, it may be necessary to apply more intense and long-lasting vestibular stimulation by irrigating each external auditory canal with up to 50 mL of ice water with the head 30 degrees above the horizontal plane (Chapter 2). An intact response in an unconscious patient consists of tonic responses with conjugate deviation toward the irrigated ear.

Note that this procedure should not be done in a patient with a suspected psychiatric presentation who may be nonresponsive but awake. A normal (awake) response includes horizontal nystagmus with the rapid phase toward the nonirrigated ear, accompanied by severe vertigo and nausea.

Corneal Responses

Responses to a cotton wisp drawn fully across the cornea or—safer—sterile saline dripped onto the cornea are recorded as present, asymmetric (describe), or absent.

Motor Responses

These should be tested and recorded in all extremities and the strength noted as normal or weak. The best score is given to patients who obey commands; care should be taken to avoid interpreting reflex grasping as obedience. If a command evokes no response, apply a noxious stimulus gently but firmly to each extremity (compression of finger or toenail beds, or of Achilles tendon) and to the supraorbital notches or temporomandibular joints. Localizing responses indicate the use of an extremity to locate or resist a remote noxious stimulus (e.g., the arm reaching toward a cranial stimulus on the face or one on the trunk). Asymmetries in sensation (neither arm moves toward stimuli on one side of the body) or motor response (one arm moves less toward both sides) may indicate lateralized damage to the ascending sensory or descending motor pathways and should be noted. A more primitive response consists of a nonstereotyped, rapid withdrawal from a noxious stimulus; this response often incorporates hip or shoulder adduction. An abnormal flexion response in the upper extremities is stereotyped, slow, and dystonic, and the thumb is often held between the second and third fingers. Abnormal flexion in the lower extremities (the reflex triple flexion response) sometimes can be difficult to distinguish from withdrawal. An abnormal extension response in the upper extremity consists of adduction and internal rotation of the shoulder and pronation of the forearm.

No response is recorded only when strong stimuli are applied to multiple sites on each side of the body and when muscle relaxants have not recently been administered.

Tendon Reflexes

These reflexes are recorded for the best limb as normal, increased, asymmetric, or absent; minimal responses are best regarded as normal. Asymmetric tendon reflexes should be described, as these may be a clue to lateralized brain or spinal cord injury.

Skeletal Muscle Tone

This should be recorded as normal, paratonic (diffuse resistance throughout the range of passive motion), flexor (spasticity), extensor (rigidity), or flaccid. Again, any asymmetries should be described.

EMERGENT TREATMENT FOR ALL PATIENTS WITH STUPOR OR COMA

Emergent interventions must be guided by history, exam findings, and basic diagnostic tests if a possible or likely cause of stupor or coma is identified. The goal of these emergent interventions is to reverse progressive medical conditions that, if untreated, will rapidly lead to further worsening of the underlying condition and accumulation of irreversible brain injury. These interventions often must be initiated even before the physician completes a comprehensive diagnostic workup.

Examples include treatment of hypoglycemia or hyperglycemia, antibiotics for infections, steps to lower ICP, antiepileptics to treat seizures, treatment of hypo- or hyperthermia, correction of acid–base abnormalities, and administration of antidotes. In addition, patients with stupor and coma may need interventions for pain and agitation. Nearly all patients with impaired consciousness will require a noncontrast head computed tomography (CT) scan, as some intracranial processes that cause coma may leave few if any clues on the neurological

examination (e.g., bilateral subdural hematomas, subarachnoid hemorrhage, acute hydrocephalus). Certainly if the patient has evidence of a supratentorial mass lesion (e.g., asymmetric sensory or motor exam, uncal herniation syndrome) or a brainstem catastrophe (e.g., due to a cerebellar hemorrhage or basilar occlusion), it may be necessary to begin attempts to reduce ICP and move immediately to a CT scan. But, for the many patients who have nonfocal exams at this point (as described in Chapter 2), it is important to perform basic diagnostic testing (e.g., finger stick glucose, oximetry, possibly arterial blood gases, drawing blood for toxicology, fluid and electrolytes, and blood counts), as well as consider the following emergent interventions before the patient is consigned to the inevitable 5- to 15-minute delay required for CT scanning (in even the best of facilities).

Hypoglycemia or Hyperglycemia

The brain depends not only on oxygen and blood flow, but also on the obligate use of glucose for energy (see Chapter 5). Both hypoglycemia and hyperglycemia have deleterious effects on the brain (see Chapter 5). If the bedside blood glucose test reveals hypoglycemia, glucose should be given. This is often done empirically along with thiamine and naloxone by paramedics, before the patient arrives at the hospital; if not, glucose and thiamine should be given after reaching the hospital. Exact recommendations vary but 50 mL of a 50% intravenous solution of glucose is frequently used. Once stabilized and in the intensive care unit, studies have shown that tight glucose control using insulin decreases morbidity in non-neurologic severely ill patients. However, patients with acute brain injury may be harmed by this approach, and more liberal glucose targets are advocated for these patients.[30] Even after a hypoglycemic patient has been treated with glucose, care must be taken to prevent recurrent hypoglycemia. Therefore, ongoing monitoring of finger stick glucose and possible infusion of glucose and water intravenously may be necessary until the situation has stabilized. The comatose patient who is diagnosed with hyperglycemia may be treated with appropriate doses of intravenous insulin and normal saline fluids containing potassium, as glucose causes potassium to move intracellularly and blood levels can drop.

Thiamine

Wernicke's encephalopathy is a rare cause of coma.[31] However, many patients admitted as emergencies in stupor or coma are chronic alcoholics or otherwise malnourished.[32,33] In such a patient, a glucose load may precipitate acute Wernicke's encephalopathy.[34] Therefore, it is important to administer 100 mg thiamine intramuscularly or to put it into the intravenous fluids at the time glucose is given or shortly thereafter. Oral thiamine is often poorly absorbed in malnourished individuals.

Antidotes

Many patients entering an emergency room in coma are suffering from drug overdose. Any of the gamut of sedative drugs, alcohol, opioids, tranquilizers, and hallucinogens may have been ingested singly or in combination. In addition, patients suffering from psychiatric disorders who attempt suicide may have ingested antidepressant or neuroleptic drugs. Most drug overdoses are best treated by the supportive measures considered in a subsequent section. Because these patients often have ingested multiple agents, specific antagonists may not be useful.[35] Even the so-called "coma cocktail"[3] (dextrose, thiamine, naloxone, and flumazenil) is rarely helpful and may be harmful.[36] However, when there is a strong suspicion that a specific agent has been ingested, certain antagonists specifically reverse the effects of several coma-producing drugs (Table 7.3).

For opioid overdose (usually signaled by pinpoint but reactive pupils), intravenous naloxone may be given at 0.4–2.0 mg every 3 minutes or by continuous intravenous infusion at 0.8 mg/kg/hr until consciousness is restored. This drug must be used with great care because in a patient physically dependent on opioids, the drug may cause acute withdrawal symptoms requiring opioid therapy.[37] (If the patient is a known or suspected opioid addict, 0.4 mg naloxone should be diluted in 10 mL of saline and given slowly.)

One should use the minimum amount necessary to establish the diagnosis, as demonstrated by pupillary dilation and reversal of the comatose state. Naloxone has a duration of action from 2 to 3 hours, much shorter than the action

of several opioid drugs, especially methadone. Thus, patients who have taken an overdose of opioids, and whose toxic reactions are reversed by naloxone, may lapse back into coma after a few hours and require further treatment.

If there is reason to suspect a benzodiazepine overdose, the patient can be treated with flumazenil, a specific competitive benzodiazepine receptor antagonist[38] (0.2 mg/min to a maximum dose of 1 mg intravenous). Flumazenil acts within minutes and has a half-life of about 40–75 minutes. However, caution is recommended as this may precipitate acute withdrawal in chronic users or seizures in patients who have ingested medications such as tricyclic antidepressants or theophylline that lower seizure thresholds.[38] In addition, flumazenil may cause nonconvulsive SE to transition into refractory SE, which has been associated with high morbidity and mortality.

Certain effects of sedative drugs that have anticholinergic properties, particularly the tricyclic antidepressants and possibly gammahydroxybutyrate, can be reversed by the intravenous injection of 1 mg physostigmine. However, its use is controversial as it may cause seizures and cardiac arrhythmias; because of its potential side effects and short duration of action, it is rarely used.[39] Specific antidotes for several other agents are discussed in Chapter 5 and indicated in Table 7.3. Extracorporeal treatments have a role in certain intoxications,

Table 7.3 **Specific Antidotes for Agents Causing Delirium and Coma**

Antidote	Indication
Naloxone	Opioid overdose
Flumazenil	Benzodiazepine overdose
Physostigmine	Anticholinergic overdose (? gamma-hydroxybutyrate toxicity)
Fomepizole	Methanol, ethylene glycol toxicity
Glucagon	? Tricyclic overdose
Hydroxocobalamin	Cyanide overdose
Octreotide	Sulfonylurea hypoglycemia
N-acetylcysteine	Acetaminophen

Data from Ries and Dart.[39]

[a] Acetaminophen overdose does not impair consciousness but is often taken as part of a polydrug overdose; if not treated promptly, it may cause liver failure that does impair consciousness.

particularly if combined with acute respiratory distress syndrome.[40]

Infections

Many different systemic or CNS infections cause delirium or coma, and infection may exacerbate coma from other causes. Systemic infections are thought to impair consciousness via systemic inflammatory mediators, including cytokines and prostaglandins, which also cause fever that may further reduce alertness. On presentation, patients may be either hyperthermic (febrile) or hypothermic, often have tachycardia, and, if they are septic, may also have hypotension. If the infection involves the CNS there may be focal neurological signs in addition to stupor or coma. Successful treatment of systemic or CNS infections to a large extent depends on rapid administration of antibiotics. Details of meningitis treatment will be discussed in Chapter 8 but a generalized approach to the patient with suspected infection will be presented here. Empiric treatment of sepsis or meningitis treatment should not be delayed by diagnostic studies if the suspicion is high. Choices of antibiotics should be guided by the likely pathogens, and local antibiograms should be taken into account when selecting the most appropriate empiric antibiotic regimen, as well as the immune competency of the patient (e.g., chemotherapy or acquired immune deficiency disorders), the clinical setting of onset of the symptoms (nursing home vs. community vs. in-hospital setting), type of infection (sepsis vs. meningitis), and age of the patient. Blood cultures should be drawn on all comatose patients who are febrile or who are hypothermic without obvious cause. For suspected bacterial meningitis, a third-generation cephalosporin together with vancomycin should be started. In elderly or obviously immunosuppressed patients, ampicillin should be added. Current evidence suggests that dexamethasone should added to the regimen[7] (see Chapter 8 for details). As discussed in Chapter 3, it is generally necessary in a comatose patient to obtain a CT scan prior to attempting lumbar puncture. If cerebrospinal fluid (CSF) cultures can be obtained within the first hour or two after antibiotics are administered, it may still be possible to identify the organism and its antibiotic sensitivities.

Intracranial Pressure

In comatose patients with suspected elevation of ICP (e.g., after head trauma), it is important first to establish cardiovascular stability and C-spine stabilization., followed by rapid-sequence intubation after premedication with lidocaine (see earlier discussion). A number of general measures to treat elevated ICP should be employed, but these should be administered simultaneous (not sequentially) to lower ICP (Figure 7.2). The head of the bed should be raised to 30 degrees and the head kept straight to allow optimal drainage of venous blood via the jugular veins. Mild hyperventilation is recommended as a temporizing measure only (never allow the PCO_2 to drop below 25 mm Hg) until more definitive treatment such as surgical evacuation of a mass lesion. Adequate oxygenation should be assured with pulse oximetry checks, and an arterial blood gas sent as soon as possible. Isotonic intravenous fluids with inotropic medications if needed should be given to maintain a mean arterial pressure (MAP) of 80 mmHg or higher to allow adequate cerebral perfusion in the setting of elevated ICP. Hypotonic fluids should be avoided and blood products given as needed. Pain needs to be controlled, ideally with short-acting analgesics with the least effect on blood pressure (fentanyl 20–200 µg/hr, alternatives in the patient without central access include intravenous morphine 2–4 mg q2–4h). Agitation should be controlled emergently, often requiring sedation with short-acting sedatives such as propofol (propofol 0.1–5 mg/kg/hr) or benzodiazepines.

If the clinical exam raises the concern for herniation, emergent pharmacologic treatments should be initiated based on the clinical exam alone and not withheld until imaging confirms the suspected diagnosis. However, a head CT needs to be obtained for all patients with suspected ICP elevation as soon as possible to allow potential treatment of the underlying cause while initial empiric therapeutics for ICP elevation are administered. Whenever possible, one should attempt to treat the underlying cause for the ICP elevation. Treatment of the underlying cause may involve placement of external ventricular drainage catheters which can be a life-saving procedure and may need to be placed in the emergency room. Other

ICP Treatment protocol

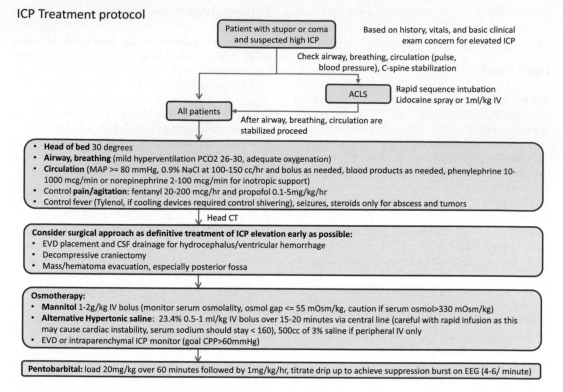

Figure 7.2 Flow diagram illustrating the initial management approach for the patient presenting with suspected elevation of intracranial pressure (ICP).

surgical interventions include emergent evacuation of space-occupying lesions such as cerebellar hemorrhages.

Emergent pharmacologic agents that lower the ICP include intravenous mannitol (typically given as 0.5–1 gm/kg total body weight over 15 minutes, with normal saline replacement of the volume lost in the subsequent diuresis). Hypertonic saline in a variety of concentrations is available as an alternative; however, data are limited and caution is warranted for patients with chronic hyponatremia, cardiac instability, and lung pathology such as pulmonary edema. Serum sodium and osmolality should be measured regularly for both patients receiving mannitol or those receiving hypertonic saline. If these interventions fail to lower the elevated ICP, barbiturate treatment may be used (pentobarbital or thiopental). Pentobarbital is given as a load 20 mg/kg over 60 minutes followed by 1 mg/kg/hr. The dose is titrated up to 3 mg/kg/hr as needed to achieve burst suppression on EEG with 4–6 bursts per minute. It is

important to observe for hypotension, which is a major side effect. The role of hypothermia in the treatment of traumatic brain injury patients with elevated ICP is not clear at this point.[41] Steroids have no role in the treatment of patients with traumatic brain injury[42] or other forms of cytotoxic edema but are given frequently for vasogenic edema, as seen in patients with brain tumors.

When treating suspected ICP elevation, it is often useful to place ICP monitors. ICP monitoring is typically performed with pressure monitors placed into the ventricles (external ventricular drainage) or brain parenchyma (typically placed in the frontal lobe ipsilateral to the injury).

In a randomized controlled trial that compared two ICP treatment protocols, in one in which ICP treatment was guided by clinical examination and serial imaging, and the other by ICP measurements exceeding 20 mm Hg,[43] the latter arm showed a trend toward more efficient delivery of care, although outcomes were similar. Experts have since suggested that the best treatment would include both ICP monitoring and clinical and imaging evaluation to take the underlying evolving pathophysiology into account,[44] but this has not been directly tested. Relating other measures of brain physiology to the elevation in ICP (Figure 7.3) may help guide management and is being tested in clinical trials (for details, please refer to the traumatic brain injury section in Chapter 8).

Seizures

Ongoing seizure activity as seen in status epilepticus (SE), of whatever etiology, can cause brain damage and must be stopped (for details please refer to Chapter 5). Important principles for the treatment of SE include early treatment at adequate dosage (80% respond to the first antiepileptic drug if treatment is initiated

within 30 minutes of onset, while only 40% respond when treatment starts 2 hours or more after seizure onset).[2] It is important to monitor the patient continuously during treatment for continuing seizure activity as well as cardiovascular or respiratory complications either from ongoing seizures or seizure treatment. In the VA cooperative study, 20% of patients in whom medication stopped the clinically visible manifestations of seizures remained in electrographic SE.[45] Hence, if the patient does not return to the pre-status baseline within 15–20 minutes after convulsions have stopped, it is important to continue monitoring using EEG to detect ongoing nonconvulsive seizure activity.

Clinical trials have established intravenous lorazepam as an acute treatment for SE (4 mg with the option of giving another 4 mg after 5 minutes if seizures continue)[45] and support intramuscular midazolam (0.2 mg/kg; max 10 mg) as an alternative.[6] Personnel and equipment

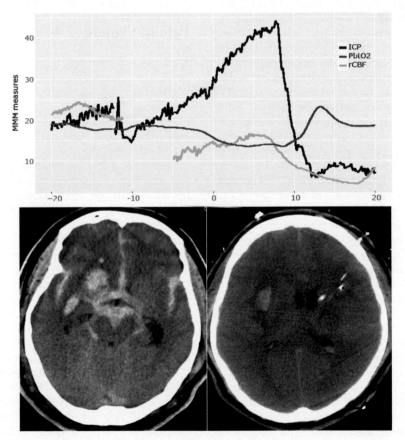

Figure 7.3 Patient with subarachnoid hemorrhage and multimodality monitoring including measures of intracranial pressure (ICP), partial brain tissue oxygenation (PbtO$_2$), and regional cerebral blood flow (rCBF).

must be available to perform emergency respiratory support if needed; because both ongoing seizure activity and many antiseizure medications may depress breathing, many patients with SE will ultimately require intubation. However, as ongoing seizure activity is more likely to cause respiratory decompensation than benzodiazepine treatment, it is still important to start the treatment of SE as soon as possible, including in the out-of-hospital setting.[5] Adding levetiracetam as a second antiepileptic agent in the pre-hospital setting was not associated with better seizure control or outcomes for patients with convulsive SE.[46]

As lorazepam typically suppresses seizures only for 20–30 minutes, it is important to begin concomitant treatment with either phenytoin/fosphenytoin (20 mg PE/kg IV administered at a rate of 50 mg/min for phenytoin and 150 mg/min for fosphenytoin; may give additional 5 mg/kg for ongoing seizures activity) or intravenous valproic acid (20–40 mg/kg; may give additional 20 mg/kg).[47] Many investigators advocate for more aggressive and rapid escalation of treatment for patients who do not respond to the initial benzodiazepine because only 7% of patients who did not respond to the first-line antiepileptic drugs responded to the second-line drug in the VA cooperative trail.[45] For example, some authorities propose going straight to continuous infusion of midazolam (initial 0.2 mg/kg; maintenance 0.05–2 mg/kg/hr)[47] but controversy regarding the early use of continuous application of antiepileptic agents at anesthetic dosages still exists.[48] The role of alternative agents such as levetiracetam or lacosamide is not clear at this point.

On the other hand, for patients with refractory SE whose seizures persist after first- and second-line treatment, most experts recommend advancing to anesthetic dosages of either midazolam or propofol because refractory SE is associated with high morbidity and mortality. Although most seizures occurring at this stage are nonconvulsive, they still should be treated in the same way as convulsive SE. No adequately powered randomized controlled trial has compared midazolam and propofol treatments, but efficacy of either treatment is highly dose dependent.[49,50] Alternatives include treatment with valproic acid or levetiracetam if not given at an earlier stage, particularly for those patients with prior directives not to intubate. Doses of anesthetics are titrated up until

seizures are controlled and typically continued for 24–48 hours, at which point weaning will start if seizures have been controlled.

Seizures that occur despite treatment with midazolam or propofol are called *super refractory SE* and carry a very high mortality rate. They are typically treated with intravenous pentobarbital infusions (load 5 mg/kg up to 50 mg/min; repeat 5 mg/kg boluses until seizures stop; maintenance, 0.5–10 mg/kg/hr).[51] A long list of additional treatments has been proposed, including ketamine, which, as an N-methyl-D-aspartate (NMDA) antagonist, may be attractive for benzodiazepine-unresponsive seizures,[52] and hypothermia, which not only suppresses seizure activity but also is neuroprotective.[53]

Focal continuous epilepsy such as epilepsia partialis continua, by contrast, frequently occurs with metabolic brain disease but is less threatening to the brain and does not require the use of anesthetic doses of anticonvulsant drugs.

Patient Vignette 7.1

A 30-year-old woman presents with sudden onset of fluctuating unresponsiveness on postpartum day six with a sudden onset of fluctuating unresponsiveness after an uncomplicated pregnancy and delivery of a healthy baby. At an outside hospital, her blood pressure was 152/88 mm Hg and she was found to have a large frontal lobe intracerebral hemorrhage; she underwent emergent placement of an external ventricular drainage catheter and an attempted clot evacuation. Post intervention she remained unconscious and was transferred to a tertiary care center. Here she was found to be unconscious, pupils were reactive to light, present corneal reflexes, present doll's eye movement, but she had no eye deviation and no motor response to stimulation. Head computed tomography (CT) scan showed persistent right frontal intracerebral hemorrhage (Figure 7.4, Panel A), but the level of consciousness was judged to be out of proportion depressed compared to the CT findings. Electroencephalogram (EEG) monitoring showed continuous right hemispheric seizure activity (Figure 7.4, Panels B and C). A digital subtraction angiogram showed beading of the arteries most consistent with postpartum reversible vasoconstriction syndrome

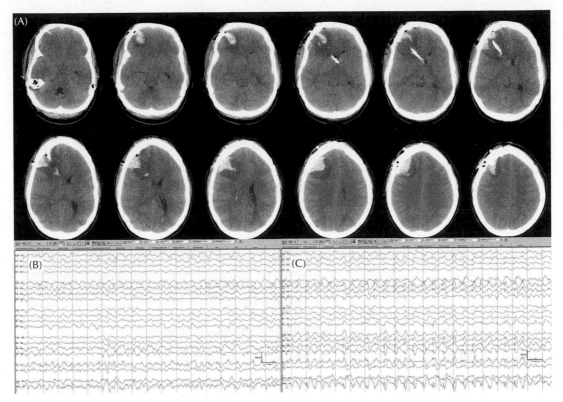

Figure 7.4 A 30-year-old woman with postpartum fluctuating unresponsiveness in setting of right frontal intracerebral hemorrhage (Panel A) and continuous right hemispheric seizure activity (Panels B and C).

(Call-Fleming syndrome). Her seizures were controlled with levetiracetam and phenytoin. Following seizure control, she had prompt recovery of consciousness and was extubated the following day.

Patient Vignette 7.2

A 39-year-old woman presented with a history of cerebral palsy and epilepsy well controlled on Tegretol. During pregnancy, Tegretol was stopped and levetiracetam started. Seizures occurred with increasing frequency despite adding Lamictal and phenobarbital. She presented with three generalized tonic-clonic seizures and subsequent frequent episodes of right arm numbness followed by head and gaze deviation to the right that evolved into nonconvulsive status epilepticus (see Figure 7.5, Panels A and B) at 30 weeks of gestational age. The obstetrics team strongly felt that eclampsia was unlikely as her blood pressure ranged from 120–130s over 70–80s mm Hg and no proteinuria was present. Despite this, with eclampsia high on the differential, the neurocritical care team treated her with magnesium infusions in addition to phenobarbital 100 every 8 hours, Lamictal 200 every 12 hours, levetiracetam 2 g every 12 hours, carbamazepine 800 mg every 12 hours, midazolam infusion up to 2.9 mg/kg/hr, and ketamine 100 mg bolus twice. Initially the fetal heart rate monitor and ultrasound showed a healthy baby. Seizures became more frequent, up to every 2 minutes and the fetal heart rate monitor showed absent decelerations and no movement on ultrasound. An emergent cesarean section was performed at the bedside (see Figure 7.5: Panel C displays quantitative EEG measures summarizing an 8-hour period initially showing increasing seizure frequency with abrupt cessation of seizures following the caesarian section). Not a single seizure was recorded subsequently, and she was

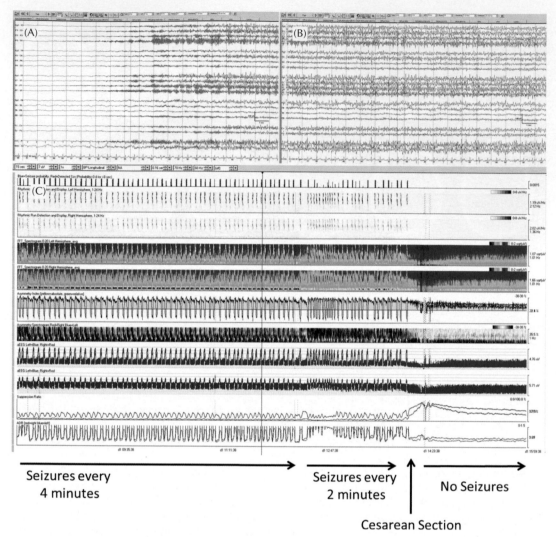

Seizures every
4 minutes

Seizures every
2 minutes

No Seizures

Cesarean Section

Figure 7.5 A 39-year-old woman with a history of cerebral palsy and epilepsy presents with nonconvulsive status epilepticus (panels A and B) that is controlled with an emergent cesarean section. Quantitative electroencephalogram (EEG) measures summarizing an 8-hour period initially showing increasing seizure frequency with abrupt cessation of seizures following the caesarian section (panel C).

rapidly titrated off the midazolam infusion. She was transitioned back to her prepregnancy antiepileptic regimen with good seizure control. Both, mother and baby recovered fully.

Hypo- and Hyperthermia

Several metabolic and structural abnormalities lead to either hyperthermia or hypothermia, and these states may exacerbate abnormalities of cerebral metabolism.[54] Hyperthermia is dangerous because it increases cerebral metabolic demands and, at extreme levels, can denature brain cellular proteins.[55] The body temperature above 38.5°C of hyperthermic patients should be reduced using antipyretics and, if necessary, physical cooling (e.g., cooling blanket). Significant hypothermia (below 34°C) can lead to pneumonia, cardiac arrhythmias, electrolyte disorders, hypovolemia, metabolic acidosis, impaired coagulation, and thrombocytopenia and leukopenia.[54] Patients should be gradually warmed to maintain a body temperature higher than 35°C.

Acid–Base Abnormalities

With severe metabolic acidosis or alkalosis, the pH should be returned to a normal level by treating the cause, as metabolic acidosis can lead to cardiovascular complications and metabolic alkalosis can depress respiration. Respiratory acidosis presages respiratory failure and warns the physician that ventilatory assistance may soon be needed. The elevated CO_2 also raises ICP. Respiratory alkalosis can cause cardiac arrhythmias and hinders weaning from ventilatory support.

Control Agitation

Many patients who are delirious or stuporous are grossly agitated. The hyperactivity is distressing to patients and family and may lead to self-injury. Sedative dosages of drugs should be avoided until the diagnosis is clear and one is certain that the problem is metabolic rather than structural. Agitation can be controlled by keeping the patient in a lighted room and asking a relative or staff member to sit at the bedside and talk reassuringly to the patient. Antipsychotic medications (i.e., haloperidol 0.5–1.0 mg orally or intramuscularly)[56] are preferred by some as benzodiazepines may complicate the examination due to sedative side effects and have been associated with the risk of developing delirium. While parenteral haloperidol is often used acutely to sedate an agitated patient, it can cause sleepiness as well as extrapyramidal side effects (dystonia, parkinsonism) that can cloud the neurological exam. Hence it should not be used prophylactically.[57] In an intensive care unit setting, if prophylactic sedation is needed and nasogastric access is available, quetiapine is the preferred neuroleptic medication as it generally does not cause extrapyramidal side effects. If benzodiazepines are chosen, small doses of short-acting medications, such as lorazepam 0.5–1.0 mg orally with additional doses every 4 hours, are preferred. In patients who have habitually abused alcohol or sedative drugs, larger doses may be necessary because of cross-tolerance. For very short-term sedation, as might be necessary to perform a CT scan, intravenous sedation with dexmedetomidine, propofol, or midazolam may be used, but ventilation and circulation must be continuously monitored as these drugs may cause respiratory arrest or hypotension. Physical restraints should be avoided whenever possible, but may be necessary for severely agitated patients to prevent self-harm. Care must be taken to ensure that body restraints do not interfere with breathing and that limb restraints do not occlude blood flow or damage peripheral nerves. The restraints should be removed as soon as the agitation is controlled.

Protect the Eyes

Corneal erosions can occur within 4–6 hours if the eyes of comatose patients remain partially or fully opened. Exposure keratitis may lead to secondary bacterial corneal ulcerations. To prevent such damage, lubricate the eyes with a lubricating artificial tears ointment every 4 hours[58] or apply a polyethylene corneal bandage.[59] Repeated testing of the corneal reflex with cotton can also damage the cornea. A safer technique is to drip sterile saline onto the cornea from a distance of 4–6 inches.[10]

MORE DEFINITIVE DIAGNOSIS AND TREATMENT OF SPECIFIC ETIOLOGIES OF STUPOR AND COMA

Initial treatment of comatose patients is most successful if a multidisciplinary team approach with well-established protocols is employed, as illustrated by the highly successful strategies commonly used for patients with traumatic brain injury. These initial efforts stabilize the patient and minimize the chances of further brain injury while more definitive diagnostic steps are taken. This workup is guided by the history and clinical examination, as well as by basic diagnostic tests (as discussed earlier) and initial response to treatment. Depending on the setting, additional workup may include imaging (CT and MRI studies; CT, MRI or digital subtraction angiography), EEG, ultrasound, or neurosurgical procedures such as placement of an intraventricular catheter. The workup and subsequent treatment for specific disorders that impair consciousness are discussed in the next chapter.

REFERENCES

1. Saver JL. Time is brain-quantified. *Stroke* 2006;37:263–266.
2. Lowenstein DH, Alldredge BK. Status epilepticus at an urban public hospital in the 1980s. *Neurology* 1993;43:483–488.
3. Emberson J, Lees KR, Lyden P, et al. Effect of treatment delay, age, and stroke severity on the effects of intravenous thrombolysis with alteplase for acute ischaemic stroke: a meta-analysis of individual patient data from randomised trials. *Lancet* 2014;384:1929–1935.
4. Campbell BC, Donnan GA, Lees KR, et al. Endovascular stent thrombectomy: the new standard of care for large vessel ischaemic stroke. *Lancet Neurol* 2015;14:846–854.
5. Alldredge BK, Gelb AM, Isaacs SM, et al. A comparison of lorazepam, diazepam, and placebo for the treatment of out-of-hospital status epilepticus. *N Engl J Med* 2001;345:631–637.
6. Silbergleit R, Durkalski V, Lowenstein D, et al. Intramuscular versus intravenous therapy for prehospital status epilepticus. *N Engl J Med* 2012;366:591–600.
7. de Gans J, van de Beek D. European dexamethasone in adulthood bacterial meningitis study I. Dexamethasone in adults with bacterial meningitis. *N Engl J Med* 2002;347:1549–1556.
8. Laureys S, Pellas F, Van Eeckhout P, et al. The locked-in syndrome: what is it like to be conscious but paralyzed and voiceless? *Prog Brain Res* 2005;150:495–511.
9. Smith WS, Weingart S. Emergency Neurological Life Support (ENLS): what to do in the first hour of a neurological emergency. *Neurocritical care* 2012;17 Suppl 1:S1–3.
10. Wijdicks EF, Bamlet WR, Maramattom BV, Manno EM, McClelland RL. Validation of a new coma scale: the FOUR score. *Annals of neurology* 2005;58:585–93.
11. Ebinger M, Winter B, Wendt M, et al. Effect of the use of ambulance-based thrombolysis on time to thrombolysis in acute ischemic stroke: a randomized clinical trial. *JAMA* 2014;311:1622–1631.
12. Seder DB, Riker RR, Jagoda A, Smith WS, Weingart SD. Emergency neurological life support: airway, ventilation, and sedation. *Neurocrit Care* 2012;17(Suppl 1):S4–20.
13. Reynolds SF, Heffner J. Airway management of the critically ill patient: rapid-sequence intubation. *Chest* 2005;127:1397–1412.
14. Yanagawa Y, Sakamoto T, Okada Y, et al. Intubation without premedication may worsen outcome for unconsciousness patients with intracranial hemorrhage. *Am J Emerg Med* 2005;23:182–185.
15. Walls RM. Rapid-sequence intubation of head trauma patients. *Ann Emerg Med* 1993;22:1071–1072.
16. Hamill JF, Bedford RF, Weaver DC, Colohan AR. Lidocaine before endotracheal intubation: intravenous or laryngotracheal? *Anesthesiology* 1981;55:578–581.
17. Davis DP, Meade W, Sise MJ, et al. Both hypoxemia and extreme hyperoxemia may be detrimental in patients with severe traumatic brain injury. *J Neurotrauma* 2009;26:2217–2223.
18. Brucken A, Kaab AB, Kottmann K, et al. Reducing the duration of 100% oxygen ventilation in the early reperfusion period after cardiopulmonary resuscitation decreases striatal brain damage. *Resuscitation* 2010;81:1698–1703.
19. Girard TD, Kress JP, Fuchs BD, et al. Efficacy and safety of a paired sedation and ventilator weaning protocol for mechanically ventilated patients in intensive care (awakening and breathing controlled trial): a randomised controlled trial. *Lancet* 2008;371:126–134.
20. Nichol G, Leroux B, Wang H, et al. Trial of continuous or interrupted chest compressions during CPR. *N Engl J Med* 2015;373:2203–14.
21. Berg RA, Hemphill R, Abella BS, et al. Part 5: adult basic life support: 2010 American Heart Association guidelines for cardiopulmonary resuscitation and emergency cardiovascular care. *Circulation* 2010;122:S685–705.
22. Aggarwal M, Khan IA. Hypertensive crisis: hypertensive emergencies and urgencies. *Cardiol Clin* 2006;24:135–146.
23. Piatt JH Jr. Detected and overlooked cervical spine injury in comatose victims of trauma: report from the Pennsylvania Trauma Outcomes Study. *J Neurosurg Spine* 2006;5:210–216.
24. Teasdale G, Knill-Jones R, van der Sande J. Observer variability in assessing impaired consciousness and coma. *J Neurol Neurosurg Psychiatry* 1978;41:603–610.
25. Lagares A, Gomez PA, Alen JF, et al. A comparison of different grading scales for predicting outcome after subarachnoid haemorrhage. *Acta Neurochir* 2005;147:5–16; discussion 16.
26. Diringer MN, Edwards DF. Does modification of the Innsbruck and the Glasgow Coma Scales improve their ability to predict functional outcome? *Arch Neurol* 1997;54:606–611.
27. Fisher CM. Oval pupils. *Arch Neurol* 1980;37:502–503.
28. Couret D, Boumaza D, Grisotto C, et al. Reliability of standard pupillometry practice in neurocritical care: an observational, double-blinded study. *Crit Care* 2016;20:99.
29. Solari D, Rossetti AO, Carteron L, et al. Early prediction of coma recovery after cardiac arrest with blinded pupillometry. *Ann Neurol* 2017;81:804–810.
30. Godoy DA, Di Napoli M, Rabinstein AA. Treating hyperglycemia in neurocritical patients: benefits and perils. *Neurocrit Care* 2010;13:425–438.
31. De Keyser J, Deleu D, Solheid C, Ebinger G. Coma as presenting manifestation of Wernicke's encephalopathy. *J Emerg Med* 1985;3:361–363.
32. Omer SM, al Kawi MZ, al Watban J, Bohlega S, McLean DR, Miller G. Acute Wernicke's encephalopathy associated with hyperemesis gravidarum: magnetic resonance imaging findings. *J Neuroimaging* 1995;5:251–3.
33. Bleggi-Torres LF, de Medeiros BC, Ogasawara VS, et al. Iatrogenic Wernicke's encephalopathy in

allogeneic bone marrow transplantation: a study of eight cases. *Bone Marrow Transplant* 1997;20:391–395.

34. Koguchi K, Nakatsuji Y, Abe K, Sakoda S. Wernicke's encephalopathy after glucose infusion. *Neurology* 2004;62:512.

35. Barnett R, Grace M, Boothe P, et al. Flumazenil in drug overdose: randomized, placebo-controlled study to assess cost effectiveness. *Crit Care Med* 1999;27:78–81.

36. Bledsoe BE. No more coma cocktails. Using science to dispel myths & improve patient care. *JEMS* 2002;27:54–60.

37. Clarke SF, Dargan PI, Jones AL. Naloxone in opioid poisoning: walking the tightrope. *Emerg Med J* 2005;22:612–616.

38. Weinbroum AA, Flaishon R, Sorkine P, Szold O, Rudick V. A risk-benefit assessment of flumazenil in the management of benzodiazepine overdose. *Drug Saf* 1997;17:181–196.

39. Ries NL, Dart RC. New developments in antidotes. *Med Clin N Am* 2005;89:1379–1397.

40. de Lange DW, Sikma MA, Meulenbelt J. Extracorporeal membrane oxygenation in the treatment of poisoned patients. *Clin Toxicol (Phila)* 2013;51:385–393.

41. Flynn LM, Rhodes J, Andrews PJ. Therapeutic hypothermia reduces intracranial pressure and partial brain oxygen tension in patients with severe traumatic brain injury: preliminary data from the Eurotherm3235 Trial. *Ther Hypothermia Temp Manag* 2015;5(3):143–151.

42. Edwards P, Arango M, Balica L, et al. Final results of MRC CRASH, a randomised placebo-controlled trial of intravenous corticosteroid in adults with head injury-outcomes at 6 months. *Lancet* 2005;365:1957–1959.

43. Chesnut RM, Temkin N, Carney N, et al. A trial of intracranial-pressure monitoring in traumatic brain injury. *N Engl J Med* 2012;367:2471–2481.

44. Chesnut R, Videtta W, Vespa P, Le Roux P, Participants in the International Multidisciplinary Consensus Conference on Multimodality M. Intracranial pressure monitoring: fundamental considerations and rationale for monitoring. *Neurocrit Care* 2014;21(Suppl 2):S64–84.

45. Treiman DM, Meyers PD, Walton NY, et al. A comparison of four treatments for generalized convulsive status epilepticus. Veterans Affairs Status Epilepticus Cooperative Study Group. *N Engl J Med* 1998;339:792–798.

46. Navarro V, Dagron C, Elie C, et al. Prehospital treatment with levetiracetam plus clonazepam or placebo plus clonazepam in status epilepticus

(SAMUKeppra): a randomised, double-blind, phase 3 trial. *Lancet Neurol* 2016;15:47–55.

47. Brophy GM, Bell R, Claassen J, et al. Guidelines for the evaluation and management of status epilepticus. *Neurocrit Care* 2012;17:3–23.

48. Sutter R, Marsch S, Fuhr P, Kaplan PW, Ruegg S. Anesthetic drugs in status epilepticus: risk or rescue? A 6-year cohort study. *Neurology* 2014;82:656–664.

49. Claassen J, Hirsch LJ, Emerson RG, Mayer SA. Treatment of refractory status epilepticus with pentobarbital, propofol, or midazolam: a systematic review. *Epilepsia* 2002;43:146–153.

50. Fernandez A, Lantigua H, Lesch C, et al. High-dose midazolam infusion for refractory status epilepticus. *Neurology* 2014;82:359–365.

51. Pugin D, Foreman B, De Marchis GM, et al. Is pentobarbital safe and efficacious in the treatment of super-refractory status epilepticus: a cohort study. *Criti Care* 2014;18:R103.

52. Gaspard N, Foreman B, Judd LM, et al. Intravenous ketamine for the treatment of refractory status epilepticus: a retrospective multicenter study. *Epilepsia* 2013;54:1498–1503.

53. Corry JJ, Dhar R, Murphy T, Diringer MN. Hypothermia for refractory status epilepticus. *Neurocrit Care* 2008;9:189–197.

54. McIlvoy LH. The effect of hypothermia and hyperthermia on acute brain injury. *AACN Clin Issues* 2005;16:488–500.

55. Minamisawa H, Smith ML, Siesjo BK. The effect of mild hyperthermia and hypothermia on brain damage following 5, 10, and 15 minutes of forebrain ischemia. *Ann Neurol* 1990;28:26–33.

56. Inouye SK. Delirium in older persons. *N Engl J Med* 2006;354:1157–1165.

57. van den Boogaard M, Slooter AJC, Bruggemann RJM, et al. Effect of haloperidol on survival among critically ill adults with a high risk of delirium: the REDUCE randomized clinical trial. *JAMA* 2018;319:680–690.

58. Lenart SB, Garrity JA. Eye care for patients receiving neuromuscular blocking agents or propofol during mechanical ventilation. *Am J Crit Care* 2000;9:188–191.

59. Korolott N, Boots R, Lipman J, Thomas P, Rickard C, Coyer F. A randomised controlled study of the efficacy of hypromellose and Lacri-Lube combination versus polyethylene/Cling wrap to prevent corneal epithelial breakdown in the semiconscious intensive care patient. *Int Care Med* 2004;30:1122–1126.

Chapter 8

Management of Frequently Encountered Causes of Unconsciousness

Chapter 7 provides a general approach to the emergency care of comatose patients. The purpose of this generalizable strategy is to stabilize the patient and prevent further brain injury while determining the specific cause of impairment of consciousness. Once the specific cause is identified, though, attention turns to dealing with the set of problems inherent to the underlying disorder. As it is not possible to cover all aspects of treatment of all possible causes of stupor and coma comprehensively, we will focus here instead on the management of frequently encountered pathologies within each of the main four categorical clinical diagnoses: (1) supratentorial or infratentorial compressive lesions; (2) supratentorial or infratentorial destructive lesions; (3) metabolic, diffuse, or multifocal coma; and (4) psychogenic coma. As treatment in psychogenic coma is mostly supportive, we will refer to Chapter 6 for the management of this topic. The focus of each of these sections will be on a discussion of the primary treatment of the cause for impaired consciousness as well as the management of frequently encountered complications, with particular attention to therapies aimed at primary and secondary processes that impair consciousness. For certain diagnoses such as trauma and ischemic stroke, systematic management protocols with clearly defined algorithms guide efforts of dedicated multidisciplinary management teams.[1–3] While these efforts are in their infancy for other acute neurological emergencies, such interdisciplinary approaches are essential as coma undermines the regulatory control of all bodily processes.[4]

STRUCTURAL LESIONS: SUPRATENTORIAL OR INFRATENTORIAL COMPRESSIVE/ DESTRUCTIVE ETIOLOGIES

The clinical signs that differentiate supra- from infratentorial compressive lesions are outlined in Table 7.1. The initial impression and concern is formed based on history and clinical examination. The most important laboratory test that allows narrowing down the differential diagnosis and guiding emergency management is an imaging study. In the emergency setting this is most often a noncontrast head computed tomography (CT) scan. If the patient is suspected from history and exam to be suffering from a supra- or infratentorial mass lesion, it is important to determine how severe the symptoms are and estimate how rapidly they are worsening as it may be necessary to intervene and stabilize the patient before the scan. For example, emergent general management of suspected elevation of intracranial pressure (ICP) or evolving herniation may require emergent treatment prior to imaging for diagnosis (see Chapter 7 for details).

If the patient is stuporous or comatose but relatively stable, then the emergency CT scan is the next step. A noncontrast head CT will rule out most significant mass lesions and usually identify subarachnoid hemorrhage (SAH). If indicated because of suspicion of a cerebrovascular occlusion, a CT angiogram can be added and will take minimal additional time. However, magnetic resonance imaging (MRI), when available, is more sensitive particularly for infratentorial lesions and may be required to identify recent cerebral infarcts,

particularly in the brainstem, and focal inflammatory lesions. Once initial imaging has ruled out a destructive or compressive lesion, other tests may be obtained to rule out nonstructural pathologies and infratentorial structural mass lesions (see Chapter 7).

Aneurysmal Subarachnoid Hemorrhage

Aneurysmal SAH is generally marked by sudden onset of a severe headache, often with impairment of consciousness. The Hunt and Hess grading system for SAH is largely based on the latter sign, with no impairment of consciousness being Grade 1 or (if there is meningismus or a cranial nerve palsy) Grade 2, mild alteration of consciousness (described as drowsiness or confusion and/or mild focal neurologic deficit) Grade 3, depressed level of consciousness (with or without moderate to severe hemiparesis) Grade 4, and coma Grade 5 (this is similarly true for the World Federation of Neurological Surgeons Scale [WFNS]). Regardless of the grade, the primary tool for identifying SAH in patients who have sudden onset of headache or impairment of consciousness is a noncontrast head CT, which has a sensitivity of at least 95%. In equivocal cases, lumbar puncture can be done to make the diagnosis (for details, please refer to Chapter 4).

Once the diagnosis of SAH is established, the initial objective of management is to stabilize vital functions while pursuing identification and potential treatment of a ruptured aneurysm, usually involving invasive angiography with possible coil embolization, or followed by intracranial surgical clipping (see Table 8.1). Meanwhile, it is important to minimize the impact of the initial injury (such as increased ICP due to the hematoma or subsequent hydrocephalus, cerebral edema, or tissue injury caused by the initial jet of blood) and proactively manage frequently encountered complications (such as rebleeding, stunned myocardium, neurogenic pulmonary edema, infarction from vasospasm, seizures, osmolar and volume disturbances, arrhythmias, central nervous system [CNS] infections, and hyperventilation). In the ensuing discussion, we will approach the management of aneurysmal SAH patients by recommending interventions as

Table 8.1 Subarachnoid Hemorrhage Management Steps

1. Emergent management steps
   a. Airway, breathing, circulation:
      i. Assess airway/breathing and intubate as needed (see Chapter 7)
      ii. Assess cardiopulmonary stability: may need central line placement, cardiopulmonary resuscitation
   b. Diagnosis of SAH: Head CT and lumbar puncture
   c. Labs: obtain platelet count, PT, PTT/INR, basic chemistry, troponin
   d. Steps to decrease the risk of rebleeding:
      i. Treat pain and anxiety: tylenol, may need morphine, fentanyl, or other opiates if pain is severe, NSAIDs are typically avoided due to the bleeding risk
      ii. Identify and treat coagulopathy: may need FFP or PCC, platelet transfusions, or vitamin K depending on the diagnosed coagulopathy
      iii. Lowering systolic blood pressure: labetalol pushes of 10 mg iv to keep SBP below 140–160 mm Hg (alternatives: hydralazine push, labetalol or nicardipine infusions)
      iv. Antifibrinolytic therapy: aminocaproic acid 4 g bolus followed by 1 g/hr infusion (caution if active myocardial infarction, history of any stents or revascularization procedure, stop 4 hours before angiography)
   e. Hydrocephalus and elevated intracranial pressure:
      i. Hydrocephalus: based on CT findings emergently place EVD
      ii. ICP: treat based on clinical findings or rarely if available based on ICP monitoring (follow protocol Figure 7.2)
   f. Seizures: load with fosphenytoin 20 mg/kg and maintained on 100 mg three times a day until the aneurysm is treated (phenytoin or levetiracetam are alternatives). If actively seizing treat also with Ativan 4 mg (may repeat once). Prolonged seizure prophylaxis is controversial.
   g. Do not feed
   h. Strict bedrest
2. Treatment of the bleeding source:
   a. Identify an aneurysm by CT of digital subtraction angiography.
   b. Treatment of the aneurysm by endovascular coil embolization or neurosurgical clipping
3. Management of neurological complications in SAH patients
   a. Admit to an ICU setting
   b. Arterial line and central line placement for all poor-grade patients, consider for all
   c. Delayed cerebral ischemia (DCI) from vasospasm:
      i. Prophylaxis: Oral nimodipine (60 mg every 4 h) for 21 days, if SBP <140 reduce dose to 30 mg (alternatively may give lower dose more frequently)
      ii. Detection of DCI: clinical exam, TCD daily, CT angiography (CT perfusion), quantitative EEG
      iii. Treatment of DCI:
         1. Equal fluid balance, raise systolic or better mean arterial blood pressure
         2. Intra-arterial (intrathecal) calcium channel blockers, balloon angioplasty
   d. Multimodality monitoring: in some comatose patients may consider invasive monitoring of the brain tissue: intracranial pressure, brain tissue oxygenation, regional cerebral blood flow, microdialysis, jugular bulb oxygenation saturation, electrical activity
4. Management of medical complications
   a. Pulmonary
      i. Mechanical ventilation, tracheostomy
      ii. Careful fluid balance
      iii. May need cardiac support for cardiogenic pulmonary edema
   b. Cardiac
      i. Tight blood pressure control, use as needed continuous infusions of vasopressors (phenylephrine or norepinephrine) and anti-hypertensives (nicardipine, labetalol, dobutamine, milrinone)
   c. Fever: achieve normothermia with Tylenol, cooling blankets, cooling pads, intravascular cooling, perform aggressive shivering control
   d. GI prophylaxis: stress ulcer prophylaxis if intubated or receiving steroids with Pepcid 20 mg po daily; for nausea give Zofran 4 mg IVSS q6h prn, bowel regime (Senna 2 tabs po/dt at bedtime and/or Colace 100 mg po/dt tid)
   e. Glucose: insulin sliding scale or continuous infusion to keep serum glucose < 200 mg/dL, avoid hypoglycemia
   f. DVT prophylaxis give heparin SC 5,000 units q12h starting typically 24 hours post-op

Table 8.1 **Subarachnoid Hemorrhage Management Steps (cont.)**

g. Anemia: transfuse to keep hemoglobin at >8 g/dL or above
h. Isotonic fluid administration: normal saline initially at 1–1.5 cc/kg/hr, later adjust based on fluid
    output, cardiac and respiratory function. Closely monitor serum and urine sodium and osmolarity

CT, computed tomography; DVT, deep venous thrombosis; EEG, electroencephalogram; EVD, external ventricular drainage; FFP, fresh frozen plasma; ICP, intracranial pressure; ICU, intensive care unit; INR, international normalized ratio; NSAID, nonsteroidal anti-inflammatory; PCC, prothrombin complex concentrate; PT, prothrombin time; PTT, partial thromboplastin time; SAH, subarachnoid hemorrhage; SBP, systolic blood pressure; TCD, transcranial Doppler.

they would be employed in a clinical scenario. Most patients with higher grade SAH marked by stupor or coma are intubated to protect the airway. If possible, intubation should be avoided as this will limit the neurological examination but the risk of aspiration pneumonia and rebleeding from elevated blood pressure need to be taken into account. In addition, SAH may cause cardiac arrhythmias and such patients may present with electrocardiographic (EKG) signs of cardiac ischemia or even in cardiac arrest. These threats to vital function need to be addressed first regardless of the underlying etiology (for details, please refer to Chapter 7). Beyond the general resuscitation steps outlined in Chapter 7, a number of complications that are specific to SAH are frequently encountered and require specific attention. Treatment of traumatic SAH will be discussed under the management of traumatic brain injury (TBI). Prognostication of long-term outcomes is challenging and clinical scales[5] are available but should be used with caution.

NEUROLOGICAL COMPLICATIONS

Rebleeding of the aneurysm within the first few weeks after the initial rupture occurs at a rate of 4–17%.[6,7] The majority of rebleeding occurs in the first 24–72 hours, is often associated with a significant sudden impairment of consciousness, and carries a major impact on functional outcome. Patients with poor clinical grade, large amounts of subarachnoid and intraventricular blood, large aneurysms, or those with external cerebrospinal fluid-drainage are at highest risk of early rebleeding.[7,8] Following the diagnosis of SAH a number of steps are initiated to reduce the risk of rebleeding. Patients are placed on strict bed rest. Pain and agitation should be treated as these may not only

increase blood pressure which enhances the risk of rebleeding but may also cause elevated ICP, which may already be elevated. Side effects of pain medications that need to be considered include sedation, which may obscure clinical worsening; hypotension seen with some of the opiates; and impaired coagulation associated with aspirin and nonsteroidal anti-inflammatory drugs (NSAIDs). Tylenol as well as opiates with less sedative and hypotensive potential, such as fentanyl, are preferred. Elective procedures that may lead to agitation such as nasogastric tube placement should be deferred, and unstable patients undergoing unavoidable procedures such as arterial line or central line placement should be adequately premedicated. Systolic blood pressure should be lowered typically below 140 or 160 mm Hg[9] using intravenous boluses of labetalol (alternatives include hydralazine or continuous infusions of labetalol or nicardipine).

The possibility of an underlying coagulopathy should be assessed based on the history, presentation, and emergency laboratory tests and, if it is found, should be addressed promptly. Coagulopathies should be treated with administration specific remedies (e.g., platelets for thrombocytopenia). Patients taking warfarin, which blocks synthesis of vitamin K-dependent clotting factors (II, VII, IX, X) should receive immediate infusion of prothrombin complex concentrate (PCC), a cryoprecipitate of the vitamin K dependent clotting factors, or recombinant factor VII. This must be followed immediately with fresh frozen plasma, approximately 2 units every 4 hours, and vitamin K, until the clotting defect is reversed. Newer oral anticoagulants, either direct thrombin (factor II) or factor Xa inhibitors, may be reversed by specific antidotes (e.g., idarucizumab is currently available for the direct thrombin inhibitor dabigatran, and andexanet for factor Xa inhibitors, such as apixaban and revaroixaban is available).[10,11]

A number of clinical trials have been conducted testing the effect of antifibrinolytic therapy on outcomes and have found that the risk of rebleeding decreased while the risk of ischemic complications increased, particularly if antifibrinolytic therapy was given for a prolonged period of time. Despite a Cochrane review concluding that currently the use of antifibrinolytic drugs cannot be recommended for the prevention of rebleeding after SAH,[12] many experts currently favor the off-label use of antifibrinolytic therapy to prevent early rebleeding (e.g., aminocaproic acid 4 g bolus followed by 1 g per hour infusion for less than 72 hours, bridging the time to emergent aneurysm treatment).[9,13]

Hydrocephalus may develop in approximately 20% of SAH victims either as a result of intraventricular blood blocking ventricular drainage (noncommunicating hydrocephalus) or because normal reabsorption of cerebrospinal fluid (CSF) over the surfaces of the hemispheres is blocked by clotted blood. In such cases, emergency placement of an external ventricular drainage (EVD) catheter is required. These patients typically have depressed arousal (Hunt and Hess grades 4 and 5) but, after placement of ventricular drainage catheters, they may show significant and rapid improvement of consciousness. EVD placement allows both direct measurements of ICP as well as treatment of raised ICP by CSF drainage. EVD placement can be done at the bedside in the emergency room or intensive care unit typically using bony skull landmarks. More advanced mechanical, magnetic, and ultrasound guiding systems are available, but because they add to the technical difficulty of the procedure, they may increase the time to successful placement and have therefore not yet been universally accepted.

Additional causes of *elevated ICP* may be encountered including intraparenchymal hematomas (which may be seen in 15% of SAH patients) or diffuse brain swelling. Diffuse brain swelling or global cerebral edema may be seen in 8% of comatose SAH patients on admission and develops during the hospital stay in 12%.[14] The underlying etiology of generalized cerebral edema in SAH is not completely clear, and therefore therapies directed at the underlying cause are lacking. In general, treatment of elevated ICP should follow recommendations previously outlined (see Chapter 7), with the caveat that administration of mannitol is controversial as it may lead to aneurysm rebleeding. Analgesia and sedation as well as very mild hyperventilation to a PCO_2 of 30–35 mm Hg may be required. If elevated ICP persists despite these measures and patients are actively herniating (see Chapter 7), emergent measures need to be taken which may include mannitol or hypertonic saline.

Seizures may be seen at the onset of the bleed or soon thereafter and may cause rising blood pressure which then may lead to either rebleeding or elevated ICP, both potentially precipitating herniation.[15] For these reasons, SAH patients should receive seizure prophylaxis until the aneurysm is definitively treated (see later discussion), and, once seizures occur, they should be treated promptly. Nonconvulsive seizures are seen in approximately 10–15% of SAH patients; the vast majority of these are in status epilepticus (SE), which may be a reversible cause of impairment of consciousness.[16] All patients who have a clinical or electrographic seizure documented should be treated with antiseizure medications and subsequently receive seizure prophylaxis, at least during the acute and subacute phase, as recurrent seizures are frequent and may be associated with worse outcome.[17] More prolonged seizure prophylaxis following successful treatment of the aneurysm is more controversial. Guidelines[9,18] do not recommend prolonged seizure prophylaxis, but practice varies widely. It is common to provide seizure prophylaxis during the perioperative period, especially in poor-grade patients or those with mass effect, but some continue the coverage throughout the intensive care unit stay. Although patients may develop seizures months or years following SAH, there is no evidence supporting efficacy of prophylactic treatment beyond the initial phase. Approximately 5–10% of all SAH patients eventually develop seizures, with risk factors including young age, intracranial surgery, cerebral ischemia due to vasospasm or thromboembolic events, poor clinical grade, or blood clot overlying the hemispheres on CT scan (Fisher grade higher than 1).[15,19,20] Most series exploring the benefits of seizure prophylaxis for SAH investigated the effects of phenytoin, which was associated with worse functional and cognitive outcomes in non controlled case series.[21,22] Phenytoin, metabolized by the hepatic cytochrome P450-3A4 system, induces more rapid metabolism of medications frequently given in patients with SAH such as the calcium channel antagonist nimodipine, thus decreasing blood levels.[23] Newer antiseizure medications such as levetiracetam, which lack this side effect, are increasingly being used for seizure prophylaxis following SAH.

Early treatment of the bleeding source is critical in aneurysmal SAH, as this removes risk of rebleeding and permits treatment of vasospasm with medications that induce hypertension. The location of a ruptured aneurysm can often be identified on the initial noncontrast head CT. However, because catheter angiography will be required for definitive identification and treatment, it is not advisable to give the dye load of CT angiography or to delay for MR angiography if aneurysmal SAH is suspected. The decision whether to treat the aneurysm definitively with coil embolization or neurosurgical clipping is generally made during the initial angiography. The International Subarachnoid Aneurysm Trial (ISAT), a large randomized controlled trial, found coil embolization superior for survival out to 7 years after the treatment for the subgroup of patients suitable for either intervention,[24] but there was a low but increased risk of late rebleeding seen in patients who underwent endovascular coiling. The choice of treatment depends on a variety of factors, including age, size and location of the aneurysm, and, perhaps most importantly, the expertise that is immediately available. SAH patients are best managed at centers that treat SAH on a regular basis, ideally offering both endovascular and surgical treatment approaches. However, the most important criterion is that the bleeding source should be secured as quickly as possible, preferably within 24 hours of hemorrhage.[25]

Vasospasm, delayed cerebral ischemia, and other infarction. Ischemic strokes can be seen following SAH in a number of scenarios, each requiring a different management approach. (1) During aneurysm rupture, ICP may rise sharply to near the levels of arterial blood pressure. This reduces cerebral blood flow, leading to loss of consciousness and at times to watershed infarcts.[26] Such events are called *ictal infarctions* and managed by supportive care. (2) Patients undergoing surgical

treatment are at risk of injury from brain retraction necessary to expose the aneurysm, which typically is near the circle of Willis at the base of the brain. These surgery-related changes appear as infarcts adjacent to the surgical site that do not respect vascular territories. Modern minimally invasive surgical techniques have made these infarcts rare and treatment is nonspecific. (3) Tissue injury or hematomas may cause the cingulate gyrus to herniate under the falx, compressing the anterior cerebral arteries, or the medial temporal lobe to herniate through the tentorial notch, compressing the posterior cerebral artery. Preventing such infarcts is best managed by measures that treat the herniation syndrome (see Chapter 7).

(4) A greatly feared complication is the delayed cerebral ischemia (DCI) due to vasospasm. Although cerebral vasospasm is seen in more than two-thirds of SAH patients, it is not always associated with morbidity. DCI, defined as a new neurologic deficit or infarction detected on imaging due to ischemia from vasospasm, is seen in about 20–25% of SAH patients and in a minority of patients with vasospasm.[27] Peak onset of DCI is between 6 and 8 days after the aneurysmal hemorrhage, and it usually does not develop before day 3 or after day 12, but outliers exist. Neurological symptoms can vary widely depending on the involved brain territory, but DCI is frequently accompanied by decreased arousal and may also affect cognitive processing. This complication, which may represent more diffuse vasospasm and prolonged inadequate cerebral blood flow, is associated with poor functional outcome, cognitive impairment, and decreased quality of life (for details on pathophysiology and diagnosis, please refer to Chapter 4).

Early detection of DCI and spasm is crucial in order for interventions to prevent infarction. Exam findings that are associated with DCI depend on the vascular territory involved. Decreasing arousal or newly developing impairment of cognitive processing may be seen as a consequence of DCI. DCI may be difficult to detect in poor-grade SAH patient (Hunt Hess grades 4 and 5), but may be as subtle as asymmetric spontaneous movements. DCI is more commonly seen after hemorrhages with substantial blood clots around the circle of Willis.[27] The development of DCI may be monitored by diagnostic techniques such as transcranial Doppler (TCD) ultrasound,[28] electroencephalogram (EEG),[29] CT angiography,[30] or CT perfusion[31]; invasive brain monitoring techniques may also be used to supplement the clinical examination.

Management starts with preventive strategies that all patients should receive, including 60 mg of oral nimodipine every 4 hours for the first 21 days after hemorrhage (in Europe, intravenous nimodipine is also available), with dose adjustments and safety margins for hypotension (see Table 8.1). This approach was approved by the US Food and Drug Administration (FDA) in 1989 based on several randomized controlled clinical trials for SAH patients with Hunt-Hess scores of 1–3 and has been recommended for all patients with SAH.[18,32,33] However, despite this improvement, nimodipine does not appear to increase cerebral blood flow after SAH,[34] and the improvement in outcome may represent a neuroprotective effect.

Once DCI has developed, treatment is aimed at maximizing cerebral blood supply and—if this fails—minimizing demand of the undersupplied brain tissue. The combination of hypertension, hypervolemia, and hemodilution, termed *triple-H therapy*, has been propagated for years with modest results in small trials and meta-analyses.[35–37] Hemodilution is not likely beneficial[18] as diluted blood will be less effective in transporting adequate oxygen or nutrients to the brain. Isotonic fluids such as normal saline are recommended, and dextrose and free water in the intravenous fluids should be avoided.

Interventional neuroradiological approaches to dilate narrowed cerebral vessels in vasospasm include balloon angioplasty and intra-arterial administration of calcium channel blockers, currently most frequently verapamil or nicardipine. These interventions are of uncertain benefit as angioplasty risks vessel rupture and provides only transient relief; if successful, it may shunt blood from areas that remain underperfused, thus worsening the ischemia elsewhere. On an experimental basis, administration of calcium channel blockers into the ventricular system and systemic administration of dantrolene have been reported. A number of interventions were not beneficial in clinical trials, including the use of magnesium,[38] statins,[39] the non-glucocorticoid aminosteroid Tirilazad,[40] and intra-arterial administration of papaverine.[41] The endothelin receptor antagonists clazosentan did reduce angiographic vasospasm but was not able to alter clinical outcomes.[42]

MEDICAL COMPLICATIONS

Patients who are comatose due to SAH are heir to a wide variety of medical complications including cardiac, pulmonary, metabolic, electrolyte imbalance, and inflammatory events that have a major impact on outcome.[43]

Respiratory failure may be encountered due to neurologic causes such as failure of airway protection in a comatose patient, but it may also be seen due to pulmonary factors including cardiogenic or neurogenic pulmonary edema.[18,44] Neurogenic pulmonary edema typically develops immediately after SAH[45] and is believed to be due to autonomically mediated increased pulmonary arterial pressure and vascular permeability.[46] Cardiogenic pulmonary edema in this setting develops within the first days following the SAH and may be related to reduced left ventricular function, especially in patients who have cardiac stunning or takotsubo cardiomyopathy (see later discussion). In addition, treatment of DCI with large volumes of fluid or treatment of elevated ICP with hypertonic saline may contribute by increasing intravascular volume and precipitating heart failure. Management depends on the underlying cause and may involve supporting cardiac function or careful fluid management, balancing the risk of ischemia that requires liberal fluid management against difficulties in oxygenation that demand restrictive fluid management.[18]

Pneumonia is frequent in comatose SAH patients and is associated with a worse prognosis. Prolonged mechanical ventilation is required particularly for those with stupor or coma, and many will need tracheostomy. Timing of tracheostomy is controversial, with some advocating for early tracheostomy. The procedure may be performed at the bedside or in the operating room. Aggressive pulmonary toilet and frequent suctioning are employed as part of intensive care measures. Antibiotics may be needed but should be given thoughtfully as they are frequently overused. Patients with acute brain injury may hyperventilate,[47] leading to hypocarbia with the potential for brain tissue hypoxia.

Cardiovascular complications include hemodynamic instability, stunned myocardium, and arrhythmias. Blood pressure needs to be tightly controlled at a low level prior to treatment of the aneurysm and at a much higher level for those patients with DCI. This tight control requires central line and arterial line placement, as well as the administration of vasopressors or antihypertensive medications. Continuous drips are preferred, as these allow more rapid up- or down-titration in patients with quickly changing requirements. Nicardipine or labetalol are antihypertensives of choice. Frequently used vasopressors include phenylephrine or norepinephrine, but positive inotropic support (dobutamine, milrinone) may be required depending on the cause of hypotension. Patients in shock may, on a case-by-case basis, benefit from transient intra-aortic balloon pump support.

Heart failure is often due to stunned myocardium, which is thought to be due to high levels of circulating catecholamines causing subendocardial ischemia with contraction band necrosis.[48] EKG abnormalities commonly associated with myocardial stunning include T wave inversions, QT prolongation, and diffuse ST segment elevation. Echocardiography may identify takotsubo cardiomyopathy, in which there is left ventricular failure and diastolic dysfunction with apical and mid-ventricular akinesis. Transient, severe hemodynamic instability may be seen, and aggressive critical care support is required. Management is challenging as a catecholamine surge is thought to be at least partially causative for the developing cardiomyopathy. Treatment with beta-blockers is recommended, but this approach is often limited by hypotension. Transient pressure support using inotropic medications is frequently attempted for hypotensive patients with takotsubo pathology,[49] but, if unsuccessful, intra-aortic balloon pump counterpulsation may be required.[50,51]

Finally, patients with SAH are at risk for thromboembolic events as well. Prevention of venous thrombosis requires prophylaxis with low-dose heparin despite the risk of repeat aneurysmal bleeding. In patients treated with antifibrinolytic therapy prior to aneurysm treatment, thrombotic events including myocardial infarction may complicate the course.

Hyperglycemia has been associated with worse prognosis, and aggressive treatment has been shown to be beneficial for medical ICU patients.[52] Concern has been raised about worsening outcomes in brain-injured patients with strict glucose control,[53–56] resulting in expert consensus recommendations to maintain serum glucose at less than 200 mg/dL. However, it is also necessary to diligently avoid hypoglycemia.[18]

Fever is frequently seen after SAH and may be associated with a primary pyretic effect of the blood breakdown products.[57] Febrile SAH patients have a worse prognosis, so it is necessary to reduce body temperature to the normal range using antipyretics such as acetaminophen, or cooling blankets. It is also necessary, when a SAH patient becomes febrile, to mount a diligent search for possible infection.

Anemia develops frequently in SAH patients, but treatment thresholds are debated. Current guidelines recommend blood transfusions to keep the hemoglobin above 8 g/dL.[18] The topic, like hemodilution to treat DCI, is highly controversial, and studies are planned to define the optimal blood hemoglobin levels specifically for SAH.[58]

Intracerebral Hemorrhage

Intracerebral hemorrhage (ICH) may present clinically with many different neurological findings, such as sudden onset of focal neurological deficits, which may or may not be associated with headache and impaired consciousness. Symptoms will depend on the location and volume of the bleed as ICH may occur in any part of the CNS. Infratentorial hemorrhages can rapidly progress from presenting with ataxia to stupor and coma when compressing the brainstem and are a surgical emergency. Similarly, patients with supratentorial hemorrhages located close to the ventricles may initially exhibit hemiparesis, and, when the hemorrhage breaks into the ventricle, this may be followed rapidly by impaired consciousness requiring emergent placement of external ventricular drainage.

Diagnosis is primarily made by noncontrast head CT. As soon as the diagnosis of ICH is established, the initial objective of management is to stabilize vital functions while pursuing identification of the likely bleeding cause. In order to direct management, location and size of the bleed need to be

334   Plum and Posner's Diagnosis and Treatment of Stupor and Coma

established as soon as possible. The volume of blood is calculated by identifying the CT slice with the largest bleed, measuring the longest axis of the bleed (in cm), then the longest axis perpendicular to this axis (in cm), and counting the number of slices on which blood appears (multiplied by the slice thickness, in cm). These three numbers are multiplied and divided by two to get the estimated ICH volume.[59] Prognosis, particularly in the acute state, is challenging. Several scores, such as the primary ICH score[60,61] or the FUNC score,[62] have been proposed and are in clinical use. These scores help give an estimate of the predicted short-term mortality and functional outcome, respectively. In addition to older age, larger volume and location of parenchymal blood (infratentorial worse than deep, worse than lobar location), the presence of intraventricular blood, a poor neurological baseline (presence of cognitive impairment), and current neurological exam (coma as defined by Glasgow Coma Score of 8 or lower) factor into these scores. Subsequent studies have shown that such scores (Table 8.2) should be treated with caution as they were developed on historical cohorts in which the investigators who had designed the

items that make up the score also provided clinical care for the subjects, raising the risk of a poor prognosis becoming a self-fulfilling prophecy.[63]

Underlying etiologies of ICH are categorized into primary and secondary causes, the latter referring to any underlying vascular causes such as arteriovenous malformations or coagulopathies. While some generalized management recommendations can be given for all patients with ICH, identifying the underlying cause is crucial because interventions for ICH secondary to vascular abnormalities or coagulopathies may need additional targeted interventions. MRI in patients with atypical hemorrhage on CT may identify an underlying cause such as tumor, amyloid angiopathy, or hemorrhagic conversion of an ischemic stroke. Digital subtraction angiography should be obtained to look for subtle evidence of a vascular malformation in patients with primary intraventricular hemorrhage (IVH) and younger patients with a lobar bleed and no history of hypertension. ICH patients with impaired consciousness should be admitted to an intensive care unit, receive central line placement, and atrial blood pressure monitoring.

Table 8.2 Scores to Prognosticate Outcome following Intracerebral Hemorrhage (ICH)

Components	Primary ICH Score[a]	FUNCT Score[b]
Glasgow Coma Score	0 if 13–15 1 if 5–12 2 if 3–4	2 if ≥9 0 if <9
ICH volume	0 if <30 mL 1 if ≥30 mL	4 if <30 mL 2 if 30–60 mL 0 if >60 mL
IVH	0 if none 1 if yes	n.a.
ICH location	0 if supratentorial 1 if infratentorial	2 if lobar 1 if deep 0 if other
Age	0 if <80 yo 1 if ≥80 yo	2 if <70 yo 1 if 70–79 yo 0 if ≥80 yo
Pre-ICH cognitive impairment	n.a.	1 if no 0 if yes
Total score: range (Poor prognosis indicated by)	0–6 (high score)	0–11 (low score)

[a]Hemphill et al. [61]

[b]Rost et al. [62]

NEUROLOGICAL COMPLICATIONS

Prevention of rebleeding or ongoing bleeding. Rebleeding in patients with primary ICH occurs in roughly a third of cases, typically within 6 hours of the initial hemorrhage.[64,65] Risk factors for rebleeding include uncontrolled hypertension, hyperglycemia, antithrombotic or antiplatelet drugs, large hemorrhage size, and liver disease. Lowering the blood pressure has been the focus of a number of clinical trials,[66–68] without clearly identifying an ideal blood pressure range for ICH patients. Elevated blood pressure is frequently seen in patients who present with ICH on hospital admission even in the absence of any prior hypertension.[69] Studies have associated ongoing hypertension with hematoma growth and increased brain swelling.[70] On the other hand, excessive blood pressure reduction[71] may worsen ischemic injury in the setting of abnormal cerebral autoregulation, which is frequently encountered in patients with acute brain injury in general and ICH patients in particular. Guidelines recommend lowering the systolic blood pressure to 140 mm Hg or lower with intravenous administration of a calcium channel blocker (i.e., nicardipine 5–15 mg/hr infusion) or beta-blocker (i.e., labetalol 20–80 mg bolus every 10 minutes up to a maximum dose of 300 mg or 0.5–2 mg/min infusion), possibly using continuous infusions, particularly for those patients who present with a systolic pressure above 220 mm Hg.[72] In critically ill patients with ICH, especially those with IVH, placement of brain multimodality monitoring, particularly ICP monitoring, may be considered.[72] For these patients a cerebral perfusion pressure goal of 50–70 mm Hg may be chosen.

Underlying coagulopathies may include taking oral anticoagulant drugs or antiplatelet medications, and those with inherited or acquired coagulation factor or platelet abnormalities need to be corrected emergently.[72,73] In the emergency setting, most of this information will be acquired via obtaining a history from patients, family, medical charts, or first responders. Patients with known coagulation factor or platelet disorders are managed by replacement of factors and platelets in consultation with the primary hematologist. Rising numbers of patients are treated with oral anticoagulant drugs such as the vitamin K antagonist warfarin and, increasingly, the novel oral anticoagulants that inhibit thrombin or factor Xa (i.e., dabigatran, rivaroxaban, and apixaban). If presenting with ICH, oral anticoagulant drugs should be held and coagulation studies be obtained. Patients with ICH while receiving a vitamin K antagonist who present with an international normalized ratio (INR) of greater than 1.4 should have their vitamin K–dependent factors replaced. Prothrombin complex concentrates (PCC) have fewer complications and correct the INR almost immediately. Fresh frozen plasma (2 units, or 500 mL) takes about an hour to thaw and transport and even longer to infuse, especially in older patients who risk congestive heart failure with the fluid load. Hence it should be ordered at the time that the PCC is infused, and then given at 4-hour intervals until the coagulation deficit is corrected. All patients on vitamin K antagonists should also be given 5–10 mg of intravenous vitamin K slowly (onset of action is at 2 hours, but it may take several days to completely reverse the deficit; therefore, while it should be given immediately, it plays little role in the emergent reversal of anticoagulation). Novel oral anticoagulants possibly have a lower risk of ICH, a short half-life, do not require frequent visits to anticoagulation clinics, and are therefore gaining popularity rapidly. A specific monoclonal antibody to reverse the activity of dabigatran (idarucizumab)[11] has recently been introduced, and agents to reverse factor Xa inhibitors (e.g., andexanet alpha-1) available.[74] Hemodialysis can also be used for patients with ICH on dabigatran, but probably is too slow in case of ICH. Nonspecific clotting promoters such as anti-inhibitor coagulant complex (FEIBA), PCCs, or recombinant activated factor VIIa can be considered in settings where specific antidotes are not available, and activated charcoal may be useful if the novel oral anticoagulant was ingested within 2 hours of presentation.

The management of ICH patients who receive antiplatelet medications is controversial, and the benefits of platelet transfusions not clear at this point.[75] However, patients who receive aspirin typically have irreversible inhibition of circulating platelets, and if the aspirin itself is given at low dosage (e.g., 81 mg/d), it is likely to be gone from the bloodstream after 8 hours. Hence, platelet transfusions at that point are an attractive alternative. If ICH occurs during intravenous heparin infusion, the infusion should be stopped, and the patient should be treated with protamine sulfate (1 mg per 100 U of heparin intravenously, maximum dose 50 mg, with adjustment based on time elapsed since heparin discontinuation; similar dosing may be used for low-molecular-weight heparin–associated ICH). Trials have explored the administration of recombinant activated factor VIIa in patients with ICH not associated with oral anticoagulants and found these to be associated with a reduction in hematoma growth but also an increase in thromboembolic events.[64,76] Overall there was no clinical benefit seen.[64] On contrast CT, images of a hyperdensity within the hemorrhage ("spot sign") may indicate ongoing bleeding and possibly warrant more aggressive interventions to stop the hematoma growth.[65] Similarly, patients receiving tranexamic acid had lower rates of hematoma expansion, but 3 months functional outcomes were unchanged.[77]

The timing of restarting anticoagulation in an ICH patient with a strong indication for anticoagulation, such as mechanical heart valves or intracranial stents, is controversial. The practitioner needs to weigh the rebleeding risk against the risk of complications due to interruption of anticoagulants and antiplatelet agents.

Treatment of the vascular cause of ICH. The initial assessment should be directed toward identifying any underlying vascular lesion as this may need to be addressed emergently to prevent rebleeding. Early angiography is required to determine whether an aneurysm is present as these may occasionally present with intraparenchymal hematomas and require treatment by coiling or surgery within the first 24 hours. In young patients, arteriovenous malformations (AVMs) are common. These have a substantial but lower risk of early rebleeding unless associated with an aneurysm and so typically are treated in a subacute fashion. Suspicion of venous sinus thrombosis is often raised from the initial CT scan as the pattern of the ICH is usually characteristic (parafalcine for superior sagittal sinus thrombosis, lateral temporal lobe for lateral sinus thrombosis). If confirmed on contrast-enhanced CT or MRI, heparinization needs to be strongly considered, weighing the risk of additional bleeding against the risk of worsening thrombosis. Endovascular thrombectomy or injection of tissue plasminogen activator (tPA or rTPA) can sometimes remove the clot and open the sinus.

Mass effect and herniation. ICH results in an immediate displacement of venous and CSF compartments followed by an exponential increase of the ICP (Monroe-Kellie doctrine) with associated compression of brain parenchyma. In addition to the mass effect from the hemorrhage itself, patients may also develop brain swelling. Brain swelling, also known as *cerebral edema*, is seen in many patients with ICH, particularly those with large bleeds. Depending on the location of the hemorrhage, this increasing mass effect will compress local neural or vascular structures and may cause herniation syndromes (Chapter 3). This increasing mass effect is most prominent within the first 72 hours but may persist into the second week. The underlying cause for brain swelling following ICH is not completely clear, but may be due to changes in perfusion as well as inflammatory responses to hemoglobin degradation products, in particular iron.[78,79]

Management of mass effect involves approaches to decrease the primary hemorrhage (i.e., clot evacuation), artificially creating more space (i.e., suboccipital craniotomy or hemicraniectomy depending on the location of the bleed) and decreasing intracranial contents (i.e., ventricular drainage or osmotic agents). Depending on the location of the bleed, emergent evaluation is required to determine the benefits from early surgical interventions as delayed surgical treatments often are less effective. In patients with cerebellar hemorrhage (Figure 8.1), there is danger of compressing the fourth ventricle or cerebral aqueduct causing acute hydrocephalus (see Chapter 4). Such patients require emergency ventricle shunting and may benefit from suboccipital craniotomy if the hematoma exceeds 3 cm in diameter. Brainstem hemorrhages are typically not felt to benefit from surgical interventions. Patients with IVH may also develop obstructive hydrocephalus particularly when completely filling the third and fourth ventricles ("casting of the ventricles"). This is frequently associated with severely depressed consciousness, often with coma. Thrombolytic therapy administered via ventricular drainage catheters for those with large third and fourth ventricular hemorrhage[80] and catheters placed in large parenchymal hemorrhages may be additional surgical interventions.[81] Supratentorial hemorrhages are generally considered for clot evacuation when there is danger of herniation and if the bleed is very superficial, but clinical trials so far are inconclusive.[82,83]

Comatose ICH patients should undergo ICP monitoring either with parenchymal or ventricular monitoring probes.[84] These measures should guide administration of mannitol 20% (0.5–1.5 g/kg body weight via peripheral or central intravenous line) or hypertonic saline solutions (given at 30 mL over 20 minutes; may be given faster only if the physician remains at the bedside as cardiovascular instability may be encountered with rapid administration) to keep ICP low (i.e., ICP lower than 20 mm Hg) or CPP within a predefined target (i.e., CPP 50–60 mm Hg). Serum osmolar gap and sodium should be followed closely if repeat doses are required.

Seizures are seen acutely in more than 10% of patients with ICH, particularly those with lobar location. Nonconvulsive seizures, which can only be diagnosed using EEG monitoring, are associated with worse outcome, mass effect, and herniation.[85,86] However, it is unclear

if prevention or treatment of seizures improves outcome. Current guidelines recommend treatment of diagnosed seizures, although in cases with large cortical bleeds in which herniation threatens, clinicians may treat prophylactically with antiepileptic medication. Recent analyses suggest that prophylaxis with levetiracetam may not be beneficial for ICH patients.[87] Late seizures often take months to years to develop after an ICH, and it is difficult to predict which patients will have them, so antiepileptic medications are not indicated until there is evidence for seizures occurring.

MEDICAL COMPLICATIONS

Many of the general ICU complications in ICH patients are similar to those encountered in SAH patients discussed earlier, such as pneumonia from intubation, the effects of fever, and hyperglycemia. However, a number of

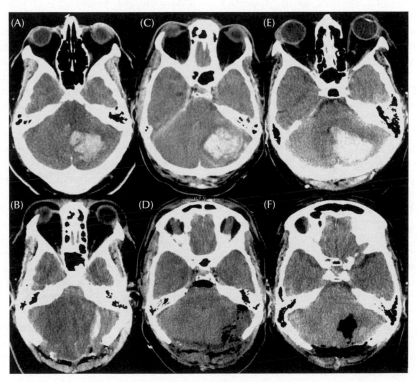

Figure 8.1 Three patients presenting with headache and initially conversant to the emergency room found to have an acute left cerebellar hemorrhage (diameter 4-5 cm) that underwent suboccipital decompression. Approximately 12 hours elapsed between onset of coma and decompression in the first patient (Figure 8.1, Panels A and B). The second patient (Figure 8.1, Panels C and D) sustained cardiac arrest at the same time of progressing to coma and had emergent suboccipital decompression within 1 hour of coma. The third patient had suboccipital decompression performed with increasing lethargy (Figure 8.1, Panels E and F). The first two patients remained comatose with myoclonus being observed in the second case. Both died after being made comfort care by the family. The third case recovered consciousness and was discharged to an acute inpatient rehabilitation program.

ICH-specific medical challenges deserve a brief discussion. Patients with ICH have a high risk of developing thromboembolic disease, and prevention has been the focus of studies.[88] All patients should receive intermittent pneumatic compression boots; after bleeding has stopped (stable CT scan on serial imaging), low-dose subcutaneous low-molecular-weight heparin or unfractionated heparin should be considered. ICH patients with documented deep venous thrombosis or pulmonary embolus should be considered for full systemic anticoagulation or placement of an inferior vena cava filter. As discussed earlier, if oral anticoagulants were stopped and reversed in initial treatment of the ICH, this may cause secondary thromboembolic complications. Patients who have medical conditions (e.g., a genetic coagulopathy or atrial fibrillation) or those with implanted cardiovascular mechanical devices (i.e., ventricular assist devices, heart valves) may be at particularly high risk of thromboembolic complications. Case-by-case multidisciplinary discussion of the risks and benefits of restarting the anticoagulants is often required.

Traumatic Brain Injury

Management of patients with trauma, including those with TBI, follows strict protocols that begin with prenotification of the emergency room prior to the patient's arrival, activating a multidisciplinary team of physicians (trauma surgery, neurosurgery, anesthesiology, neurology, and emergency physicians, as well as mobilizing nursing, respiratory technician and pharmacy resources).[89,90] The approach follows a prescribed path, with an initial focus on identification and management of acute life-threatening injuries requiring emergent interventions (primary survey), followed by a more detailed clinical exam combined with imaging (secondary survey), and then screening for missed injuries and identification of complications which may be done after hospital admission (tertiary survey). Impairment of consciousness at the time of injury as well as secondary development of unconsciousness are common, particularly in multisystem trauma, and are clearly major determinants of outcome. There are specific complications for the trauma patient that result in impaired consciousness that need to be identified and treated emergently to prevent permanent brain injury. Diagnosis of trauma is often obvious based on the history and external signs of trauma, but in some patients neurological emergencies, such as a cerebral infarct due to arterial occlusion or ICH, may have been the primary event precipitating accidents, and the subsequent trauma may be secondary to the primary brain disorder.

The *primary survey* should be completed within a few minutes and focuses on identification and treatment of acutely life-threatening conditions. For comatose patients, this process follows the strategies for initial management of patients with stupor and coma outlined in Chapter 7. The following discussion focuses on special considerations for the trauma patient. Importantly for the patient with trauma, special attention should be paid to potential cervical spine instability. Cervical spine injury, including fractures and ligamentous injury, should be assumed until ruled out, so that, in the field, the neck must be stabilized prior to moving the trauma patient.[91] This includes in-line manual stabilization and placement of a hard neck collar. Techniques for patients requiring airway or ventilator support are controversial, but "chin lift" or "head-tilt" maneuvers are contraindicated as these may cause further cervical spine injury and in-line stabilization is mandatory. Rapid sequence intubation is recommended because all trauma patients requiring intubation are at high risk of aspiration. Nasotracheal intubation is typically recommended in the spontaneously breathing patient and orotracheal intubation in patients who are not breathing. However, blind nasal intubation is relatively contraindicated in patients with a potential for skull base fractures or unstable midface injuries, and alternate techniques such as laryngeal mask airways should be considered.

Tension pneumothorax may be present or develop as a result of blunt or penetrating trauma, resulting in mediastinal shift causing decreased venous return and severe hypotension. Patients with pneumothorax will have absence of breath sounds and hyperresonance on the affected side, hemodynamic shock, tachypnea, tracheal deviation, and jugular venous distention. Emergent treatment includes needle decompression (large-bore needle inserted into the midclavicular second intercostal space above the third rib) followed by chest tube insertion. Open pneumothorax is less frequent, but the chest opening should be occluded emergently initially using a semi-occlusive dressing that allows air to exit but not to enter the chest.

Hemodynamic compromise may occur from a myriad of causes in the trauma patient, but conceptually etiologies can be stratified into low circulating volume (e.g., most importantly from hemorrhage), inadequate myocardial function (e.g., cardiac contusion), and sympathetic failure (e.g., spinal cord injury). For general assessment and management, please refer to Chapter 7. Hemorrhagic shock is particularly frequent in trauma patients and may occur from external or internal bleeding such as that encountered with pelvic fractures. Initially, crystalloid infusions are given for hypotension, and compression of bleeding sites is performed. Blood loss needs to be estimated to guide replacement strategies. Proactive replacement of blood products is recommended to prevent a state of acute coagulopathy of trauma and shock, which is driven by tissue injury and inflammation and may be exacerbated by crystalloid infusions.[92] Current replacement strategies advocate replacing equal ratios of red blood cells, plasma, and platelets; activation of institutional "massive transfusion protocols" may be required.[93] If given within 3 hours of trauma, administration of tranexamic acid, an antifibrinolytic synthetic analog of the amino acid lysine, may be an option.[94] On arrival to the hospital, sources of bleeding must be identified rapidly as part of the primary survey. This includes clinical screening supported by chest radiograph (thoracic hemorrhage, hematothorax, cardiac tamponade), pelvic radiograph (pelvic and retroperitoneal hemorrhage), and focused assessment by sonography for trauma (FAST; screens pericardium, the right and left upper quadrants, and the pelvis for fluid collections indicating bleeding).[95] Identification of active hemorrhage prompts both replacement of the lost volume as outlined earlier and emergent surgical intervention.

As part of the primary survey and further risk stratification, neurological assessment to guide diagnostics and treatment for the trauma victim is crucial.[96] Part of this assessment is to obtain the Glasgow Coma Scale (GCS), which was developed as a standardized assessment for the initial neurological examination of trauma patients in an effort to identify patients who were likely to require a neurosurgical intervention[97] and to predict their long-term outcome. It categorizes eye opening (spontaneous, to voice, to pain, none), best motor response (obeys commands, localizes to pain, withdraws, flexor posturing, extensor posturing, none), and best verbal response (oriented, disoriented, inappropriate, incomprehensible, none) to generate a composite score. In addition, the components of the coma exam laid out in Chapter 2, including examining spontaneous eye movements, pupillary response to light, corneal reflexes, cough and gag reflex, and motor or sensory deficits or posturing, should be determined and documented serially. Do not perform a doll's-eye (vestibulo-ocular) maneuver in the trauma patient until cervical spine injury has been ruled out (but warm or cold water caloric responses can be obtained if the tympanic membrane is intact). The presence of blood behind the tympanic membrane, in the area behind the ear (Battle sign), or surrounding the eyes (raccoon eyes) suggests a basilar skull fracture and requires CT scan of the head with bone windows.

TBI patients are categorized into mild, moderate, and severe cases based on history and clinical characteristics, as well as general and neurological examination. Patients with mild TBI are those who have a normal neurological examination and do not have a history of neurological impairment after the head injury (concussion). It is important to take into account bystander reports in determining this, as anterograde amnesia is a common sign of concussion and may result in the patient being unable to recall transient or even more prolonged loss of consciousness or other neurological impairment. Intoxication with alcohol or other drugs, which is common in these patients, should also be identified, and taken into account. Patients with normal neurological examination, no concussion, and no intoxication are in the low-risk category that may be discharged from the hospital without a CT scan if a reliable observer is available to monitor for the development of headache, vomiting, or neurological symptoms and bring the patient back to the hospital if these occur.

The moderate-risk group of TBI patients includes those who sustained a concussion, have a GCS of 9 to 14, or have any of the following: basilar or depressed skull fracture, other general (i.e., nausea, vomiting) and neurological findings (i.e., seizures, posttraumatic amnesia), alcohol or drug intoxication, or are less than 2 or older than 65 years of age. Management and need for hospital admission of mild to moderate TBI patients depends on the presence of abnormalities on CT imaging or neurological examination (it is recommended to admit any patient for observation with a GCS of less than 15, or, in other words, with any impairment of consciousness or motor or eye opening abnormalities).

Severe TBI patients have a much higher morbidity and mortality and are characterized by coma (defined as a GCS 8 or less) or progressive decline of consciousness, focal neurological abnormalities such as hemiparesis, or penetrating skull injury or palpable depressed skull fracture. All severe TBI patients need to be managed in an ICU setting and emergently evaluated by neurosurgical experts to identify those who require emergent neurosurgical interventions (i.e., epidural hematoma [EDH] evacuation, ICP monitor placement, hemicraniectomy, bifrontal craniotomy).

The *secondary survey* involves further physical examination, focused diagnostic procedures, and imaging studies to identify all injuries. Treatments given as part of the secondary survey include additional operations, pain relief, splinting, dressings, and antibiotic administration.

The *tertiary survey* follows and includes management of all injuries and developing complications of trauma patients. Care should be taken to search for missed injuries; this involves a thorough general and neurological examination supplemented by a detailed review of acquired imaging and ongoing laboratory evaluation. All extremities demonstrating deformation or with limitations in range of motion should be imaged using plain radiographs. CT imaging has replaced virtually all spine radiographs as the imaging modality of choice, and MRI should be chosen to screen for cervical spine ligamentous injury (these need to be obtained within 48 hours of the injury as the specificity of MRI for ligamentous injury decreases after this time).

Prognostication is challenging and, in particular, prediction of recovery of consciousness is often inaccurate. The 10 strongest predictive variables were identified based on data collected as part of two large trials (International Mission for Prognosis and Clinical Trial [IMPACT] and the Corticosteroid Randomization After Significant Head Injury [CRASH]). These included age, clinical severity, head CT abnormalities, systemic insults (hypoxia and hypotension), and laboratory variables and were used to build a prognostic online calculator[98,99] which is available at http://www.tbi-impact.org/?p=impact/calc.

NEUROLOGICAL COMPLICATIONS

ICP, epidural and subdural hemorrhages, and cerebral edema. All comatose TBI patients need to have an ICP monitor placed because 10–20% of all these patients, particularly those with intracranial hemorrhage or cerebral edema, will have ICP elevations. Please refer to Chapter 7 for general principles of TBI management. Following TBI, management of suspected or documented ICP elevation involves rapid identification of intracranial masses that may require surgical interventions. ICHs (occurring in approximately 40% of cases due to tearing of small or medium-sized vessels),[100] subdural hematomas (SDHs), and, less frequently, EDHs (occurring in less than 1% from tearing of meningeal arteries) may be seen on CT scan. Patients with EDH may have a period during which they regain consciousness (a "lucid interval") followed by rapid subsequent deterioration of consciousness (referred to by Adams and Jennett as patients who "talk and die"). EDH is associated with a high mortality unless addressed emergently by surgical evacuation. Management of acute subdural, epidural, and parenchymal hematomas with mass effect involves open craniotomy, while subacute or chronic SDHs may be managed with burr-hole or twist-drill evacuation. Prophylactic decompressive craniectomy in the absence of a hematoma is not recommended for TBI based on the results of a randomized clinical trial.[101] Parenchymal contusions often associated with parenchymal hemorrhages are seen underlying the impact to the skull (coup lesion) with a contralateral contre-coup lesion at the opposite pole where the brain hits the inner table of the skull. Contusional lesions may worsen within 24 hours of the injury and rarely beyond that time frame. Cerebral edema may be severe and not necessarily correlate well with the severity of the injury. Abnormal vasoreactivity with vascular dilatation is implicated in the pathophysiology of cerebral edema following acute brain injury.

Treatment of elevated ICP should follow a preset protocol (see Chapter 7). Hypertonic saline is likely equally effective as mannitol in TBI patients with demonstrated elevation of ICP. Hyperventilation is used as a temporizing emergent measure for patients with ICP elevation. However, hyperventilation below a level of PCO_2 of 28 mm Hg or used in a prolonged or prophylactic measure may cause ischemia and will not benefit TBI patients.[102] Similarly, barbiturates (i.e., pentobarbital) are used to treat refractory ICP elevations but have been associated with worse outcome when given prophylactically.[103] Mild to moderate hypothermia does reduce the ICP, but in TBI patients it was not found to be beneficial[104–106] in a series of clinical trials. High-dose steroids in the first week after TBI have been associated with higher mortality and should not be given.[107–109] Targeting cerebral perfusion pressure (CPP) to promote adequate brain perfusion is advised, but the target threshold is controversial.[110] Current guidelines recommend to keep CPP above 60 mm Hg[111] as liberal use of pressors and fluids to keep CPP elevated above this level may be associated with increased risk of pulmonary edema and worse outcome.[112] Invasive multimodal monitoring may help identify individualized perfusion pressures based on brain oxygenation, metabolic measurements such as microdialysis, and EEG activity. Noninvasive measurement of CPP may be generated using arterial line blood pressure monitoring, transcranial Doppler measurement, and the use of a simple linear circuit model.[113] Preferentially infusions of short-acting antihypertensive agents (e.g., labetalol and nicardipine) and vasopressors (e.g., norepinephrine and phenylephrine) are used to keep arterial pressure and CPP within the desired range. Management protocols to prevent ICP crises and brain tissue hypoxia using multimodal invasive brain monitoring may be promising.[114]

Subarachnoid hemorrhage. Trauma is the most common cause of SAH and can be detected in the CSF in most cases of TBI. SAH following trauma is predominantly located in the sulci of the convexity and only secondarily in the basal cisterns, whereas most of the blood is located around the circle of Willis following aneurysmal rupture. Vasospasm may develop in approximately a third of severe TBI patients within 3 days of trauma but is much less studied and often underappreciated when compared to vasospasm following aneurysmal rupture. Underlying mechanisms are poorly understood, but mechanical stretching, inflammation, endothelin, calcium dysregulation, contractile proteins, and cortical spreading depolarization have been implicated. Management may include prophylaxis with nimodipine based on a number of randomized controlled trials and case series[115] but this is highly controversial.[116]

Diffuse axonal injury (DAI). The underlying pathogenetic mechanisms of DAI are discussed in Chapter 4. Fundamentally the acceleration-deceleration movements of the head during trauma lead to shearing and stretching of axons, particularly those in the ascending arousal system that connect the forebrain with the brainstem. In addition, in patients with prolonged loss of consciousness, there is often damage to the neurons of origin of the ascending arousal system in the dorsal pons, which sits just under the unyielding sharp edge of the tentorium. Neurological impairment, and particularly the severity of impaired consciousness, is often out of proportion when compared to routine imaging findings, particularly on CT. Small hemorrhages may be seen particularly on gradient echo sequences when obtaining MRIs. Damage to white matter tracts can best be visualized subacutely on MRI diffusion tensor sequences, and this may evolve into white matter tract atrophy. Management of DAI is supportive as there are no specific interventions available to date, but detection of DAI does affect the prognosis of the comatose TBI victim.[117]

Skull fractures. The majority of skull fractures are linear and nondepressed and generally do not require specific interventions. However, depressed, open, or basilar skull fractures may need specific management. Depressed skull fractures are almost always open and may cause infection, CSF leaks, dural sinus thrombosis, or refractory seizures. Most depressed skull fractures require surgical exploration. Open (or compound) skull fractures have to be differentiated from closed skull fractures. Skin lacerations in association with skull fractures and pneumocephalus on head CT may indicate open skull fractures. Basilar skull fractures are identified on CT and may require dedicated sequences, such as fine cuts through the skull base. They may be associated with cranial nerve deficits (particularly involving the facial or oculomotor nerves). Deficits in ocular motility due to nerve injury must be differentiated from those due to entrapment of the ocular muscles in the fracture. If the eye cannot be moved by forced duction (i.e., anesthetizing the sclera and pulling on it with a fine-toothed forceps), then entrapment must be sought. Signs of basilar skull fracture include ecchymosis over the mastoid (Battle's sign), blood behind or perforation of the tympanic membrane, CSF otorrhea, or hearing loss. Involvement of the carotid canal can lead to stroke or hemorrhage, and a dural tear with CSF leak can result in delayed bacterial meningitis. Antibiotic prophylaxis for open skull fractures is controversial and not universally recommended at this time.[118] Other intracranial infections may occur in patients with skull fractures, including meningitis, subdural empyema, osteomyelitis, or brain abscess. These may develop within weeks of the injury, may be identified with contrast CT or MRI, and may require prolonged antibiotics and surgical exploration and drainage.

Seizures. Acute prophylaxis with phenytoin reduces the frequency of early (from 14% to 4%) but not late seizures following TBI.[119] Based on these data, unless seizures are encountered in the first week after injury, antiepileptics should be stopped after 7 days. Many experts advocate for alternative antiseizure medications such as levetiracetam, but no adequately powered clinical trial has compared these agents head to head. Nonconvulsive seizures and nonconvulsive SE are frequent (10–20% of comatose patients) after TBI, but can only be identified using continuous EEG monitoring. Nonconvulsive SE is associated with metabolic crisis[120] and hippocampal atrophy on long-term follow-up MRI and worse functional outcome.[121] If detected, nonconvulsive seizures should be treated similar to convulsive seizures or SE. Long-term epilepsy develops in 15–25% of patients with severe TBI.[122] These seizures typically develop up to a year after initial injury, and mechanisms underlying epileptogenesis are poorly understood,[123] although patients who have intracranial hemorrhages or more severe brain damage are at greater risk.

Cervical spine injury. As discussed earlier for all TBI patients, an unstable spine should be assumed and a hard collar placed until C-spine instability is ruled out. Standardized protocols such as those proposed by the Canadian C-Spine Rules or the National Emergency X-Radiography Utilization Study (NEXUS) should be followed[124-126] to identify C-spine fractures, ligamentous injury, and spinal cord injury. These mandate a successive series of imaging modalities followed by clinical examination. This will allow identification of injuries that need to be addressed without subjecting the patient to the risk of additional injury from the examination. In the context of patients with impaired consciousness, clinical evaluation alone is not possible and imaging of the C-spine by CT scans must be done. MRI may also be needed to identify ligamentous injury, and CT angiography is necessary for those with suspected blunt cerebrovascular injuries.[127]

Other neurological complications. Cerebrovascular injuries may include arterial dissection of either the carotid or vertebral arteries. Strokes may develop from thrombosis of the dissected artery as well as by emboli distal to the dissection. There is no evidence to support anticoagulation over antiplatelet drugs for preventing stroke or death in patients with symptomatic carotid or vertebral dissection.[128] Aneurysms and pseudoaneurysms which may form have been successfully treated with stent deployment.

Carotid cavernous fistulas present with orbital bruits, ocular chemosis, and pulsating exophthalmus (other cranial nerves such as II, IV, V, and VI may be involved) and can be seen with trauma or rupture of an internal carotid artery aneurysm. CSF fistulas may develop as a result of dura, and arachnoid membranes rupture in 5–10% of basilar skull fractures and 3% of closed head injuries. In most cases, CSF leaks stop with head elevation for several days, but a few may require lumbar drains or surgical repair.

Neuroprotective strategies. A complex series of secondary cellular and biochemical cascades is triggered following initial injuries, which have a major impact on neurologic outcome. Despite multiple attempts so far no neuroprotective agent has been able to improve outcome after TBI in clinical trials.

MEDICAL COMPLICATIONS

Medical complications have a major impact on outcomes in patients with acute brain injury, including those with TBI.[129] General critical care measures including deep venous thrombosis (DVT) prophylaxis should be followed. Typically, mechanical thromboembolism prevention devices (e.g., intermittent pneumatic compression) are initiated within 24 hours of injury.[130] Unfractionated or low-molecular-weight heparin is recommended within 24–48 hours for all patients even with any intracranial bleeding or craniotomy (typically as long as the initial traumatic bleeding is stable on follow-up imaging). Routine placement of prophylactic inferior vena cava filters is not recommended.

Fever is frequent following TBI, and an increased fever burden is associated with worse outcome.[131] Fever and leukocytosis are seen in a number of noninfectious causes in these patients, such as neurological injury, systemic inflammatory response syndrome, atelectasis, and pulmonary contusions. However, in addition to general critical care infections, such as aspiration pneumonia, urinary tract infections, and any catheters associated infections, a number of trauma-specific infectious scenarios are worth considering.[132] These include infections related to open fractures, intra-abdominal or thoracic abscesses, and burn injuries. Infections may require surgical intervention, and frequently antibiotics are given perioperatively. Post trauma, an overwhelming inflammatory reaction with immune dysfunction resulting in multiorgan failure may occur requiring aggressive management strategies.

Secondary pulmonary deterioration may occur due to acute respiratory distress syndrome as well as transfusion-related acute lung injury (TRALI). Ischemia-reperfusion injury from hemorrhagic shock may result in acute kidney and liver failure of the trauma patient. Abdominal compartment syndrome is a feared complication in polytrauma patients as it may also exacerbate ICP and should be monitored with serial assessments of bladder pressures.

Hematology. Neither higher transfusion thresholds (keeping the hemoglobin greater than 10 g/dL instead of 7 g/dL) nor the administration of erythropoietin were shown to be beneficial for patients with closed head injury who were unable to follow commands.[133] Adverse events such as thromboembolic events were more frequent for patients with more liberal transfusion administration (more than 10 g/dL).

Fluids and nutrition. D5W and half normal saline should be avoided as the excess free water may worsen brain swelling. Preferential fluids are isotonic, such as normal saline (0.9% sodium) and plasmalyte solutions. Careful monitoring of serum sodium should be done as sudden drops in sodium may precipitate brain swelling. Negative fluid balances are associated with worse outcome and should be avoided; however, assessment of fluid status is challenging and supportive measures in addition to urine output measurements, such as central venous pressure, arterial pulse contour analysis, and ultrasound-guided inferior vena cava collapsibility, are used. The hypermetabolic and catabolic state following acute brain injury with increased caloric needs (50–100% above normal) necessitates early initiation of feeding (via nasogastric or nasoduodenal feeding tubes within 24–48 hours of injury), but parenteral feeding is typically not recommended. Stress ulcer prevention should be started for all intubated patients and those with coagulopathy (pantoprazole 40 mg/d or famotidine 20 mg/d).

Subdural and Epidural Hematoma

Both SDH and EDH are primarily seen in the setting of trauma (discussed earlier), but particularly SDHs may also occur spontaneously, such as in the elderly, patients with brain atrophy (i.e., due to chronic alcoholism), and in patients receiving anticoagulation, and rarely as a presentation of vascular abnormalities or malignancies. Management will depend on the presumed underlying etiology. Spontaneous SDHs are more prevalent in the elderly or those with brain atrophy due to stretching of bridging veins. The chronicity of the hemorrhage as determined by history and imaging appearance dictates to a large extent the management of these patients. Fresh blood quickly forms clots, but in the more chronic state membranes may form, isolating different pockets of blood within the hematoma. Management approaches include monitoring without neurosurgical intervention, burr-hole or twist-drill evacuation, and open craniotomy (Figure 8.2).[134] Frequently, these hemorrhages show a mixture of differently aged blood, such as acute on chronic or acute on subacute, and surgical approaches for these patients have to be individualized. The extent of neurological deficits and mass effect (i.e., midline shift), acuity of the blood, perioperative risk profile, and likelihood of reaccumulation should be taken into account when choosing between therapeutic approaches. Chronic SDHs often liquefy, and burr-hole or twist-drill evacuation may be successful for drainage, sparing the often fragile elderly patient a large open craniotomy procedure. Major acute SDHs will require open craniotomy.

Management otherwise mirrors that of the trauma patient. Often patients with spontaneous SDHs are placed on 1 week of seizure prophylaxis at least perioperatively.[135,136] Decisions on whether or when to restart antiplatelet agents or anticoagulation are often challenging in patients who developed SDHs or EDHs while receiving one of these mediations. The issues are similar to those in the patient who suffers from an ICH in the context of antiplatelet or anticoagulant therapy: the risk of hemorrhage reaccumulation has to be weighed against the risk of complications due to interruption of these medications.

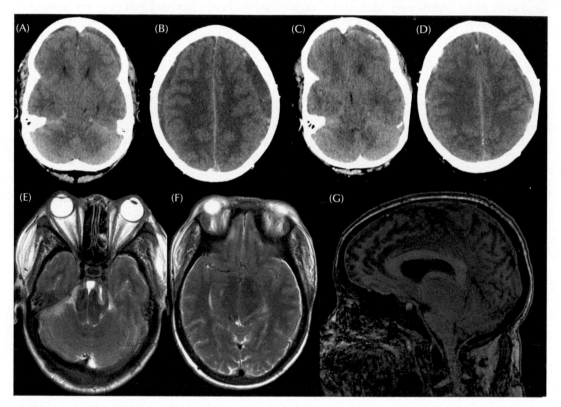

Figure 8.2 A 29-year-old woman with congenital HIV on highly active retroviral therapy and hemodialysis, superior vena cava syndrome after tunneled dialysis catheter with chronic left sided internal jugular vein thrombus on anticoagulation with coumadin. She presented with nausea, vomiting, and headache and was found to have a subtherapeutic INR of 1.4 with thrombus in the tunneled dialysis catheter. She was anticoagulated using a heparin drip and developed a severe headache three days later. Despite developing lethargy heparin drip was continued for another day and a Head CT obtained only after the patient developed loss of consciousness with elevation of systolic blood pressure to 240 mmHg. Head CT demonstrated bilateral acute on chronic subdural hematoma (Figure 8.2: panel A and B). Heaprin drip was stopped and Vitamin K 10 mg IV, fresh frozen plasma, and cryoprecipitate were administered emergently. She was transferred to the Neuro ICU and bedside evacuation of the subdural blood collections via burholes was performed (Figure 8.2, panel C and D post drainage). Despite good resolution of the subdural blood she developed recurrent headaches with loss of consciousness following each session of hemodialysis. MRI immediately following hemodialysis demonstrated central downward herniation likely explained the symptoms (Figure 8.2, panel E and G), which resolved together with the symptoms after switching the patient to continuous venovenous hemodialysis. After repeat drainage of the hygromas she tolerated hemodialysis without headache or loss of consciousness. The impression was that she had intracranial pressure changes precipitating reversible herniation as a severe manifestation of dialysis disequilibrium syndrome.[137,138]

Arterial Ischemic Stroke

Emergent management of patients with ischemic stroke has undergone major changes over the past two decades, first with the arrival of systemically administered intravenous thrombolysis and more recently with intra-arterial thrombolysis and mechanical clot removal. In addition, control of blood pressure and prevention and management of secondary neurological (e.g., hemicraniectomy for brain swelling) and medical complications (e.g., infections) remain important areas of management. Neuroprotective strategies, while promising in the laboratory and preclinical stages, have largely failed in the clinical setting but remain an active area of research. Additionally, secondary stroke prophylaxis such as lipid, glucose, and blood pressure modifications are a major focus of subacute and chronic management of the stroke patient. As in other acute neurological emergencies, revascularization and delivery of neuroprotective strategies are highly time-sensitive.[139] Much effort and success in improving outcomes of stroke victims has been directed toward improving workflow and thereby optimizing the emergency care of the stroke patient. Development of these clinical pathways have been spurred by regulatory mandates that govern certification of stroke centers and stroke units, including nationally accepted stroke protocols and time lines.

Emergency presentation of the stroke patient. Stroke may present with numerous neurological signs and symptoms depending on the affected vascular territory. Standardized stroke screening by first responders is a fundamental building block in triaging the suspected stroke patient to the appropriate facility, such as a certified stroke center.[3] This will increase the patient's chance of receiving intravenous tPA, one of the major interventions for acute ischemic stroke (discussed later) as only one-quarter of patients arrive at the hospital within the therapeutic window to be eligible for this intervention. Similar to the trauma patient, prenotification of the stroke team allows providers to reduce time to treatment administration. All time points for obtaining diagnostic information and delivering therapeutic interventions need to be documented and compared to national benchmarks. In an effort to shorten the time from suspected acute ischemic stroke to thrombolysis, some studies have explored the feasibility of ambulances that are equipped with a mobile CT scanner. These are specifically deployed to patients with a suspected stroke and can rule out hemorrhage or other potential contraindications, thus allowing administration of intravenous thrombolysis in the field.[140]

Systemic thrombolysis. Intravenous administration of thrombolytic medication is a cornerstone of the acute ischemic stroke treatment. A number of thrombolytic medications were explored and given at various time points following stroke onset, with mixed results. Intravenous administration of tPA (0.9 mg/kg, given 10% as a bolus and the remainder over 1 hour; serum half-life of tPA is 4–10 minutes) was FDA approved for treatment of eligible stroke patients in 1996, following the publication of the results of the NINDS rtPA stroke study group.[141]

The key risk identified in that early NINDS study of thrombolysis with rTPA was that it causes intracranial hemorrhage in approximately 6% of patients (compared to 0.6% in controls). Subsequent studies have identified specific risk factors which, once excluded, can minimize this risk. It is therefore critical to obtain the following information that might bring to light contraindications, including (1) the time that the patient was last seen normal; (2) the specifics of the neurological syndrome (i.e., is it typical of stroke or does it suggest some other cause, such as seizure?); (3) a brief previous medical history, including prior hemorrhages and medications such as blood thinners; (4) a brief neurological examination using the National Institutes of Health Stroke Scale (NIHSS, range 0–42; higher numbers indicating a worse deficit;[142] and (5) obtaining imaging to rule out a lesion that would prevent rTPA treatment.

In most centers, a noncontrast head CT is the most rapid imaging study available. It can rule out ICH and can reveal early infarct signs such as loss of gray–white differentiation (especially in the insular region), loss of sulci, hypodensity in the basal ganglia region, and the "dense MCA sign," which may be seen with a thrombus in the proximal middle cerebral artery (MCA). CT findings may be summarized using the Alberta Stroke Prognosis of acute ischemia Early CT Score (ASPECTS).[143] On the other hand, a large area of edema can suggest an alternative pathology, such as a tumor, or that the infarction may have occurred substantially hours earlier than suspected clinically.

The main concern with intravenous tPA administration is intracranial bleeding, which was symptomatic in 6% of patients[141] in the initial National Institutes of Health (NIH) trial. With increasing time from stroke onset, the benefit from tPA decreases and the risk of hemorrhage increases.[144] Patients younger than 80 years, with a NIHSS of 25 or less, without a history of diabetes or prior stroke, and not on anticoagulation benefitted also from intravenous tPA given up to 4.5 hours after the stroke onset.[145,146] Risk factors for hemorrhagic conversion include older age, increased time from stroke symptom onset to medication administration, early infarct or dense MCA signs on CT, higher stroke severity (higher NIHSS), hyperglycemia, and hypertension. Predictions can be made using the SEDAN score.[147] Worsening of the neurologic exam during tPA infusion should prompt stopping the tPA infusion immediately, administering clotting factor cryoprecipitate, and obtaining a noncontrast head CT for suspected intracranial hemorrhage. Depending on the CT findings, including size and location of the hematoma, neurosurgical evacuation may be considered. Additionally, administration of tPA may rarely be complicated by anaphylaxis and angioedema with respiratory compromise in 1–5% of cases, potentially requiring intubation, antihistamines, steroids, and epinephrine.

Intravenous tPA should be given as rapidly as possible and within 3 hours to all eligible patients with arterial ischemic stroke.[141,145] This has been shown to improve functional outcome at 3 months in 13% of stroke patients. Current guidelines indicate that absolute contraindications for intravenous tPA are cerebral hemorrhage on CT, early infarction involving one-third or more of the MCA territory, recent major surgery, and time elapse of more than 4.5 hours between stroke onset and administration of the medication. Hypertension needs to be lowered to less than 185/110 mm Hg prior to administration of intravenous tPA, preferentially using a short-acting medication given as an infusion (i.e., nicardipine). On a case-by-case basis, a risk-benefit evaluation should inform the decision to administer tPA, particularly in the case of minor or rapidly resolving stroke symptoms, minimal anticoagulation (relative contraindication

if INR is 1.7–2.0; if no history to suggest coagulopathy, do not wait for INR or platelet tests), or thrombocytopenia (relative contraindication if 50,000–100,000). Intravenous tPA is discouraged and typically intra-arterial approaches—discussed later—are preferred in patients receiving novel anticoagulants (i.e., dabigatran), but, as specific antibody-based reversal strategies are becoming available,[9,10] intravenous tPA may be reconsidered in these cases. Seizures and hypo- and hyperglycemia should be treated and considered as potential stoke mimics but are no longer considered contraindications for administration of tPA. Ultrasound-augmented administration of intravenous tPA has been shown to be effective in small clinical trials,[148] but due to high operator variability and dependency has not gained general acceptance.

Interventional neuroradiology. Patients with large vessel occlusions who do not respond to intravenous tPA may still benefit from endovascular revascularization approaches. Identification of the patient with a suspected large vessel occlusion starts with the neurological examination suggesting a typical stroke syndrome for occlusion of a specific large artery; a high NIHSS by itself is not a reliable guide.[149] Hence, understanding the vascular deficit patterns discussed in Chapter 4 is essential to identifying which patients may benefit from endovascular approaches. It is necessary to make this determination early in the course as endovascular procedures are not universally available and may require transporting the patient to an appropriate facility as well as activation of the interventional radiology team to perform the procedure. Presence of a dense opacification of a large cerebral vessel on initial noncontrast head CT scan can also help identify such patients. In institutions where rapid CT angiography is also done routinely, this confirmation of large vessel occlusion can minimize organizational challenges as well as risk to the patient.

Intra-arterial thrombolysis. Although mechanical thrombectomy techniques are now generally approved, when this is not available intra-arterial tPA or prourokinase may be administered locally off-label by catheter to the occluded vessel. This approached increased recanalization rates from 18% to 66% in MCA patients treated within 6 hours of stroke onset using IA prourokinase (PROACT II)[150] but has marginal benefits on functional outcomes (40% vs. 25% good functional outcome) and higher ICH rates (10% vs. 2%).

Mechanical thrombectomy. Several clinical trials published within a short time showed the benefit of stent retriever-assisted thrombectomy for occlusion of the basilar artery, carotid terminus, and middle cerebral arteries (Multicenter Randomized Clinical Trial of Endovascular Treatment for Acute Ischemic Stroke in the Netherlands [MR CLEAN],[151] Extending the Time for Thrombolysis in Emergency Neurological Deficits-Intra-Arterial [EXTEND-IA],[152] Evaluation Study of Congestive Heart Failure and Pulmonary Artery Catheterization Effectiveness [ESCAPE],[153] Endovascular Revascularization with Solitaire Device Versus Best Medical Therapy in Anterior Circulation Stroke Within 8 Hours [REVASCAT],[154] Solitaire with the Intention for Thrombectomy as Primary Endovascular Treatment [SWIFT PRIME]) (Figure 8.3).[155] These trials, when pooled together,[156,157] showed that, in contrast to previous studies using earlier-generation devices, there was[158,159] not only a neuroradiological benefit but also an improvement in functional outcome as measured by the modified Rankin scale. Device

development progressed from corkscrew-like (MERCI), to suction (Penumbra), and, most recently, stent-retriever devices (TREVO, Solitaire). The newer devices were shown to have a much higher revascularization rate and are becoming increasingly user-friendly. Apart from using these newer technologies, the more recent successful trials applied stringent patient selection criteria in order to identify only those patients who still had a large vessel occlusion and would benefit from the intervention. These selection algorithms are important to remember when trying to generalize the findings of these clinical trials. Selection criteria most frequently included maximum elapsed time between stroke onset and procedure (in between 4.5 and 12 hours), varying cutoffs for minimum or maximum NIHSS levels, and imaging preselection (CT angiography with or without CT perfusion studies). Benefit for mechanical thrombectomy appears to persist in select patients in the 6- to 24-hour time window after last known normal for those who had a mismatch between clinical deficit and infarct volume[160,161] using an automated imaging-based quantification of the mismatch.[153] Endovascular approaches are particularly promising for patients with contraindications

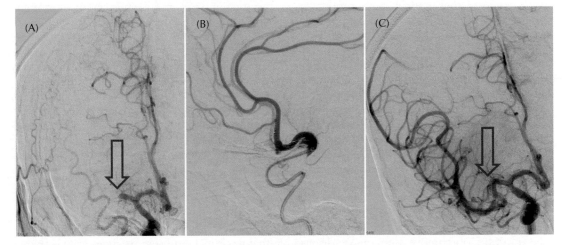

Figure 8.3 A 33-year-old healthy truck driver presented with sudden onset of acute left hemiparesis. On examination he was found to have fluent dysarthric speech without aphasia, left sided neglect, mild right gaze preference, no blink to threat on the left, with a left sided facial droop and plegia of the left arm and leg. His NIH Stroke Scale was calculated as 11. Head CT did not show any early infarct signs or hemorrhage (ASPECT score 10). CT angiogram showed a right proximal cut off of the middle cerebral artery (M1) with distal reconstitution without evidence for intra- or extracranial dissection. He received intravenous tPA at 2 hours and 28 minutes with persistent neurological deficits. He underwent emergent intra-arterial clot evacuation with TICI III achieved at 4 hours and 45 minutes (Figure 8.3, panel A showing right middle cerebral artery cut off at the M1 level pre clot evacuation, panel B showing deployment of the stent retriever device, panel C shows the radiograph demonstrating revascularization of the right middle cerebral artery obtained 3 minutes after panel A). His neurological deficits rapidly resolved without any detectable neurological deficits 12 hours post stroke onset.

for intravenous thrombolysis and may offer some hope for patients presenting in a delayed fashion. Recanalization rates appear to be higher in patients who received tenecteplase instead of alteplase, possibly due to higher fibrin-specificity and longer activity.[162]

Intraprocedural management. Anesthesia management of the acute stroke patient is not well studied, and both medications such as anesthetics as well as derangements of vitals signs (particularly blood pressure, oxygenation, and temperature) may have major impact on neuronal survival in this scenario. During the procedure, the patient may be kept under general anesthesia, but, increasingly and supported by practices in recent clinical trials, it is recommended to keep patients awake and undergo an approach called *monitored anesthesia care.* General anesthesia, while more controlled, may be associated with hypotension during induction, leading to deleterious drops in cerebral perfusion pressure. There is some evidence suggesting that general anesthesia may be associated with higher morbidity and mortality of stroke patients undergoing endovascular procedures.[163–165] This was also supported by post hoc analyses of the anesthetic regimen in one of the large clinical trials.[151,166] However, most recently, a small study suggests that patients undergoing general anesthesia did have similar outcomes to those with conscious sedation.[167] Blood pressure goals are controversial, but permissive hypertension is allowed prior to the procedure and typically lowered after revascularization to systolic blood pressure of 120–140 mm Hg to minimize reperfusion injury.

Medical management of the acute stroke patient. Patients should be managed following a strict protocol and admitted to specialized stroke units; those with concern for herniation or with hemorrhage should be admitted to specialized intensive care units.[3] Patients with stroke frequently have concomitant cardiac disease (i.e., arrhythmias) or pulmonary disease (i.e., chronic obstructive pulmonary disease [COPD]), which need to be kept in mind when stabilizing the stroke patient.

Blood pressure. Both hypo- and hypertension following acute ischemic stroke are associated with poor outcome (U-shaped relationship).[168] The ideal blood pressure is controversial and subject to a number of completed and ongoing clinical trials.[169] Currently, permissive hypertension is allowed (up to 220/120 mm Hg, with stricter cutoffs for patients who have received thrombolysis or developed hemorrhagic conversion; preferred agents are labetalol or nicardipine infusions, followed subacutely by more strict blood pressure control. *Hypercholesteremia* increases the risk of stroke, and lipid-lowering medications such as statins are part of primary or secondary stroke prophylaxis.[170] Reduced cardiovascular events with statin treatment, even in subjects with normal lipid levels, has suggested that they may also have some neuroprotective effect.[171]

Secondary stroke prevention. Patients with acute ischemic stroke are at risk of recurrent strokes, and secondary stroke prevention should start during the acute hospitalization.

Aspirin. For the purposes of secondary stroke prevention stroke patients should be started on aspirin 325 mg/d within 24–48 hours following the stroke onset. Contraindications include hemorrhagic conversion on follow-up CT scans obtained 24 hours after administration of thrombolysis or 24 hours after stroke onset if thrombolysis was not given. Patients do not appear to benefit from adding clopidogrel to aspirin for secondary stroke prophylaxis.[172]

Anticoagulation. Patients with atrial fibrillation should be considered for anticoagulation to prevent stroke recurrence. Long-term management in appropriate candidates includes oral warfarin once the acute stroke period is over (typically 3–7 days post stroke onset; aspirin should be stopped once warfarin is therapeutic). Acutely bridging with heparin infusions or full-dose low-molecular-weight heparin is controversial. Additionally, patients should undergo rate control of atrial fibrillation but rhythm control is not beneficial.[173]

Carotid disease. Patients with anterior circulation cerebral strokes should undergo screening of the ipsilateral carotid artery to determine the degree of stenosis and to evaluate the patient for possible carotid endarterectomy or carotid stenting. Dissections of the major cranial arteries are increasingly being recognized as a cause of stroke. Hence MRI imaging of these arteries, with fat saturation, is recommended, particularly in younger patients without a clear cause of stroke. However, treating these patients with anticoagulation remains controversial.

Vertebrobasilar disease. Aggressive blood pressure management is recommended for stroke patients, but distal quantification of perfusion is associated with subsequent strokes in patients with atherosclerotic vertebrobasilar occlusive disease. These measures may guide more aggressive interventions in the future.[174] Angioplasty and stenting are considerations in isolated cases for patients with symptomatic vertebrobasilar disease.[3]

Management of acute stroke patients should involve strict protocols that dictate tight blood pressure control (monitoring of vital signs and neurological deficits, kept at lower than 220/120 for all, and for 24 hours at lower than 180/105 for patients post tPA), aspirin 325 mg by mouth or rectally or subcutaneous enoxaparin 40 mg (both contraindicated for 24 hours post tPA), glucose (target 140–180 mg/dL), high-dose statin, sequential compression devices, dysphagia screening, and workup of the underlying etiology (EKG, transthoracic and possibly transesophageal echocardiogram, telemetry, hypercoagulable screen, urine toxicology screen, lipid panel, hemoglobin A1c, carotid Dopplers; consider other imaging studies).

Special considerations for those with impaired consciousness. Consciousness is often impaired in stroke patients with brainstem strokes; stroke due to basilar artery occlusion may directly damage the ascending arousal system, while cerebellar or large hemispheric infarction may cause swelling that compresses the brainstem (see Chapter 3). The dismal prognosis of patients with basilar artery occlusion requires more aggressive management.[175] Endovascular interventions including mechanical clot extraction and also angioplasty or stenting are considered on a case-by-case basis up to 24 hours after stroke onset. Edema caused by cerebellar infarction may both compress the brainstem directly as well as cause obstructive hydrocephalus due to compression of the fourth ventricle. Symptoms of fourth ventricular compression include decreasing alertness as well as hyperreflexia, particularly in the lower extremities; brainstem compression may produce eye movement abnormalities as well as hemiparesis or even quadriparesis. The progression of clinical symptoms may be rapid and lead to coma and irreversible brain injury. Emergency management of patients with fourth ventricular compression may begin with hyperventilation and mannitol or hypertonic saline, followed

by placement of an extraventricular drain in the lateral ventricle. However, this may lead to upward herniation of the brainstem or cerebellum through the tentorial opening, so if the swelling is extensive or there are brainstem signs, suboccipital decompression is the treatment of choice.

Patients with large MCA infarctions are at risk of cerebral edema leading to subfalcine and uncal herniation with strikingly increased morbidity and mortality. This risk is directly related to the size of the infarcted territory (approaching 95% for those with two-thirds or more of the MCA territory affected). Predictors of herniation and malignant brain edema include worse neurological function (reflected in a higher baseline NIHSS score), more involved ischemic territories (reflected in a lower ASPECTS[143]), poor collaterals (reflected in the Collateral Score), and revascularization failure.[176] Neurological symptoms will depend on the herniation syndrome, but often progressive depression of consciousness is seen. Cortical spreading depression may be part of the pathophysiology and an early sign of brain swelling and impending herniation.[177,178] Intracranial monitoring is, however, for most of these patients not part of the management protocol as herniation may occur prior to any ICP elevations. Medical management strategies are similar to other patients with elevated ICP, including mild temporary hyperventilation for those in extremis and hypertonic saline and mannitol (see Chapter 7 for details). Hemicraniectomy is the definitive treatment, but timing of this treatment remains somewhat controversial. Three trials have shown the potential of prophylactic decompressive hemicraniectomy to improve outcomes for patients with large hemispheric MCA infarction.[179] The pooled analysis[180] of these trials showed an absolute reduction of the risk for death or severe disability in patients 60 years or younger by 51% compared to medical management alone (from 78% to 29%; additionally, among survivors, the likelihood of moderate disability or the chance to require no more than some help and to be able to walk without assistance increased from 32% to 43%). For patients older than 60 years, the risk of death decreased (from 70% to 33%) although most of those who were salvaged had severe disability.[179,181,182] Timing of this surgical intervention is controversial, but in these trials enrollment was within 48 hours and performed prior to the development of herniation symptoms. Post hemicraniectomy physicians need to be aware of the rare *sinking flap syndrome*,[183] which may present with paradoxical herniation.

Secondary neurological deterioration, with or without development of impaired consciousness, may be seen in any stroke patient, and the underlying cause needs to be established rapidly. The differential is vast and includes expansion of the stroke, development of a new stroke, hemorrhagic conversion, and seizures. Hemorrhagic conversion is diagnosed by noncontrast CT scan and requires aggressive blood pressure control (systolic BP lower than 140 mm Hg), reversal of anticoagulation or platelet medication, and consideration for surgical evacuation of the bleed or hemicraniectomy. In patients with critical stenosis of a major cerebral blood vessel, fluctuation in the neurological examinations may be due to marginal cerebral perfusion, which requires carefully monitored attempts to raise perfusion pressure by placing the patient in reverse Trendelenburg position or administering fluids or pressors until either a vascular intervention is performed or collateral blood vessels have matured. Seizures are less frequent than in patients with hemorrhagic strokes but, depending on the study design, may be seen in 10–15% of ischemic stroke patients.[184] Seizure prophylaxis is not recommended, but, if diagnosed, seizures should be treated similar to other acute brain injury ictal events (see Chapter 7).

Medical complications. Fever is associated with worse outcome after stroke and should be managed aggressively. While recent trials have not found hypothermia to be neuroprotective,[185] the current goal is to maintain normothermia. In patients without identifiable infection, acetaminophen and possibly external cooling devices to achieve normothermia may be used to treat high fevers. Aspiration pneumonia is frequent in patients with strokes as dysphagia and speech difficulties are common in these patients. All stroke patients should remain NPO until they can undergo standardized speech and swallow evaluations to determine the safest mode of food administration (per mouth, per nasogastric or nasoduodenal tube, or percutaneous endoscopic gastrostomy tube) and choice of diet (consistency). Avoidance and early

removal of urinary catheters are most effective in preventing urinary tract infections. Hyper- as well as hypoglycemia may worsen outcome after ischemic stroke.[186] Serum glucose levels are controversial, but a target of 140–180 mg/dL is recommended and may be achieved with insulin administered by infusions or on a sliding scale. Patients with strokes, particularly those with hemiparesis, are at extremely high risk of DVT and pulmonary embolism. All patients should get pneumatic compression devices when in bed and undergo early mobilization whenever possible. Enoxaparin (40 mg/d) should be started on stroke patients unless a contraindication exists (hemorrhagic conversion, within 24 hours of receiving intra-arterial or intravenous thrombolysis).[187]

Neuroprotection. In an attempt to translate the promise of neuroprotective agents from animals to the bedside, several clinical trials of neuroprotection were attempted, but so far most have failed to show an effect on outcomes in humans.[188,189] On the other hand, drugs that were introduced for other reasons (e.g., statins to control lipids and nimodipine after SAH to prevent vasospasm) may ironically improve outcomes by having a neuroprotective effect. Currently, neuroprotective agents continue to be an area of active research and hold potential as future interventions. Pathomechanisms of the ischemic cascade are complex, and it is likely that approaches combining novel strategies to achieve reperfusion with agents targeting multiple mechanisms hold most promise.[190]

Venous Sinus Thrombosis

Thrombosis of the cerebral venous sinuses may cause ischemic or hemorrhagic strokes. Symptoms depend on the involved territory (see Chapter 4), but headache and impaired consciousness are not infrequent and may be a symptom of elevated ICP, or occasionally of inclusion of the deep cerebral veins with impaired perfusion and edema of the diencephalon. Treatment must be individualized, but anticoagulation is the cornerstone to prevent progression of thrombosis even in the presence of intracranial hemorrhage. Additional treatment should be directed at the management of secondary effects such as elevated ICP, headaches, and seizures. Prophylactic use of antiepileptic agents is not recommended, but seizures should be treated and sinus thrombosis patients with seizures should receive long-term antiseizure medication. For management of elevated ICP, please refer to Chapter 7. Definitive treatment requires identifying the underlying cause of the venous sinus thrombosis. Although a proximate cause is not apparent in approximately a third of cases, common etiologies include thrombophilia and oral contraceptive pills. Additionally, other medications (i.e., chemotherapy) or hematologic diseases or coagulopathies (i.e., factor V Leiden or prothrombin mutations), infections (i.e., encephalitis) or inflammatory diseases (i.e., vasculitis), malignancy (i.e., local invasion or coagulopathy), trauma, or obstetric history (elevated coagulability in the weeks before and after delivery) account for a large number of cases. Any of these underlying causes may need to be addressed as the thrombosis can progress if the cause of thrombosis is not addressed.

Thrombosis treatment. In a small randomized controlled trial, full-dose anticoagulation using unfractionated heparin was shown to be superior to placebo in preventing progression of thrombosis.[191] Interestingly, anticoagulated patients did not have a higher risk of hemorrhage than those who received placebo. Subsequently, studies found treatment with low-molecular-weight heparin to be a viable alternative to unfractionated heparin.[192,193] Endovascular approaches including local thrombolysis and mechanical thrombectomy are typically reserved for cases with clinical deterioration despite anticoagulation or contraindications for anticoagulation. Prolonged microcatheter-based local thrombolytic infusion may be offered on a case-by-case basis.[194] Open surgical interventions such as sinus clot removal or hemicraniectomy may be offered in select cases. For sinus venous thrombosis patients without contraindications, anticoagulation for 3 months or longer, followed by antiplatelet therapy, is recommended.[195]

Brain Tumor

Management of brain tumors is a rapidly evolving, highly specialized field beyond the scope of this book. Here we will focus on the causes and treatment of acute deterioration

in consciousness of the brain tumor patient. Acute or progressive deterioration of consciousness may be seen due to tumor invasion of specific brain structures, direct tissue compression or herniation from edema caused by the tumor, hemorrhage into the tumor, seizures, paraneoplastic effects, or as a side effect of the tumor treatment (i.e., radiation necrosis). The first principle of management is to identify the cause of impaired consciousness in the brain tumor patient. Following a careful neurological examination, typically imaging studies are obtained. Acutely, CT scans are often obtained but most brain tumor patients will undergo MRI studies with contrast to better delineate margins of the tumor from surrounding edema and help preoperative planning (see Patient Vignette 8.1). The majority of patients will not need to be intubated, but safety to protect the airway should be assessed carefully.

Patient Vignette 8.1

An 85-year-old professor of medicine developed a left frontal glioblastoma. He was treated with surgical resection, radiation therapy, and dexamethasone to reduce swelling of the tumor. He had some difficulty finding words but was otherwise alert and took care of all activities of daily living in his home environment. Two months later, his family noted that his cognitive function was failing, and he was less interactive and had more trouble speaking. This was attributed to progression of his tumor. Over several days, he became stuporous and was unable to eat, so he was admitted to the hospital, where he was put on comfort measures and died a few days later. Because he was a strong advocate of autopsies, his will mandated that a postmortem examination be done. At autopsy it was found that his tumor progression had been minimal but that he had a thick coating of pus over his cerebral hemispheres. Cultures grew out *Streptococcus pneumonia*, sensitive to penicillin.

Comment

There is often a strong tendency in patients who have a known fatal illness to attribute cognitive deterioration to the underlying illness.

However, even patients with terminal illnesses can have intercurrent and reversible processes that can rob them of their faculties. In this case, the sympathetic colleagues and students of the professor wanted to spare him the pain of a lumbar puncture, which might have discovered his Strep infection at an early enough time to treat it effectively. And because the tumor had not progressed, they might have spared him for several more months of independent living.

Treatment of tumor progression will be highly dependent on the tumor type, but surgical resection may be chosen for debulking of the tumor mass even when total resection is not an option. Mass effect may also be decreased by evacuation of hemorrhages that may occur within tumors. Brain swelling from the tumor or in the perioperative period is traditionally treated with steroids (doses are controversial but frequently an initial bolus of 10–20 mg of dexamethasone is followed by 4–24 mg/d in divided doses).[196] Recent studies suggest that corticosteroids may actually cause gliomas to progress,[197] so that they are generally reduced after surgery and radiation therapy to the minimal dose required to maintain good function.

Seizures are frequent presenting symptoms of tumors or may develop in the subsequent clinical course. Prophylactic administration of antiepileptic medications is generally not recommended,[198] but, importantly, these data are primarily based on trials using older medications such as phenytoin[199,200] or valproic acid.[199,201] These drugs may have more side effects, more interactions with chemotherapeutic agents, and lead to worse cognitive performance. In addition, phenytoin may interact with radiation therapy, so that levetiracetam is currently preferred.[202] Patients with brain tumors may have impaired consciousness due to nonconvulsive seizures, which were extensively discussed earlier (see Chapter 7). Nonconvulsive seizures in brain tumor patients should be treated similarly to other patients, but when choosing antiepileptic drugs (AEDs), coadministration of other medications such as chemotherapeutic agents should be taken into account. AEDs, especially those affecting the cytochrome P450 system, may affect the metabolism of chemotherapeutic agents used for the treatment of metastatic or primary brain tumors.

Paraneoplastic syndromes. Impaired consciousness in the context of paraneoplastic syndromes is most frequently encountered secondary to autoantibody-mediated encephalitis. Treatment most importantly involves identification and treatment of the primary tumor as the paraneoplastic symptoms may be the presenting findings of the malignancy (although a substantial percentage of patients presenting with autoantibody-mediated limbic encephalitis have no known primary tumor, and indeed some may have the antibodies in response to a non-neoplastic antigen). Paraneoplastic syndromes with antibodies against cell surface antigens are potentially reversible and more responsive to immunomodulatory therapy than other paraneoplastic syndromes. Most prominently, this includes anti-NMDA receptor or voltage-gated calcium channel–mediated encephalitis,[203] which is primarily treated with identification of the primary malignancy (frequently ovarian teratomas requiring ovariectomy), intravenous immunoglobulin infusions (0.4 mg/kg for 5 days), plasmapheresis, and early immunosuppressive therapy as second-line therapy (rituximab,[204] a monoclonal antibody against B cells).[204] Additionally anti–voltage gated potassium channel encephalitis as a cell surface antibody type encephalitis is primarily treated with high-dose steroid therapy (methylprednisolone 1,000 mg/d for 5 days).

Complication of tumor therapy. Impaired consciousness may be encountered as a complication of tumor therapy. Early side effects of radiation (occurring within 1 week) are predominantly related to brain swelling, while delayed effects are mostly caused by injury of small blood vessel, demyelination, and immunologic effects. Corticosteroids are used primarily to manage the early effects of radiation (dexamethasone 4 mg given every 4 hours or less by mouth or intravenously). N-methyl-D-aspartate (NMDA) receptor blockers have shown some promise to delay cognitive decline following radiation therapy (memantine 20 mg/d given within 3 days of radiotherapy).[205]

Side effects of chemotherapeutic agents are frequent but depend largely on the dose, agent, and class that is administered. Impaired consciousness and seizures are frequently encountered, but other findings such as cerebellar syndromes, posterior reversible encephalopathy syndrome, and neurocognitive changes are seen. Management depends on the offending agent and encountered symptoms, but stopping the presumed offender is generally recommended when encountering CNS side effects. Ifosfamide-induced encephalopathy may be treated with methylene blue (50 mg intravenous four times daily). Monoclonal antibodies and other immunomodulatory treatments are increasingly and successfully used in cancer treatment but may be associated with thromboembolic and hemorrhagic strokes and posterior reversible encephalopathy syndrome. Management primarily involves discontinuation of the offending agent.

Brain Abscess

Bacterial abscess of the CNS may be located in the brain parenchyma or in the subdural or epidural space. Depending on the location and size, presenting symptoms may vary but headache, fever, focal neurological findings seizures, and raised ICP are common. Impaired consciousness is rarely a presenting sign for a patient with brain abscess but may develop in the clinical course if either the abscess is large enough to cause brain herniation or if it spills its contents intraventricularly or into the subarachnoid space. Diagnosis is based on clinical presentation and examination followed by imaging studies (contrast enhanced CT, MRI showing high signal on diffusion-weighted imaging and low apparent diffusion coefficient sequences [Figure 8.4]). Lumbar puncture should be avoided because the change in pressure across the abscess wall may cause rupture of the abscess. In case of spinal epidural abscesses, the lumbar puncture may track infectious organisms into the subarachnoid space. Management is categorized into surgical, medical, and identification of a possible underlying infectious source. Surgical excision is generally recommended for abscesses greater than 2.5 cm in diameter and for all causing significant mass effect. The procedure of choice will depend on the location of the abscess but CT-guided aspiration is attempted if feasible. Broad-spectrum antibiotics (such as vancomycin, metronidazole, and cefotaxime) are the medical alternative in cases where surgical aspiration is not possible, as in patients with meningitis or inaccessible abscesses.

Antibiotics are given at least for 6–8 weeks and success is closely monitored using serial imaging. Subdural or epidural empyemas are primarily treated neurosurgically by placing burr holes or performing a craniotomy or laminectomy in the case of spinal epidural abscess. Frequent causes of abscess are hematogenous spread such as from a lung source, and part of the management includes identification and treatment of possible underlying systemic infectious sources for abscesses.

NONSTRUCTURAL LESIONS: METABOLIC, DIFFUSE, OR MULTIFOCAL COMA

The clinical presentation of patients with nonstructural lesions leading to coma varies based on the precipitating cause, but making the diagnosis requires careful assessment of the past medical history and history of present illness as well as a focused neurological assessment. As described in Chapter 3, the neurological examination in metabolic coma is marked by depressed levels of consciousness in the absence of focal neurological signs (other than a few nonspecific findings described in that chapter). Because SDHs or multifocal brain processes can occasionally present in a nonfocal manner, early imaging is necessary. There is not a single most important laboratory test to make the diagnosis and narrow down the differential diagnosis in patients with nonstructural causes of coma, but, guided by the initial history and examination, screening laboratory tests may be sent (Table 8.3). All management starts with general resuscitative efforts outlined in Chapter 7. Emergent management of suspected ICP elevation and evolving herniation may require emergent treatment prior to starting an extended workup (see Chapter 7 for details).

Central Nervous System Infections

A low index of suspicion should place CNS infections on the differential for any patient presenting with abnormal consciousness particularly if associated with fever or leukocytosis. Additional symptoms may include meningismus, rash, focal neurological findings,

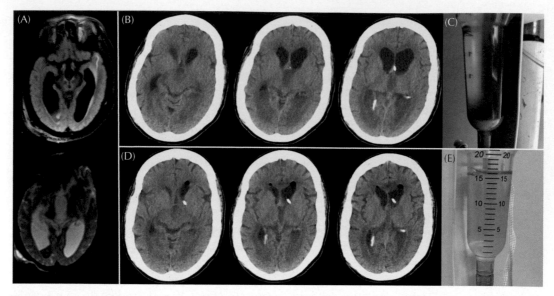

Figure 8.4 66 year old woman with a history of "normal pressure hydrocephalus" underwent ventiriculo-peritoneal shunt placement 16 years prior to admission. She presented to an outside hospital with confusion, agitation, impaired upward gaze, and gait instability. Head CT showed hydrocephalus and when she did not improve she underwent a large volume lumbar puncture. The CSF was unremarkable with zero white and red blood cells, glucose of 62 and protein of 12. With increasing obtundation, abdominal distension, and fever, a CT of her abdomen was done revealing a large pneumoperitoneum as well as subcutaneous emphysema. There were also a possible abdominal wall abscess and bowel ischemia as well as an enterocutaneous fistula from enterotomy. She underwent an exploratory laparotomy with extensive bowel resection, and removal of the VP shunt. The patient was started on broad spectrum antibiotics (vancomycin and ertapenem later switched to meropenem). An MRI was performed which shows a possible brain abscess (Figure 8.4, Panel A: restricted diffusion on lower image). After shunt revision she continued to be febrile, tachypnic, tachycardic, and diaphoretic. She was transferred in a state of unconsciousness, pupils were fixed 4mm bilaterally and she had forced downward gaze. Muscle tone was normal tone throughout although she was hyperreflexic and had a positive Babinski sign. Her Head CT was unchanged and the EEG did not show any seizures. On exam she remained obtunded. Her level of consciousness fluctuated and she was intermittently febrile. On serial CSF studies her white blood cells increased to 85 (97% neutrophils), glucose dropped to 7, and protein rose to 200. Urine culture grew E Coli. On admission head CT showed persistent hydrocephalus and isodense fluid collection in the 3rd and lateral ventricles (Figure 8.4, Panel B). Her eyes were open but deviated to left and downward, with pupils minimally reactive bilaterally, and she did not following commands. She became tachypneic to painful stim and withdrew to pain on right arm, right leg, and left leg; the left arm was flaccid. CSF (Figure 8.4, Panel C) showed 1000 red blood cells, 445 white cells, 96% neutrophils, protein 243, glucose 7, lactate 11, CSF cultures were positive for multi-drug resistant E. Coli. She went to the OR for endoscopic third ventriculostomy, and trans-septal EVD placement and ventricular washout. Post operatively the Head CT showed reduced hydrocephalus (Figure 8.4, Panel D) and the CSF (Figure 8.4, Panel E) had 10,000 red cells, 6,437 white cells, glucose 15 (peripheral 125), protein352, lactate 12, gram stain positive for Gram negative rods, CSF cultures grew E coli. The patient was extubated and started following commands and eye movements returned to normal except for a mild sixth nerve palsy.

and new-onset seizures. As a number of CNS infections can be treated extremely successfully if management is started urgently, empiric treatment may need to be started prior to firmly establishing the diagnosis.[206] The management of these patients includes empiric broad-spectrum antibiotics and steroids, making the diagnosis to narrow down the empiric management, treatment of secondary effects of CNS infection such as seizures and brain edema, and management of medical complications.

EMPIRIC MANAGEMENT

Many different infections cause delirium or coma, and infection may exacerbate coma from other causes. Any patient presenting acutely and suspected of possibly harboring a CNS infection should be started on broad-spectrum antibiotics typically including a third-generation cephalosporin (i.e., ceftriaxone) and vancomycin with doses adequate for CNS penetration. In patients who are immune suppressed, it is necessary to add ampicillin for the possibility of *Listeria monocytogenes*. The goal for this broad

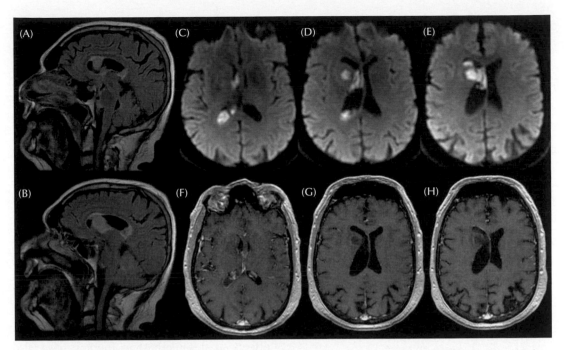

Figure 8.5 A 71-year-old active man with hypertension, hyperlipidemia, and a history of thromboembolism found to have a positive lupus anticoagulant. He presented to an outside hospital with two days of lethargy, fatigue, fever, meningism, and headaches. On examination he was febrile, mildly lethargic but fully oriented with nuchal rigidity. The impression of the physicians was likely meningitis and a lumbar puncture was performed revealing 1260 /µL white blood cells (81% polymorphonuclear cells), 9 /µL red blood cells, glucose 27 mg per dL, protien 531 mg/dL. Opening pressure, how much fluid was drained, and macroscopic appearance of the CSF were not documented. The patient became acutely very lethargic and an emergent Head CT showed an ill-defined 3cm hypodensity in the right frontal lobe with 4 mm right to left midline shift interpreted as a possible acute infarct. MRI of the brain demonstrated a 1.4 x 1.4 x 1.4 cm ring enhancing lesion in the R frontal lobe with intraventricular expansion. This was most consistent with an abscess that had ruptured into the ventricles as there was hyperintensity on T2 (Figure 8.5, Panel A-B), homogenous restricted diffusion on diffusion weighted imaging (Figure 8.5, Panel C-E), and ring-enhancement seen on T1 post gadolinium enhanced images (Figure 8.5, Panel F-H). Further history revealed that the patient had an ulcer on his great toe for several months that was infected and required antibiotics. Transthoracic echo showed a vegetation on the aortic valve. He was started on broad spectrum antibiotics and steadily improved neurologically without any residual deficits. Imaging studies should be considered prior to lumbar puncture to minimize the risk of abscess rupture which is most frequently associated with significant morbidity and mortality.

antibiotic regimen is to cover most bacterial CNS infections as these are potentially treatable and have a very high morbidity and mortality if not treated emergently (Figure 8.4). Treatment with acyclovir (10 mg/kg every 8 hours) should also be considered for all patients unless CNS infection with herpes simplex virus (HSV) can be excluded or deemed extremely unlikely to be the cause of the acute presentation. It is important to provide adequate fluids as the risk of renal injury from acyclovir increases in hypovolemic patients. Steroids should be given for any patients with suspected bacterial meningitis, particularly *Streptococcus pneumoniae* meningitis. Intravenous dexamethasone 10 mg is given emergently and ideally prior to or at the start of antibiotic therapy and continued with

repeat doses every 6 hours.[207] For patients with suspected fungal meningitis (prior history of the disease or systemic fungal infections) and rapidly progressing clinical deterioration, empiric Amphotericin B may be considered.

All of these management steps should be initiated as soon as the diagnosis is suspected as any delay in treatment initiation may worsen the outcome.[208,209] All patients should also undergo a lumbar puncture unless contraindicated, and urine and blood cultures should be sent. Head CT is recommended prior to lumbar puncture to determine safety of the procedure as, rarely, herniation or abscess rupture may occur.[210] CSF culture is still likely to grow out the organism until at least 6 hours after starting antibiotics even in the most sensitive organisms. Additionally, patients with suspected CNS infection must have intravenous access inserted and be started on intravenous fluids because febrile patients may have a fluid deficit. Considering brain biopsies earlier in the clinical course may be helpful as delayed biopsies often only show nonspecific reactive changes.[211] Increasingly, an unbiased approach of using a metagenomic next-generation deep sequencing approach that detects all nucleic acids in a specimen is gaining traction.[212] This approach will likely identify causative pathogens in a number of cases that are classified currently as infections of unclear etiology, but the clinical benefit for patients remains to be shown. All staff in contact with patients harboring suspected meningococcal infection need to be placed on exposure prophylaxis due to the highly contagious nature of the disease.

NARROWING DOWN THE EMPIRIC TREATMENT

In bacterial CNS infection, the CSF typically has a very high leukocytosis (100–1,000 or higher), low glucose (less than two-thirds serum glucose, but rarely normal), elevated protein (more than 50 mg/dL), and elevated CSF lactate, C-reactive protein or procalcitonin, while red blood cells may be absent (Figures 8.4 and 8.5). Organisms may be seen on Gram stain. Based on the CSF Gram stain, antibiotics may at times be narrowed, but typically culture growth data will allow changing the broad antibiotic approach to a targeted one that is tailored to the specific cultured organisms. Further information is gained from determining resistance and sensitivities to specific antibiotics, which allows choosing optimal antibiotics. Dexamethasone should to be started as soon as possible,[207] ideally prior to the first dose of antibiotics and continued for 4 days (10 mg given every 6 hours). ICP monitoring in these patients is controversial, but routine treatment for elevated ICP in the absence of monitoring is not justified and may even be harmful.[213]

Viral CNS infection. Although a number of viral pathogens need to be considered as viral causes of CNS infection, HSV encephalitis is by far the most common spontaneous viral encephalitis, and, if not treated promptly, it is often fatal or associated with severe morbidity. Alteration of consciousness is frequent as is fever, changes in personality, focal cortical abnormalities such as aphasia or neglect, and seizures. Diagnosis is based on clinical pretest probability, elevated CSF white blood cell count (10–2,000 cells/mm^3) with lymphocytic predominance, elevated red cells (10s to 1000s/mm^3) possibly with xanthochromia, mild to moderately elevated CSF protein, and normal to slightly reduced CSF glucose. HSV polymerase chain reaction in the CSF is highly sensitive and specific for HSV but may be falsely negative, particularly early in the disease. MRI may show characteristic temporal lobe hyperintensities on T2, and EEG may demonstrate slowing as well as lateralized periodic discharges. In controversial cases, brain biopsy may be required. Acyclovir is the drug of choice (10 mg/kg given intravenously every 8 hours for 21 days).[214] Impaired consciousness on presentation is associated with worse outcome.

Other CNS infections. These are generally more difficult to diagnose, but beneficial effects of dexamethasone therapy have also been shown for tuberculous meningitis.[215]

NEUROLOGIC COMPLICATIONS

Seizures. Acute brain injury seizures appear to be associated with inflammation[216] and therefore are particularly frequent in patients with CNS infections. Seizure prophylaxis is not recommended, and treatment is similar to other acute brain injury seizures.

Brain edema. Invasive ICP monitoring is controversial but elevated ICP is likely underdiagnosed in this patient population. Confirmed or suspected ICP elevations can be treated with mannitol or hypertonic saline. Induced hypothermia to treat brain swelling or as a neuroprotectant is contraindicated for patients with bacterial meningitis as this was shown in a randomized controlled trial to cause more harm than benefit.[217] Infarcts may occur with CNS infections, particularly in patients with syphilis, varicella zoster virus infection, and other types of meningitis.

Acute Disseminated Encephalomyelitis

Acute disseminated encephalomyelitis (ADEM) is characterized by a widespread inflammatory attack of the brain and spinal cord often following a viral infection or immunization. Impaired consciousness possibly with coma is a common feature in ADEM, and MRI often shows widespread white matter demyelination. The mainstay of treatment is suppression of the inflammatory reaction (e.g., with high-dose corticosteroids; i.e., intravenous methylprednisolone 1 g/d for 5 days,[218] followed by oral corticosteroids, which may need to be continued at lower levels for months). Additional treatment with plasmapheresis or intravenous immunoglobulin may also be considered early on.[219]

Hypoxic Brain Injury/Cardiac Arrest

Cardiac arrest is a common condition leading to acute onset of impaired consciousness and requires a focused management approach. In Chapter 7, the steps necessary to provide cardiopulmonary resuscitation were outlined in detail. Once spontaneous circulation has been restored, management can be categorized into steps necessary to minimize ongoing brain injury in the aftermath of the no-flow situation (neuroprotection), steps to prevent recurrence of cardiac arrest, and management of neurological and medical complications.

Management of the underlying cause. A 12-lead EKG should be performed immediately after resuscitation. Arterial and central lines, naso- or orogastric tubes, and urinary catheters should be placed if not present already. Hemodynamic stability needs to be maintained using intravenous fluids and vasopressors (norepinephrine is frequently used, but choice of vasopressors depends on the clinical presentation). The goal for systolic blood pressure is controversial, but it is typically kept greater than 90 mm Hg (mean arterial blood pressure greater than 60 mm Hg). Higher perfusion may be beneficial particularly in patients with elevated ICP or stenosis of intracranial vessels, but it may in the reperfusion situation also cause more harm than benefit. Rarely, mechanical assist devices such as intra-aortic balloon counterpulsation, cardiopulmonary bypass, ventricular assist devices, or extracorporeal membrane oxygenation may be required for appropriate candidates. Oxygen saturation of no higher than 94–98% should be targeted as hyperoxia may be harmful,[220–223] and an elevated burden of cumulative exposure to oxygen

tension has been associated with a higher likelihood of poor functional outcomes.[224]

Patients should undergo noncontrast head CT scanning if at all possible as several acute neurological emergencies, such as ischemic and hemorrhagic strokes and, most importantly, SAH, may present with cardiac arrest. Emergent cardiac catheterization is recommended for survivors of cardiac arrest with ST elevation myocardial infarction.[225]

Neuroprotection. The most important determinant of functional outcome for cardiac arrest patients is the degree of brain injury sustained as a consequence of the transient lack of cerebral blood flow. Particularly vulnerable areas include the CA1 region of the hippocampus, globus pallidus, and neocortex, all of which are involved in circuitry crucial to promote consciousness. Targeted temperature management is currently the primary measure applied with the goal of neuroprotection and should be applied following a strict institutional protocol. Although therapeutic hypothermia for comatose survivors of cardiac arrest, including those with initial rhythms of asystole or pulseless electrical activity,[226] was initially found to be beneficial,[226–228] attempts to identify the ideal temperature range have more recently found similar functional, quality of life, and cognitive outcomes[229,230] for patients treated with a temperature goal of 33°C when compared to 36°C. It is important and often overlooked that this trial did not compare cooling to no cooling as both treatment arms required active temperature modulation to maintain the target temperature. These data may suggest that the primary effect is achieved by preventing fever, which is frequently encountered after cardiac arrest and which was prevented in either treatment arm of the study. Few patients have absolute contraindications for hypothermia, but most providers would currently not offer it for arrest due to refractory bleeding at a noncompressible site and severe and recurrent symptomatic bradycardia. Relative contraindications relate to baseline neurologic function, multiorgan system failure, infections (sepsis, meningitis), trauma, and pregnancy. Some physicians will still treat these patients with a temperature control goal of 36°C. The benefits of hypothermia for in-hospital cardiac arrests is even more controversial.[231]

Temperature modulation can be achieved in a number of ways including physical surface cooling (e.g., cold baths, ice packs, pads that stick to the skin, helmets), intravenous infusion of chilled fluids, and endovascular temperature control devices (e.g., balloons with circulating ice cold fluid). Modern surface or intravascular temperature control devices have a built-in temperature feedback loop that provides the machine with real-time information about the patient's current core temperature. Temperature control should be achieved as soon as possible, and initial infusion of cooled fluids, administration of paralytics, and ice packs may be helpful; however, initiation of hypothermia in the out-of-hospital setting is much more difficult and controversial.[230,232] Typically, hypothermia is maintained for 24 hours and then controlled rewarming is achieved over the next 24 hours (0.1–0.5°C/hr). Currently there is no evidence to support hypothermia for longer than 24 hours.[233] Rewarming is complicated by rebound fever in about 40% of patients, which typically initially is treated with Tylenol but may require further workup and additional interventions.[234]

Side effects of hypothermia include shivering, pneumonia, sepsis, bleeding, electrolyte abnormalities, cardiac arrhythmias, and glucose dysregulation. The body's natural defense to induced hypothermia is high-frequency muscle contractions (i.e., shivering). In healthy individuals, this sets in at around 35.5°C and stops below 34°C, while acutely injured patients do not follow this rule and shivering is very prominent in most patients who undergo temperature modulation. Absence of any shivering response to induced hypothermia is an ominous prognostic sign.[235] Shivering needs to be controlled as the increase in metabolic demand is likely highly detrimental.[234] A staged approach utilizes skin counter-warming (which targets highly sensitive temperature sensors particularly in the hands and feet), acetaminophen (650 mg given every 4 hours by mouth), buspirone (30 mg given every 8 hours by mouth), sedation (propofol infusions are most widely used, benzodiazepines may serve as alternatives), and analgesia (preferred are opiate infusions such as fentanyl).[236] Dexmedetomidine infusions may be a very potent additional agent to fight shivering and are used instead or in addition to other sedatives. Magnesium sulphate may be given to achieve serum magnesium levels of 3–4 mg/Eq (0.5–0.1 g/hr). Meperidine (25 mg given every 6 hours intravenously for shivering) can

be successful, but the associated lowering of the seizure threshold limits its use. Rarely is it necessary to apply full neuromuscular blockade, such as with non-depolarizing neuromuscular blocking agents (such as vecuronium 0.1 mg/kg given intravenously each hour (titrate to a goal of 0 out of 4 on the train-of-four monitoring).

Neurological complications. Seizures and myoclonus are frequently encountered, alone or together, following cardiac arrest. Seizures are seen in 10–30% of comatose cardiac arrest patients, and most of these will have SE. These are encountered at any point after cardiac arrest, particularly during rewarming.[237–241] Very early seizures are associated with worse outcome. Although older guidelines warned that recovery was rare in patients with myoclonus post-arrest, more modern studies suggest that the prognosis may be less bleak in the era of temperature modulation and aggressive critical care.[239] Continuous EEG monitoring is crucial as seizures may be intermittent and nonconvulsive.[242] Seizures are aggressively managed as for other acute neurological injuries (see Chapter 7). Subcortical myoclonus may be seen without any associated EEG seizure activity. As both seizures and myoclonus may respond to levetiracetam, valproic acid, and benzodiazepines (such as clonazepam), many prefer these agents in the cardiac arrest patient.

ICP. Brain swelling may occur in up to a third of patients after cardiac arrest[243] and is managed similarly to other patients with elevated ICP (see Chapter 7), except that brain swelling and ICP elevation are poor prognostic signs in cardiac arrest patients as they are evidence of extensive injury to cortical neurons, and so craniectomy is generally not indicated. Cardiac arrest patients undergoing induced hypothermia need to be carefully monitored during rewarming for possible herniation.

Medical complications. Low tidal volume lung-protective ventilation strategies (tidal volumes of 6 mL/kg of ideal body weight) are initiated for cardiac arrest patients with acute respiratory distress syndrome (ARDS). Cardiac arrest and hypothermia have major effects on hemodynamics, liver and renal function, electrolytes, and the immune system. Electrolytes (particularly potassium, magnesium, and phosphate) should be monitored and replaced judiciously as cold diuresis, intracellular displacement during hypothermia (which reverses during rewarming), and administered resuscitative fluids have to be accounted for. Avoid administration of hypotonic intravenous fluids. Normoglycemia should be maintained with insulin infusions (serum glucose goal 140–180 mg/dL). Patients undergoing hypothermia are at higher risk of infections and should be screened aggressively for pneumonia and urinary tract or catheter-associated infections. Prophylactic antibiotics are not recommended at this time. DVT prophylaxis with pneumatic compression devices and subcutaneous heparin or enoxaparin is recommended.

Metabolic Coma

The many causes of metabolic coma are covered in Chapter 5. These generally fall into four categories: lack of substrate for metabolism (hypoxia [Figure 8.6], hypoglycemia), excess substances (hypercarbia, hyperglycemia), disturbance of internal milieu (high or low sodium, calcium, or magnesium; low levels of thyroid or corticosteroid hormones), or toxic substances that normally are not present (seen in liver or renal failure; abnormal cells in the CSF, including red cells, white cells, or microorganisms; or exogenous toxins ranging from prescription to street drugs and including toxins such as methanol or propylene glycol). The following discussion will cover general aspects of metabolic coma followed by a more focused presentation on fulminant hepatic failure and electrolyte imbalances. Metabolic coma is usually characterized by a history of confusion and disorientation having preceded the onset of stupor or coma, usually in the absence of any motor signs. When motor signs

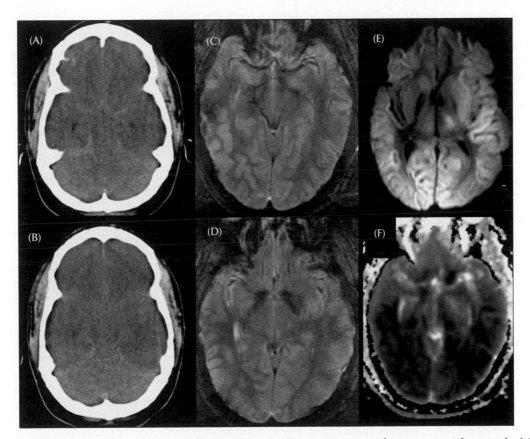

Figure 8.6 A 35-year-old man with history of asthma that suffered a respiratory arrest due to a severe asthma attack while bathing his girlfriend's dog. The Head CT (Figure 8.6, panels A and B) was originally interpreted as consistent with subarachnoid hemorrhage but as are, confirmed by MRI (panels C and D show gradient echo sequences without evidence of subarachnoid blood, panels E and F show widespread anoxic injury on diffusion weighted images and apparent diffusion coefficient images, respectively), most consistent with pseudo subarachnoid hemorrhage. This phenomenon is seen in patients with diffuse hypoxic brain injury often as a result of respiratory arrest.

(decorticate or decerebrate rigidity, usually in hepatic or hypoglycemic coma) appear, they are usually symmetric. If the patient is stuporous rather than comatose, asterixis, myoclonus, and tremor are common, and, in comatose patients, the presence of repetitive seizures, either focal or generalized, provide presumptive evidence of metabolic dysfunction. Unlike in structural seizures, a major part of the treatment of metabolic seizures includes the reversal of the metabolic abnormality.

Some patients with metabolic coma either hyperventilate (hepatic or septic coma) or hypoventilate (which may either cause the coma or be due to exogenous sedative drugs), but it is rare to see the abnormal respiratory patterns that characterize infratentorial mass or destructive lesions (see Chapters 2 and 3). There are two common errors in the diagnosis of metabolic coma. The first is in differentiating patients with the diencephalic stage of supratentorial masses from those with metabolic coma. In the absence of focal motor signs, one may initially suspect metabolic coma even in patients who have a supratentorial mass lesion with early central herniation. The second error occurs in those occasional patients with metabolic coma (e.g., hepatic coma or hypoglycemia) who have strikingly asymmetric motor signs with hyperventilation and deep coma. In this instance, the preservation of intact and symmetric pupillary and oculovestibular responses provides strong presumptive evidence for metabolic rather than structural disease.

It is stupor and coma caused by metabolic brain disease that most challenges the internist, neurologist, or general physician likely to be reading this monograph. If patients suffer from major damage caused by supra- or infratentorial mass lesions or destructive lesions, specific treatment often involves a surgical or intravascular procedure. If psychogenic unresponsiveness is the problem, the ultimate management of the patient rests with a psychiatrist. In metabolic brain disease, however, the task of preserving the brain from permanent damage rests with the physician of first contact. The physician should first evaluate the vital signs, provide adequate ventilation and arterial pressure, check a fingerstick glucose level, and then draw blood for metabolic studies. Metabolic studies that should be secured from the first blood drawing are

Table 8.3 Emergency Laboratory Evaluation of Metabolic Coma

1. Stat tests
   A. Venous blood
      1. Glucose
      2. Electrolytes
      3. Urea or creatinine
      4. Osmolality
      5. Complete blood count
      6. Coagulation studies
   B. Arterial blood
      1. Check color
      2. pH
      3. PO_2
      4. PCO_2
      5. Carboxyhemoglobin (if available, especially if blood is bright red)
   C. Cerebrospinal fluid
      1. Cells
      2. Gram stain
      3. Glucose
   D. Electrocardiogram
2. Additional tests[a]
   A. Venous blood
      1. Liver function tests
      2. Thyroid and adrenal function
      3. Blood cultures
      4. Viral titers
   B. Urine
      1. Culture
   C. Cerebrospinal fluid
      1. Protein
      2. Culture
      3. Viral and fungal antibodies, polymerase chain reaction

[a]These tests are "additional," because in most hospitals it will take hours to days to get the results. The blood and cerebrospinal fluid for these tests, however, is drawn at the same time as the stat tests.

indicated in Table 8.3. Because drug ingestion is a common cause of coma, procure blood and urine for toxicologic study on all patients (see Table 8.4). Those metabolic encephalopathies that are most likely to produce either irreversible brain damage or a quick demise but are potentially treatable include drug overdose, hypoglycemia, metabolic or respiratory acidosis (from several causes), hyperosmolar states, hypoxia, bacterial meningitis or sepsis, and severe electrolyte imbalance.

It is important to secure an arterial sample for blood gas analysis, although emergency management may have to begin even before laboratory results are returned. Both acidosis and alkalosis can cause cardiac arrhythmias,

Table 8.4 **Stat Toxicology Assays Required to Support an Emergency Department**

Quantitative serum toxicology assays	Qualitative urine toxicology assays
Acetaminophen (paracetamol)	Cocaine
Lithium	Opiates
Salicylate	Barbiturates
Co-oximetry for oxygen saturation, carboxyhemoglobin, and methemoglobin	Amphetamines
	Propoxyphene
Theophylline	Phencyclidine (PCP)
Valproic acid	Tricyclic antidepressants (TCAs)
Digoxin	
Phenobarbital (if urine barbiturates are positive)	
Iron	
Transferrin (or unsaturated iron-binding capacity [UIBC] assay if transferrin is not available)	
Ethyl alcohol	
Methyl alcohol	
Ethylene glycol	

From Wu et al.,[244] with permission.

but acute metabolic acidosis is more likely to be lethal; however, pH is not an independent predictor of mortality in critically ill patients with metabolic acidosis.[245] Whether sodium bicarbonate should be given to treat severe acidosis is controversial.[246–248] The agent is not indicated in the treatment of diabetic acidosis and may not be helpful in treating acidosis from other causes (severe acidosis may be associated with hemodynamic collapse and intravenous sodium bicarbonate may be required as part of the resuscitation). Instead, urgent treatment of the underlying cause of the acidosis is probably the best approach. Relieve hypoxia immediately by ensuring an adequate airway and delivering sufficient oxygen to keep the blood fully oxygenated. Even in the presence of a normal PaO_2, blood oxygen content may be insufficient to supply the brain's needs for several reasons: (1) the hemoglobin may be abnormal (carboxyhemoglobinemia, methemoglobinemia, or sulfhemoglobinemia). Methemoglobin or sulfhemoglobin are diagnosed by the typical chocolate appearance of oxygenated blood, and cyanide poisoning by blue color of arterial blood; patients are treated with methylene blue (1–2 mg/kg intravenous over 5 minutes).[249,250] Topical anesthetic agents such as benzocaine used in endoscopy can cause acute methemoglobinemia.[251] (2) Carbon monoxide binds hemoglobin with 200 times the affinity of oxygen and thus displaces oxygen and yields carboxyhemoglobin. The PaO_2 is

normal and the patient's color is pink or "cherry red," but he or she is hypoxic because insufficient hemoglobin is available to deliver oxygen to the tissue. Such patients should be given 100% oxygen and hyperventilated to increase blood oxygenation. Hyperbaric oxygenation may improve the situation, and if a hyperbaric chamber is available, it should probably be utilized for patients with life-threatening exposure.[252] (3) Severe anemia itself generally does not cause coma but lowers the oxygen-carrying capacity of the blood even when the PaO_2 is normal and thus decreases the oxygen supply to the brain. In patients with other forms of hypoxia, anemia may exacerbate the symptoms. Severe anemia (hematocrit less than 25) in a comatose patient should be treated with transfusion of whole blood or packed red cells. (4) Tissues can be hypoxic even when the PaO_2 and O_2 content is normal if they cannot metabolize the oxygen (e.g., cyanide poisoning). Intravenous hydroxocobalamin administered as a one-time dose of 4–5 g is a safe and effective method of treating poisoning.[253] In any comatose or stuporous patient who is febrile, whether or not nuchal rigidity and/or other signs of meningeal irritation (e.g., positive Kernig or Brudzinski signs or jolt accentuation) are present, consider acute bacterial meningitis (see earlier discussion).

Drug overdose is a common cause of coma in patients brought to an emergency room. Many emergency departments can provide a rapid assessment of toxic drugs (Table 7.6).[244] Most of these drugs are not rapidly lethal but, because they are respiratory depressants, they risk producing respiratory arrest or circulatory depression at any time. Therefore, no stuporous or comatose patient suspected of having ingested sedative drugs should ever be left alone. This is particularly true in the minutes immediately following the initial examination; the stimulation delivered by the examining physician may arouse the patient to a state in which he or she appears relatively alert or his or her respiratory function appears normal, only to lapse into coma with depressed breathing when external stimulation ceases. The management of specific drug poisonings is beyond the scope of this chapter,[250] but certain general principles apply to all patients suspected of having ingested sedative drugs. The type of medication influences the treatment and its duration. Accordingly, search the patient and ask relatives or the police to search the patient's living quarters for potentially toxic agents or empty medication vials that might have contained sedative drugs. Both respiratory and cardiovascular failure may occur with massive sedative drug overdose. Anticipation and early treatment of these complications often smooth the clinical course. Insert an endotracheal tube in any stuporous or comatose patient suspected of drug overdose and be certain that an apparatus for respiratory support is available in case of acute respiratory failure. The placement of a central venous line allows one to maintain an adequate blood volume without overloading the patient. Give generous amounts of fluid to maintain blood volume and blood pressure, but avoid overhydrating oliguric patients. Place a pulse oximeter on the finger, but also measure arterial blood gases; a difference between the two (oxygen saturation gap) may indicate poisoning. Carbon monoxide, methemoglobin, cyanide, and hydrogen sulfide cause an increased oxygen saturation gap.

Once the vital signs have been stabilized, thought should be given to attempting to remove, neutralize, or reverse the effects of the drug. This is rarely necessary for sedative or hypnotic drugs, the most common cause of coma due to drug overdose, because once the patient is stabilized, with time, the drug will be eliminated and the patient will wake up. Attempts to remove sedatives from the gastrointestinal tract and thus prevent absorption, such as inducing vomiting with syrup of ipecac[254] or gastric lavage,[255] run the risk of causing aspiration pneumonia, particularly in a patient who is obtunded but has not yet been intubated, and should be avoided.

However, in case of ingestion of a toxin that affects other systems, such as the heart or liver, it may be necessary to attempt to remove the poison. Position papers from the American Academy of Clinical Toxicology and the European Association of Poison Centers and Clinical Toxicologists indicate a lack of evidence that inducing vomiting is helpful[256–258]; it is contraindicated in patients with a decreased level or impending loss of consciousness.[259] They concluded that gastric lavage should not be employed routinely, but could be considered in patients who have ingested a potentially life-threatening amount of a poison within an hour of the time they are to be treated.[260] However, aspiration is a common complication, and so patients with impaired consciousness should be intubated first. Cathartics have no role in the management of the poisoned patient.[256] A single dose of activated charcoal (50 g) can be administered to a patient with an intact or protected airway, but it will not efficiently adsorb acid, alkali, ethanol, ethylene glycol, iron, lithium, or methanol. Multiple doses of charcoal administered at an initial dose of 50-100 g, and then at a rate of not less than 12.5 g/hour via nasogastric tube, may be indicated when patients have ingested a life-threatening amount of carbamazepine, dapsone, phenobarbital, quinine, or theophylline. In addition to eliminating drugs from the small bowel, the agents may interrupt the enteroenteric and, in some cases, the enterohepatic circulation of drugs.[261] Whole-bowel irrigation using polyethylene glycol electrolyte solutions may decrease the bioavailability of ingested drugs, particularly enteric-coated or sustained-release drugs.[257]

Intravenous sodium bicarbonate in amounts sufficient to produce a urine pH of 7.5 promotes the elimination of salicylate, phenobarbital, and chlorpropamide.[262] For very severe poisoning with barbiturates, glutethimide, salicylates, or alcohol, hemodialysis or hemoperfusion may be necessary.[261,262] Although acetaminophen does not by itself cause impaired consciousness, it may be included in opioid combinations (e.g., acetaminophen with codeine or oxycodone) and is often included in polydrug overdoses. Doses of greater than 5 g in adults may cause acute hepatic injury (see later discussion) and thereby cause impaired consciousness, especially if combined with other hepatotoxins such as ethanol; when acetaminophen overdose is suspected, the patient should be treated with N-acetylcysteine as well.[263]

ELECTROLYTE IMBALANCE AND NUTRITION

Hyponatremia. Electrolyte abnormalities are frequent and may be found on admission in the patient with impaired consciousness or develop during the hospital stay. The most commonly encountered electrolyte abnormality is hyponatremia, which must be managed carefully as rapid correction in chronic hyponatremia may lead to central pontine or extrapontine myelinolysis.[264] Based on history, clinical exam, and laboratory studies, it should be determined if the electrolyte abnormality developed acutely or has been present chronically. Hyponatremia may develop during the hospital stay, particularly in patients with acute brain injury or meningitis.[265] The most prominent syndromes that need to be differentiated are cerebral salt wasting (CSW) and syndrome of inadequate secretion of antidiuretic hormone (SIADH). Both may develop in a number of acute brain injuries, most characteristically in patients with SAH but also with infectious etiologies such as tuberculosis. Classically, patients with CSW are hypovolemic while those with SIADH are not. Serum sodium is decreased and urine sodium increased in either disorder. Treatment of CSW focusses on replacement with isotonic fluids while patients with SIADH are classically treated with water restriction.

Chronic hyponatremia of other causes should be slowly corrected using hypernatremic fluids, correcting the serum sodium at no more than 0.5 mEq/L/hr. Acute derangements may be more rapidly corrected, but if unsure, slow correction should be chosen. Patients with acute brain injury and hyponatremia may have a combination of the two syndromes and, given frequent fluid replacements and diuretic administration, the syndromes may be difficult to tease apart. Fluid restriction in the acute state may be dangerous (e.g., as in patients with vasospasm following SAH who may develop DCI). In practice, most patients with

acute presentation of hyponatremia are treated with isotonic fluid replacement. Particularly in the subacute or chronic state administration of a selective vasopressin V_2 receptor antagonist given orally or intravenously may be considered for the hyponatremic patient.[266]

Hypernatremia may develop in the setting of diabetes insipidus, an inappropriate excretion of free water with massively increased output of diluted urine (in excess of 300 mL/hr, urinary specific gravity is 1,000–1,005, and urinary osmolality 50–150 mOsm/L). The underlying cause is either central, in which there is impaired secretion of arginine vasopressin due to TBI, brain surgery, or brain tumors; or nephrogenic, due to failure of the kidney to respond to arginine vasopressin (which is often inherited). When impaired consciousness is seen in patients with central diabetes insipidus, treatment with vasopressin is usually recommended.

Other electrolyte abnormalities. Hypercalcemia can present as impaired consciousness and may be the first sign of a tumor with osteoblastic metastases. If serum albumin is also low, the total calcium level may appear to be deceptively normal, but ionized serum calcium may be elevated. Hypercalcemia is usually treated with diuresis and fluid replacement. It is also important to monitor phosphate and magnesium levels in such patients. Hypomagnesemia may cause impaired consciousness and even coma paired with tremors, myoclonic jerks, and seizures. Magnesium is given intravenously to a goal of greater than 2 mEq/L. Severe potassium imbalance usually affects the heart more than the brain. Accordingly, an EKG often suggests the diagnosis before serum electrolytes are returned from the laboratory. It usually is advisable to adjust both electrolyte and acid–base imbalances slowly, since too rapid correction often leads to overshoot or intracellular-extracellular imbalances and worsens the clinical situation.[267]

Refeeding syndrome needs to be carefully screened for in malnourished patients. Starvation may be seen in the chronically or acutely critically ill patient and in those with severe anorexia. Following a period of starvation, feeding may cause cells to take up glucose, potassium, phosphate, and magnesium leading to severe hypoglycemia, hypophosphatemia, hypokalemia, and hypomagnesemia. This may cause alteration of consciousness and be life-threatening. Vigilance for detection and prevention of the syndrome is key. Caloric restriction together with careful electrolyte replacement is recommended to guide feeding in critically ill patients who develop refeeding syndrome.[268]

FULMINANT AND ACUTE HEPATIC FAILURE

Liver failure is frequently associated with impaired consciousness, particularly when it develops rapidly. This hepatic encephalopathy is particularly prominent when rapid deterioration of liver function occurs in patients without preexisting liver disease. Patients with liver failure often have jaundice, evidence of coagulation abnormality (INR 1.5 or higher), and, if it is acute, may have elevated liver function enzymes. However, in patients with slowly progressive liver failure, these accompanying signs may be minimal, but the patient may still have hepatic encephalopathy,[269] which often fluctuates over time, often depending on whether the patient has recently ingested a protein load. Diagnosing the cause of the encephalopathy can be challenging in such patients in the outpatient clinic or on the general medical ward (see Chapter 5).

Chronic liver failure patients may develop slowly progressive cognitive deficits and may acutely decompensate due to infections, gastrointestinal bleeding, or ingestion of hepatotoxic medications. Subtle alterations of consciousness are seen in more than 80% and hepatic encephalopathy in a third or every other patient with chronic liver failure. Identifying and addressing the underlying cause for liver failure and precipitating factors are the primary focus of the workup. Decreasing serum levels of ammonia by reducing production, increasing metabolism, and increasing excretion are key concepts. Lactulose may be given to achieve diarrhea; rifaximin (550 mg by mouth twice daily for 5–10 days), L-ornithine-L-aspartate, and specific hepatic diets are part of the management in the chronic state. Chronic hyponatremia should be replaced slowly (no more than 8–12 meq/L/d) to avoid central pontine myelinolysis.

On the other hand, in the emergency setting, acute liver failure is more often seen. Liver failure is categorized into fulminant if developing within 8 weeks and hyperacute if developing within 1 week. Acute fulminant liver failure is associated with high morbidity and mortality, and much of the following discussion is focused on this spectrum of the disease.

Acute liver failure. Management of the patient with acute liver failure depends on the underlying etiology, time course of development, and presence of neurologic and medical complications. The degree of impaired consciousness is a major determinant of outcome in these patients and affects transplant status. The differential diagnosis of impaired consciousness in the patient with liver failure is broad. Apart from the interlinked complications of hyperammonemia, brain swelling, and elevated ICP, other frequently encountered phenomena that depress consciousness, such as electrolyte imbalance (i.e., hyponatremia), intracranial hemorrhage due to coagulopathy, uremia from renal failure, hypotension, infections possibly with septic encephalopathy, and hypoglycemia, need to be considered.

Identification and management of the precipitating cause. The most frequent cause of fulminant and acute liver failure is acetaminophen intoxication mostly in suicidal intention; other causes include accidental or nonaccidental non-acetaminophen intoxication, ingestion of hepatotoxic mushrooms, side effects of medications and recreational drugs, hepatitis B and A, autoimmune causes, Wilson's disease, and pregnancy; when the cause is unknown, the liver failure is said to be cryptogenic. In order to identify the precipitating cause, a careful history of present illness, past medical history including currently ingested medications and unusual foods, family and social history, and careful examination are key. Diagnostic workup should be broad unless the precipitating cause is obvious and may include blood tests (liver function tests, GGT, amylase, lipase, full coagulation profiles, basic chemistries including magnesium and phosphate, complete blood count, acetaminophen level, viral hepatitis serologies and viral loads [antibodies and antigen tests for hepatitis A, B, C, and E, varicella zoster, herpes simplex, and HIV testing], autoimmune screen [ANA, liver kidney microsome-1 antibody, rheumatoid factor, anti-smooth muscle antibody, antimitochondrial antibody], ceruloplasmin level, ferritin, iron, total iron binding capacity), ammonia levels on ice, urinalysis for toxicology, and a pregnancy test. Doppler ultrasound may also be useful in detecting cryptogenic cirrhosis, liver metastases, or bile duct disease as a cause of liver failure.

Management of liver failure in the setting of acetaminophen toxicity includes administration of activated charcoal 1 g/kg given orally if diagnosed within 4 hours of ingestion. N-acetylcysteine should be initiated immediately after activated charcoal is given (140 mg/kg dose orally diluted to 5% solution, followed by 70 mg/kg q4h × 17 doses; or intravenous loading dose of 150 mg/kg in 5% dextrose over 15 minutes, followed by 50 mg/kg given over 4 hours and then 100 mg/kg administered over 16 hours). N-acetylcysteine may still be considered even more than 48 hours after suspected acetaminophen ingestion. When the dose of acetaminophen ingested is not known, standard acetaminophen toxicity nomograms may be helpful in determining whether blood levels at a certain time after ingestion predict hepatotoxicity, but these are not accurate in cases of multiple acetaminophen doses or metabolic abnormalities (e.g., starvation/fasting, alcoholism). Duration of N-acetylcysteine administration is controversial, but some argue that dosing past 72 hours may be beneficial.[270]

Etiology-specific treatment of patients with acute or fulminant liver failure includes nucleoside and nucleotide analogs (e.g., lamivudine) for hepatitis B, intravenous acyclovir for VZV or HSV, and prednisone (40–60 mg/d) for early stages of liver failure (avoid in patients with multiorgan failure and may depend on the underlying etiology); penicillin G may be considered for mushroom poisoning (*Amanita phalloides*). Supportive care only is the treatment of choice for cases of hepatic failure in the setting of hepatitis A and E. It is useful to contact the Poison Control Centers for any suspected cases of intoxication. Immediate evaluation for transplantation is required for cases of Wilson's disease. It may be necessary to consult ob-gyn for consideration of early delivery for patients with acute fatty liver of pregnancy/hemolysis, elevated liver enzymes and low platelets (HELLP) syndrome.

Management of neurological complications. The development and management of hepatic encephalopathy is the most important neurological complication of the liver failure patient and needs to be discussed together with the related phenomena of global cerebral edema and elevation of ICP.

Hepatic encephalopathy. The exact mechanisms underlying hepatic encephalopathy are not completely understood, but a number of studies have implicated excessive ammonia levels.[271] Ammonia is a byproduct of nitrogenous and glutamine metabolism in enterocytes and colonic bacteria. Normally, ammonia is converted to glutamine in the liver, but capacity for this reaction may be limited in liver failure. Neurotoxic effects of ammonia and excessive gamma-aminobutyric acid (GABA) ergic inhibition causing astrocyte swelling are thought to be the primary causes of hepatic encephalopathy.[272] Acute declines in serum osmolality are associated with brain swelling and neurologic deterioration in severe hepatic encephalopathy.[273] Brain swelling may further be exacerbated by cerebral vasodilation triggered by NMDA receptor-mediated nitric oxide release, breakdown of cerebral autoregulation, activation of astrocytic aquaporin-4 water channel proteins, and inflammation.

The West Haven Criteria[274] are the most widely used scheme to categorize hepatic encephalopathy. It assigns four levels based on the impairment of different components of arousal and awareness. Patients in Grade 1 show euphoria or anxiety, with decreased attention and ability to perform simple calculations. Grade 2 patients have decreased arousal and apathy, when spoken to have minimal disorientation, and have subtle personality changes. With increasing difficulty to arouse, confusion, and disorientation, patients are labeled as Grade 3. All comatose patients are categorized as Grade 4. A head CT should be obtained even for West Haven Grade 1 patients and for those with any focal neurologic findings to eliminate confounding causes for impaired awareness and arousal, such as intraparenchymal, subarachnoid, or subdural hemorrhages, as these patients often have coagulopathy and tend to fall, causing head trauma. Sedative medications should be avoided as transitions to higher grades are crucial to guide management and prognosis, and many sedatives are metabolized by the liver, thus causing excessive and prolonged sedation.

ICP and cerebral edema. Patients should be monitored for signs of cerebral edema, which is the leading cause of death for patients with acute liver failure.[275] All patients with acute liver failure should undergo very close monitoring with hourly neurological examinations. ICP elevations may be frequent and severe, and detection of ICP rises is challenging in the absence of ICP monitoring.[276] Head CT may appear unremarkable even with elevated ICP, particularly in patients who had premorbid brain atrophy (e.g., with age or alcoholism). The decision to place an invasive ICP monitor is complicated by the fact that patients with liver failure, particularly those with impaired consciousness, frequently have severe coagulopathy, thus raising the risks of ICP monitor placement.

All basic measures to decrease ICP (see Chapter 7) such as head elevation and treatment of pain and agitation, shivering, and fever should be instituted but prophylactic administration of ICP-lowering medications is not recommended. Prescribing oral or rectal lactulose in an effort to lower ammonia levels is controversial, but if given should be titrated to achieve diarrhea. If used, it is important to monitor for megacolon and bowel ischemia, which are feared complications of lactulose. Due to the risk of renal failure, nephrotoxic drugs such as neomycin, which may decrease ammonia production, should be avoided. Some experts recommend using osmotic agents to target a serum sodium level between 150 and 155 mEqu/L for West Haven Grade 3 to 4 patients. Boluses of hypertonic saline or mannitol are given for documented ICP elevation, clinical worsening, or imaging evidence of herniation. Serum sodium goals can also be achieved by adjusting the dialysate in those on renal replacement therapy. Continuous veno-venous hemofiltration may reduce brain edema, particularly in patients with renal failure. Patients with refractory ICP elevation may be managed with hypothermia, barbiturates, and mild hyperventilation (pCO_2 goal 28–30 mm Hg). Corticosteroids should not be used to manage elevated ICP.

Noninvasive methods to measure ICP are not matured at this point but would be particularly helpful in the coagulopathic acute liver failure patient with cerebral edema. A number of potentially interesting surrogate measures include quantifying pupillary reactivity (i.e., reaction and latency time),[277] optic nerve sheath diameter assessments using ultrasound (i.e., diameters greater than 5 mm correlate to ICPs greater than 20 mm Hg),[278] and transcranial Doppler (i.e., suggestive of high ICP are low systolic blood flow velocities in the MCA, pulsatility index greater 1.6, loss of vessel recoil or sharpening of the peak systolic wave, and loss of vasoreactivity).[279] None of these measures allows exact determination of ICP values and are better used as trend measures over time in a patient with a known baseline measure. If chosen, it is advised to obtain a baseline measure prior to the patient developing any encephalopathy symptoms.

Guidelines recommend placement of invasive ICP monitors for Grade 3 and 4 patients who are candidates for liver transplantation.[269] However, in an observational, prospective study, patients with ICP monitoring were more likely to receive ICP-lowering agents and undergo liver transplantation, and had hemorrhagic complications in 7% of cases, but 3-week mortality did not differ from those without ICP monitoring.[280] At this time, no definitive recommendations for or against placement of an invasive ICP monitor can be made. Reversal of coagulopathy is necessary prior to surgical procedures (recommendations on the management of coagulopathy in these patients are given later). Blood pressure goals should take ICP into account if available and then target CPP of 60 mm Hg or higher.

Seizures occur in approximately a quarter to a third of patients and are predominantly nonconvulsive[281,282] necessitating EEG monitoring for detection. Seizures may cause further ICP elevation and should be treated aggressively. Prophylactic AEDs are not indicated,[282] possibly with the exception of patients with intracranial hemorrhages in the setting of acute liver failure. Patients who do have seizures are treated with levetiracetam, topiramate, and zonisamide as these agents have minimal hepatic metabolism. Metabolic and electrolyte imbalance needs to be ruled out for those with new-onset seizures as both are encountered frequently.

Management of medical complications. Acute liver failure that is not managed aggressively may progress rapidly to multiorgan failure.

Airway and breathing. West Haven Grade 3–4 patients generally need to be intubated, and, if required, small doses of propofol are the sedative agent of choice. Lidocaine spray or 1 mL/kg intravenous bolus before laryngoscopy may blunt increases in ICP in the peri-intubation period. Permissive hypercapnia should be avoided as this may elevate ICP and is one of the risks of delayed intubation. Frequently, patients will have spontaneous hyperventilation as part of an autoregulatory response, which should generally be allowed. Initial diagnostics include arterial puncture for arterial blood gas analysis, arterial lactate, and obtaining a chest radiograph.

Hemodynamics and renal function. Patients with liver failure may have dramatically low systemic vascular resistance and additionally are frequently volume depleted. Management includes placement of arterial blood pressure monitors, fluid resuscitation, and possibly vasopressor support. Careful monitoring of renal function is required as renal failure is common in patients with acute liver failure and may limit the ability of fluid resuscitation unless dialysis is started. The initial fluid of choice is normal saline. Initial mean arterial blood pressure goals should aim for a mean perfusion pressure of 75 mm Hg or higher, and for those patients with ICP monitoring, blood pressure should be titrated to achieve a goal cerebral perfusion pressure of 60–80 mm Hg. Vasopressors of choice include norepinephrine and vasopressin, particularly for those with sepsis. Stress doses of hydrocortisone (200–300 mg/d, given in divided doses) may be considered for patients with adrenal insufficiency.

About half of all patients with acute liver failure may also develop renal failure, which is also related to the development of hepatic encephalopathy, as discussed earlier. Renal replacement therapy may be required possibly using continuous modes of hemodialysis, depending on hemodynamic stability of the patient. Continuous veno-venous hemofiltration has been shown to lower ammonia in acute liver failure patients even in the absence of renal failure.[283,284] Frequent thrombosis of the dialysis circuit may complicate renal replacement therapy despite laboratory evidence of coagulopathy due to decreased production of natural anticoagulants (i.e., antithrombin III, protein S, protein C).

Electrolyte and metabolic abnormalities. Hyponatremia may develop rapidly and can be associated with confusion, seizures, and impaired arousal. If persistent, then careful, slow repletion is recommended. Hypoglycemia is common as hepatic glycogen is depleted and gluconeogenesis and insulin degradation are impaired. Close monitoring for detection of hypoglycemia is crucial, but corrective therapy with dextrose drips should only be done in isotonic solutions to prevent further brain swelling. Hypokalemia, hypophosphatemia, and hypomagnesemia can develop and should be repleted carefully. Repletion should take renal function and other medications, particularly diuretic administration, into account. Feeding should be initiated early if possible. Enteral feedings are preferred over total parenteral nutrition, but specific formulations such as branched chain amino acids have not been shown to be superior.

Hematology. Coagulopathy frequently accompanies development of liver failure. Patients should receive at least one dose of 10 mg vitamin K if coagulopathic in the setting of acute liver failure. Unless surgical procedures (i.e., liver biopsy) are planned or the patient is spontaneously bleeding, coagulopathy in the acute liver failure patient should not be reversed. Active blood typing and screens should be kept to allow rapid transfusion of blood products should this be needed. As a general rule, placement of intracranial ICP monitors is considered when INR is lower than 1.4, platelets are greater than 50,000/mm³, fibrinogen is greater than 100 mg/dL, and the partial thromboplastin time (PTT) normalized. If it is necessary to stop bleeding or to perform a procedure, prothrombin complex concentrates may be provided if fibrinogen is below 100 mg/dL. This only lasts for a few hours, though, and is usually followed with fresh frozen plasma, repeated every 4–6 hours, to keep the INR in the required range.

Infection. Patients with acute liver failure are at increased risk for infections including sepsis. Prophylactic parenteral or nonabsorbable enteral antibiotics have not been shown to confer a survival benefit. Surveillance cultures may allow earlier detection of bacterial and fungal infections. When signs of infection develop, broad-spectrum antibiotics may need to be started empirically and be narrowed down based on culture results.

Liver transplantation is the definitive treatment for acute liver failure and achieves survival rates up to 80% at 1 year post transplant.[285,286]

368   Plum and Posner's Diagnosis and Treatment of Stupor and Coma

GENERAL MANAGEMENT CONSIDERATIONS APPLYING TO ALL OR MOST BRAIN-INJURED PATIENTS

Hospitalized patients are at high risk of developing fluctuating states of attention, agitation, and arousal, and impaired content processing.[287] This phenomenon is labeled as *delirium* and is particularly common in intensive care unit patients. Pathophysiologically, inflammation, endothelial dysfunction,[288] melatonin dysregulation,[289] hypothalamic-pituitary adrenal axis dysfunction,[290] pain, and other mechanisms have been proposed to play a role in the development of delirium.[291] In large observational studies, delirium has been associated with poor outcome, including mortality[292] and cognitive decline.[293–296]

Treatment of delirium is challenging as no specific treatments have been developed, but a number of risk factors have emerged. These include old age,[294] infections, sleep deprivation, use of benzodiazepines and opiates, and stress. Management of patients at risk of delirium requires preventive strategies including nonpharmacologic strategies such as reorientation to day–night cycles, limiting nighttime exams and interruptions in sleep, early mobilization, and occupational and physical therapy. Physical restraints should be minimized as these may cause further agitation and worsened delirium.[297] Minimizing sedation may be supportive. Importantly, underlying causes need to be identified as delirium may be the presenting symptom of undertreated pain, infections, metabolic derangements, and neurological complications such as strokes. Prophylactic administration of haloperidol (Haldol) is not beneficial.[298] Once developed, agitated delirium is often managed with antipsychotic agents, but it is important to note that a randomized controlled trial did not find differences in duration of delirium or longer term outcomes in patients randomized to receive a dopamine D_2 antagonists, haloperidol, or ziprasidone when compared to placebo.[299]

GOALS OF CARE

As the ability to allow patient survival increases with sophisticated critical care and surgical interventions, the goals of care for each patient should always be kept in mind. Unfortunately, despite advances in the acute management of patients with devastating neurological injury, survival may still be easier to achieve than full functional recovery. Factors to consider when determining goals of care include the patient's known or—if wishes are not clear—the patient's presumed wishes based on the healthcare proxy or next of kin, the degree of injury, and the likelihood of recovery. Goals of care choices include full medical support (the default until goals are of care are changed), comfort care measures only, and end of life care. Additionally, providing appropriate palliative care and consultation is an important aspect of neurocritical care of patients with devastating neurological injury.[300] Maybe most importantly, physicians should be aware of the many biases that cloud or at a minimum affect their ability to provide guidance to healthcare decision-makers of acutely brain-injured patients.[301] These biases are important to recognize in order to best participate in the goals of care decision-making process.

A FINAL WORD

This chapter has presented an etiology-specific approach to the emergency management of the stuporous and comatose patient. The approach is based on the belief that, after a history and a general physical and neurologic examination, the informed physician can, with reasonable confidence, place the patient into one of four major groups of illnesses that cause coma and guide the initial approach. The specific group into which the patient is placed directs the rest of the diagnostic evaluation and treatment. At times, however, the diagnosis is uncertain even after the examination is completed, and it is necessary to defer even the preliminary categorization of patients until the imaging or metabolic tests are carried out and the most serious infections or metabolic abnormalities have been considered. If there is any suspicion of a mass lesion, immediate imaging is mandatory despite the absence of focal signs. Conversely, the presence of hemiplegia or other focal signs does not rule out metabolic disease, especially hypoglycemia.

A number of etiologies may present supra- and infratentorially, and much of the management overlaps regardless of the location of the pathology. At all times during the diagnostic evaluation and treatment of a patient who is stuporous or comatose, the physician must ask him- or herself whether the diagnosis could possibly be wrong and whether he or she needs to seek consultation or undertake other diagnostic or therapeutic measures. Fortunately, with constant attention to the changing state of consciousness and a willingness to reconsider the situation minute by minute, few mistakes should be made.

REFERENCES

1. Fakhry SM, Trask AL, Waller MA, Watts DD, Force INT. Management of brain-injured patients by an evidence-based medicine protocol improves outcomes and decreases hospital charges. *J Trauma* 2004;56(3):492–499; discussion 499–500.
2. Powers WJ, Derdeyn CP, Biller J, et al. 2015 American Heart Association/American Stroke Association focused update of the 2013 guidelines for the early management of patients with acute ischemic stroke regarding endovascular treatment: a guideline for healthcare professionals from the American Heart Association/American Stroke Association. *Stroke* 2015;46(10):3020–35.
3. Jauch EC, Saver JL, Adams HP Jr, et al. Guidelines for the early management of patients with acute ischemic stroke: a guideline for healthcare professionals from the American Heart Association/American Stroke Association. *Stroke* 2013;44(3):870–947.
4. Miller CM, Pineda J, Corry M, Brophy G, Smith WS. Emergency neurologic life support (ENLS): evolution of management in the first hour of a neurological emergency. *Neurocrit Care* 2015;23(Suppl 2):S1–4.
5. Witsch J, Frey HP, Patel S, et al. Prognostication of long-term outcomes after subarachnoid hemorrhage: the FRESH score. *Ann Neurol* 2016;80(1):46–58.
6. Starke RM, Connolly ES Jr. Participants in the International Multi-Disciplinary Consensus Conference on the critical care management of Subarachnoid H. Rebleeding after aneurysmal subarachnoid hemorrhage. *Neurocrit Care* 2011;15(2):241–246.
7. Naidech AM, Janjua N, Kreiter KT, et al. Predictors and impact of aneurysm rebleeding after subarachnoid hemorrhage. *Arch Neurol* 2005;62(3):410–416.
8. van Donkelaar CE, Bakker NA, Veeger NJ, et al. Predictive factors for rebleeding after aneurysmal subarachnoid hemorrhage: rebleeding aneurysmal subarachnoid hemorrhage study. *Stroke* 2015;46(8):2100–2106.
9. Connolly ES Jr, Rabinstein AA, Carhuapoma JR, et al. Guidelines for the management of aneurysmal subarachnoid hemorrhage: a guideline for healthcare professionals from the American Heart Association/American Stroke Association. *Stroke* 2012;43(6):1711–1737.
10. Siegal DM, Curnutte JT, Connolly SJ, et al. Andexanet alfa for the reversal of factor Xa inhibitor activity. *N Engl J Med* 2015;373(25):2413–2424.
11. Pollack CV, Jr., Reilly PA, Eikelboom J, et al. Idarucizumab for dabigatran reversal. *N Engl J Med* 2015;373(6):511–520.
12. Baharoglu MI, Germans MR, Rinkel GJ, et al. Antifibrinolytic therapy for aneurysmal subarachnoid haemorrhage. *Cochrane Database Syst Rev* 2013;(8):CD001245.
13. Schuette AJ, Hui FK, Obuchowski NA, et al. An examination of aneurysm rerupture rates with epsilon aminocaproic acid. *Neurocrit Care* 2013;19(1):48–55.
14. Claassen J, Carhuapoma JR, Kreiter KT, Du EY, Connolly ES, Mayer SA. Global cerebral edema after subarachnoid hemorrhage: frequency, predictors, and impact on outcome. *Stroke* 2002;33(5):1225–1232.
15. Hasan D, Schonck RS, Avezaat CJ, Tanghe HL, van Gijn J, van der Lugt PJ. Epileptic seizures after subarachnoid hemorrhage. *Ann Neurol* 1993;33(3):286–291.
16. Claassen J, Hirsch LJ, Frontera JA, et al. Prognostic significance of continuous EEG monitoring in patients with poor-grade subarachnoid hemorrhage. *Neurocrit Care* 2006;4(2):103–112.
17. De Marchis GM, Pugin D, Meyers E, et al. Seizure burden in subarachnoid hemorrhage associated with functional and cognitive outcome. *Neurology* 2016;86(3):253–260.
18. Diringer MN, Bleck TP, Claude Hemphill J 3rd, et al. Critical care management of patients following aneurysmal subarachnoid hemorrhage: recommendations from the Neurocritical Care Society's Multidisciplinary Consensus Conference. *Neurocrit Care* 2011;15(2):211–240.
19. Claassen J, Peery S, Kreiter KT, et al. Predictors and clinical impact of epilepsy after subarachnoid hemorrhage. *Neurology* 2003;60(2):208–214.
20. Rhoney DH, Tipps LB, Murry KR, Basham MC, Michael DB, Coplin WM. Anticonvulsant prophylaxis and timing of seizures after aneurysmal subarachnoid hemorrhage. *Neurology* 2000;55(2):258–265.
21. Naidech AM, Kreiter KT, Janjua N, et al. Phenytoin exposure is associated with functional and cognitive disability after subarachnoid hemorrhage. *Stroke* 2005;36(3):583–587.
22. Rosengart AJ, Huo JD, Tolentino J, et al. Outcome in patients with subarachnoid hemorrhage treated with antiepileptic drugs. *J Neurosurg* 2007;107(2):253–260.
23. Wong GK, Poon WS. Use of phenytoin and other anticonvulsant prophylaxis in patients with aneurysmal subarachnoid hemorrhage. *Stroke* 2005;36(12):2532; author reply 2532.
24. Molyneux AJ, Kerr RS, Yu LM, et al. International subarachnoid aneurysm trial (ISAT) of neurosurgical clipping versus endovascular coiling in 2143 patients with ruptured intracranial aneurysms: a randomised comparison of effects on survival, dependency, seizures, rebleeding, subgroups, and aneurysm occlusion. *Lancet* 2005;366(9488):809–817.
25. Phillips TJ, Dowling RJ, Yan B, Laidlaw JD, Mitchell PJ. Does treatment of ruptured intracranial aneurysms within 24 hours improve clinical outcome? *Stroke* 2011;42(7):1936–1945.
26. Schmidt JM, Wartenberg KE, Fernandez A, et al. Frequency and clinical impact of asymptomatic cerebral infarction due to vasospasm after subarachnoid hemorrhage. *J Neurosurg* 2008;109(6):1052–1059.

27. Claassen J, Bernardini GL, Kreiter K, et al. Effect of cisternal and ventricular blood on risk of delayed cerebral ischemia after subarachnoid hemorrhage: the Fisher scale revisited. *Stroke* 2001;32(9):2012–2020.

28. Frontera JA, Fernandez A, Schmidt JM, et al. Defining vasospasm after subarachnoid hemorrhage: what is the most clinically relevant definition? *Stroke* 2009;40(6):1963–1968.

29. Claassen J, Hirsch LJ, Kreiter KT, et al. Quantitative continuous EEG for detecting delayed cerebral ischemia in patients with poor-grade subarachnoid hemorrhage. *Clin Neurophysiol* 2004;115(12):2699–2710.

30. Sanelli PC, Pandya A, Segal AZ, et al. Cost-effectiveness of CT angiography and perfusion imaging for delayed cerebral ischemia and vasospasm in aneurysmal subarachnoid hemorrhage. *AJNR Am J Neuroradiol* 2014;35(9):1714–1720.

31. Malinova V, Dolatowski K, Schramm P, Moerer O, Rohde V, Mielke D. Early whole-brain CT perfusion for detection of patients at risk for delayed cerebral ischemia after subarachnoid hemorrhage. *J Neurosurg* 2016 Jul;125(1):128–136. doi:10.3171/2015.6.JNS15720. Epub 2015 Dec 18.

32. Dorhout Mees SM, Rinkel GJ, Feigin VL, et al. Calcium antagonists for aneurysmal subarachnoid haemorrhage. *Cochrane Database Syst Rev* 2007;(3):CD000277.

33. Pickard JD, Murray GD, Illingworth R, et al. Effect of oral nimodipine on cerebral infarction and outcome after subarachnoid haemorrhage: British aneurysm nimodipine trial. *BMJ* 1989;298(6674):636–642.

34. Choi HA, Ko SB, Chen H, et al. Acute effects of nimodipine on cerebral vasculature and brain metabolism in high grade subarachnoid hemorrhage patients. *Neurocrit Care* 2012;16(3):363–367.

35. Rosenwasser RH, Delgado TE, Buchheit WA, Freed MH. Control of hypertension and prophylaxis against vasospasm in cases of subarachnoid hemorrhage: a preliminary report. *Neurosurgery* 1983;12(6):658–661.

36. Egge A, Waterloo K, Sjoholm H, Solberg T, Ingebrigtsen T, Romner B. Prophylactic hyperdynamic postoperative fluid therapy after aneurysmal subarachnoid hemorrhage: a clinical, prospective, randomized, controlled study. *Neurosurgery* 2001;49(3):593–605; discussion 606.

37. Treggiari MM, Walder B, Suter PM, Romand JA. Systematic review of the prevention of delayed ischemic neurological deficits with hypertension, hypervolemia, and hemodilution therapy following subarachnoid hemorrhage. *J Neurosurg* 2003;98(5):978–984.

38. Dorhout Mees SM, Algra A, Wong GK, et al. Early magnesium treatment after aneurysmal subarachnoid hemorrhage: individual patient data meta-analysis. *Stroke* 2015;46(11):3190–3193.

39. Liu J, Chen Q. Effect of statins treatment for patients with aneurysmal subarachnoid hemorrhage: a systematic review and meta-analysis of observational studies and randomized controlled trials. *Intl J Clin Exp Med* 2015;8(5):7198–7208.

40. Zhang S, Wang L, Liu M, Wu B. Tirilazad for aneurysmal subarachnoid haemorrhage. *Cochrane Database Syst Rev* 2010;(2):CD006778.

41. Badjatia N, Topcuoglu MA, Pryor JC, et al. Preliminary experience with intra-arterial nicardipine as a treatment for cerebral vasospasm. *AJNR Am J Neuroradiol* 2004;25(5):819–826.

42. Macdonald RL, Higashida RT, Keller E, et al. Clazosentan, an endothelin receptor antagonist, in patients with aneurysmal subarachnoid haemorrhage undergoing surgical clipping: a randomised, double-blind, placebo-controlled phase 3 trial (CONSCIOUS-2). *Lancet Neurol* 2011;10(7):618–625.

43. Wartenberg KE, Schmidt JM, Claassen J, et al. Impact of medical complications on outcome after subarachnoid hemorrhage. *Critical care medicine* 2006;34(3):617–623; quiz 624.

44. Mayer SA, Fink ME, Homma S, et al. Cardiac injury associated with neurogenic pulmonary edema following subarachnoid hemorrhage. *Neurology* 1994;44(5):815–820.

45. Mutoh T, Kazumata K, Ueyama-Mutoh T, Taki Y, Ishikawa T. Transpulmonary thermodilution-based management of neurogenic pulmonary edema after subarachnoid hemorrhage. *The American journal of the medical sciences* 2015;350(5):415–419.

46. Simon RP. Neurogenic pulmonary edema. *Neurol Clin* 1993;11(2):309–323.

47. Carrera E, Schmidt JM, Fernandez L, et al. Spontaneous hyperventilation and brain tissue hypoxia in patients with severe brain injury. *J Neurol Neurosurg Psychiatry* 2010;81(7):793–797.

48. Lee VH, Oh JK, Mulvagh SL, Wijdicks EF. Mechanisms in neurogenic stress cardiomyopathy after aneurysmal subarachnoid hemorrhage. *Neurocrit Care* 2006;5(3):243–249.

49. Lee VH, Connolly HM, Fulgham JR, Manno EM, Brown RD Jr, Wijdicks EF. Tako-tsubo cardiomyopathy in aneurysmal subarachnoid hemorrhage: an underappreciated ventricular dysfunction. *J Neurosurg* 2006;105(2):264–270.

50. Taccone FS, Lubicz B, Piagnerelli M, Van Nuffelen M, Vincent JL, De Backer D. Cardiogenic shock with stunned myocardium during triple-H therapy treated with intra-aortic balloon pump counterpulsation. *Neurocrit Care* 2009;10(1):76–82.

51. Lazaridis C, Pradilla G, Nyquist PA, Tamargo RJ. Intra-aortic balloon pump counterpulsation in the setting of subarachnoid hemorrhage, cerebral vasospasm, and neurogenic stress cardiomyopathy. Case report and review of the literature. *Neurocrit Care* 2010;13(1):101–108.

52. Van den Berghe G, Wilmer A, Hermans G, et al. Intensive insulin therapy in the medical ICU. *N Engl J Med* 2006;354(5):449–461.

53. Naidech AM, Levasseur K, Liebling S, et al. Moderate hypoglycemia is associated with vasospasm, cerebral infarction, and 3-month disability after subarachnoid hemorrhage. *Neurocrit Care* 2010;12(2):181–187.

54. Vespa P, Boonyaputthikul R, McArthur DL, et al. Intensive insulin therapy reduces microdialysis glucose values without altering glucose utilization or improving the lactate/pyruvate ratio after traumatic brain injury. *Crit Care Med* 2006;34(3):850–856.

55. Oddo M, Schmidt JM, Carrera E, et al. Impact of tight glycemic control on cerebral glucose metabolism after severe brain injury: a microdialysis study. *Crit Care Med* 2008;36(12):3233–3238.

56. Helbok R, Schmidt JM, Kurtz P, et al. Systemic glucose and brain energy metabolism after subarachnoid hemorrhage. *Neurocrit Care* 2010;12(3):317–323.

57. Fernandez A, Schmidt JM, Claassen J, et al. Fever after subarachnoid hemorrhage: risk factors and impact on outcome. *Neurology* 2007;68(13):1013–1019.
58. Naidech AM, Shaibani A, Garg RK, et al. Prospective, randomized trial of higher goal hemoglobin after subarachnoid hemorrhage. *Neurocrit Care* 2010;13(3):313–320.
59. Kothari RU, Brott T, Broderick JP, et al. The ABCs of measuring intracerebral hemorrhage volumes. *Stroke* 1996;27(8):1304–1305.
60. Hemphill JC 3rd, Bonovich DC, Besmertis L, Manley GT, Johnston SC. The ICH score: a simple, reliable grading scale for intracerebral hemorrhage. *Stroke* 2001;32(4):891–897.
61. Hemphill JC 3rd, Farrant M, Neill TA Jr. Prospective validation of the ICH Score for 12-month functional outcome. *Neurology* 2009;73(14):1088–1094.
62. Rost NS, Smith EE, Chang Y, et al. Prediction of functional outcome in patients with primary intracerebral hemorrhage: the FUNC score. *Stroke* 2008;39(8):2304–2309.
63. Morgenstern LB, Zahuranec DB, Sanchez BN, et al. Full medical support for intracerebral hemorrhage. *Neurology* 2015;84(17):1739–1744.
64. Mayer SA, Brun NC, Begtrup K, et al. Efficacy and safety of recombinant activated factor VII for acute intracerebral hemorrhage. *N Engl J Med* 2008;358(20):2127–2137.
65. Goldstein JN, Fazen LE, Snider R, et al. Contrast extravasation on CT angiography predicts hematoma expansion in intracerebral hemorrhage. *Neurology* 2007;68(12):889–894.
66. Qureshi AI, Palesch YY, Martin R, et al. Effect of systolic blood pressure reduction on hematoma expansion, perihematomal edema, and 3-month outcome among patients with intracerebral hemorrhage: results from the antihypertensive treatment of acute cerebral hemorrhage study. *Arch Neurol* 2010;67(5):570–6.
67. Anderson CS, Heeley7 E, Huang Y, et al. Rapid blood-pressure lowering in patients with acute intracerebral hemorrhage. *N Engl J Med* 2013;368(25):2355–2365.
68. Qureshi AI, Palesch YY, Barsan WG, et al. Intensive blood-pressure lowering in patients with acute cerebral hemorrhage. *N Engl J Med* 2016;375(11):1033–1043.
69. Qureshi AI, Ezzeddine MA, Nasar A, et al. Prevalence of elevated blood pressure in 563,704 adult patients with stroke presenting to the ED in the United States. *Am J Emerg Med* 2007;25(1):32–38.
70. Anderson CS, Huang Y, Wang JG, et al. Intensive blood pressure reduction in acute cerebral haemorrhage trial (INTERACT): a randomised pilot trial. *Lancet Neurol* 2008;7(5):391–399.
71. Vemmos KN, Tsivgoulis G, Spengos K, et al. U-shaped relationship between mortality and admission blood pressure in patients with acute stroke. *J Intern Med* 2004;255(2):257–265.
72. Hemphill JC 3rd, Greenberg SM, Anderson CS, et al. Guidelines for the management of spontaneous intracerebral hemorrhage: a guideline for healthcare professionals from the American Heart Association/American Stroke Association. *Stroke* 2015;46(7):2032–2060.
73. Frontera JA, Lewin JJ 3rd, Rabinstein AA, et al. Guideline for reversal of antithrombotics in intracranial hemorrhage: a statement for healthcare professionals from the Neurocritical Care Society and Society of Critical Care Medicine. *Neurocrit Care* 2016;24(1):6–46.
74. Siegal DM, Curnutte JT, Connolly SJ, et al. Andexanet alfa for the reversal of factor Xa inhibitor activity. *N Engl J Med* 2015;373(25):2413–2424.
75. Baharoglu MI, Cordonnier C, Al-Shahi Salman R, et al. Platelet transfusion versus standard care after acute stroke due to spontaneous cerebral haemorrhage associated with antiplatelet therapy (PATCH): a randomised, open-label, phase 3 trial. *Lancet* 2016;387(10038):2605–2613.
76. Mayer SA, Brun NC, Begtrup K, et al. Recombinant activated factor VII for acute intracerebral hemorrhage. *N Engl J Med* 2005;352(8):777–785.
77. Sprigg N, Flaherty K, Appleton JP, et al. Tranexamic acid for hyperacute primary IntraCerebral Haemorrhage (TICH-2): an international randomised, placebo-controlled, phase 3 superiority trial. *Lancet* 2018;391(10135):2107–2115.
78. Selim M, Yeatts S, Goldstein JN, et al. Safety and tolerability of deferoxamine mesylate in patients with acute intracerebral hemorrhage. *Stroke* 2011;42(11):3067–3074.
79. Yeatts SD, Palesch YY, Moy CS, Selim M. High dose deferoxamine in intracerebral hemorrhage (HI-DEF) trial: rationale, design, and methods. *Neurocrit Care* 2013;19(2):257–266.
80. Ziai WC, Tuhrim S, Lane K, et al. A multicenter, randomized, double-blinded, placebo-controlled phase III study of Clot Lysis Evaluation of Accelerated Resolution of Intraventricular Hemorrhage (CLEAR III). *Int J Stroke* 2014;9(4):536–542.
81. Mould WA, Carhuapoma JR, Muschelli J, et al. Minimally invasive surgery plus recombinant tissue-type plasminogen activator for intracerebral hemorrhage evacuation decreases perihematomal edema. *Stroke* 2013;44(3):627–634.
82. Mendelow AD, Gregson BA, Rowan EN, et al. Early surgery versus initial conservative treatment in patients with spontaneous supratentorial lobar intracerebral haematomas (STICH II): a randomised trial. *Lancet* 2013;382(9890):397–408.
83. Mendelow AD, Gregson BA, Fernandes IIM, et al. Early surgery versus initial conservative treatment in patients with spontaneous supratentorial intracerebral haematomas in the International Surgical Trial in Intracerebral Haemorrhage (STICH): a randomised trial. *Lancet* 2005;365(9457):387–397.
84. Helbok R, Olson DM, Le Roux PD, Vespa P, Participants in the International Multidisciplinary Consensus Conference on Multimodality M. Intracranial pressure and cerebral perfusion pressure monitoring in non-TBI patients: special considerations. *Neurocrit Care* 2014;21(Suppl 2): S85–94.
85. Vespa PM, O'Phelan K, Shah M, et al. Acute seizures after intracerebral hemorrhage: a factor in progressive midline shift and outcome. *Neurology* 2003;60(9):1441–1446.
86. Claassen J, Jette N, Chum F, et al. Electrographic seizures and periodic discharges after intracerebral hemorrhage. *Neurology* 2007;69(13):1356–1365.
87. Naidech AM, Beaumont J, Muldoon K, et al. Prophylactic seizure medication and health-related quality of life after intracerebral hemorrhage. *Crit Care Med* 2018;46(9):1480–1485.

88. Paciaroni M, Agnelli G, Venti M, Alberti A, Acciarresi M, Caso V. Efficacy and safety of anticoagulants in the prevention of venous thromboembolism in patients with acute cerebral hemorrhage: a meta-analysis of controlled studies. *J Thromb Haemost* 2011;9(5):893–898.

89. Miller D, Crandall C, Washington C, 3rd, McLaughlin S. Improving teamwork and communication in trauma care through in situ simulations. *Acad Emerg Med* 2012;19(5):608–612.

90. Sumann G, Kampfl A, Wenzel V, Schobersberger W. Early intensive care unit intervention for trauma care: what alters the outcome? *Curr Opin Crit Care* 2002;8(6):587–592.

91. Inaba K, Byerly S, Bush LD, et al. Cervical spinal clearance: a prospective Western Trauma Association multi-institutional trial. *J Trauma Acute Care Surg* 2016;81(6):1122–1130.

92. Kasotakis G, Sideris A, Yang Y, et al. Aggressive early crystalloid resuscitation adversely affects outcomes in adult blunt trauma patients: an analysis of the Glue Grant database. *J Trauma Acute Care Surg* 2013;74(5):1215–1221; discussion 1221–1222.

93. Murphy CH, Hess JR. Massive transfusion: red blood cell to plasma and platelet unit ratios for resuscitation of massive hemorrhage. *Curr Opin Hematol* 2015;22(6):533–539.

94. CRASH-2 collaborators, Roberts I, Shakur H, et al. The importance of early treatment with tranexamic acid in bleeding trauma patients: an exploratory analysis of the CRASH-2 randomised controlled trial. *Lancet* 2011;377(9771):1096–1101.

95. Rozycki GS, Ballard RB, Feliciano DV, Schmidt JA, Pennington SD. Surgeon-performed ultrasound for the assessment of truncal injuries: lessons learned from 1540 patients. *Ann Surg* 1998;228(4):557–567.

96. Masters SJ, McClean PM, Arcarese JS, et al. Skull x-ray examinations after head trauma. Recommendations by a multidisciplinary panel and validation study. *N Engl J Med* 1987;316(2):84–91.

97. Jennett B, Teasdale G. Aspects of coma after severe head injury. *Lancet* 1977;1(8017):878–881.

98. Lingsma HF, Roozenbeek B, Steyerberg EW, Murray GD, Maas AI. Early prognosis in traumatic brain injury: from prophecies to predictions. *Lancet Neurol* 2010;9(5):543–554.

99. Steyerberg EW, Mushkudiani N, Perel P, et al. Predicting outcome after traumatic brain injury: development and international validation of prognostic scores based on admission characteristics. *PLoS Med* 2008;5(8):e165; discussion e165.

100. Cepeda S, Gomez PA, Castano-Leon AM, Martinez-Perez R, Munarriz PM, Lagares A. Traumatic intracerebral hemorrhage: risk factors associated with progression. *Journal of neurotrauma* 2015;32(16):1246–1253.

101. Cooper DJ, Rosenfeld JV, Murray L, et al. Decompressive craniectomy in diffuse traumatic brain injury. *N Engl J Med* 2011;364(16):1493–1502.

102. Muizelaar JP, Marmarou A, Ward JD, et al. Adverse effects of prolonged hyperventilation in patients with severe head injury: a randomized clinical trial. *J Neurosurg* 1991;75(5):731–739.

103. Ward JD, Becker DP, Miller JD, et al. Failure of prophylactic barbiturate coma in the treatment of severe head injury. *J Neurosurg* 1985;62(3):383–388.

104. Andrews PJ, Sinclair HL, Rodriguez A, et al. Hypothermia for Intracranial Hypertension after Traumatic Brain Injury. *N Engl J Med* 2015;373(25):2403–2412.

105. Clifton GL, Miller ER, Choi SC, et al. Lack of effect of induction of hypothermia after acute brain injury. *N Engl J Med* 2001;344(8):556–563.

106. Clifton GL, Valadka A, Zygun D, et al. Very early hypothermia induction in patients with severe brain injury (the National Acute Brain Injury Study: Hypothermia II): a randomised trial. *Lancet Neurol* 2011;10(2):131–139.

107. Alderson P, Roberts I. Corticosteroids for acute traumatic brain injury. *Cochrane Database Syst Rev* 2005;(1):CD000196.

108. Roberts I, Yates D, Sandercock P, et al. Effect of intravenous corticosteroids on death within 14 days in 10008 adults with clinically significant head injury (MRC CRASH trial): randomised placebo-controlled trial. *Lancet* 2004;364(9442):1321–1328.

109. Edwards P, Arango M, Balica L, et al. Final results of MRC CRASH, a randomised placebo-controlled trial of intravenous corticosteroid in adults with head injury-outcomes at 6 months. *Lancet* 2005;365(9475):1957–1959.

110. Chesnut RM, Bleck TP, Citerio G, et al. A consensus-based interpretation of the benchmark evidence from South American trials: treatment of intracranial pressure trial. *Journal of neurotrauma* 2015;32(22):1722–1724.

111. Carney N, Totten AM, O'Reilly C, et al. Guidelines for the management of severe traumatic brain injury, fourth edition. *Neurosurgery* 2017 Jan 1;80(1):6–15. doi:10.1227/NEU.0000000000001432. PMID:27654000.

112. Contant CF, Valadka AB, Gopinath SP, Hannay HJ, Robertson CS. Adult respiratory distress syndrome: a complication of induced hypertension after severe head injury. *J Neurosurg* 2001;95(4):560–568.

113. Kashif FM, Verghese GC, Novak V, Czosnyka M, Heldt T. Model-based noninvasive estimation of intracranial pressure from cerebral blood flow velocity and arterial pressure. *Sci Transl Med* 2012;4(129):129ra44.

114. Okonkwo DO, Shutter LA, Moore C, et al. Brain oxygen optimization in severe traumatic brain injury. Phase-II: a phase II randomized trial. *Crit Care Med* 2017;45(11):1907–1914.

115. Langham J, Goldfrad C, Teasdale G, Shaw D, Rowan K. Calcium channel blockers for acute traumatic brain injury. *Cochrane Database Syst Rev* 2003;(4):CD000565.

116. Vergouwen MD, Vermeulen M, Roos YB. Effect of nimodipine on outcome in patients with traumatic subarachnoid haemorrhage: a systematic review. *Lancet Neurol* 2006 Dec;5(12):1029–1032. Review. PMID: 17110283.

117. Moen KG, Brezova V, Skandsen T, Haberg AK, Folvik M, Vik A. Traumatic axonal injury: the prognostic value of lesion load in corpus callosum, brain stem, and thalamus in different magnetic resonance imaging sequences. *Journal of neurotrauma* 2014;31(17):1486–1496.

118. Ratilal BO, Costa J, Pappamikail L, Sampaio C. Antibiotic prophylaxis for preventing meningitis

in patients with basilar skull fractures. *Cochrane Database Syst Rev* 2015;(4):CD004884.

119. Temkin NR, Dikmen SS, Wilensky AJ, Keihm J, Chabal S, Winn HR. A randomized, double-blind study of phenytoin for the prevention of post-traumatic seizures. *N Engl J Med* 1990;323(8):497–502.

120. Vespa P, Tubi M, Claassen J, et al. Metabolic crisis occurs with seizures and periodic discharges after brain trauma. *Ann Neurol* 2016;79(4):579–590.

121. Vespa PM, McArthur DL, Xu Y, et al. Nonconvulsive seizures after traumatic brain injury are associated with hippocampal atrophy. *Neurology* 2010;75(9):792–798.

122. Lowenstein DH. Epilepsy after head injury: an overview. *Epilepsia* 2009;50(Suppl 2):4–9.

123. Frey LC. Epidemiology of posttraumatic epilepsy: a critical review. *Epilepsia* 2003;44(Suppl 10):11–17.

124. Hoffman JR, Mower WR, Wolfson AB, Todd KH, Zucker MI. Validity of a set of clinical criteria to rule out injury to the cervical spine in patients with blunt trauma. National Emergency X-Radiography Utilization Study Group. *N Engl J Med* 2000;343(2):94–99.

125. Stiell IG, Clement CM, McKnight RD, et al. The Canadian C-spine rule versus the NEXUS low-risk criteria in patients with trauma. *N Engl J Med* 2003;349(26):2510–2518.

126. Bandiera G, Stiell IG, Wells GA, et al. The Canadian C-spine rule performs better than unstructured physician judgment. *Ann Emerg Med* 2003;42(3):395–402.

127. Bonatti M, Vezzali N, Ferro F, Manfredi R, Oberhofer N, Bonatti G. Blunt cerebrovascular injury: diagnosis at whole-body MDCT for multi-trauma. *Insights Imaging* 2013;4(3):347–355.

128. CADISS trial investigators, Markus HS, Hayter E, et al. Antiplatelet treatment compared with anticoagulation treatment for cervical artery dissection (CADISS): a randomised trial. *Lancet Neurol* 2015;14(4):361–367.

129. Muehlschlegel S, Carandang R, Ouillette C, Hall W, Anderson F, Goldberg R. Frequency and impact of intensive care unit complications on moderate-severe traumatic brain injury: early results of the Outcome Prognostication in Traumatic Brain Injury (OPTIMISM) Study. *Neurocrit Care* 2013;18(3):318–331.

130. Nyquist P, Bautista C, Jichici D, et al. Prophylaxis of venous thrombosis in neurocritical care patients: an evidence-based guideline: a statement for healthcare professionals from the Neurocritical Care Society. *Neurocrit Care* 2016;24(1):47–60.

131. Bao L, Chen D, Ding L, Ling W, Xu F. Fever burden is an independent predictor for prognosis of traumatic brain injury. *PloS One* 2014;9(3):e90956.

132. Rabinowitz RP, Caplan ES. Management of infections in the trauma patient. *Surg Clin N Am* 1999;79(6):1373–1383, x.

133. Robertson CS, Hannay HJ, Yamal JM, et al. Effect of erythropoietin and transfusion threshold on neurological recovery after traumatic brain injury: a randomized clinical trial. *JAMA* 2014;312(1):36–47.

134. Busl KM, Prabhakaran S. Predictors of mortality in nontraumatic subdural hematoma. *J Neurosurg* 2013;119(5):1296–1301.

135. Radic JA, Chou SH, Du R, Lee JW. Levetiracetam versus phenytoin: a comparison of efficacy of seizure prophylaxis and adverse event risk following acute or subacute subdural hematoma diagnosis. *Neurocrit Care* 2014;21(2):228–237.

136. Rabinstein AA, Chung SY, Rudzinski LA, Lanzino G. Seizures after evacuation of subdural hematomas: incidence, risk factors, and functional impact. *J Neurosurg* 2010;112(2):455–460.

137. Lin CM, Lin JW, Tsai JT, et al. Intracranial pressure fluctuation during hemodialysis in renal failure patients with intracranial hemorrhage. *Acta Neurochir Suppl* 2008;101:141–144.

138. Kopitnik TA Jr, de Andrade R Jr, Gold MA, Nugent GR. Pressure changes within a chronic subdural hematoma during hemodialysis. *Surg Neurol* 1989;32(4):289–293.

139. Saver JL. Time is brain: quantified. *Stroke* 2006;37(1):263–266.

140. Ebinger M, Winter B, Wendt M, et al. Effect of the use of ambulance-based thrombolysis on time to thrombolysis in acute ischemic stroke: a randomized clinical trial. *JAMA* 2014;311(16):1622–1631.

141. The National Institute of Neurological Disorders and Stroke rt-PA Stroke Study Group. Tissue plasminogen activator for acute ischemic stroke. *N Engl J Med* 1995;333(24):1581–1587.

142. Lyden P, Brott T, Tilley B, et al. Improved reliability of the NIH Stroke Scale using video training. NINDS TPA Stroke Study Group. *Stroke* 1994;25(11):2220–2226.

143. Barber PA, Demchuk AM, Zhang J, Buchan AM. Validity and reliability of a quantitative computed tomography score in predicting outcome of hyperacute stroke before thrombolytic therapy. ASPECTS Study Group. Alberta Stroke Programme Early CT Score. *Lancet* 2000;355(9216):1670–1674.

144. Lees KR, Bluhmki E, von Kummer R, et al. Time to treatment with intravenous alteplase and outcome in stroke: an updated pooled analysis of ECASS, ATLANTIS, NINDS, and EPITHET trials. *Lancet* 2010;375(9727):1695–1703.

145. Del Zoppo GJ, Saver JL, Jauch EC, Adams HP Jr.; American Heart Association Stroke Council. Expansion of the time window for treatment of acute ischemic stroke with intravenous tissue plasminogen activator: a science advisory from the American Heart Association/American Stroke Association. *Stroke* 2009;40(8):2945–2948.

146. Hacke W, Kaste M, Bluhmki E, et al. Thrombolysis with alteplase 3 to 4.5 hours after acute ischemic stroke. *N Engl J Med* 2008;359(13):1317–1329.

147. Strbian D, Engelter S, Michel P, et al. Symptomatic intracranial hemorrhage after stroke thrombolysis: the SEDAN score. *Ann Neurol* 2012;71(5):634–641.

148. Alexandrov AV, Molina CA, Grotta JC, et al. Ultrasound-enhanced systemic thrombolysis for acute ischemic stroke. *N Engl J Med* 2004;351(21):2170–2178.

149. Smith WS, Lev MH, English JD, et al. Significance of large vessel intracranial occlusion causing acute ischemic stroke and TIA. *Stroke* 2009;40(12):3834–3840.

150. Furlan A, Higashida R, Wechsler L, et al. Intra-arterial prourokinase for acute ischemic stroke. The

PROACT II study: a randomized controlled trial. Prolyse in Acute Cerebral Thromboembolism. *JAMA* 1999;282(21):2003–2011.

151. Berkhemer OA, Fransen PS, Beumer D, et al. A randomized trial of intraarterial treatment for acute ischemic stroke. *N Engl J Med* 2015;372(1):11–20.

152. Campbell BC, Mitchell PJ, Kleinig TJ, et al. Endovascular therapy for ischemic stroke with perfusion-imaging selection. *N Engl J Med* 2015;372(11):1009–1018.

153. Goyal M, Demchuk AM, Menon BK, et al. Randomized assessment of rapid endovascular treatment of ischemic stroke. *N Engl J Med* 2015;372(11):1019–1030.

154. Jovin TG, Chamorro A, Cobo E, et al. Thrombectomy within 8 hours after symptom onset in ischemic stroke. *N Engl J Med* 2015;372(24):2296–2306.

155. Saver JL, Goyal M, Bonafe A, et al. Stent-retriever thrombectomy after intravenous t-PA vs. t-PA alone in stroke. *N Engl J Med* 2015;372(24):2285–2295.

156. Chen CJ, Ding D, Starke RM, et al. Endovascular vs medical management of acute ischemic stroke. *Neurology* 2015;85(22):1980–1990.

157. Badhiwala JH, Nassiri F, Alhazzani W, et al. Endovascular Thrombectomy for Acute Ischemic Stroke: A Meta-analysis. *JAMA* 2015;314(17):1832–1843.

158. Broderick JP, Palesch YY, Demchuk AM, et al. Endovascular therapy after intravenous t-PA versus t-PA alone for stroke. *N Engl J Med* 2013;368(10):893–903.

159. Kidwell CS, Jahan R, Gornbein J, et al. A trial of imaging selection and endovascular treatment for ischemic stroke. *N Engl J Med* 2013;368(10):914–923.

160. Nogueira RG, Jadhav AP, Haussen DC, et al. Thrombectomy 6 to 24 hours after stroke with a mismatch between deficit and infarct. *N Engl J Med* 2018;378(1):11–21.

161. Albers GW, Marks MP, Kemp S, et al. Thrombectomy for stroke at 6 to 16 hours with selection by perfusion imaging. *N Engl J Med* 2018;378(8):708–718.

162. Campbell BCV, Mitchell PJ, Churilov L, et al. Tenecteplase versus alteplase before thrombectomy for ischemic stroke. *N Engl J Med* 2018;378(17):1573–1582.

163. Jumaa MA, Zhang F, Ruiz-Ares G, et al. Comparison of safety and clinical and radiographic outcomes in endovascular acute stroke therapy for proximal middle cerebral artery occlusion with intubation and general anesthesia versus the nonintubated state. *Stroke* 2010;41(6):1180–1184.

164. Nichols C, Carrozzella J, Yeatts S, Tomsick T, Broderick J, Khatri P. Is periprocedural sedation during acute stroke therapy associated with poorer functional outcomes? *J Neurointerv Surg* 2010;2(1):67–70.

165. Abou-Chebl A, Lin R, Hussain MS, et al. Conscious sedation versus general anesthesia during endovascular therapy for acute anterior circulation stroke: preliminary results from a retrospective, multicenter study. *Stroke* 2010;41(6):1175–1179.

166. van den Berg LA, Koelman DL, Berkhemer OA, et al. Type of anesthesia and differences in clinical outcome after intra-arterial treatment for ischemic stroke. *Stroke* 2015;46(5):1257–1262.

167. Simonsen CZ, Yoo AJ, Sorensen LH, et al. Effect of general anesthesia and conscious sedation during endovascular therapy on infarct growth and clinical outcomes in acute ischemic stroke: a randomized clinical trial. *JAMA Neurol* 2018;75(4):470–477.

168. He J, Zhang Y, Xu T, et al. Effects of immediate blood pressure reduction on death and major disability in patients with acute ischemic stroke: the CATIS randomized clinical trial. *JAMA* 2014;311(5):479–489.

169. Tikhonoff V, Zhang H, Richart T, Staessen JA. Blood pressure as a prognostic factor after acute stroke. *Lancet Neurol* 2009;8(10):938–948.

170. Willey JZ, Elkind MS. Stroke: do statins improve outcomes after acute ischemic stroke? *Nat Rev Neurol* 2011;7(7):364–365.

171. Yusuf S, Bosch J, Dagenais G, et al. Cholesterol Lowering in Intermediate-Risk Persons without Cardiovascular Disease. *N Engl J Med* 2016;374(21):2021–2031.

172. Johnston SC, Easton JD, Farrant M, et al. Clopidogrel and aspirin in acute ischemic stroke and high-risk TIA. *N Engl J Med* 2018;379(3):215–225.

173. Roy D, Talajic M, Nattel S, et al. Rhythm control versus rate control for atrial fibrillation and heart failure. *N Engl J Med* 2008;358(25):2667–2677.

174. Amin-Hanjani S, Pandey DK, Rose-Finnell L, et al. Effect of hemodynamics on stroke risk in symptomatic atherosclerotic vertebrobasilar occlusive disease. *JAMA Neurol* 2016;73(2):178–185.

175. Raymond S, Rost NS, Schaefer PW, et al. Patient selection for mechanical thrombectomy in posterior circulation emergent large-vessel occlusion. *Interv Neuroradiol* 2018;24(3):309–316.

176. Jo K, Bajgur SS, Kim H, Choi HA, Huh PW, Lee K. A simple prediction score system for malignant brain edema progression in large hemispheric infarction. *PloS One* 2017;12(2):e0171425.

177. Dohmen C, Sakowitz OW, Fabricius M, et al. Spreading depolarizations occur in human ischemic stroke with high incidence. *Ann Neurol* 2008;63(6):720–728.

178. Drenckhahn C, Winkler MK, Major S, et al. Correlates of spreading depolarization in human scalp electroencephalography. *Brain* 2012;135(Pt 3):853–868.

179. Hofmeijer J, Kappelle LJ, Algra A, et al. Surgical decompression for space-occupying cerebral infarction (the Hemicraniectomy After Middle Cerebral Artery infarction with Life-threatening Edema Trial [HAMLET]): a multicentre, open, randomised trial. *Lancet Neurol* 2009;8(4):326–333.

180. Vahedi K, Hofmeijer J, Juettler E, et al. Early decompressive surgery in malignant infarction of the middle cerebral artery: a pooled analysis of three randomised controlled trials. *Lancet Neurol* 2007;6(3):215–222.

181. Juttler E, Unterberg A, Woitzik J, et al. Hemicraniectomy in older patients with extensive middle-cerebral-artery stroke. *N Engl J Med* 2014;370(12):1091–1100.

182. Schwab S, Steiner T, Aschoff A, et al. Early hemicraniectomy in patients with complete middle cerebral artery infarction. *Stroke* 1998;29(9):1888–1893.

183. Sarov M, Guichard JP, Chibarro S, et al. Sinking skin flap syndrome and paradoxical herniation after hemicraniectomy for malignant hemispheric infarction. *Stroke* 2010;41(3):560–562.

184. Bladin CF, Alexandrov AV, Bellavance A, et al. Seizures after stroke: a prospective multicenter study. *Arch Neurol* 2000;57(11):1617–1622.

185. Lyden P, Hemmen T, Grotta J, et al. Results of the ICTuS 2 trial (Intravascular Cooling in the Treatment of Stroke 2). *Stroke* 2016;47(12):2888–2895.

186. Bruno A, Durkalski VL, Hall CE, et al. The Stroke Hyperglycemia Insulin Network Effort (SHINE) trial protocol: a randomized, blinded, efficacy trial of standard vs. intensive hyperglycemia management in acute stroke. *Int J Stroke* 2014;9(2):246–251.

187. Sherman DG, Albers GW, Bladin C, et al. The efficacy and safety of enoxaparin versus unfractionated heparin for the prevention of venous thromboembolism after acute ischaemic stroke (PREVAIL Study): an open-label randomised comparison. *Lancet* 2007;369(9570):1347–1355.

188. Saver JL, Starkman S, Eckstein M, et al. Prehospital use of magnesium sulfate as neuroprotection in acute stroke. *N Engl J Med* 2015;372(6):528–536.

189. Ginsberg MD, Palesch YY, Hill MD, et al. High-dose albumin treatment for acute ischaemic stroke (ALIAS) Part 2: a randomised, double-blind, phase 3, placebo-controlled trial. *Lancet Neurol* 2013;12(11):1049–1058.

190. Chamorro A, Dirnagl U, Urra X, Planas AM. Neuroprotection in acute stroke: targeting excitotoxicity, oxidative and nitrosative stress, and inflammation. *Lancet Neurol* 2016;15(8):869–881.

191. Einhaupl KM, Villringer A, Meister W, et al. Heparin treatment in sinus venous thrombosis. *Lancet* 1991;338(8767):597–600.

192. Misra UK, Kalita J, Chandra S, Kumar B, Bansal V. Low molecular weight heparin versus unfractionated heparin in cerebral venous sinus thrombosis: a randomized controlled trial. *Eur J Neurol* 2012;19(7):1030–1036.

193. de Bruijn SF, Stam J. Randomized, placebo-controlled trial of anticoagulant treatment with low-molecular-weight heparin for cerebral sinus thrombosis. *Stroke* 1999;30(3):484–488.

194. Qureshi AI, Grigoryan M, Saleem MA, et al. Prolonged microcatheter-based local thrombolytic infusion as a salvage treatment after failed endovascular treatment for cerebral venous thrombosis: a multicenter experience. *Neurocrit Care* 2018;29(1):54–61.

195. Kernan WN, Ovbiagele B, Black HR, et al. Guidelines for the prevention of stroke in patients with stroke and transient ischemic attack: a guideline for healthcare professionals from the American Heart Association/American Stroke Association. *Stroke* 2014;45(7):2160–2236.

196. Roth P, Wick W, Weller M. Steroids in neurooncology: actions, indications, side-effects. *Curr Opin Neurol* 2010;23(6):597–602.

197. Pitter KL, Tamagno I, Alikhanyan K, et al. Corticosteroids compromise survival in glioblastoma. *Brain* 2016;139(Pt 5):1458–1471.

198. Glantz MJ, Cole BF, Forsyth PA, et al. Practice parameter: anticonvulsant prophylaxis in patients with newly diagnosed brain tumors. Report of the Quality Standards Subcommittee of the American Academy of Neurology. *Neurology* 2000;54(10):1886–1893.

199. Beenen LF, Lindeboom J, Kasteleijn-Nolst Trenite DG, et al. Comparative double blind clinical trial of phenytoin and sodium valproate as anticonvulsant prophylaxis after craniotomy: efficacy, tolerability, and cognitive effects. *J Neurol Neurosurg Psychiatry* 1999;67(4):474–480.

200. North JB, Penhall RK, Hanieh A, Frewin DB, Taylor WB. Phenytoin and postoperative epilepsy. A double-blind study. *J Neurosurg* 1983;58(5):672–677.

201. Glantz MJ, Cole BF, Friedberg MH, et al. A randomized, blinded, placebo-controlled trial of divalproex sodium prophylaxis in adults with newly diagnosed brain tumors. *Neurology* 1996;46(4):985–991.

202. Milligan TA, Hurwitz S, Bromfield EB. Efficacy and tolerability of levetiracetam versus phenytoin after supratentorial neurosurgery. *Neurology* 2008;71(9):665–669.

203. Graus F, Titulaer MJ, Balu R, et al. A clinical approach to diagnosis of autoimmune encephalitis. *Lancet Neurol* 2016;15(4):391–404.

204. Titulaer MJ, McCracken L, Gabilondo I, et al. Treatment and prognostic factors for long-term outcome in patients with anti-NMDA receptor encephalitis: an observational cohort study. *Lancet Neurol* 2013;12(2):157–165.

205. Brown PD, Pugh S, Laack NN, et al. Memantine for the prevention of cognitive dysfunction in patients receiving whole-brain radiotherapy: a randomized, double-blind, placebo-controlled trial. *Neuro-oncology* 2013;15(10):1429–1437.

206. Venkatesan A, Geocadin RG. Diagnosis and management of acute encephalitis: a practical approach. *Neurol Clin Pract* 2014;4(3):206–215.

207. de Gans J, van de Beek D. European Dexamethasone in Adulthood Bacterial Meningitis Study I. Dexamethasone in adults with bacterial meningitis. *N Engl J Med* 2002;347(20):1549–1556.

208. Glimaker M, Johansson B, Grindborg O, Bottai M, Lindquist L, Sjolin J. Adult bacterial meningitis: earlier treatment and improved outcome following guideline revision promoting prompt lumbar puncture. *Clin Infect Dis* 2015;60(8):1162–1169.

209. Sheu JJ, Hsu CY, Yuan RY, Yang CC. Clinical characteristics and treatment delay of cerebral infarction in tuberculous meningitis. *Intern Med J* 2012;42(3):294–300.

210. Hasbun R, Abrahams J, Jekel J, Quagliarello VJ. Computed tomography of the head before lumbar puncture in adults with suspected meningitis. *N Engl J Med* 2001;345(24):1727–1733.

211. Thakur KT, Motta M, Asemota AO, et al. Predictors of outcome in acute encephalitis. *Neurology* 2013;81(9):793–800.

212. Wilson MR, O'Donovan BD, Gelfand JM, et al. Chronic Meningitis Investigated via Metagenomic Next-Generation Sequencing. *JAMA Neurol* 2018;75(8):947–955.

213. Ajdukiewicz KM, Cartwright KE, Scarborough M, et al. Glycerol adjuvant therapy in adults with bacterial meningitis in a high HIV seroprevalence setting in Malawi: a double-blind, randomised controlled trial. *Lancet Infect Dis* 2011;11(4):293–300.

214. Whitley RJ, Alford CA, Hirsch MS, et al. Vidarabine versus acyclovir therapy in herpes simplex encephalitis. *N Engl J Med* 1986;314(3):144–149.

215. Critchley JA, Young F, Orton L, Garner P. Corticosteroids for prevention of mortality in people with tuberculosis: a systematic review and meta-analysis. *Lancet Infect Dis* 2013;13(3):223–237.

216. Claassen J, Albers D, Schmidt JM, et al. Nonconvulsive seizures in subarachnoid hemorrhage link inflammation and outcome. *Ann Neurol* 2014;75(5):771–781.

217. Mourvillier B, Tubach F, van de Beek D, et al. Induced hypothermia in severe bacterial meningitis: a randomized clinical trial. *JAMA* 2013;310(20):2174–2183.

218. Straub J, Chofflon M, Delavelle J. Early high-dose intravenous methylprednisolone in acute disseminated encephalomyelitis: a successful recovery. *Neurology* 1997;49(4):1145–1147.

219. Bennetto L, Scolding N. Inflammatory/postinfectious encephalomyelitis. *J Neurol Neurosurg Psychiatry* 2004;75(Suppl 1): i22–i28.

220. Janz DR, Hollenbeck RD, Pollock JS, McPherson JA, Rice TW. Hyperoxia is associated with increased mortality in patients treated with mild therapeutic hypothermia after sudden cardiac arrest. *Crit Care Med* 2012;40(12):3135–3139.

221. Kuisma M, Boyd J, Voipio V, Alaspaa A, Roine RO, Rosenberg P. Comparison of 30 and the 100% inspired oxygen concentrations during early postresuscitation period: a randomised controlled pilot study. *Resuscitation* 2006;69(2):199–206.

222. Kilgannon JH, Jones AE, Shapiro NI, et al. Association between arterial hyperoxia following resuscitation from cardiac arrest and in-hospital mortality. *JAMA* 2010;303(21):2165–2171.

223. Kilgannon JH, Jones AE, Parrillo JE, et al. Relationship between supranormal oxygen tension and outcome after resuscitation from cardiac arrest. *Circulation* 2011;123(23):2717–2722.

224. Youn CS, Park KN, Kim SH, et al. The cumulative partial pressure of arterial oxygen is associated with neurological outcomes after cardiac arrest treated with targeted temperature management. *Crit Care Med* 2018;46(4): e279–e285.

225. Dumas F, Cariou A, Manzo-Silberman S, et al. Immediate percutaneous coronary intervention is associated with better survival after out-of-hospital cardiac arrest: insights from the PROCAT (Parisian Region Out of hospital Cardiac Arrest) registry. *Circ Cardiovasc Interv* 2010;3(3):200–207.

226. Nolan JP, Morley PT, Vanden Hoek TL, et al. Therapeutic hypothermia after cardiac arrest: an advisory statement by the advanced life support task force of the International Liaison Committee on Resuscitation. *Circulation* 2003;108(1):118–121.

227. Bernard SA, Gray TW, Buist MD, et al. Treatment of comatose survivors of out-of-hospital cardiac arrest with induced hypothermia. *N Engl J Med* 2002;346(8):557–563.

228. Hypothermia after Cardiac Arrest Study Group. Mild therapeutic hypothermia to improve the neurologic outcome after cardiac arrest. *N Engl J Med* 2002;346(8):549–556.

229. Nielsen N, Wetterslev J, Cronberg T, et al. Targeted temperature management at 33 degrees C versus 36 degrees C after cardiac arrest. *N Engl J Med* 2013;369(23):2197–2206.

230. Cronberg T, Lilja G, Horn J, et al. Neurologic function and health-related quality of life in patients following targeted temperature management at 33 degrees C vs 36 degrees C after out-of-hospital cardiac arrest: a randomized clinical trial. *JAMA Neurol* 2015;72(6):634–641.

231. Chan PS, Berg RA, Tang Y, Curtis LH, Spertus JA, American Heart Association's get with the guidelines—Resuscitation I. Association between therapeutic hypothermia and survival after in-hospital cardiac arrest. *JAMA* 2016;316(13):1375–1382.

232. Moler FW, Silverstein FS, Holubkov R, et al. Therapeutic hypothermia after out-of-hospital cardiac arrest in children. *N Engl J Med* 2015;372(20):1898–1908.

233. Kirkegaard H, Soreide E, de Haas I, et al. Targeted temperature management for 48 vs 24 hours and neurologic outcome after out-of-hospital cardiac arrest: a randomized clinical trial. *JAMA* 2017;318(4):341–350.

234. Leary M, Grossestreuer AV, Iannacone S, et al. Pyrexia and neurologic outcomes after therapeutic hypothermia for cardiac arrest. *Resuscitation* 2013;84(8):1056–1061.

235. Benz-Woerner J, Delodder F, Benz R, et al. Body temperature regulation and outcome after cardiac arrest and therapeutic hypothermia. *Resuscitation* 2012;83(3):338–342.

236. Choi HA, Ko SB, Presciutti M, et al. Prevention of shivering during therapeutic temperature modulation: the Columbia anti-shivering protocol. *Neurocrit Care* 2011;14(3):389–394.

237. Rittenberger JC, Popescu A, Brenner RP, Guyette FX, Callaway CW. Frequency and timing of nonconvulsive status epilepticus in comatose postcardiac arrest subjects treated with hypothermia. *Neurocrit Care* 2012;16(1):114–122.

238. Mani R, Schmitt SE, Mazer M, Putt ME, Gaieski DF. The frequency and timing of epileptiform activity on continuous electroencephalogram in comatose post-cardiac arrest syndrome patients treated with therapeutic hypothermia. *Resuscitation* 2012;83(7):840–847.

239. Rossetti AO, Oddo M, Logroscino G, Kaplan PW. Prognostication after cardiac arrest and hypothermia: a prospective study. *Ann Neurol* 2010;67(3):301–307.

240. Rossetti AO, Oddo M, Liaudet L, Kaplan PW. Predictors of awakening from postanoxic status epilepticus after therapeutic hypothermia. *Neurology* 2009;72(8):744–749.

241. Legriel S, Bruneel F, Sediri H, et al. Early EEG monitoring for detecting postanoxic status epilepticus during therapeutic hypothermia: a pilot study. *Neurocrit Care* 2009;11(3):338–344.

242. Alvarez V, Sierra-Marcos A, Oddo M, Rossetti AO. Yield of intermittent versus continuous EEG in comatose survivors of cardiac arrest treated with hypothermia. *Crit Care* 2013;17(5):R190.

243. Naples R, Ellison E, Brady WJ. Cranial computed tomography in the resuscitated patient with cardiac arrest. *Am J Emerg Med* 2009;27(1):63–67.

244. Wu AH, McKay C, Broussard LA, et al. National academy of clinical biochemistry laboratory medicine practice guidelines: recommendations for the use of laboratory tests to support poisoned patients who present to the emergency department. *Clin Chem* 2003;49(3):357–379.

245. Gunnerson KJ, Saul M, He S, Kellum JA. Lactate versus non-lactate metabolic acidosis: a retrospective

outcome evaluation of critically ill patients. *Crit Care* 2006;10(1): R22.

246. Forsythe SM, Schmidt GA. Sodium bicarbonate for the treatment of lactic acidosis. *Chest* 2000;117(1):260–267.

247. Gunnerson KJ, Kellum JA. Acid-base and electrolyte analysis in critically ill patients: are we ready for the new millennium? *Curr Opin Crit Care* 2003;9(6):468–473.

248. Swenson ER. Metabolic acidosis. *Respir Care* 2001;46(4):342–353.

249. Clifton J 2nd, Leikin JB. Methylene blue. *Am J Ther* 2003;10(4):289–291.

250. Mokhlesi B, Corbridge T. Toxicology in the critically ill patient. *Clin Chest Med* 2003;24(4):689–711.

251. Bayard M, Farrow J, Tudiver F. Acute methemoglobinemia after endoscopy. *J Am Board Fam Pract* 2004;17(3):227–229.

252. Weaver LK, Hopkins RO, Chan KJ, et al. Hyperbaric oxygen for acute carbon monoxide poisoning. *N Engl J Med* 2002;347(14):1057–1067.

253. Sauer SW, Keim ME. Hydroxocobalamin: improved public health readiness for cyanide disasters. *Ann Emerg Med* 2001;37(6):635–641.

254. Position paper: Ipecac syrup. *J Toxicol Clin Toxicol* 2004;42(2):133–143.

255. Benson BE, Hoppu K, Troutman WG, et al. Position paper update: gastric lavage for gastrointestinal decontamination. *Clin Toxicol* 2013;51(3):140–146.

256. Barceloux D, McGuigan M, Hartigan-Go K. Position statement: cathartics. American Academy of Clinical Toxicology; European Association of Poisons Centres and Clinical Toxicologists. *J Toxicol Clin Toxicol* 1997;35(7):743–752.

257. Tenenbein M. Position statement: whole bowel irrigation. American Academy of Clinical Toxicology; European Association of Poisons Centres and Clinical Toxicologists. *J Toxicol Clin Toxicol* 1997;35(7):753–762.

258. Chyka PA, Seger D, Krenzelok EP, et al. Position paper: Single-dose activated charcoal. *Clin Toxicol* 2005;43(2):61–87.

259. Meadows-Oliver M; American Academy of Pediatrics. Syrup of ipecac: new guidelines from the AAP. *J Pediatr Health Care* 2004;18(2):109–110.

260. Vale JA. Position statement: gastric lavage. American Academy of Clinical Toxicology; European Association of Poisons Centres and Clinical Toxicologists. *J Toxicol Clin Toxicol* 1997;35(7):711–719.

261. Bradberry SM, Vale JA. Poisons. Initial assessment and management. *Clin Med* 2003;3(2):107–110.

262. Proudfoot AT, Krenzelok EP, Vale JA. Position Paper on urine alkalinization. *J Toxicol Clin Toxicol* 2004;42(1):1–26.

263. Rowden AK, Norvell J, Eldridge DL, Kirk MA. Updates on acetaminophen toxicity. *Med Clin N Am* 2005;89(6):1145–1159.

264. Burcar PJ, Norenberg MD, Yarnell PR. Hyponatremia and central pontine myelinolysis. *Neurology* 1977;27(3):223–226.

265. Adrogue HJ, Madias NE. Hyponatremia. *N Engl J Med* 2000;342(21):1581–1589.

266. Schrier RW, Gross P, Gheorghiade M, et al. Tolvaptan, a selective oral vasopressin V2-receptor antagonist, for hyponatremia. *N Engl J Med* 2006;355(20):2099–2112.

267. Weiss-Guillet EM, Takala J, Jakob SM. Diagnosis and management of electrolyte emergencies. *Best Pract Res Clin Endocrinol Metab* 2003;17(4):623–651.

268. Doig GS, Simpson F, Heighes PT, et al. Restricted versus continued standard caloric intake during the management of refeeding syndrome in critically ill adults: a randomised, parallel-group, multicentre, single-blind controlled trial. *Lancet Respir Med* 2015;3(12):943–952.

269. Stravitz RT, Kramer AH, Davern T, et al. Intensive care of patients with acute liver failure: recommendations of the US Acute Liver Failure Study Group. *Crit Care Med* 2007;35(11):2498–2508.

270. Lee WM, Stravitz RT, Larson AM. Introduction to the revised American Association for the Study of Liver Diseases Position Paper on acute liver failure 2011. *Hepatology* 2012;55(3):965–967.

271. Tofteng F, Hauerberg J, Hansen BA, Pedersen CB, Jorgensen L, Larsen FS. Persistent arterial hyperammonemia increases the concentration of glutamine and alanine in the brain and correlates with intracranial pressure in patients with fulminant hepatic failure. *J Cereb Blood Flow Metab* 2006;26(1):21–27.

272. Albrecht J, Norenberg MD. Glutamine: a Trojan horse in ammonia neurotoxicity. *Hepatology* 2006;44(4):788–794.

273. Liotta EM, Romanova AL, Lizza BD, et al. Osmotic shifts, cerebral edema, and neurologic deterioration in severe hepatic encephalopathy. *Crit Care Med* 2018;46(2):280–289.

274. Ferenci P, Lockwood A, Mullen K, Tarter R, Weissenborn K, Blei AT. Hepatic encephalopathy: definition, nomenclature, diagnosis, and quantification: final report of the working party at the 11th World Congresses of Gastroenterology, Vienna, 1998. *Hepatology* 2002;35(3):716–721.

275. Ostapowicz G, Fontana RJ, Schiodt FV, et al. Results of a prospective study of acute liver failure at 17 tertiary care centers in the United States. *Ann Intern Med* 2002;137(12):947–954.

276. Raschke RA, Curry SC, Rempe S, et al. Results of a protocol for the management of patients with fulminant liver failure. *Crit Care Med* 2008;36(8):2244–2248.

277. Yan S, Tu Z, Lu W, et al. Clinical utility of an automated pupillometer for assessing and monitoring recipients of liver transplantation. *Liver Transplant* 2009;15(12):1718–1727.

278. Rajajee V, Vanaman M, Fletcher JJ, Jacobs TL. Optic nerve ultrasound for the detection of raised intracranial pressure. *Neurocrit Care* 2011;15(3):506–515.

279. Figaji AA, Zwane E, Fieggen AG, Siesjo P, Peter JC. Transcranial Doppler pulsatility index is not a reliable indicator of intracranial pressure in children with severe traumatic brain injury. *Surg Neurol* 2009;72(4):389–394.

280. Karvellas CJ, Fix OK, Battenhouse H, et al. Outcomes and complications of intracranial pressure monitoring in acute liver failure: a retrospective cohort study. *Crit Care Med* 2014;42(5):1157–1167.

281. Ellis AJ, Wendon JA, Williams R. Subclinical seizure activity and prophylactic phenytoin infusion in acute liver failure: a controlled clinical trial. *Hepatology* 2000;32(3):536–541.

282. Bhatia V, Batra Y, Acharya SK. Prophylactic phenytoin does not improve cerebral edema or survival in

acute liver failure: a controlled clinical trial. *J Hepatol* 2004;41(1):89–96.

283. Banares R, Nevens F, Larsen FS, et al. Extracorporeal albumin dialysis with the molecular adsorbent recirculating system in acute-on-chronic liver failure: the RELIEF trial. *Hepatology* 2013;57(3):1153–1162.

284. Slack AJ, Auzinger G, Willars C, et al. Ammonia clearance with haemofiltration in adults with liver disease. *Liver Intl* 2014;34(1):42–48.

285. Lidofsky SD. Liver transplantation for fulminant hepatic failure. *Gastroenterol Clin N Am* 1993;22(2):257–269.

286. Caldwell C, Werdiger N, Jakab S, et al. Use of model for end-stage liver disease exception points for early liver transplantation and successful reversal of hepatic myelopathy with a review of the literature. *Liver Transplant* 2010;16(7):818–826.

287. Ely EW, Inouye SK, Bernard GR, et al. Delirium in mechanically ventilated patients: validity and reliability of the confusion assessment method for the intensive care unit (CAM-ICU). *JAMA* 2001;286(21):2703–2710.

288. Hughes CG, Morandi A, Girard TD, et al. Association between endothelial dysfunction and acute brain dysfunction during critical illness. *Anesthesiology* 2013;118(3):631–639.

289. Bellapart J, Boots R. Potential use of melatonin in sleep and delirium in the critically ill. *Br J Anaesth* 2012;108(4):572–580.

290. Cerejeira J, Batista P, Nogueira V, Vaz-Serra A, Mukaetova-Ladinska EB. The stress response to surgery and postoperative delirium: evidence of hypothalamic-pituitary-adrenal axis hyperresponsiveness and decreased suppression of the GH/IGF-1 Axis. *J Geriatr Psychiatry Neurol* 2013;26(3):185–194.

291. Maldonado JR. Neuropathogenesis of delirium: review of current etiologic theories and common pathways. *Am J Geriatr Psychiatry* 2013;21(12):1190–1222.

292. Ely EW, Shintani A, Truman B, et al. Delirium as a predictor of mortality in mechanically ventilated patients in the intensive care unit. *JAMA* 2004;291(14):1753–1762.

293. Fong TG, Jones RN, Shi P, et al. Delirium accelerates cognitive decline in Alzheimer disease. *Neurology* 2009;72(18):1570–1575.

294. Inouye SK, Westendorp RG, Saczynski JS. Delirium in elderly people. *Lancet* 2014;383(9920):911–922.

295. Girard TD, Jackson JC, Pandharipande PP, et al. Delirium as a predictor of long-term cognitive impairment in survivors of critical illness. *Crit Care Med* 2010;38(7):1513–1520.

296. Pandharipande PP, Girard TD, Jackson JC, et al. Long-term cognitive impairment after critical illness. *N Engl J Med* 2013;369(14):1306–1316.

297. Inouye SK, Zhang Y, Jones RN, Kiely DK, Yang F, Marcantonio ER. Risk factors for delirium at discharge: development and validation of a predictive model. *Arch Intern Med* 2007;167(13):1406–1413.

298. van den Boogaard M, Slooter AJC, Brüggemann RJM, et al. Effect of haloperidol on survival among critically ill adults with a high risk of delirium: the REDUCE randomized clinical trial. *JAMA* 2018;319:680–690.

299. Girard TD, Exline MC, Carson SS, et al. Haloperidol and Ziprasidone for treatment of delirium in critical illness. *N Engl J Med.* 2018;27;379(26):2506–2516.

300. Blinderman CD, Billings JA. Comfort care for patients dying in the hospital. *N Engl J Med* 2015;373(26):2549–2561.

301. Rohaut B, Claassen J. Decision making in perceived devastating brain injury: a call to explore the impact of cognitive biases. *Br J Anaesth* 2018;120(1):5–9.

Chapter 9

Prognosis in Coma and Related Disorders of Consciousness and Mechanisms Underlying Outcomes

INTRODUCTION

It is much more difficult to predict the outcome for patients with severe brain damage than to make the usually straightforward diagnosis of brain death. Brain death, in principle, is conceptually a single biologic state with an unequivocal future, while severe brain injuries span a wide range of outcomes depending on a number of variables that include not only the degree of neurologic injury, but also the presence and severity of medical complications. Scientific, philosophic, and emotional uncertainties that attend predictions of outcome from severe brain injuries can intimidate even the most experienced physicians. Nevertheless, the problem must be faced: physicians are frequently called upon to treat patients with severe degrees of neurologic dysfunction. To do the job responsibly, the physician must organize available information to anticipate as accurately as possible the likelihood that the patient will either recover or remain permanently disabled. The physician's role as a translator of medical knowledge is essential in counseling families who must make the ultimate decisions concerning the care of an unconscious patient. The financial and emotional costs of caring for patients who will not recover can exhaust both family and medical staff. Physicians must attempt to reduce those burdens while at the same time retaining an unwavering commitment to do everything possible to treat those who can benefit. Equally important, the rendering of accurate information about the potential levels of recovery and expected time course of evolution of functional recovery after serious brain injuries is essential for informed decision-making by patient surrogates. A present conundrum remains that prognostication is generally accepted as being very imprecise in many instances, yet nevertheless the vast majority of patients with brain injuries currently die as a result of withdrawal of care based on such prognostic assessments.[1-3]

Many groups of neurologists and neurosurgeons have continued to advance studies to identify and quantify early clinical, neurophysiological, radiological, and biochemical indicants that might predict outcome in comatose patients. In addition, large population studies have examined the natural history of recovery in disorders of consciousness (DOC) arising after coma.[4] Several changes

in expectations for outcome following coma have resulted most notably in the area of post–cardiac arrest coma. Several limitations, as discussed later, continue to place stringent demands on physicians to carefully consider all available historical details and the reliability of clinical and laboratory evaluations in their consideration of prognosis for an individual patient. Prospective studies of prognosis in adults and children indicate that within a few hours or days after the onset of coma, neurologic signs and electrophysiological markers in many patients differentiate, with a high degree of probability, the extremes of no improvement or good recovery. Unfortunately, radiologic and biochemical indicators have generally provided less accurate predictions of outcome, with some exceptions discussed later. While accurate coma prognostication continues to improve over time, there is increasing complexity evident in developing accurate predictions for other DOC that mark the initial recovery from coma (e.g., vegetative state [VS] versus minimally conscious state [MCS]) as recently emphasized in cross-disciplinary consensus guidelines[5] reviewed below from the American Academy of Neurology (AAN), American Congress of Rehabilitation Medicine (ACRM), and National Institute of Disability, Independent Living, and Rehabilitation Research (NIDILRR).

The first section of this chapter details what we now know about prognosis, emphasizing broad outcome categories, and both short- and long-term outcomes. To assess the reliability of the data presented in this section, consider the following levels of evidence:

- Level I: Data from randomized trials with low false-positive (α) and low false-negative (β) errors
- Level II: Data from randomized trials with high false-positive (α) or high false-negative (β) errors
- Level III: Data from nonrandomized concurrent cohort studies
- Level IV: Data from nonrandomized cohort studies using historical controls
- Level V: Data from anecdotal case series (modified from Broderick et al.)[6]

The second section addresses mechanisms that may underlie patterns of recovery, or lack thereof, following coma. In this section we discuss advances in neuroimaging and electro-physiological assessments aimed at uncovering the biological distinctions that underlie VS, MCS, and related enduring DOC following coma. The third section frames an integrative approach to the diagnosis and initial assessment of patients with enduring DOC following recovery from coma. This section includes an algorithm for conducting pharmacologic time trials to aid both the evaluation of accurate diagnosis and care of patients at any time point in their recovery.

Figure 9.1 shows a conceptual organization of functional outcomes following severe brain injuries, placing the DOC along a continuum of recovery function on the horizontal axis. As indicated by the interrupted red and green lines intersecting the vertical axis representing level of recovery of motor function, a very wide range of cognitive capacities may be present in the setting of very limited or no observable motor function; this range includes in principle the level of normal cognition typically demonstrated in the locked-in state (LIS) where patients retain some narrow motor output channel.

PROGNOSIS IN COMA

Coma has a grave prognosis. For the two most carefully studied etiologies of coma, traumatic brain injury (TBI) and cardiopulmonary arrest, mortality ranges from 40% to 50%[7] and from 54% to 88%,[8] respectively. Statistics continue to improve since the last edition of this book because of better acute management both in the field and in the intensive care unit (ICU), as well as institution of novel interventions such as targeted temperature management for coma following cardiac arrest.[9–11] While improvements in mortality following common etiologies of coma have been demonstrated,[12–14] morbidity continues to remain highly challenging. Beyond mortality statistics, very few studies of prognosis in coma have looked at large numbers of patients for careful evaluation of outcomes other than survival or death. These studies indicate that patients comatose from TBI have a significantly better prognosis than patients with anoxic injuries. For example, of 1,000 trauma patients in coma for at least 6 hours, 39% recovered independent function at

6 months,[15] whereas only 16% of 500 patients suffering nontraumatic coma made similar recoveries at 1 year.[16]

Statistics such as these, however, are too coarse to guide individual patient management. That step requires clinical judgment combined with accurate knowledge of the medical literature, as applied specifically to the patient's history and with an awareness of common diagnostic pitfalls. This section reviews efforts to predict outcome from coma for different etiologies. The reader will find that the literature continues to provide little specific information about the kind of outcome enjoyed or suffered by patients (cf. Jennett and Bond[17]). As a result, except where specified, descriptions of recovery from coma often connote little more than survival and fail to tell one about the social, vocational, or emotional outcome (i.e., the human qualities) of the life that followed.

The Glasgow Outcome Scale (GOS, Table 9.1), originates from a study of outcome following nontraumatic coma in 500 patients. The definitions attempted to identify fairly precisely what was meant by each grade of outcome. Only a small number of outcomes were chosen in the hope that sufficient numbers of patients would fall into each class to allow statistical analysis but that important differences in medical and social recovery would not be excessively blurred. A shortcoming of this classification is that the category of severe disability (3) is too broad in that it includes all patients who cannot function independently, from those minimally conscious to those almost independent. Most of the reported literature in coma outcomes utilizes the GOS, which requires further subdivision and consideration of outcomes in the severely disabled group as discussed later; this general problem of coarse graining of outcomes arises with many other instruments (e.g., the Cerebral Performance Category Score, CPC, see later) used to assess coma outcomes. Another measure the Glasgow Outcome Scale Extended (GOSE)[18] has improved upon the GOS, and more recent long-term follow up studies of comatose patients have begun to employ the GOSE measure.[4] Another important limitation in evaluating the prognostic data in the literature is that some studies conflate death, VS, and severely disabled but conscious outcomes of coma survivors. For example, when using the prognostic data provided herein, care should be taken to distinguish indicators of death from

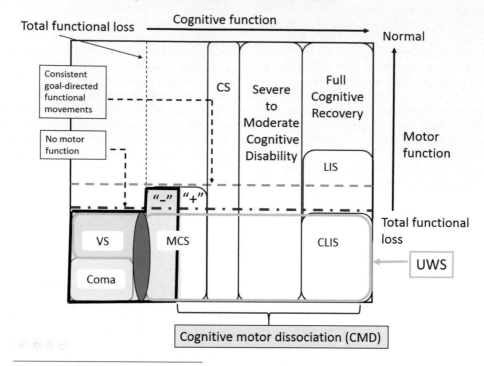

Figure 9.1 Recovery of consciousness following severe brain injuries is represented on a two-dimensional axis plotting degree of expressed cognitive function against degree of measured motor function. The functional equivalence of coma and vegetative state (VS) is marked by their aligned vertical placement to the left of the interrupted vertical line; both are defined as unconscious brain states in which no behavioral evidence of consciousness is present and both cognitive and motor function are absent (VS differing from coma by presence of intermittent eyes open periods). A dark gray oval between coma/ VS and minimally conscious state (MCS) indicates a transition zone where fragments of behavior untied to sensory stimuli may be observed prior to the unequivocal but potentially intermittent behavioral evidence of consciousness demonstrated by MCS patients (see below and Figure 9.5). MCS spans a wide range of expressed behaviors from nonreflexive movements such as visual tracking to inconsistent gestural communications. Recovery of consistent goal-directed behaviors marks the emergence from MCS above the interrupted green line into the range of the confusional state (CS), in which patients are disoriented and exhibit a limited range of cognitive function. CS patients cannot be formally tested using standard neuropsychometric measures. To the extreme right of the figure, locked-in state (LIS) designates conditions typically associated with brainstem strokes in which normal conscious awareness and cognitive function are present, but severe motor impairment limits communication channels typically to vertical eye movements. UWS designates the term "unresponsive wakefulness," which operationally applies to the entire range of patients within the "yellow" lined region. This designation has been suggested by a European consortium to be used in place of VS[19] and appears increasingly in the published literature. While the AAN/ACRM/NIDILRR Guidelines[5] use the term VS/UWS, they note that it is not endorsed. Bernat[20] has provided strong arguments against the adoption of this term. The light gray zone encompassing coma, VS, and the left half of the MCS region (corresponding to the subset of MCS patient who do not show evidence of language comprehension, also known as MCS−; see Bruno et al.[21]) indicates the range of behaviors associated with the proposed designation of cognitive motor dissociation (CMD). CMD patients show behavioral examinations consistent with coma, VS, or limited nonreflexive behaviors seen in MCS− patients, but nonetheless demonstrate command-following as assessed using neuroimaging or electrophysiological techniques.[22] As marked by inverted bracket below the axes, CMD marks the wide range of uncertainty regarding the underlying cognitive capacity present in such patients without any behavioral response to allow for direct assessments.[22] CMD patients may retain a level of cognitive function across a range consistent with that observed in MCS+ (the subset of MCS patients with evidence of language comprehension) to the complete locked-in state (CLIS) in which no communication is evident. Determination of level of cognitive capacity in a CMD patient requires methods allowing the patient to both initiate and respond to communication.

Table 9.1 **Glasgow Outcome Scale (GOS) and the Glasgow Outcome Scale Extended (GOSE)**

Glasgow Outcome Scale (GOS):	
Good Recovery (5)	Patients who regain the ability to conduct a normal life or, if a preexisting disability exists, to resume the previous level of activity.
Moderate disability (4)	Patients who achieve independence in daily living but retain either physical or mental limitations that preclude resuming their previous level of function.
Severe disability (3)	Patients who regain at least some cognitive function but depend on others for daily support.
Vegetative state (2)	Patients who awaken but give no sign of cognitive awareness.
No recovery (1)	Patients who remain in coma until death.
Glasgow Outcome Scale Extended (GOSE):	
Upper Good Recovery (8)	
Lower Good Recovery (7)	
Upper Moderate Disability (6)	
Lower Moderate Disability (5)	
Upper Severe Disability (4)	
Lower Severe Disability (3)	
Vegetative State (2)	
Death (1)	

From Jennett and Bond,[17] with permission

those indicating outcomes including severe disability, which remains a very broad category. Moreover, many outcome studies to do not provide sufficient follow-up of subjects to assess outcomes of chronic VS. To allow comparisons across studies, this chapter indicates the GOS cutoff or other outcome score used in each report here and does not categorize outcomes as "good" or "bad" or "favorable" or "unfavorable." Perhaps even more importantly, many studies do not account for the role of withdrawal of life-sustaining therapies in the statistical outcomes provided.

Another fundamental issue in determining a prognosis for any individual patient is the etiology of injury. It must be recognized that the overwhelming weight of medical knowledge for prognosis in coma falls into two large categories: TBI and anoxic-ischemic brain injury. Unfortunately, there are many additional etiologies that can produce coma and related DOC, and it is often not possible simply to place an individual patient with another etiology into the context of TBI or anoxic-ischemic brain injury. Where possible, information specific to other etiologies is provided herein, but the physician should recognize this general limitation when formulating a prognosis for a comatose patient who has not suffered a TBI or a cardiac arrest.

Finally, it should be emphasized that across the range of etiologies of severe brain injuries producing coma there is recognized uncertainty about the underlying determinants of outcome. Specifically, cellular and circuit-level mechanisms that in principle might allow the restoration of communication or other clinical endpoints that may be meaningful if still co-existent with significant motoric or sensory impairments remain unknown. A mix of recent advances in novel ICU interventions now allow for wide rescue of neuronal viability after varying insults. In this context, demonstrations that neuronal activity may remain deeply suppressed for long periods despite later recovery,[23] and of very delayed recovery of cerebral network function with significant functional restoration,[24] impact our rapidly evolving understanding of prognosis after coma. Improved understanding of the long-term outcome potentials for the individual severely brain-injured subject will eventually require a predictive, mechanistic model of graded capacity to restore cortico-thalamic function which is not yet available; evidence and pointers in direction of such an approach are suggested by the studies reviewed at the end of this chapter.

PROGNOSIS BY DISEASE STATE

Traumatic Brain Injury

More effort has been directed at trying to predict outcome from TBI than from any other cause of coma. This emphasis reflects the high prevalence of TBI (estimated at 1.5–2.0 million persons/year in the United States),[25] the young age of most patients (peak 15–24 years old), and the enormous financial, social, and emotional impact of the illness that may persist for decades. Additionally, more recent initiatives have been triggered by governmental support for the many young veterans with different types of TBI resulting from direct or indirect TBI, such as blast injury. Coma arising from TBI has a better prognosis than nontraumatic coma, likely because patients are usually younger and the pathophysiology differs from other types of coma. Recovery after prolonged traumatic coma is well described, and unconsciousness for 1 month does not necessarily preclude good recovery. Severe head injury causing 6 hours or more of coma still carries a 40% probability of recovering to a level of moderate disability or better.[26] A comprehensive literature review by the Brain Trauma Foundation (BTF) in 2000[7] organizes evidenced-based data for early prognostic signs in TBI. Class I prognostic evidence is listed in Table 9.2. A multivariate statistical model based on these BTF findings, the IMPACT model, has been successfully used to predict mortality and functional outcomes at 6 months following TBI[27,28]; see later discussion.

Table 9.2 Class I Evidence for Early Prognosis in Coma due to Traumatic Brain Injury

I.   Glasgow Coma Scale (see Chapter 1): worsening outcome grades in continuous stepwise manner with lower GCS score

II. Age: 70% positive predictive value (PPV) with increasingly worse outcome in continuous and stepwise manner associated with increasing age

III. Absent pupillary responses: 70% positive predictive value of an outcome less than 4 on the GOS

IV. Hypotension/hypoxia: systolic blood pressure less than 90 mmHg has 67% PPV for an outcome less than 4 on the GOS outcome, and 79% PPV when combined with evidence of hypoxia

V.   CT imaging abnormalities: 70% positive predictive value of an outcome less than 4 on the GOS with initial abnormalities including compression, effacement or blood within the basal cisterns, or extensive traumatic subarachnoid hemorrhage

Developed from Brain Trauma Foundation Guidelines for Management and Prognosis of Severe Traumatic Brain Injury (2000).[7]

The Glasgow Coma Score (GCS) has at least a 70% positive predictive value for an outcome of less than 4 on the GOS. Evaluations done after cardiopulmonary resuscitation were performed after sedative and paralytic agents had been metabolized. Gennarelli et al.[29] found a progressive increase in mortality for patients with descending GCS scores in the 3–8 range in 46,977 head-injured patients. Two studies provide Class I evidence for the predictive value of the GCS. Narayan et al.[30] prospectively studied 133 patients of all age ranges and found that 62% of patients with a GCS of 3–5, when examined either in the emergency room or on admission to an ICU, at later evaluation had a GOS of 1 (Table 9.1). Braakman et al.[31] prospectively studied 305 patients and correlated GOS level 1 outcomes in 100% of patients with a GCS of 3, 80% with a GCS of 4, and 68% with a GCS of 5, respectively. The several studies examined in the BTF review support a survival rate of 20% for patients with the lowest GCS scores and an outcome above the level of severe disability (GOS 4 or 5) in 8–10% of the patients, limiting the use of the GCS alone for prognosis.

MOTOR FINDINGS

A reasonably good indication of outcome can be predicted by testing motor responses to noxious stimulation.[32,33] Abnormal flexor (decorticate), abnormal extensor (decerebrate), or predominantly flaccid responses in patients with severe head injury denote an outcome of less than 4 on the GOS in every reported series. By 6 hours, motor responses no better than abnormal flexor were associated with a mortality of 63%, while abnormal extensor or flaccid responses predicted an 83% mortality.[15] Unfortunately, the European Brain Injury Consortium found that the motor score of the GCS was untestable in 28% of 1,005 patients at the time of admission to a neurosurgery service, and that the full GCS could not be assessed in 44% patients due to prehospital medications and management with intubation.[33] Testing of the motor response by application of nail bed or supraorbital pressure is considered most reliable but may be complicated by tissue injury (e.g., periorbital swelling or quadriplegia, or risk of elevation of intracranial pressure [ICP] in severe TBI patients).[34,35]

AGE

Advanced age unfavorably influences outcome in traumatic coma. Paradoxically, elderly patients may require a much longer recovery time, so it is risky to predict ultimate recovery early in the course. Of 700 patients with severe head injury causing coma, 56% of those less than age 20 recovered to a GOS of 4 or 5. This number fell to 39% between age 20 and 59 years and to only 5% among those older than 60 years.[36] In a prospective study of 372 patients with GCS of less than 13, age greater than 50 and lower GCS scores correlated with higher mortality.[37] A prospective series with 2,664 patients found an essentially linear correlation of age and outcome following severe brain injury.[38] The odds of an outcome less than 4 on the GOS increased 40–50% for every 10 years of age as a continuous variable. A meta-analysis of 5,600 patients identified a continuously worsening prognosis without a sharp step-wise drop at any point.[38] One potential criticism of these studies is that because older individuals may require much longer to recover (in some cases they continue to improve for 6 or 12 months), the assessment times may have been set too early or care may have been withdrawn in elderly individuals, thus truncating their recovery curve. Several factors, other than age alone, may play a role in the association of age with outcome in TBI. Data from the Traumatic Coma Data Bank[7] reveal an increased incidence of intracranial hemorrhage with age and premorbid medical illnesses but did not demonstrate a significant statistical association.

NEURO-OPHTHALMOLOGIC SIGNS

The BTF review identified Class I evidence that loss of pupillary light reflexes has at least a 70% positive predictive value for a poor prognosis following TBI. Bilateral absence of pupillary or oculocephalic responses or both at any point in the illness predict an outcome less than 4 on the GOS. In one series, 95% of patients who had either bilaterally nonreactive pupils or absent oculocephalic responses at 6 hours after injury died.[37]

SECONDARY INJURIES

Hypotension, hypoxia, and uncontrolled intracranial hypertension are independent predictors of poor outcome. Class I evidence supports a high likelihood of an outcome less than 4 on the GOS in comatose TBI patients who suffer either hypoxia or hypotension (defined as a supine systolic blood pressure of less than 90 mm Hg) early in the course. A single episode of hypotension (arterial line reading) is associated with a doubling of mortality and significant increase in morbidity.[7]

NEUROIMAGING

Several neuroimaging findings correlate with outcome following TBI. Class I and strong Class II evidence identifies several computed tomography (CT) findings that predict outcome[7]; accurate interpretation requires consideration of the type of brain injury (e.g., focal brain injuries versus diffuse axonal injury). The majority of patients with TBI have an abnormal CT scan, but certain findings carry a stronger predictive value for an outcome less than 4 on the GOS. Compression of the basal cisterns, a reliable indicator of increased ICP, is a strong negative predictor in several studies[39] (see BTF[7] for review). Midline shift of brain structures, another indicator of increased ICP, is also a predictor of an outcome less than 4 on the GOS.[40] A midline shift of greater than 1.5 cm has a 70% positive predictive value of death.[7] Other CT findings that predict an outcome less than 4 on the GOS include traumatic subarachnoid hemorrhage (SAH) in the suprasellar or ambient cisterns and mass lesions (intracerebral hematoma, variable density CT abnormalities, epidural and subdural hematomas).

DURATION OF COMA

Figure 9.2 reproduces Carlsson's[41] classic diagram (1968) of the effect of duration of TBI-induced coma on outcomes at different ages. Not surprisingly, the longer the coma, the worse the outcome. Although length of coma provides a good indication of severity of brain damage, it can be determined only retrospectively when the patient awakens and thus cannot be used for early prognosis of outcome. On the other hand, it can be predicted with some confidence that a patient in prolonged coma is unlikely to recover. (The same limitation applies to efforts to correlate outcomes of recovery of cognitive functions with the duration of posttraumatic amnesia).

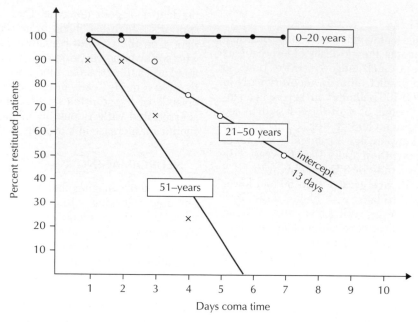

Figure 9.2 Percentage of patients recovered full consciousness as a function of duration of coma for several age groups. From Carlsson et al.,[41] with permission.

ELECTROPHYSIOLOGICAL MARKERS

Electrophysiological measures have limited effectiveness in assessing TBI outcome. Several electroencephalographic (EEG) abnormalities are seen following TBI,[42] and although EEG is useful for the identification of treatable complications of head trauma such as seizures, it does not predict outcome. Somatosensory evoked potentials (SSEPs) are a better indicator.[43] Bilateral absence of cortical components of SSEPs strongly correlates with a GOS below 4[44]; in one small study, bilateral loss of SSEPs predicted outcomes of death or VS in all patients,[45] but other reports indicate that bilateral loss of cortical response in posttraumatic coma may on rare occasions be associated with favorable outcome.[46,47] In these published reports, the measurements may have been confounded by sedating medications or the very early testing of the evoked potentials. Logi et al.[44] prospectively studied 131 comatose patients of varying etiologies including head trauma patients (n = 22) and found 100% specificity for bilateral absence of cortical responses predicting nonawakening when sedating medications had been withdrawn and there were no other metabolic disturbances. However, a more recent study of patients with bilateral loss of SSEPs in initial measurements but able to survive to enter long-term rehabilitation reported a 50% recovery rate of SSEPs late (mean interval 66–55.8 days) on re-examination. A retrospective analysis of outcome in these patients showed that nearly half of the subjects achieved good functional long-term outcomes.[48] Other electrophysiological markers, including cognitive event-related potentials,[49] might provide better prognostic value in future studies. Lew et al.[45] suggested that the P300 response elicited by spoken words such as "mommy" may find use as an early predictor of outcomes greater than 3 on the GOS for comatose TBI patients. However, Perrin et al.[50] found that similar P300 paradigms could not differentiate patients remaining in VS studied months after injury from other patients recovering to higher functional levels. Several studies have examined the mismatch negative (MMN) signal as a candidate to indicate favorable outcome in posttraumatic coma; the presence of the MMN in patients who do not survive coma and slow evolution of dynamic changes in auditory evoked responses require that further refinement of these approaches be considered.[51]

BIOCHEMICAL MARKERS

Elevated serum levels of glial fibrillary acidic protein (GFAP), part of the astroglial skeleton, and S100B, an astroglial protein, have been reported to predict mortality.[52] A recent systematic review found strong evidence for the statistical association of S100B protein concentration and outcomes measured after severe TBI at less than 3-month, 3- to 6-month, and more than 6-month time points. Serum concentration of S100B showed correlation; in a meta-analysis, serum thresholds of 2.16–14 µg/L were associated with 100% specificity for outcomes of 3 or less on the GCS.[53] Another biochemical marker, neuron specific enolase, demonstrated a positive association with outcomes of 3 or less on the GCS, but threshold values for unfavorable prognosis could not be determined.[54] In 42 severely injured adults studied within 7 days of injury, the ratio of glutamate/glutamine and choline was significantly elevated in occipital gray and parietal white matter in patients who showed long-term (6- to 12-month) outcomes of less than 4 on the GOS.[55] Other serum markers have been examined for correlation with prognosis in TBI but have not been studied with similarly large numbers of patients (see Sharma and Stevens[56] for review).

MULTIVARIATE MODELING

Several efforts have been made to establish multivariate predictive models for outcomes of coma following TBI.[28,57,58] No multivariable method has demonstrated prediction at the individual subject level. However, these modeling studies generally support the data reviewed earlier that identify common clinical and neuroimaging features relevant to outcomes (see Sharma and Stevens[56] for review). The IMPACT model is based on the BTF data reviewed earlier.[27,28]

Nontraumatic Coma

PROSPECTIVE ANALYSES OF OUTCOME FROM NONTRAUMATIC COMA

In the late 1960s, a team of investigators at the New York Hospital, led by Plum and co-workers in close association with Jennett and colleagues in Glasgow, undertook prospective studies of the outcome from coma as caused by medical disorders.[16] Collaborating with the Royal Victoria Hospital, Newcastle upon Tyne, United Kingdom, and the San Francisco General Hospital, the investigators ultimately evaluated 500 patients in acute nontraumatic coma. All patients over 12 years old, save those with head trauma or exogenous intoxication in acute coma, were identified and repeatedly examined. Meticulous efforts were made to examine every patient in coma using examining techniques that guaranteed consistency of observation. To avoid bias, the examiners refrained from either making recommendations for therapy or disclosing preliminary results to the treating staffs. The patients were followed for a minimum of 12 months (unless death occurred first) and many for much longer (only 2 of the 500 patients were lost to follow-up). This large population provided landmark data on substantial numbers of individuals in each of the major disease categories, permitting correlations between outcome and both the severity of early signs of neurologic dysfunction and the specific etiology of coma. Subsequent studies have largely confirmed the conclusions drawn from this patient population, including larger prospective studies of coma following cardiac arrest.[59]

The results of the medical coma study indicated that loss of consciousness lasting 6 hours or more bestows a poor prognosis. Of the 500 patients, 379 (76%) died within the first month and 88% had died by the end of a year. Three-quarters of those dying by 1 month never regained consciousness, and, within that month, only 15% of the entire 500 recovered to a GOS of 4 or 5.

Table 9.3 charts the best 1-month recovery by disease state. It should noted that these numbers are likely influenced by practices of withdrawal of life-sustaining therapies.[60] Some of the patients died during that first month of non-neurologic causes, but the table is constructed to indicate the highest possible chance of recovery by the brain. The overall distribution provides some intuition about the relative outcomes of different etiologies of coma. (Actual outcome from the illness in many instances was worse than this best neurologic state because some patients who temporarily recovered neurologically died from complicating conditions, such as

Table 9.3 Best 1-Month Outcome Related to Cause of Coma

Cause of coma	Best 1-month outcome (%)				
	No recovery	Vegetative state	Severe disability	Moderate disability	Good recovery
All patients (500)	61	12	12	5	10
Subarachnoid hemorrhage (38)	74	5	13	5	3
Other cerebrovascular disease (143)[a]	74	7	11	4	4
Hypoxia ischemia (210)[a]	58	20	11	3	8
Hepatic encephalopathy (51)	49	2	16	10	23
Miscellaneous (58)[a]	45	10	14	5	6

[a]Hypoxia ischemia includes 150 patients with cardiac arrest, 38 with profound hypotension, and 22 with respiratory arrest. Other cerebrovascular diseases include 76 with brain infarcts and 67 with brain hemorrhage. Miscellaneous includes 19 patients with mixed metabolic disturbances, 16 with infection.

recurrent cardiac arrhythmias, infections, and pulmonary embolism.)

Nontraumatic coma, while always serious, has a better outcome in some diseases than in others. About 30% of patients with hepatic and miscellaneous causes of coma recovered to a GOS of 4 or 5, three times the recovery rate of patients with vascular ischemic neurologic injuries (SAH, cerebral vascular diseases, and hypoxia ischemia). The difference is explained by most of the hepatic and miscellaneous patients having reversible biochemical, infectious, or extracerebral intracranial (e.g., subdural hematoma) lesions that may have transiently depressed the brain function, but nevertheless left the structure of the brain intact. By contrast, many patients with stroke or global cerebral ischemia suffered destruction of brain structures crucial for consciousness. Reflecting this difference, the metabolic miscellaneous group of patients showed significantly fewer signs of severe brainstem dysfunction than did those with vascular ischemic disorders. For example, corneal responses were absent in fewer than 20% of the metabolic group but in more than 30% of the remaining patients. Furthermore, when patients with hepatic and miscellaneous causes of coma did show abnormal neuro-ophthalmologic signs (see later discussion), their prognosis was as poor as that of patients in the other disease groups with similar signs.

Patients who survived nontraumatic coma had achieved most of their improvement by the end of the first month. Among the 121 patients still living at 1 month, 61 died within the next year, usually from progression or complication of the illness that caused coma in the first place. There were seven moderately disabled patients who improved to a good recovery. Of 39 patients severely disabled at 1 month, nine later improved to a good recovery or moderate disability rating. At the end of the year, three patients remained vegetative and four severely disabled. While current patients may have a greater chance of survival with modern therapies, it is unfortunately not likely that they would have a significantly different natural history after 1 month, suggesting that the data from this series remain relevant.

The outcome was influenced by three major clinical factors: the duration of coma, neuro-ophthalmologic signs, and motor function. Of somewhat lesser importance was the course of recovery; a history of steady improvement was generally more favorable than was initially better function that remained unchanged for the next several days. Only one patient who remained in coma for a week recovered to a GOS of 5 at 1 month. Conversely, the earlier consciousness returned, the better was the outcome. Among patients who awakened and regained their mental faculties within 1 day, nearly half achieved a GOS of 4 or 5, compared with only 14% among those who at 1 day remained vegetative or in coma. Among patients who survived 3 days, 60% of those who were awake and talked made a satisfactory recovery within the first month, compared with only 5% of those still vegetative or in a coma. Contrary to initial expectations, no consistent relationship emerged between age and prognosis either for the study as a whole or for individual illnesses. The sex of the patient had no apparent influence on outcome. Coma of 6 hours or more turned out to be such an innately serious state that in most cases it became difficult to predict accurately who would do well (i.e., make a moderate or good recovery) much before the third day of illness. By contrast, about one-third of patients destined to a GOS of 1 or 2 showed overwhelmingly strong indications of that outcome on admission.

Earlier editions of this book relied on the studies of Levy, Plum, and colleagues who provided specific algorithms and expectations for clinical variables to predict outcomes in nontraumatic coma with high accuracy. Subsequent prospective evaluations of outcome in medical coma have generally confirmed the accuracy of these original studies; however, as changes in a wide range of acute care practices have shifted outcome statistics this 5th edition does not reproduce the original decision-making algorithms. A prospective cohort study of 596 patients with nontraumatic coma identified five clinical variables that predicted 2-month mortality (Table 9.4).[61] This population reflected mostly patients in coma following cardiac arrest (31%), post-cerebral infarction, or intracerebral hemorrhage (ICH) (36%) (other etiologies included SAH, sepsis, neoplasm, infections). Patients with four of five clinical findings of abnormal brainstem responses (absent pupillary responses, absent corneal reflexes, absent or dysconjugate roving eye movements), absent verbal response, absent withdrawal to pain, age greater than 70 years, or a creatinine of 1.5 mg/d or greater (132 mmoles/L), had a 97% mortality at 2 months. An age-related worsening of prognosis was identified in distinction from the Plum and Levy study,[20] but may be partly confounded by comorbid systemic conditions. A prospective study of 169 patients older than

10 years with nontraumatic coma admitted to the ICU found that 75% of those with hypoxic or ischemic injuries had died or remained comatose at 2 weeks (Table 9.5).[62]

Greer et al.[63] undertook a recent effort to reevaluate the utility of the neurological examination in nontraumatic coma in a prospective observational study of 500 patients at a single site. Etiologies included cardiac arrest, SAH, ICH, hepatic encephalopathy, and others. Observations in this study occurred on Days 0, 1, 3, and 7 with outcome assessment utilizing the modified Rankin Scale at 6 months. Clinical examination variables demonstrated strong predictive validity with absence of pupillary reflex providing a significant odds ratio of poor prognosis independent of the day of measurement.

How is one to act on these predictions? The physician, together with the patient's healthcare proxy and the patient's family must decide. A patient who has been in coma for 6 hours from a known nonpharmacologic cause, without pupillary responses or eye movements, has a likely very poor prognosis which will deter many physicians from applying heroic and extraordinary measures of care. (Nevertheless such patients may be candidates for well-controlled new or unconventional treatments, since conventional therapy offers such a dismal outcome.) Conversely, a seriously ill and still unresponsive patient who shows normal eye or motor signs at 1–3 days following cardiac arrest has about a 50% chance of recovering to a GOS of 4 or 5. This information should provide strong encouragement to intensive care staff. The latter individuals often feel they are working blindly and with little chance of success when caring for patients who have suffered brain

Table 9.4 **Variables Correlated with 2-Month Mortality**

Risk factor present on day 3	Two-month mortality, num (%)	
	If factor present	If factor not present
Abnormal brainstem function	88/99 (89)	83/136 (61)
Absent verbal response	151/175 (86)	23/57 (40)
Absent withdrawal to pain	122/136 (90)	52/96 (54)
Creatinine ≥ 132.6 micromol/L (1.5 mg/dL)	82/94 (87)	99/153 (65)
Age ≥70	93/111 (84)	88/136 (65)

From Hamel et al.,[61] with permission

Table 9.5 Two-Week Outcome of Nontraumatic Coma and Coma Etiology

Coma etiology	No. (%)	Awake (%)	Dead (%)	Coma (%)
Hypoxic/ischemic	61 (36.1)	21.3	54.1	24.6
Metabolic or septic	37 (21.8)	32.4	48.7	18.9
Focal cerebral injury	38 (22.5)	34.2	47.4	18.4
Generalized cerebral injury	22 (13.0)	45.4	36.4	18.2
Drug-induced	11 (6.5)	72.7	0	27.3
All	169 (100)	33.1	44.4	21.5

From Sacco et al.,[62] with permission

injury. Knowledge of a potentially favorable outcome greatly improves morale and the associated level of care. Ultimately, survival and level of outcome may depend on the prognosis perceived by the family and caretakers.

CARDIOPULMONARY ARREST/HYPOXIC-ISCHEMIC ENCEPHALOPATHY

The Greer et al.[63] study noted earlier enrolled more than 200 patients with hypoxic-ischemic encephalopathy and found a consistent prediction of negative outcomes for these patients linked to an absent pupillary reflex; some statistical driving of outcome originated from loss of oculocephalic and corneal reflexes as well, supporting the earlier data from Levy et al.[16] Several other large studies have examined outcome in coma specifically following cardiac arrest subsequent to the Levy et al. data. Data from 942 patients prospectively enrolled in the Brain Resuscitation Clinical Trials[64] (circa 1979–1994) demonstrated that loss of any of the cranial nerve reflexes following cardiac arrest significantly predicted poor outcome. Booth et al.[59] reviewed all available large studies of coma following cardiac arrest from 1966 to 2003 to assess the precision and accuracy of the physical examination in prognosis. They found that five clinical signs were strongly predictive of death, VS, or severe disability (GOS 1, 2, or 3): absent corneal reflexes, absent pupillary reflexes, absent withdrawal to painful stimuli, or absent motor response at 24 hours, and absent motor response at 72 hours (Table 9.6). Notably, no clinical examination finding strongly predicted a GOS of 4 or 5. It should be recognized that the Booth et al.[59] predictors aggregate severely disabled outcomes (GOS 3) with outcomes of death or permanent VS (GOS 1 and 2). Thus, careful

explanation of the predicted outcomes is required if the physician uses these data to counsel families as choices concerning severe disability may differ widely (see Fins chapter 11).

Since the publication of the 4th edition of this book, the broad institution of therapeutic hypothermia (TH) and targeted temperature management (TTM) for treatment of post-cardiac arrest coma has resulted in significant shifts in the effectiveness of these early predictive models. It should be first noted that the statistics and approach to formulating a prognostic judgment remain sound in instances in which TTM has not been instituted; the Greer et al.[63] study has verified that similar criteria to that observed by Levy et al.[16] remain consistent in an out-of-sample group treated with modern intensive care methods outside of TTM. Post-cardiac arrest patients treated with TTM, however, must be considered as a separate group.

Recent AAN Practice Guidelines[65] identified strong (Level A) evidence for the use of TH (defined as cooling of the body core temperature to 32–34°C for 24 hours) in comatose patients following cardiac arrest who present with either pulseless ventricular tachycardia or ventricular fibrillation. Additionally, the use of TTM (defined as cooling to 36°C for 24 hours followed with 8 hours of rewarming to 37°C and maintenance of core temperature of less than 37.5°C over 72 hours) showed moderate (Level B) evidence of similar efficacy for such patients and those with asystole or pulseless electrical activity at the time of cardiac arrest. The improved neurological outcomes with TH and TTM have been closely associated with changes in the predictive value of many clinical signs. Rosetti and colleagues[11] organized a comparison of positive and negative predictors of neurological outcomes of coma following cardiac arrest treated with TTM, as shown in

Table 9.6 Useful Clinical Findings in the Prognosis of Post-Cardiac Arrest Coma Organized by Likelihood Ratios (LRs) for Poor Neurological Outcome and Time after Onset of Coma

Clinical finding	Study	LR of poor neurological outcome (95% confidence interval)	
		Positive	Negative
At time of coma onset			
Absent pupillary reflex	Earnest et al.	7.2 (1.9–28,0)	0.5 (0.4–0.6)
Absent motor response	Levy et al.[16]	3.5 (1.4–8.6)	0.6 (0.4–0.7)
Absent corneal reflex	Levy et al.[16]	3.2 (1.1–9.5)	0.7 (0.6–0.8)
Absent oculocephalic reflex	Earnest et al.	2.5 (1.3–4.8)	0.4 (0.3–0.6)
Absent spontaneous eye movement	Levy et al.[16]	2.2 (1.3–4.0)	0.4 (0.3–0.6)
ICS <4	Berek et al.	2.2 (1.1–4.5)	0.2 (0.1–0.6)
GCS <5	Madl et al.[70]	1.4 (1.1–1.6)	0.3 (0.2–0.5)
Absent verbal effort	Levy et al.[16]	1.2 (0.9–1.6)	0.1 (0.0–0.7)
At 12 hours			
Absent cough reflex	Sasser[64]	13.4 (4.4–40.3)	0.3 (0.2–0.4)
Absent corneal reflex	Sasser[64]	9.1 (3.9–21.1)	0.3 (0.2–0.4)
Absent gag reflex	Sasser[64]	8.7 (4.0–18.9)	0.4 (0.4–0.5)
Absent pupillary reflex	Sasser[64]	4.0 (2.5–6.6)	0.5 (0.5–0.6)
GCS <5	Sasser[64]	3.5 (2.4–5.2)	0.4 (0.3–0.4)
Absent motor response	Sasser[64]	3.2 (2.2–4.6)	0.4 (0.3–0.5)
Absent withdrawal to pain	Sasser[64]	2.4 (1.9–3.1)	0.2 (0.1–0.2)
Absent verbal effort	Sasser[64]	1.6 (1.4–1.9)	0.1 (0.0–0.1)
At 24 hours			
Absent cough reflex	Sasser[64]	84.6 (5.3–1342.0)	0.4 (0.3–0.5)
Absent gag reflex	Sasser[64]	24.9 (6.3–98.3)	0.5 (0.4–0.5)
GCS <5	Sasser[64]	8.8 (5.1–15.1)	0.4 (0.3–0.4)
Absent eye opening to pain	Sasser[64]	5.9 (3.9–9.0)	0.3 (0.3–0.4)
Absent spontaneous eye movement	Levy et al.[16]	3.5 (1.4–8.8)	0.5 (0.4–0.7)
Absent eye opening to pain	Levy et al.[16]	3.0 (1.5–6.2)	0.4 (0.3–0.5)
Absent oculocephalic reflex	Sasser[64]	2.9 (1.8–4.6)	0.5 (0.5–0.6)
Absent spontaneous eye movement	Sasser[64]	2.7 (2.1–3.4)	0.3 (0.2–0.3)
Absent verbal effort	Sasser[64]	2.4 (2.0–2.9)	0.1 (0.0–0.1)
At 48 hours			
GCS <6	Madl et al.[66]	2.8 (1.3–5.9)	0.3 (0.1–0.5)
GCS <10	Madl et al.[66]	1.3 (1.0–1.7)	0.0 (0.0–0.7)
At 72 hours			
Absent withdrawal to pain	Levy et al.[16]	36.5 (2.3–569.9)	0.3 (0.2–0.4)
Absent spontaneous eye movement	Levy et al.[16]	11.5 (1.7–79.0)	0.6 (0.5–0.7)
Absent verbal effort	Levy et al.[16]	7.4 (2.0–28.0)	0.3 (0.2–0.5)
Absent eye opening to pain	Levy et al.[16]	6.9 (1.8–27.0)	0.5 (0.4–0.6)
At 7 days			
Absent withdrawal to pain	Levy et al.[16]	29.7 (1.9–466.0)	0.4 (0.3–0.6)
Absent verbal effort	Levy et al.[16]	14.1 (2.0–97.7)	0.4 (0.2–0.6)

In patients not treated with therapeutic hypothermia or targeted temperature management.[59]

From Booth et al.[59] with permission.

Table 9.7. As seen in Table 9.7, the loss of pupillary and corneal reflexes within the first 72 hours remains a strong predictor with a false-positive rate including zero in their confidence intervals. Similarly, bilateral loss of SSEPs remained a strong negative predictor. While no signs predict good outcomes with confidence, several findings showed strong positive predictive value, including the presence of pupillary and corneal responses within 72 hours, the presence of a "continuous" EEG background (i.e., nonepileptiform, nonbursting record with a mix of frequency content), and the absence of reduced diffusion on magnetic resonance imaging (MRI).[11] Notably, the loss of motor responses within the first 72 hours has become an unreliable predictor of outcome in patients treated with TTM or TH.[11] It should also be noted that several of the physiological measures associated with strong negative prediction in Table 9.7 have counterexamples in the published literature. Importantly, a burst suppression EEG pattern which is identified with a very strong negative prediction of outcome if present at 24 hours (0%, FPR confidence interval of 0–17) has been associated with very late good recovery.[23,67] A general problem in the present literature is the lack of available information about the natural history of postcardiac arrest coma lasting more than 5 days as most studies are strongly confounded by institution of withdrawal of life-sustaining therapy after 1 week in a large fraction of patients (Table 9.7).

ELECTROPHYSIOLOGICAL TESTING IN HYPOXIC/ISCHEMIC ENCEPHALOPATHY

Although the physical examination gives a strong prediction of poor outcome, it does not accurately assess the extent of cortical injury in a comatose patient. Electrophysiological testing adds valuable data. SSEPs provide the best predictors of poor outcomes and are relatively insensitive to metabolic derangements and drug effects.[68] Bilateral loss of primary cortical somatosensory responses has been repeatedly confirmed to have virtually 100% specificity for outcomes no better than a chronic VS following anoxic injuries[66,69,70] in patients without TH or TTM treatments (although there may be very rare exception[71,72]). One review found that of 176

patients with absent bilateral primary somatosensory responses (N20), none recovered beyond a persistent VS (Table 9.7).[43] The robust correlation of bilateral loss of SSEPs and poor outcome reflects a close connection with the underlying degree of anoxic injury as indicated by autopsy studies.[73] Of 10 patients examined at autopsy who had SSEP measurements obtained within 48 hours of cardiac arrest, all 7 with bilateral absence of the SSEPs had extensive anoxic-ischemic destruction of the cerebral cortex (with acute ischemic changes in patients with short survival and frank necrosis of the pseudolaminar type in those patients with longer survival times). Two additional patients (one with delayed SSEPs and one with normal latency SSEPs) showed patchy neuronal loss in the cerebral cortex. Importantly, although an index of better outcomes, preservation of normal latency SSEPs following cardiac arrest is not a definite predictor of positive outcomes. Death or vegetative outcomes may occur in as many as 40% of cases where a normal N20 response is measured.[74]

Other electrophysiological techniques including EEG, brainstem auditory evoked responses (BAERs), and transcranial motor evoked responses also have predictive value (see Young et al.[43] for detailed review). EEG patterns are often suppressed early following anoxic injuries, and a variety of signal abnormalities correlate with poor outcomes[42]; these include burst-suppression, alpha-theta patterns, and generalized suppression or periodic patterns. The BAER test can identify severe brainstem injury but does not address the outcome of cerebral cortical injury. Preservation of longer latency auditory evoked responses that involve contributions from larger cerebral cortical networks may predict with greater specificity recovery of cerebral function. Both a late auditory response (N100) and the MMN response have value in predicting outcome from coma following anoxic injury.[75] Other longer latency evoked responses such as the P300 and N400 have also been studied (see Young et al.[43] for review).

BIOCHEMICAL MARKERS

Among several serum biochemical markers evaluated for prognosis of coma following

Table 9.7 Prognosticators in Adult Patients given Targeted Temperature Management

	Feature related to good outcome	PPV (95% CI)	Feature related to poor outcome	FPR (95% CI)
Clinical examination				
Pupillary light reflex	Bilaterally present at >72 h	61% (50–71)	Bilaterally absent at >72 h	0–5% (0–2)
Corneal reflex	Bilaterally present at >72 h	62% (51–72)	Bilaterally absent at >72 h	5% (0–25)
Early myoclonus	NA	NA	Present at <48 h with epileptiform EEG (status myoclonus)	0% (0–3)
Early myoclonus	NA	NA	Present at <48 h with continuous reactive EEG	5–11% (3–26)
Motor reaction to pain	Flexion or better at >72 h	81% (66–91)	Absent or extension posturing at >72 h	10–24% (6–48)
EEG				
Background	Continuous at 12–24 h	92% (80–98)	Diffuse suppression or kw voltage at 24 h	0% (0–17)
	Normal voltage at 24 h	72% (53–86)	Burst suppression at 24 h	0% (0–11)
Reactivity to stimuli	Present during hypothermia	86% (76–92)	Absent during hypothermia	2% (0–9)
	Present after return of normothermia	78% (64–88)	Absent after return of	7% (1–15)
SIRPIDs	NA	NA	Present at any time	2% (0–11)
Repetitive epileptiform transients	NA	NA	Present during hypothermia	0% (0–30)
			Present after return of normothermia	9% (2–21)
SSEP				
SSEP recording	Bilaterally present	58% (49–68)	Bilaterally absent after return of normothermia	0–5% 0–21
NSE				
Serum NSE concentration	<33 μg/L at 48 h	63% (52–83)	>120 μg/L at 48 h	0% (0–1)
			>68 μg/L at 48 h	1% (1–3)
Imaging				
Brain CT	Normal gray–white matter at 2–48 h	37% (9–75)	Reduced gray–white matter ratio at 2–48 h	0% (0–12)
Brain M	Absence of reduced diffusion at 24 h to 7 days	73% (45–92)	Reduced diffusion at 24 h Reduced diffusion 7 days	54% (26–80)

From Rosetti et al.,[11] with permission.

FPR, false positive rate; PIN, positive predictive value; NA, not applicable; SIRPID, stimulus-induced rhythmic, periodic, or ictal discharge; SSEP, somatosensory evoked potential; NSE, neuron-specific enolase.

cardiac arrest, neuron specific enolase (NSE) has shown the most consistent evidence of predictive value (Table 9.7).[11,57] NSE serum concentrations of less than 33 µg/L when assessed at less than 48 hours have shown correlation with good outcomes, whereas NSE concentrations of greater than 120 µg/L within the same time frame have been correlated with a zero false-positive rate of prediction of poor outcome.[11] A recent follow-up of a large sample of 689 post-cardiac arrest comatose patients all treated with TTM showed that serum tau protein significantly predicted CPC 3–5 with high sensitivity and low false-positive rates that outperformed NSE measures in this study.[76] Patients with poor outcomes demonstrated an interquartile range of 5.7–245 ng/L of serum tau levels, whereas good outcome was reliably associated with an interquartile range of 0.7–2.4 ng/L with $p < 0.0001$.

PITFALLS IN THE EVALUATION OF COMA FOLLOWING CARDIOPULMONARY ARREST

Prognosis in coma following cardiopulmonary arrest is susceptible to a range of pitfalls given the narrow time window for decision-making, which usually begins at 5 days and rarely extends beyond 1–2 weeks. Patient Vignette 9.1 illustrates one example from the literature.[77]

Patient Vignette 9.1

A 25-year-old asthmatic man collapsed at home and stopped breathing. The patient received cardiopulmonary resuscitation (CPR) from a family member for 6 minutes until emergency medical technicians arrived to find the patient without respiratory effort or palpable pulse. An electrocardiogram (EKG) showed a rate of 24 bpm; CPR and tracheal intubation were performed. Three minutes later, the pulse was 107 bpm and spontaneous respirations were noted. Initial Glasgow Coma Scale was 3. In the emergency room, the patient was unresponsive with dilated pupils that were responsive to light; spontaneous decorticate posturing was noted. The patient was sedated with propofol, given atracurium, and transferred to the intensive care unit (ICU).

In the ICU, the patient required minimal pressor support and was noted to exhibit frequent myoclonic jerks of the head and all four limbs. Electroencephalogram (EEG) recordings revealed generalized status epilepticus. Theophylline levels were within the normal therapeutic range. Seizures were uncontrolled with phenytoin, midazolam, clonazepam, valproate, and $MgSO_4$, resulting in thiopental infusion producing burst. After cessation of the thiopental drip, generalized alpha frequency activity was noted. On the sixth day, the patient was extubated, given a Do Not Resuscitate status, and transferred to the general neurology floor still with a GCS of 3. He subsequently gradually improved and had a GCS of 10 by day 16 with the recovery of head nodding and verbalization. His GCS reached 15 by the 19th week following the respiratory arrest. While EEG examinations showed progressive improvements, the patient continued to exhibit frequent myoclonic jerks and epileptiform activity despite multiple antiepileptic medication trials. Ultimately, this patient regained independent function.

Comment

This patient's case highlights the potential complexity of prognosis in coma even in circumstances that appear to predict poor outcome following cardiac arrest and severe hypoxic injury. A retrospective review of the history suggests several points for consideration. While the patient's young age, initial presence of pupillary light responses, and early return of spontaneous respiration were positive predictors, the presence of myoclonus and seizures with no history of epilepsy suggested severe hypoxic injury. As reviewed earlier, postanoxic myoclonus has in some studies been associated with poor outcomes,[78] but this is not invariably the case.[79] More recent studies indicate that good outcomes can occur with postanoxic myoclonus of all types.[80–82] The early sedation and paralysis of the patient due to the seizure activity may have masked improvement in level of consciousness within the first 6 hours, and the extensive use of different antiepileptic medications may have mimicked the pattern of alpha coma, a finding that otherwise carries a greater than 90% mortality in the setting of anoxic injury.[83]

This patient demonstrates the limitations of obtaining complete information from events in the field and unequivocal separation of the effects of primary injury versus potential confounds introduced by methods of treatment. A pulseless patient may still have some undetected circulatory activity or have lost perfusion just prior to evaluation, making accurate estimate of duration of hypoxic ischemia problematic. A similar case involving seizures and myoclonus following a cardiac arrest has been reported in literature with late improvement on day 16 after remaining at a GCS of 5 until that point.[84]

Finally, a postictal state can severely depress brainstem function, and tonic seizures can simulate flexion or extension posturing, whereas single epileptic jerks can be difficult to distinguish from myoclonus. Cardiac arrest from a seizure-induced cardiac arrhythmia can further complicate the picture.

Further complicating the early stage of formulating a prognosis in post-cardiac arrest coma are well-documented cases of late (>2 weeks, up to 6 weeks) emergence from coma that progress to good outcomes.[23,66,85] Such observations indicate that intrinsic neuronal dysfunction may not return for variable periods of time following cardiac arrest; the underlying mechanisms producing such enduring depressed neuronal function are not as yet characterized.

Vascular Disease

ISCHEMIC STROKE

Prognosis in coma following stroke depends on the arterial territory affected by the stroke that produces bilateral hemispheric dysfunction, as detailed in Chapter 2. Wijdicks and Rabinstein surveyed the literature of prognostic factors for severe stroke from 1966 to 2003.[86] They found no evidence-based studies better than Class 3 to indicate prognosis, although several suggestive clinical and radiological features were identified. Large proximal vessel occlusions causing diffuse hemispheric edema and midline shift carry a grave prognosis, with a nearly 90% mortality when the shift of the septum pellucidum was greater

than 12 mm.[87] Patients with coma caused by acute basilar occlusions may recover[88] (see Chapter 2), whereas those with coma due to hypertensive pontine hemorrhages usually do not.[89]

INTRACEREBRAL HEMORRHAGE

ICH typically results in impairment of consciousness if bleeding or the associated mass effect involves deeper structures (i.e., bilateral thalami or the midbrain), large cortical areas with possible herniation, or if associated with intraventricular extension of the often periventricular deeper hemorrhages. Morbidity and mortality in patients with ICH are driven by hemorrhage volume and location, presence of ventricular hemorrhage, neurological function on admission (GCS), and patient pre-hemorrhage baseline (age, cognitive impairment). Outcome prediction scores like the primary ICH score and the FUNC score incorporate these measures.[90,91]

SUBARACHNOID HEMORRHAGE

Coma resulting from spontaneous SAH has a grave prognosis. The World Federation of Neurological Surgeons (WFNS) grades SAH using the GCS[92] (see also Table 9.8).[93] Although brief loss of consciousness is common, coma is a relatively uncommon sign in patients who reach the hospital with SAH; two-thirds present with WFNS Grade III examinations or better. However, as many as one-half of the patients presenting with grades I or II deteriorate from vasospasm, rebleeding, hydrocephalus, or brain edema. About 10% (range 3–17%) of patients die before reaching medical attention, and another 10% die prior to hospital evaluation. The overall mortality is 40–50%.[94] Grade V SAH associated with GCS 3 at presentation, however, has been associated in one study with a 22% rate of good outcome.[95]

Loss of consciousness at the time of hemorrhage was strongly associated with death following SAH.[96] GCS is a good predictor of outcome from SAH if the patient's age, the amount of blood on CT scan, the location of the aneurysm (worst for posterior circulation sites compared with anterior circulation),[94] and secondary complications following the initial rupture are also factored in. A high percentage of patients with grades IV and V die

Table 9.8 **Somatosensory Evoked Potentials (SSEPs) in Anoxic-Ischemic Encephalopathy: Absent N20 Response**

Series	Day	Proportion with sign	Proportion recovering
Brunko and Zegers De Byl, 1987	<8 h	30/50	0/30
Rothstein, 2000	<2 h	19/40	0/19
Madl et al., 2000	<2 h	22/66	0/22
Chen et al., 2000	1–3	12/34	0/12
Total	<3	83/190	0/83

From Young et al.,[43] with permission.

from secondary complications if they remain in coma for 2 weeks or more. Prognostication tools that combine clinical (Hunt Hess or WFNS score which are heavily driven by the level of consciousness, aneurysmal rebleeding), medical (acute physiology and chronic health evaluation), imaging (intraventricular hemorrhage), and premorbid measures (age, education level, premorbid GOS) may assist in predicting patients' functional, cognitive, and quality of life outcomes following aneurysmal SAH.[97,98]

In addition to demographic variables (i.e., age) and clinical presentation (i.e., loss of consciousness) discussed earlier, direct effects of the primary hemorrhage (aneurysm size and bleeding size and location), aneurysm rebleeding, and medical complications were primary factors associated with death following SAH.[99] Rebleeding of an aneurysm causing coma and depression or loss of brainstem reflexes carries a mortality of 50%. In one study, bilateral loss of pupillary responses carried a 95% mortality rate. Electrophysiological measurements have also shown some utility in the prognosis of SAH; loss of brainstem auditory evoked potentials and SSEPs correlate with poor grades on examination.[100,101]

Central Nervous System Infection

Coma was present on admission in 14% of 696 patients with bacterial meningitis[102] (see also Chapter 5). Obtundation on admission was a significant risk factor for death or a GOS less than 4, as were age over 60 years, hypotension, seizures within 24 hours (often associated with a low serum sodium), and cerebrospinal fluid (CSF) abnormalities including decreased glucose concentration or elevation of the CSF protein (250 mg/dL or higher). In most cases death was a result of herniation, occasionally following an ill-advised lumbar puncture. Some

investigators have suggested that the presence of coma is the best predictor of morbidity from acute meningitis.[103] Coma is often the result of increased ICP resulting from alteration of the blood–barrier by toxins (vasogenic edema), impaired resorption of CSF (interstitial edema), or venous or arterial occlusions (infarction with cytotoxic edema).[104] Recent studies of coma in the setting of fulminant bacterial meningitis nonetheless underscore that if aggressive medical management is successful in bringing patients to hospital discharge, the majority of patients can have an excellent neurological recovery.[105] Depth of coma as measured by the GCS in one study showed inverse correlation with the odds ratio of death or major disability consistent with earlier studies.[105] Cognitive slowing has been reported in survivors of bacterial meningitis, which may slowly improve over years.[106] A brain abscess causing coma also has a poor prognosis (GOS less than 4);[107] herniation is the principal cause of coma, with a 60% mortality.[104]

Viral encephalitis and meningitis may be associated with coma particularly when the course is complicated by bleeding, seizures, or herniation. Particularly, herpes virus–related infections need to be diagnosed rapidly as effective treatment is available (for details regarding the management, please refer to Chapters 7 and 8). Coma in patients with herpes simplex encephalitis carries a poor prognosis.[109]

Autoimmune Encephalitis and Encephalomyelitis

Acute disseminated encephalomyelitis(ADEM) is a monophasic autoimmune demyelinating disease most commonly affecting children and young adults that follows viral or bacterial illnesses or may arise post-vaccination.[110]

(See also Chapter 5) Although prognosis for ADEM has historically been considered poor, current experience reflects that most patients (range 55–90% across studies) will recover fully or with minor neurological disabilities. The improved prognosis may reflect either the increased frequency of diagnosis of relatively mild cases, which often can be demonstrated on MRI, or perhaps the tendency to treat patients with corticosteroids. Most patients with ADEM improve within 6 months although many documented cases showed longer recovery times. In a retrospective multicenter study over 7 medical ICUs, 20 patients with ADEM presented with a mean GCS of 7; of this cohort 5 died, 1 remained partially dependent, and 14 patients gained independent ambulation.[111] Compared to the patients with independent ambulation, patients who died or remained severely disabled had lower significantly lower GCS scores and increased seizure activity.

Recent advances in diagnosis and management of autoimmune encephalitis, including more aggressive autoimmune modulatory approaches, have resulted in striking improvements in outcomes, particularly for patients with N-methyl-D-aspartate (NMDA)-mediated encephalitis.[112] When diagnosed and treated early and aggressively, patients may survive with no or minimal deficits, but diagnosis remains challenging.

Hepatic Coma

Hepatic coma develops either as an inexorable stage in progressive hepatic failure or as a more reversible process in patients with portal-systemic shunts when increased loads of nitrogenous substances are suddenly presented to the circulation (see Chapter 5). Prognosis in hepatic coma depends on the cause, the acuteness and severity of the liver failure, and the presence of cerebral edema, as well as dysfunction of other organs. Patients with cerebral edema and increased ICP typically are in fulminant hepatic failure and have a much worse prognosis, with more than 50% dying, although many of these die of systemic complications.[113] Patients with chronic cirrhosis or portacaval shunting typically have a better prognosis, and, among all patients with nontraumatic coma, those with hepatic encephalopathy demonstrated the best chance for recovery (33%).[16]

Survival also correlates with age in patients with infectious and serum hepatitis. Patients with chronic hepatocellular disease often drift in and out of encephalopathy, a situation that can be managed by correction of intercurrent processes such as infection or reduction of circulating nitrogenous load. If no exogenous factor can be identified, the presence of encephalopathy is far more ominous and correlates with high mortality; approximately 50% of patients with cirrhosis die within 1 year of demonstrating encephalopathy.[114] A risk model for deterioration in hepatic encephalopathy has been developed to assess triaging of hepatic encephalopathy for liver transplantation, which may nonetheless be associated with persistent cognitive dysfunction in severe cases.[115]

Prolonged Hypoglycemia

Few studies have looked at coma associated with prolonged hypoglycemia.[116–118] While short-term alteration of consciousness and coma associated with hypoglycemia is common as a result of diabetes (see Chapter 5), coma in the setting of prolonged hypoglycemia is generally considered a grave illness with a uniformly poor prognosis. A small number of studies have examined outcomes in the setting of prolonged coma resulting from sustained hypoglycemia. In a multicenter study of 49 patients in coma for more than 24 hours following hypoglycemia, overall outcomes were poor (63%, 22 nonsurvivors, 9 survivors); however, in this study 6 patients discharged with poor functional status improved at 1 year, with 5 reaching a good outcome (on Modified Rankin Scale[119]). Prolonged hypoglycemia of greater than 480 minutes duration was associated with uniformly poor prognosis in this cohort; good premorbid function and normal brain imaging appeared as potential factors associated with good outcomes. The presence of early-onset seizures showed a statistical association with poor outcome. A separate small retrospective study demonstrated similar outcomes.[116]

Depressant Drug Poisoning

Most fatal intentional depressant drug poisonings occur outside the hospital. Once such patients reach treatment, experienced centers worldwide generally report an overall mortality among intoxicated patients with altered consciousness of less than 1% (cf. Table 9.5). The death rate climbs to approximately 5% in those with grade 3 to 4 coma. The mortality can be substantially higher when institutions treat only small numbers of patients or lack experience or proper facilities. Adverse prognostic factors in depressant drug coma include an advanced age, the presence of complicating medical illnesses (especially systemic infections, hepatic insufficiency, and heart failure), and lengthy coma. Alkaline diuresis (for phenobarbital), hemodialysis, and charcoal hemoperfusion all have been reported to shorten coma and improve prognosis for patients with severe poisoning, especially from phenobarbital. Barring unexpected complications, patients recovering from depressant drug poisoning suffer no residual brain damage even after prolonged coma lasting 5 days or more. Rare exceptions to this rule occur in overdose patients who suffer aspiration pneumonia or cardiac arrest (e.g., during tracheal or gastric intubation). A small number of patients develop cutaneous pressure sores or pressure neuropathies from prolonged periods of immobility during the period of immobile coma before the victim is found and brought to hospital; this may be particularly common with barbiturate overdoses.

PROGNOSIS IN DISORDERS OF CONSCIOUSNESS

Vegetative State

The *vegetative state* (also called *coma vigil* or *apallic state* in the past, and most recently, *unresponsive waking state* or *UWS*, see below) denotes the recovery of a crude cycling of arousal states heralded by the appearance of "eyes-open" periods in an unresponsive patient.[120] Very few patients remain in eyes-closed coma for more than 10–14 days; vegetative behavior usually replaces coma by that time. Patients in the VS, like comatose patients, show no evidence of awareness of self or their environment but do retain brainstem regulation of cardiopulmonary function and visceral autonomic regulation. The term *persistent vegetative state* (PVS) introduced by Plum and Jennett in 1972 to refer to patients

who remained in that state for prolonged periods of time, is generally commonly reserved for patients remaining in that state for at least 30 days (see ANA Committee on Ethical Affairs 1993).[121] However, the term had initially gone into disuse following the suggestion of Jennett,[122] who has pointed out that of those patients who were vegetative at 1 month, 43% awakened by 1 year, and that, even after 6 months, 13% eventually regained consciousness. As indicated in the following paragraphs, there are no clear criteria for determining when VS becomes permanent. Moreover, the recent AAN/ACRM/NIDILRR Guidelines (see later discussion) have established a US practice guideline for the removal of this term and its replacement with "chronic vegetative state" in place of "permanent" for patients remaining in VS at 3 months after nontraumatic brain injuries and 12 months following TBI.[5]

One reason for the inability to predict permanence early in the course of VS is that patients usually have badly damaged cerebral hemispheres combined with a relatively intact brainstem. Such a combination during the early days of illness causes coma with relatively good brainstem function, a picture similar to patients with reversible cerebral injury. Another important factor is that even prolonged VS in the setting of very severely deafferented brains may in some instance be responsive to interventions[123] and thus harbor a potential substrate for behaviorally identifiable changes in responsiveness. Nonetheless, there is general evidence that prolonged VS is associated with typically no further recovery or very limited recovery when correlated with clear evidence of very extensive multifocal cerebral deafferentation.

Minimally Conscious State

The minimally conscious state, MCS,[124] identifies a condition of severely impaired consciousness with minimal but definite behavioral evidence of self- or environmental awareness. Table 9.11 provides the criteria for the diagnosis of MCS. Like VS, MCS often exists as a transitional state arising during recovery from coma or during the worsening of progressive neurological disease. In some patients, however, it may be a chronic condition.

MCS also includes some forms of the clinical syndrome of akinetic mutism (Box 9.1 and Figure B9.1) and other less well-characterized

Box 9.1 Akinetic Mutism Versus "Slow Syndrome"

The term "akinetic mutism" originated with Cairns et al.[129] They described a young woman who, although appearing wakeful, became mute and rigidly motionless when a craniopharyngiomatous cyst expanded to compress the walls of her third ventricle and the posterior medial-ventral surface of the frontal lobe. The patient appeared to be unconscious; there was no spasticity. After the cyst was drained, she recovered full awareness but possessed no memory of the "unconscious" period. Eye movements were not described in this woman, but most documented cases of this type reveal seemingly attentive, conjugate eye movements.

Subsequent observations have shown that similar findings can be produced by lesions of the medial-basal prefrontal area, the anterior cingulate cortex, the medial prefrontal regions supplied by the anterior cerebral arteries, and the rostral basal ganglia. A similar syndrome can rarely be a feature of untreated, rigid Parkinson's disease, or prion disease.[130]

The hyperattentive form of akinetic mutism is typically seen in patients with bilateral lesions of the anterior cingulate and medial prefrontal cortices, as occurs after rupture of an anterior communicating artery aneurysm.[131] The associated injury may sometimes be accompanied by injury to the hypothalamus and anterior pallidum. Castaigne et al.[132] and Segarra[133] introduced "akinetic mutism" to

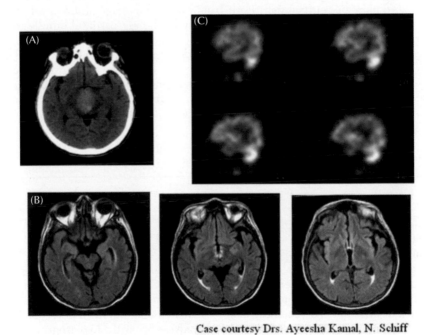

Case courtesy Drs. Ayeesha Kamal, N. Schiff

Figure B9.1 Akinetic mutism. (A) CT scan demonstrating large mesencephalic mass with surrounding edema. (B) Series of MRI axial images following treatment with steriods and reduction of mesencephalic lesion. Middle image shows high signal abnormalities in the ventral midbrain. (C) SPECT imaging demonstrates diffuse cerebral hypoperfusion with relative sparing of cerebellar blood flow.

Box 9.1 Akinetic Mutism Versus "Slow Syndrome" (cont.)

describe the behavior of patients suffering structural injuries affecting the medial-dorsal thalamus extending into the mesencephalic tegmentum. The patients suffered severe memory loss and demonstrated apathetic behavior. Although such patients exhibit severe global disturbances of consciousness, they are not categorized as minimally conscious because they are capable of communication. To mitigate confusion, we use the term "slow syndrome"[126] to describe patients who appear apathetic and hypersomnolent but are able to move and may speak with understandable words.[134] Unlike akinetic mute patients, they are not semi-rigid, and they lack the appearance of vigilance. Subcortical lesions that may produce the slow syndrome include bilateral lesions of the paramedian anterior or posterior thalamus and basal forebrain, the mesencephalic reticular formation including periaqueductal gray, caudate nuclei (or left caudate in isolation), globus pallidus interna, or selective interruption of the medial forebrain bundle (reviewed in Schiff and Plum[124]).

A common denominator of akinetic mute states may be damage to the cortico-striato-pallidal-thalamocortical loops that are critical for the function of the frontal lobes.[135,136] The distinction between hypervigilant akinetic mutism and "slow" syndrome/abulic states may reside in the degree of available frontal cortical systems maintaining a capacity for sensorimotor integration and emitted behaviors although no studies have specifically addressed a functional boundary between these conditions. The prefrontal cortex is served by a loop including the ventral striatum, ventral pallidum, and mediodorsal nucleus of the thalamus, and akinetic mutism can result from bilateral damage at any level of this system.[135] Similarly, bilateral injury that includes the nigrostriatal bundle in the lateral hypothalamus may produce a state of akinetic mutism that is similar to severe parkinsonism and is reversible with dopaminergic agonists.[137] Similarly, patients with VS and MCS clinical exams with traumatic brainstem injuries showing evidence of damage to the ventral tegmental tract may also demonstrate responsiveness to L-dopa.[138] At least partial cognitive function can be recovered following restricted bilateral injuries to the paramedian thalamus and mesencephalon.[132,133,139,140]

DOC. At least two different identifiable groups of patients are considered exemplars of akinetic mutism: those with a hypervigilant appearance and nearly motionless state and another group of patients with very slowed behaviors and apathy.[125,126] Although occasionally confused with the VS, classical akinetic mutism resembles a state of constant hypervigilance. The patients appear attentive and vigilant but remain motionless, with robust preservation of visual tracking in the form of smooth pursuit movements (or optokinetic responses). Limited preservation of brief visual fixation can be accepted in the VS, but robust and consistent visual tracking as seen in akinetic mutism is absent in VS.[122]

Patient Vignette 9.2

A 47-year-old right handed man was brought to the ICU with progressive somnolence and unresponsiveness. Neurological examination revealed bilateral third nerve palsy, fluctuating bradycardia with hypertension and extensor posturing to pain. The initial CT scan (Figure B9.1A) revealed a large mass lesion centered on the mesencephalon with surrounding edema. Intracranial lymphoma was suspected and confirmed by biopsy. The patient received cranial irradiation, IV steroids and chemotherapy. A post-treatment MRI (Figure B9.1B) demonstrated resolution of mass effect with

high signal abnormalities within the upper mesencephalon and hypothalamus. The patient
appeared alert but did not intiate communication. He occasionally displayed sudden periods
of agitated behavior. Responses to simple
questions were markedly delayed, but correct
using yes and no answers. Physical examination
was notable for waxy flexibility and as well as rigidity and spontaneous movements were minimal and limited to the left upper extremity.

EEG showed periods of frontal intermittent
rhyhmic delta activity and mild generalized
slowing. An HmPAO SPECT revealed diffuse
profound frontal bihemispheric hypoperfusion
(left greater right, see Figure B9.1C). The
patient's clinical state did not improve prior to
death from a systemic infection.

Autopsy of brain was normal except for the
midbrain, hypothalamus and left paramedian
thalamus which showed infiltration of lymphoma
cells and necrosis in the midline of the midbrain
extending rostrally into the left thalamus to involve
the intralaminar nuclei and surrounding tissue.

Since the publication of the fourth edition
of this book, new guidelines[5] issued jointly by
the AAN/ACRM/NIDILRR have re-examined
earlier guidelines developed in 1995 based on
the Multisociety Task Force on PVS,[127,128] a
joint commission composed of neurologists,
neurosurgeons, and other specialists who organized a comprehensive review of outcomes
of patients with prolonged VS using GOS
criteria. In the original task force guidelines,
outcomes of 434 adult and 106 pediatric
patients with TBI and 169 adult and 45 pediatric patients with nontraumatic etiologies
of VS were assessed. Table 9.11 displays data
from the TBI group for adults. For patients in
VS for at least 1 month, 52% had recovered
consciousness at 1 year post-injury (some 33%
of the patients had recovered earlier than
3 months from the time of injury). If adult
TBI patients remained in VS at 3 months, the
percentage recovering consciousness at 1 year
dropped to 35%, and to 16% for VS lasting
at least 6 months. For pediatric patients with
TBI-induced VS for 1 month, 62% recovered
consciousness at 1 year; if VS persisted for
3 months, this percentage dropped only to
56% and to 32% for patients in VS for at least
6 months. The outcome of "conscious" per se

**Table 9.9 Grading System
for Subarachnoid Hemorrhage,
World Federation of Neurological
Surgeons (WFNS)**

Grade	GCS Score	Presence of any motor deficit
I	15	None
II	14–15	None
III	14–13	Present
IV	12–7	Present or Absent
V	6–3	Present or Absent

WFNS score is indexed by Glasgow Coma Score (GCS) and
evidence of identifiable motor deficits.

From Report of World Federation of Neurological Surgeons
Committee,[92] with permission.

does not reflect level of disability. However,
the Task Force review indicated that, for
adults, within the 52% of patients recovering
consciousness after 1 month in VS, only
24% became independent by GOS criteria.
This figure dropped to 16% for VS lasting
3 months and to only 4% if taken out to at
least 6 months.

Not surprisingly, nontraumatic VS carried a
far less optimistic prognosis. Table 9.12 shows
comparison percentages for adult and pediatric patients with nontraumatic VS. For adult
VS patients remaining in VS at 1 month, only
15% regained consciousness (with only 4%
independent by GOS). These percentages
worsened to 8% and 0% for patients remaining
in a nontraumatic VS for 3 or 6 months,
respectively.

Based on these data, the Task Force paper
suggested that VS after 12 months following
TBI or 3 months following an anoxic injury should be considered essentially permanent. However, as noted in the new AAN
Guidelines,[5] only a very limited segment of
patients had longitudinal follow-up driving
these recommendations. In the current
guidelines, the denotation of "permanent"
for either VS or MCS is not recommended,
in favor of "chronic" modifying either condition. It is important to recognize that some patients may recover from VS beyond these time
points.[145–147] Such late recovery past the cutoffs
for permanent VS from both anoxic and traumatic etiologies has generally been to levels
of severe disability including the MCS.[145–147]
Nevertheless, application of these statistics

Table 9.10 Aspen Working Group Criteria for the Clinical Diagnosis of the Minimally Conscious State

Evidence of limited but clearly discernible self or environmental awareness on a reproducible or sustained basis, as demonstrated by one or more of the following behaviors:
1. Simple command-following
2. Gestural or verbal "yes/no" responses (independent of accuracy)
3. Intelligible verbalization
4. Purposeful behavior including movements or affective behaviors in contingent relation to relevant stimuli: examples include:
   a. Appropriate smiling or crying to relevant visual or linguistic stimuli
   b. Response to linguistic content of questions by vocalization or gesture
   c. Reaching for objects in appropriate direction and location
   d. Touching or holding objects by accommodating to size and shape
   e. Sustained visual fixation or tracking as response to moving stimuli

From Giacino et al.,[124] with permission.

to individual cases can be risky unless independent evidence of the mechanism of brain injury is available, as rare cases of late recovery continue to be reported. The uncertainty in prognosis in such cases highlights the need for better methods, such as direct measurements of cerebral function, to help identify cases where recovery is likely.

Mortality is very high within the first year; approximately one-third of patients die.[127,128] If patients remain alive after a year, mortality per year is low, and some patients may continue to live for many years.[122] Plum and Schiff studied one patient who had remained in PVS for 25 years (Figure 9.5).[148] Most patients in VS die from infection of the pulmonary system or urinary tract.

The new AAN, ACRM, and NIDILRR Guidelines expand on these earlier statistics and provide some corrections to the earlier Task Force findings in VS as well as providing the first guidance on prognostic distinctions between VS and MCS of varying etiologies.[5] The guidelines have addressed the question of whether any features or tests are helpful for prognosis in patients remaining in a posttraumatic or nontraumatic VS or MCS at least 4 weeks post-injury. In the Guidelines, univariate analyses were considered separately from predictive models with multivariable analyses; a total of 99 out of 266 articles met initial inclusion criteria for the systematic review process.[5]

Comparison of diagnostic subtypes between VS/UWS and MCS demonstrated an etiologic difference in prognosis. When secondary to TBI, a diagnosis of MCS as opposed to VS/UWS is "probably associated with increased odds of better than severe disability at 12 months (moderate confidence in the evidence, 1 Class II study with increased confidence in the evidence due to magnitude of effect)." This conclusion was driven in the Guidelines review by four Class II studies that

Table 9.11 Prognosis in Vegetative State (VS) following Traumatic Brain Injury at 1 Month, 3 Months, and 1 Year

Prognosis VS in traumatic brain injury

Age	n	Dead (%) CI (99%)	VS (%) CI (99%)	Conscious (%) CI (99%)	Independent (%) CI (99%)
VS at 1 month					
Adults	434	33	15	52	24
Children	106	9	29	62	27
VS at 3 months					
Adults	218	35(27–43)	30(22–38)	35(27–44)	16(10–22)
Children	50	14(1–27)	30(13–47)	56(37–74)	32(15–49)
VS at 6 months					
Adults	123	32(40–64)	52(40–64)	16(9–27)	4(0–9)
Children	28	14(30–78)	54(30–78)	32(12–58)	11(0–26)

examined the prognostic value of diagnoses of MCS versus VS/UWS. A single Class II study[149] considered the prognostic value of MCS versus VS/UWS separately in patients with traumatic and nontraumatic DOC followed for 12 months. The odds ratio for an outcome better than severe disability for patients in MCS compared to VS/UWS of traumatic etiology (n = 60) was 13.75 (95% CI 3.9–48.3). In patients with a nontraumatic disorder of consciousness (n = 25), MCS was also associated with a positive odds ratio for an outcome for better than severe disability of 9.1 (95% CI 0.4–212.7). The clear distinction between MCS and VS/UWS prognosis has resulted in a Level B practice recommendation to counsel that MCS is associated with more favorable outcomes. Some clinicians are misled to think that occurrence of outcomes better than severe disability are similar for both MCS and VS/UWS patients; in fact, patients remaining in MCS for 1 month have a 10% chance of zero disability at 1 year[149] and on average up to 25% of patients entering rehabilitation in MCS months after injuries may return to employment.[4] The establishment of firm practice guidelines with an evidence-based foundation will hopefully advances attitudes and correct common misunderstandings about outcomes in MCS.

Beyond the 12-month time point, prolonged DOC (either MCS or VS/UWS) had insufficient evidence to support or refute the prognostic value of diagnostic category for outcomes better than severe disability at 12 months when confined to nontraumatic injuries. A behavioral profile consistent with MCS in the setting of mixed etiologies of injury (traumatic and nontraumatic) was "possibly associated with increased odds of improvement versus VS/UWS."[150] Additionally, for prolonged DOC resulting from a mixed etiology that remained unchanged at 1 year, patients in VS/UWS showed a possible association with an increased odds of future deterioration. The significance of recovery after 1 year of remaining in MCS may include restoration of functional communication, which in one study occurred in a majority of patients followed for 5 years.[150]

One study[151] of the prognostic value of EEG for VS/UWS and MCS examined subjects upon admission to a rehabilitation unit and then re-examined them 6 months after the baseline

EEG. The outcome of interest was "improvement." For the VS group, improvement indicated advance to MCS or better diagnostic category, whereas for the MCS group improvement indicated shift to a diagnostic category better than MCS. Patient were divided into two groups, with and without "severe disturbances" on EEG. The group without severe disturbances on EEG (as defined by the study) (n = 76: MCS = 38, VS/UWS = 38) showed no difference in outcome between MCS and VS/UWS (OR for "improvement" with MCS 1.0, 95% CI 0.28–3.57). In contrast, in those patients with a severe disturbance of the EEG (n = 12), the OR for improvement with MCS versus VS/UWS was 1.56 (95% 0.46–5.23). These data underscore the fundamental role of underlying biological substrate in outcomes following coma (see the later "Mechanism" section).

The guidelines also identified evidence for better outcomes associated with traumatic versus nontraumatic etiologies of injury for patients with a diagnosis of either VS/UWS or MCS. Traumatic etiology was "probably associated with increased odds of better than severe disability at 12 months (OR 11.0, 95% CI 1.9–63.2, moderate confidence in the evidence, 1 Class II study with increased confidence in the evidence due to magnitude of effect)"[150] when compared with nontraumatic etiologies. Insufficient evidence supported evidence of differential impact of etiology on VS/UWS when present for a duration of 6 months.

For patients with traumatic etiologies of injury, two Class II studies of patients with traumatic VS/UWS demonstrated evidence for a prognostic impact of age. No evidence of prognostic impact of gender emerged in the review. Several factors were identified for patients in posttraumatic VS/UWS for at least a month that indicated a "probably (moderate confidence) associated increased chance of recovery of consciousness or improvement in degree of disability within 12 months"[5] in posttraumatic VS/UWS for at least a month. Measured factors associated with the increase chance of recovery. These included higher level activation of the associated auditory cortex when measured with blood oxygen-level dependent (BOLD) signal/functional MRI (fMRI) responses to a familiar voice speaking the patient's name (OR 18.0, 95% CI 2.2–162.7) (moderate confidence in the evidence, 1 Class I study)[152]; Disability

Rating Scale (DRS) scores of less than 26 present within 2–3 months post-injury (OR 30.67, 95% CI 2.52–373.6) (1 Class II with increased confidence in the evidence due to magnitude of benefit)[153]; a detectable P300 (an electrical evoked potential elicited by infrequent sensory stimuli) within 2–3 months post-injury (OR 114.1, 95% CI 5.3–2447.4) (1 Class II study with increased confidence in the evidence due to magnitude of effect)[154]; and the presence of a reactive EEG within 2–3 months post-injury (OR 19.0, 95% CI 1.97–183.4) (1 Class II study with increased confidence in the evidence due to magnitude of effect).[155]

For patients with nontraumatic VS/UWS, a combination of certain behavioral and electrodiagnostic prognostic factors were predictive of outcome. Specifically, it is "probable that that a "CRS-R scores of ≥6 more than 1 month after onset (OR 4.61, 95% CI 1.05–11643.58) and the presence of SEPs (OR 17.88, 95% CI 1.37–6511.41) are important predictors of recovery of responsiveness by 24 months post-injury (moderate confidence in the evidence, 1 Class I study)."[156] Although several neuroimaging and electrodiagnostic methods were reviewed for the AAN/ACRM/ NIDILRR Guidelines, there was insufficient evidence to support or refute the prognostic significance of any other variables reviewed for patients with nontraumatic VS/UWS across a wide range of measures studied.[5] The major prognostic recommendations of the Guidelines are listed in Table 9.12.

LATE RECOVERIES FROM MCS

Word-of-mouth stories and news reports sometimes claim dramatic recovery from prolonged coma or a VS. Invariably, these reports generate wide public interest and much confusion concerning the difference between coma and VS, as well as between diagnosis and prognosis. The original Multisociety Task Force[127,128] examined 14 cases from the media and found that the majority of these "late" recoveries from VS fell within their guidelines (i.e., less than 3 months following an anoxic injury or 12 months following a TBI in an adult). However, as noted earlier, the recent AAN/ACRM/NIDILRR Guidelines reviewed the evidence base for supporting a diagnosis of permanent VS and found that the term should no longer be used and instead

be replaced by "chronic VS."[5] However, most reports of very late recovery from coma or VS involve very late transition of MCS patients to emergence. There are no data to allow guidelines for the expected duration of MCS. Some MCS patients harbor significant residual capacities, as demonstrated by wide fluctuation of cognitive function.[157] The term "minimally conscious state" seems most appropriate; alternatives include "minimal responsive state" and "minimal awareness state."[158] Minimal responsiveness as assessed at the bedside may belie considerable cognitive capacities without further evaluation of etiologic mechanisms, including normal cognitive function as present in the LIS or less well-defined but higher level cognitive function in patients with cognitive motor dissociation (CMD), discussed later.

Locked-In State

A related and important issue is late recovery of consciousness in patients with severe motor and sensory impairment leading to the locked-in or partial LIS (a condition with severe motor disability approximating the traditional definition). As reviewed in Chapter 1, the LIS is not a disorder of consciousness. Nonetheless, because most cases of the LIS are due to a pontine injury, it is common for patients to experience an initial coma,[159] a brief period of unresponsiveness, or to respond inconsistently during the initial period of the injury similar to MCS. In a survey of 44 LIS patients, the mean time of diagnosis was 2.5 months after onset; in more than one-half of these cases, a family member and not a physician first recognized the condition.[160] Furthermore, investigators working with LIS patients often report early counseling of withdrawal of care either because of an incorrect diagnosis or based on physician attitudes without a careful and vetted informed consent process that includes a review of the available information on quality of life obtained from surveys of patients in this condition.[160,161] While it is quite reasonable to doubt that most people would want to trade a normal existence for that of a locked-in patient, the important question is whether a LIS patient would rather live or die. Quality of life assessments administered to LIS patients provide a source of information for patients and families, as do written first-person accounts, several of which have become well-known.[162] Doble et al. reported on 5-, 10-, and 20-year survival (83%, 83%, and 40%, respectively) and quality of life in 29 patients.[161] Among several notable findings, these investigators found that 12 patients remained living 11 years after the study onset; 7 of these patients described "satisfaction with life," 5 were noted to exhibit occasional depressive symptoms, but none held a DNR order. Leon-Carrion et al.[160] described quality of life measures in more detail in their survey of 44 LIS patients (see Table 9.14). The majority of these patients (86%) described a good capacity to maintain attention, nearly half (47%) described their mood as "good," most (81%) met with friends at least twice a month, and 30% could maintain sexual relations (see Table 9.10).

Quality of life was also assessed in 17 chronic (i.e., more than 1 year) locked-in patients who used eye movements or blinking as the principal mode of communication, lived at home, and had a mean duration of LIS of 6 years (range 2–16 years).[163,164] Self-scored perception of mental health (evaluating mental well-being and psychological distress) and personal general health were not significantly lower than values from age-matched French control subjects. Importantly, perception of mental health and the presence of physical pain correlated with the frequency of suicidal thoughts (r = –0.67 and 0.56 respectively, $p <$ 0.05), indicating the importance of proper pain

management in chronic LIS patients who are frequently undertreated. At present, there are three European societies for locked-in patients with a membership exceeding 300 persons http://alis-asso.fr/.

MECHANISMS UNDERLYING OUTCOMES OF COMA: INVESTIGATIONAL STUDIES OF DISORDERS OF CONSCIOUSNESS

In the aggregate, the clinical neurological exam, standard assessments of structural brain integrity, resting electroencephalographic activity, and clinical evoked potentials provide only limited insight into the neurophysiological mechanisms of coma, VS, or MCS. The functional impairment of distributed neuronal populations of the cerebral cortex, basal ganglia, thalamus, basal forebrain, and brainstem underlying these conditions often cannot be adequately assessed by these methods. Neuroimaging and more advanced electrophysiological techniques that can directly assess functional changes across cerebral networks hold significant promise to ultimately improve diagnostic accuracy and understanding of the pathophysiology of the severely injured brain (see Laureys and Schiff and Giacino et al.[165,166] for review).

Expanded use of neuroimaging and electrophysiological techniques for evaluating functional outcomes of patients recovering from

Table 9.12 **Prognosis in Vegetative State following Nontraumatic Brain Injury at 1 Month, 3 Months, and 1 Year**

Prognosis VS in anoxic brain injury					
Age	n	Dead (%) CI (99%)	VS (%) CI (99%)	Conscious (%) CI (99%)	Independent (%) CI (99%)
VS at 1 Month					
Adults	169	53	32	15	4
Children	45	22	65	13	6
VS at 3 Months					
Adults	77	46(31–61)	47(32–62)	8(2–19)	1(0–4)
Children	31	3(0–11)	94(83–100)	3(0–11)	0
VS at 6 Months					
Adults	50	28(12–44)	72(56–88)	0	0
Children	30	0	97(89–100)	3(0–11)	0

From Jennett and The Multi-Society Task Force on PVS, [127,128] with permission.

Table 9.13 **Recommendation Statements for Prognosis for Adults with a Prolonged Disorder of Consciousness (DOC)**[5]

Recommendation number	Recommendation statement and level
3	When discussing prognosis with caregivers of patients with a DOC during the first 28 days postinjury,[a] clinicians must avoid statements that suggest these patients have a universally poor prognosis (Level A).
4	Clinicians caring for patients with prolonged DOC should perform serial standardized behavioral evaluations to identify trends in the trajectory of recovery that are important for establishing prognosis (Level B).
5	PosttraumaticVS/UWS: Clinicians should perform the DRS at 2–3 months postinjury (Level B) and may assess for the presence of P300 at 2–3 months postinjury (Level C based on feasibility) or assess EEG reactivity at 2–3 months postinjury (Level C based on feasibility) to assist in prognostication regarding 12-month recovery of consciousness for patient in traumatic VS/UWS. Clinicians should perform MRI 6–8 weeks postinjury to assess for corpus callosal lesions, dorsolateral upper brainstem injury, or corona radiata injury in order to assist in prognostication regarding remaining in PVS at 12 months for patient in traumatic VS/UWS (Level B). Clinicians should perform a SPECT scan 1–2 months postinjury to assist in prognostication regarding 12-month recovery of consciousness and degree of disability/recovery for patients in traumatic VS/UWS (Level B). Clinicians may assess for the presence of higher level activation of the auditory association cortex using BOLD fMRI in response to a familiar voice speaking the patient's name to assist in prognostication regarding 12-month (postscan) recovery of consciousness for patient in traumatic VS/UWS 1–60 months postinjury (Level C based on feasibility, cost).
6	Nontraumatic, postanoxic VS/UWS: Clinicians should perform the CRS-R (Level B) and may assess SEPs (Level C based on feasibility) to assist in prognostication regarding recovery of consciousness at 24 months for patients in nontraumatic postanoxic VS/UWS.
7	Given the frequency of recovery of consciousness after 3 months in patients in nontraumatic VS/UWS, and after 12 months in patients with traumatic VS/UWS (including some cases emerging from MCS), use of the term "permanent VS" should be discontinued. After these time points, the term "chronic VS" (UWS) should be applied, accompanied by the duration of the VS/UW'S (Level B).

Prognostic counseling recommendations

8	Clinicians should counsel families that MCS diagnosed within 5 months of injury and traumatic etiology are associated with more favorable outcomes and VS/UWS and nontraumatic DOC etiology are associated with poorer outcomes, but individual outcomes vary and prognosis is not universally poor (Level B based on importance of outcomes).
9	In patient with a prolonged DOC, once a prognosis has been established that indicates a likelihood of severe long-term disability, clinicians must counsel family members to seek assistance in establishing goals of care and completing state-specific forms regarding medical decision-making (e.g., MOLST forms), if not already available, applying for disability benefit, and starting estate, caregiver, and long-term care planning (Level A).
10	When patients enter the chronic phase of VS/UWS (i.e., 3 months after non-TBI and 12 months after TBI), prognostic counselling should be provided that emphasizes the likelihood of permanent severe disability and the need for long-term assistive care (Level B).

BOLD, blood oxygen level-dependent; CRS-R, Coma Recovery Scale-Revised; DRS, Disability Rating Scale; fMRI, functional magnetic resonance imaging; MCS, minimally conscious state; MOLST, medical orders for life-sustaining treatment; PVS, persistent vegetative state; SEP, somatosensory evoked potential; TBI, traumatic brain injury; UWS, unresponsive wakefulness syndrome; VS, vegetative state.

[a]This recommendation pertains to individuals in a DOC for less than 28 days. While patients with an acute DOC are not the primary population covered by this guideline, the results of the systematic review and review of related evidence showing the potential for long-term recovery in individuals with DOC lasting longer than 28 days also apply when counseling the families of patients who are less than 28 days from injury.

coma will likely have the greatest impact on the category of severe disability. This broad category includes within its limits patients who, while not permanently unconscious as in the chronic VS, may nonetheless never regain a capacity to communicate, as well as other patients near the functional borderline of independence in activities of daily living. The significance of identifying the physiological mechanisms underlying different functional outcomes within the category of severe disability is that this knowledge will lead to a better understanding of the necessary and sufficient neurologic substrates to recover consciousness and varying levels of cognitive capacity. Just as the concept of brain death clarified the concept of death, MCS and other future subdivisions of the category of severe disability will continue to force us to consider the concept of consciousness more precisely.

The identification of severely brain-injured patients with covert evidence of cognitive capacities not evident on bedside examination has rapidly accumulated. The published literature demonstrates that in some patients with VS or MCS− (patients with only nonreflexive behaviors and no evidence of language comprehension), behavioral profiles may demonstrate command-following using fMRI or electrophysiological assessments (reviewed in Laureys and Schiff[165]). The mental imagery tasks typically used in such assessments place strong demands on sustained attention, working memory, and a range of frontal executive functions; as such, successful completion of tasks requiring typically eight bouts or more of sustained cognitive work for 30 seconds at a time reveals capacities not evident in VS or MCS− and perhaps in some MCS+ as well, in which motoric responses are limited and inconsistent.[167–171] The term "cognitive motor dissociation" (CMD) has been proposed to label that group of patients with the sharp distinction of VS or MCS− behavioral profiles and fMRI or similar proxy evidence of command-following.[22] CMD patients show a potential readiness to establish communication as a result of demonstrating both definite command-following potential but also a range of important cognitive resources that are required to enable consistent communication. Establishing efforts to systematically identify their capacities and work with CMD

patients is an important forward goal for neurology and neurorehabilitation.[172]

Several studies have begun to elucidate the mechanistic distinctions between CMD patients and other patients with coma, VS, or MCS behavioral profiles. In Figure 9.3 we organize the neuroimaging and electrophysiological studies within the context of a broadly drawn picture of the physiological correlates and underlying differences anticipated among VS, MCS, the confusional state, and the more fully recovered cognition in patients with evidence of CMD.

Functional Imaging of the Vegetative State

Levy et al.[173] provided the first experimental evidence supporting the clinical hypothesis that patients in the VS were unconscious. Using FDG-PET, seven patients in PVS were compared to three patients in LIS and 18 normal subjects. In the PVS patients, cerebral metabolic rates were globally reduced by 50% or more. Regional cerebral blood flow measurements showed a similar but more variable pattern of global reduction. Subsequent studies have confirmed these findings, with an average of less than 50% of normal metabolic rates in most VS patients studied (reduced further to 30–40% in cases of hypoxic-ischemic etiology).[174–178] Comparable reductions are identified during generalized anesthesia[179,180] and in deep slow-wave sleep in normal individuals.[181] The small number of patients in LIS (3) in the Levy et al. study had a low average metabolic rate, but recent quantitative FDG-PET studies have demonstrated essentially normal resting metabolic rates in the cerebrum even acutely.[182] Cerebellar metabolic rates were low, consistent with the lack of motor outflow in LIS.[183]

More sensitive imaging techniques have recently been applied to the evaluation of PVS patients. They reveal a marked loss of distributed network processing in the VS.[177,184,185] Elementary auditory and somatosensory stimuli fail to produce brain activation outside of primary sensory cortices (Figure 9.4). These data suggest multiple functional disconnections along the auditory or somatosensory cortical pathways and support the inference that the residual cortical activity seen

Table 9.14 **Neuropsychological Functioning in a Cohort of Locked-in Patients (n = 44)**

Neuropsychological functioning of patients with LIS.

Variable	%
Cognitive functioning	
Level of attention	
• Good	86.0
• Tends to sleep	9.0
• Normally awake	2.3
• Sleeps most of the time	2.3
Can pay attention >15 minutes	95.3
Can watch and follow a film on TV	95.3
Can say what day it is	97.6
Can read	76.7
Visual deficit	14.0
Memory problems	18.6
Emotions and feelings	
Mood state	
• Good	47.5
• Bad	5.0
• Depressed	12.5
• Other	35.0
More sensitive since onset	85.0
Laughs or cries more easily	87.8
Sexuality	
Sexual desire	61.1
Can maintain sexual relations	30.0
Communication	
Can emit sounds	78.0
Can communicate without technical aid	65.8
Social activities	
Enjoys going out	73.2
Participates in social activities	14.3
Watches television normally	23.8
Other family activities	61.9
Is accompanied out once or twice a week	61.9
Meets with friends at least twice a month	81.0

From Leon-Carrion et al.,[160] with permission.

in the PVS patients does not reflect awareness. The findings are consistent with evidence of early sensory processing in PVS patients as measured by evoked potential studies, but loss of later components[165]; they suggest that VS/PVS correlates with failure of sensory information to propagate beyond the earliest stages of cortical processing. Preliminary studies discussed later indicate that MCS patients show wider activation of cortical networks, findings that may help ultimately distinguish

the conditions among patients with severe sensory and motor impairments limiting behavioral assessments (e.g., spastic contractions and blindness).

Atypical Behavioral Features in PVS

Stereotyped behavior, typically limbic displays of crying, smiling, or other emotional patterns that are not related to environmental stimuli, occur in some patients in VS. Occasionally, other fragments of behavior that may appear semi-purposeful or inconsistently related to environmental stimuli arise in VS/PVS patients. Neuroimaging studies, including FDG-PET, magnetoencephalography (MEG), and fMRI have identified residual cerebral circuits underlying such isolated behavioral fragments.[148,186,187] One remarkable patient studied had remained in PVS for 20 years but infrequently expressed single words (typically epithets) not related to environmental stimulation (see Figure 9.5). Two other VS patients revealed similar isolated regions of preserved metabolic activity that could be correlated with unusual behavioral patterns.[187] These data provide novel evidence for the modular organization of the brain and suggest that preservation of residual cerebral activity following severe brain injuries may be associated with behavioral fragments. Regional preservation of cerebral metabolic activity likely reflects both preservation of anatomical connectivity and endogenous neuronal firing patterns of remnant, but incomplete, networks.

Further study of this patient showed that islands of higher resting brain metabolism included Herschel's gyrus (Figure 9.5), Broca's area, Wernicke's area, and the left anterior basal ganglia (caudate nucleus, possibly putamen). Despite limited amounts of remaining left thalamus identified by MRI that expressed a very low metabolic rate, incompletely preserved MEG patterns of spontaneous and evoked gamma-band responses were seen. Taken together, these imaging data suggest the modular sparing of cortical networks associated with language functions.[187] Nevertheless, despite this patient, any verbal output suggests function better than vegetative until proved otherwise.

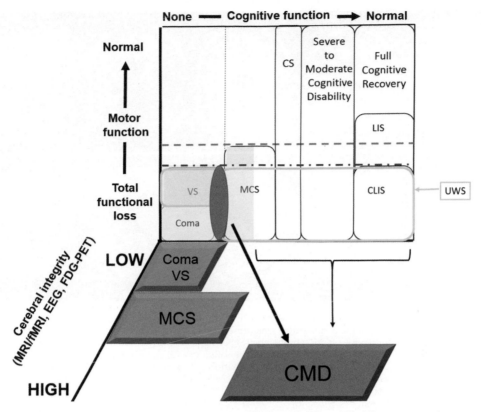

Figure 9.3 Dissociations of behavioral and physiological measures in recovery patterns following severe brain injuries. Patterns of recovery of consciousness and cognition following severe brain injuries are represented on a three-dimensional coordinate system. Dimensions illustrate the dissociations of behavioral and physiological measurements observed in the assessment of patients with DOC, as seen in both the chronic recovery phase and the acute ICU setting.[141] A light gray zone encompassing coma, VS, and the left half of the MCS identifies patients with CMD. The dark gray oval between coma/VS and MCS indicates a transition zone in which behavioral fragments may be present in patients otherwise fulfilling the criteria for VS; an interrupted vertical line indicates the boundary of evidence for awareness as judged behaviorally (none to the left of the line). CMD is a clinical syndrome operationally defined as having a bedside examination consistent with coma, VS, or the limited nonreflexive behaviors seen in MCS patients who are unable to follow commands and the concurrent demonstration of command-following utilizing fMRI, EEG, or similar technologies alone. A wide range of uncertainty exists regarding the ultimate underlying cognitive capacity in CMD as patients may span the range from command-following to higher integrative function (as indicated by the brackets to the right of the light gray region). Many studies now show that CMD is associated with highly preserved cerebral integrity,[22,142,143] suggesting that CMD patients are likely closer in preservation of cerebral function to patients in LIS or complete LIS (CLIS) but distinct from such patients because of multiple injuries across the corticothalamic systems. Quantitative measurements of behavioral function smoothly span recovery of cognitive function when expressed through observable behaviors using the Coma Recovery Scale-Revised (CRS-R) to measure recovery from coma through emergence from MCS, the use of the Confusion Assessment Protocol (CAP) to measure function in the confusional state, and a wide array of standardized measures to capture the emerging recovery of normative neuropsychological function. Because motor impairments following severe brain injuries may mask even full cognitive recovery, the search for reliable correlative physiological measures to identify levels of cognitive function is critical. Research reviewed later in this chapter demonstrates that functional neuroimaging with MRI and position emission tomography (PET) tools (fMRI, fluorodeoxyglucose PET [FDG-PET]) and the EEG correlate high degrees of preservation of cerebral functional integrity in CMD.[144] Adapted from Schiff, 2017.

Isolated Neuroimaging of Cortical Responses in PVS Patients

In a widely discussed *Lancet* paper, Menon et al.[188] described selective cortical activation patterns using an ^{15}O-PET subtraction paradigm in a 26-year-old woman described as being in a PVS 4 months following an attack of ADEM. MRI studies of the patient's brain showed evidence of both diffuse cortical and subcortical (brainstem and thalamic) lesions. Although the patient inconsistently demonstrated visual

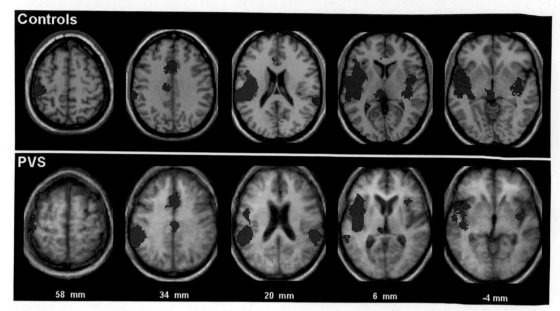

Figure 9.4 Somatosensory stimulation in vegetative state (VS). Top row: Brain activation patterns from normal subjects, shown in red, that is elicited by noxious stimulation (superthreshold electrical stimulation experienced as "painful"; subtraction stimulation-rest). Bottom row: Brain activation patterns from patient in permanent VS (PVS), again shown in red, elicited by same noxious stimulation method (subtraction stimulation-rest). Blue regions indicate areal differences in network activation showing region less active in patients than in controls (interaction [stimulation versus rest] × [patient versus control]). All regions of activation are projected onto transverse sections of a normalized brain magnetic resonance imaging (MRI) template in controls and on the mean MRI of the patients (distances are relative to the bicommissural plane) From Laureys et al.[185] with permission.

tracking (leading to some debate as to whether her condition at the time of study reflected PVS or MCS), no other features of her examination were inconsistent with the diagnosis of VS. Improvements in responsiveness unequivocally consistent with the MCS level were noted by 6 months, with emergence from MCS occurring sometime after 8 months. As noted earlier, it is now generally recognized that prognosis in ADEM includes later recoveries at time periods 6 months or longer after the injury. Thus, patients with ADEM, which tends to damage axons but spare cortical neurons, may harbor residual integrative capacities despite a long convalescence. By contrast, similar clinical examination findings in a patient 6 months following cardiac arrest, which would be expected to correlate with widespread neocortical, striatal, thalamic, and hippocampal cell death, would not portend such a cerebral reserve. The patient with ADEM eventually made a full cognitive recovery.[189] Imaging studies in this patient at 4 months, at a time when she was described as being in a PVS, demonstrated selective activations of right occipital-temporal regions (in a subtraction paradigm comparing familiar faces and scrambled images). The investigators interpreted activation of the right fusiform gyrus and extrastriate visual association areas as indicating a recovery of minimal awareness without behavioral manifestation. The findings in this patient, however, point out a significant limitation of brain imaging techniques in this clinical context and have been extensively debated.[188,190,191]

The selective identification of relatively complex information processing associated with visual processing of faces may not by itself provide an index of recovery of cognitive function or even potential for recovery. Specific cortical responses to faces are obtainable in anesthetized animals,[192] and, if found in isolation of any other imaging evidence or bedside demonstration of awareness, do not guarantee that these patterns of activation represent cognitive function per se. Without further clinical evidence, the present state of imaging technologies cannot provide alternative markers of awareness. While neuroimaging studies hold the promise of elucidating underlying differences between VS/PVS and MCS patients, at present no techniques are able to identify awareness in such patients unambiguously.

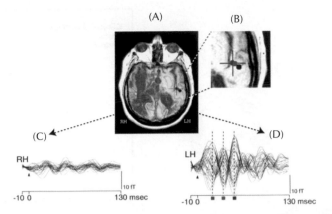

Figure 9.5 (A) An MRI (1.5T) reveals destruction of the right basal ganglia and thalamus as well as severe damage to most of the cerebral cortex of the right hemisphere. Additional areas of damage include the left posterior thalamus and posterior parietal cortex with moderately severe atrophy of the rest of the left hemisphere. Resting FDG-PET measurements of the patient's brain demonstrated a widespread and marked reduction in cerebral metabolism to <50% of normal across most brain regions. Several isolated and relatively small regions in the left hemisphere, however, expressed higher levels of metabolism (yellow color indicates values greater than 55% of normal). Magnetoencephalographic (MEG) analysis of responses to bilateral auditory stimulation (C and D) demonstrated a time-locked response in the high-frequency (20-50 Hz) range restricted to the left hemisphere reduced in amplitude, coherence and duration compared with normal controls.[187] Source localization of the time-varying magnetic field obtained from the averaged response identified sources in the left (D) but not right (C) temporal lobe, consistent with preservation of a response from Heschl's gyrus.

Functional Neuroimaging of Minimally Conscious State

An exceptionally large number of neuroimaging and electrophysiological studies have emerged examining the physiological distinctions of brain function in MCS patients versus that measurable in VS patients (see Laureys and Schiff; Giacino et al.[165,166] for review). Several studies have developed successful frameworks for identifying distinctions between VS and MCS patients utilizing a variety of measures, including machine learning algorithms utilizing the patterns of resting activity measured in the BOLD signals of the fMRI[193] (see Figure 9.6), EEG evoked and spontaneous activity patterns,[194,195] and the complexity of high-density EEG waves recorded after stimulation by transcranial magnetic coils.[196,197]

Similarly strong discrimination of VS and MCS patients has also been established utilizing quantitative measures of the resting EEG signal. Figure 9.7A shows the results of a study by King et al.[198] employing a novel technique, "weighted symbolic mutual information," to quantify the information sharing present across brain regions in the resting EEG. Increases in information sharing correlated with behavioral diagnosis, with increasing values of this measure indicating recovery to a more normal pattern, and VS responses showing statistical separation

from other conditions. Using a related approach, Chennu et al.[194] have shown that the density mathematical graphs formed using the resting EEG signal can be correlated with behavioral diagnosis, measured cerebral metabolic activity, and outcome at 1 year post-study. Figure 9.7B shows the top 30% of connections of the cortical areas with the strongest functional connectivity in a three-dimensional network of alpha frequency EEG (8–13 Hz by definition within this study) across cohorts of patients (VS/UWS, MCS+, MCS−, EMCS, LIS) and controls. VS/UWS patients in this study showed statistical separation from other categories.

A related method of EEG evaluation is that of Massamini and colleagues,[196,197] who have developed a theoretically based measurement of resting brain activity that combines use of high-density EEG to measure the electrocortical responses of the brain induced by transcranial magnetic stimulation (TMS) pulses. The perturbational complexity index (PCI) derives from a theoretical framework that proposes that wakeful consciousness reflects an integration of information across multiple brain regions with a high degree of differentiation of the activity. To calculate PCI, many short segments of an EEG after each TMS pulse are averaged, the underlying sources of the resulting EEG pattern are modeled, and a matrix of binary values summarizing the significant activation

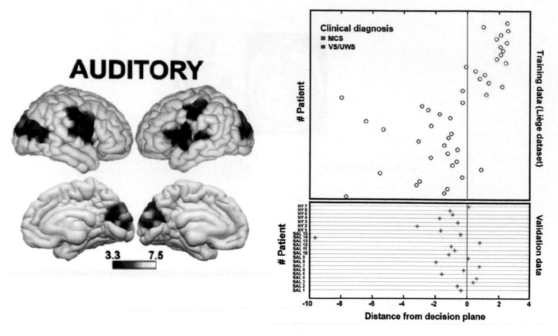

Figure 9.6 Figure shows the results of the Demertzi et al.[193] study that employed machine learning algorithms to the resting signal blood oxygen level-dependent (BOLD) signal measured using functional magnetic resonance imaging (fMRI). In this study, a total of 73 patients were studied, using 51 patients imaged from one center to establish a classifier to discriminate vegetative state (VS) from minimally conscious state (MCS) on the basis of patterns of resting state networks. Using a sample of 22 patients as a validation cohort from data acquired at two different centers demonstrated classification of greater than 80% accuracy in discrimination for the measure; the auditory resting state network provided the best classification performance.

of different modeled sources is analyzed with algorithmic complexity measures to produce the single nominal value of the PCI index. High PCI values indicate that the initial TMS perturbation alters activity across a large set of interacting brain regions. A unique feature of this EEG/TMS/PCI approach is that it is applied directly to the brain, and the assessment does not depend on the integrity of specific sensory pathways or motor efferent systems.

Figure 9.8 shows the results of time-averaging the EEG signal after repetitive TMS pulses, which generate reproducible wave patterns of activity that are then subjected to an algorithmic analysis to produce a single value, the PCI, to quantify the TMS EEG response. As shown in Figure 9.8, the PCI index shows a 94.7% sensitivity in discriminating MCS from VS and provides reliable separations for MCS-level versus VS-level behavioral function.[193] In addition, temporary and reversible brain states that correlate with unconsciousness, including non-rapid eye movement (NREM) sleep and pharmacologically induced coma, show similar PCI values to VS.

Conceptualizing Patterns of Restoration of Cerebral Network Activity in Disorders of Consciousness Following Coma

Collectively, the prior chapters of this volume have drawn the consistent observation that coma arises as the result of either (1) relatively diffuse structural lesions producing bihemispheric dysfunction, (2) relatively discrete bilateral lesions within the rostral pontine or paramedian midbrain tegmentum or diencephalon, or (3) metabolic or toxic encephalopathies producing widespread neuronal dysfunction. The final common pathway of cerebral dysfunction in all instances of coma (as detailed in Chapters 1–5) can be thus understood as a broad bilateral dysfunction of neuronal populations across the corticothalamic system and their allied connections with basal ganglia and limbic structures. In instances of nonselective cerebral hemispheric injuries or global cellular functional impairment arising

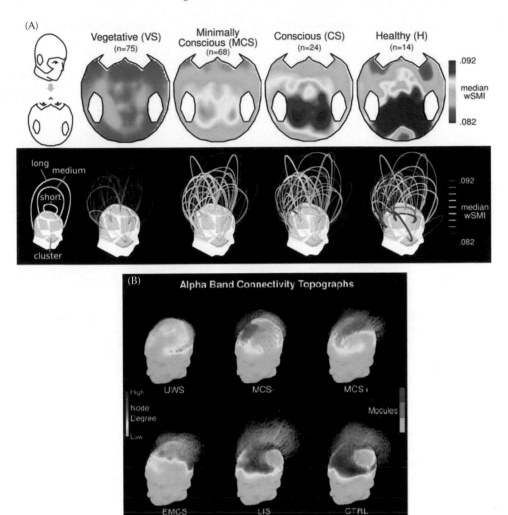

Figure 9.7 The results of two studies utilizing electroencephalographic (EEG) signals as classifiers of behavioral state. (A) King et al.[198] used weighted symbolic mutual information (wSMI) to quantify the degree of information sharing and correlate it with behavioral diagnosis. Increasing values of wSMI graded with behavioral recovery; in this study, wSMI in vegetative state (VS) patients showed statistical separation from other conditions. (B) Chennu et al.[194] used a related but different approach to the EEG, calculating the density of mathematical graphs formed from the resting EEG signal. Graph density correlated with behavioral diagnosis, measured cerebral metabolic activity, and outcome at 1 year post-study.

with loss of critical metabolic substrates (e.g., oxygen), the physiological mechanism underlying coma is dominated by the effects of a broad withdrawal of excitatory synaptic activity.[199] The strong downregulation of neuronal firing rates produced by either structurally deafferented or dysfunctional neocortical and thalamic neurons results from a process known as "disfacilitation" as the neuronal membrane potentials passively hyperpolarize as excitatory inputs are withdrawn due to a dominance of potassium leakage currents.[200,201] A very slow, less than 1 Hertz rhythm then typically

arises across the corticothalamic system under these conditions.[199] A very similar rhythm also emerges in fully connected, healthy brains when excitation is broadly suppressed under all types of general anesthesia.[202]

Discrete lesions within the upper brainstem producing coma also create widespread disfacilitation by a combined effect of direct functional deafferentation and specific circuit mechanisms. Discrete bilateral lesions within the upper tegmental brainstem or limited unilateral involvement of the upper tegmental brainstem combined with bilateral central

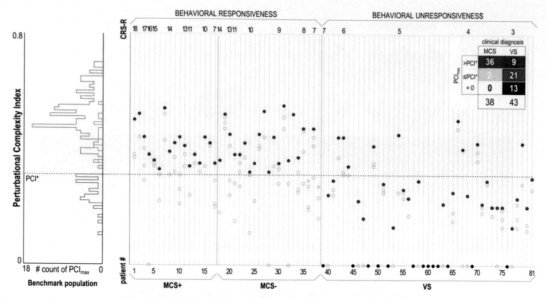

Figure 9.8 Massamini and colleagues[196,197] innovated a theoretically based measurement of resting brain activity in the electroencephalogram (EEG) that combined the use of high-density EEG to measure response induced across the EEG by transcranial magnetic stimulation (TMS) pulses. The investigators constructed a measure, the perturbational complexity index (PCI), by time-averaging the EEG signal after repetitive TMS pulses which generate reproducible wave patterns of activity; the wave patterns were compressed using an algorithmic analysis to produce a PCI single value to quantify the TMS EEG. The PCI index demonstrated a 94.7% sensitivity in discriminating minimally conscious state (MCS) from vegetative state (VS) and also provided reliable separations for MCS-versus VS-level behavioral function.[196]

thalamic injuries may present with coma in the acute phase of injury.[132,139,203] Typically, a similar low-frequency pattern of activity is initially seen across the EEG consistent with other etiologies of coma, although in some instances spike-and-wave activity similar to that of primary generalized seizures may occur.[139] When combined, such lesions affect both the brainstem arousal projection systems[204] and the central thalamic arousal regulation pathways.[205,206] Differences in the natural history of lesions restricted to either the brainstem or the central thalami provide mechanistic insight into their distinct contributions to the initial comatose state. In the subset of patients who survive isolated brainstem lesions associated with coma, while coma may persist for several days, recovery is typically rapid.[204] Conversely, when a limited component of upper brainstem infarction and wide bilateral central thalamic lesions produce coma, the coma rarely lasts more than 24–48 hours but typically gives way to a much slower and uncertain recovery process.[132,139,203] When large combined lesions exist within both the brainstem and central thalamus with some bilateral involvement, recovery is less

likely. This distinction illustrates the separate contributions of the central thalamus to arousal regulation of the corticothalamic system during wakefulness,[207] provided by its powerful modulation of the frontostriatal systems.[208,209] Importantly, the lack of evidence for isolated paramedian thalamic lesions producing coma demonstrates a functional distinction for these neurons in not providing an essential foundation for the overall state of wakefulness, but rather the support of activation of frontal executive resources within wakefulness that require powerful excitatory inputs to frontostriatal regions.[207] Nonetheless, the emergence of coma with only limited extension of upper brainstem injuries when large bilateral paramedian thalamic infarcts are present emphasizes the impact of immediate withdrawal of these glutamatergic afferents.[132,139,203] Disruption of projections emanating from the basal forebrain have been demonstrated to produce a coma-like state in rodents.[210] An important distinction of the experimentally derived state in these animals, however, is the preservation of the righting response, which is the standard demonstration of comatose-like behavior in the rodent. As such, this model appears to bear a stronger resemblance to the hypervigilant form of akinetic mutism (see earlier discussion).

Generally, both cellular and circuit mechanisms play a role in the recovery from coma as excitatory neurotransmission is restored across the corticothalamic system. Accordingly, reversible coma is the result of a wide range of possible underlying mechanisms that may globally alter neuronal function or disable specific circuits (as discussed in other chapters; see Edlow et al.[211] for a short review of reversible mechanisms). Following structural brain injuries, patterns of recovery from coma appear to be strongly influenced by the degree of distributed structural deafferentation and the impact of structural injuries on functional activity of specific large-scale networks, as reviewed later.

However, even very severe multifocal structural brain injuries and diffuse cellular functional alteration (e.g., hypoxia) producing coma present increasing challenges for linking potential recovery to underlying mechanisms. Marked structural deafferentation associated with severe TBI is rarely associated with late recovery from prolonged DOC after coma.[212] On the other hand, protracted but reversible diffuse cellular impairment secondary to hypoxia can rarely permit recovery.[23] Understanding the cellular and circuit mechanisms supporting recovery in such instances is needed to better track the impact of acute treatment and interventions as well as improve the precision of prognosis.

Functional Imaging of Recovery of Consciousness: Linked Roles of the Anterior Forebrain Mesocircuit and Default Mode Network/Posterior Medial Complex

Studies over the past two decades have consistently implicated the role of two large-scale networks in the recovery from DOC[165]: the anterior forebrain mesocircuit[213,214] and the frontoparietal network.[165,215] The anterior forebrain mesocircuit includes the frontal/prefrontal cortices and the striatopallidal modulatory system that regulates thalamic outflow back to the cortex and striatum. As described later, this network is uniquely

vulnerable to multifocal brain injuries based on its widespread anatomical connections; the functional impact of direct injuries or deafferentation of the central thalamic neurons that provide broad afferent excitation across the frontostriatal system has a fundamental role in recovery from DOC. The frontoparietal network is composed largely of two experimentally defined subnetworks. One is the *default mode network* (DMN) comprised of medial cortical structures including the anterior cingulate cortex (ACC), medial frontal cortices, and posterior cingulate (PCC)/precuneus cortical regions that have been linked to internal awareness or self-related processes; the other involves more lateral areas of prefrontal and posterior parietal cortex which are experimentally linked to attention and awareness of the environment.[165,215] Moreover, these networks have strong interconnections, and evidence supports their joint role in the recovery process following coma as patients transition from VS to MCS to emergence into higher levels of recovery.

Raichle and colleagues first proposed that the normal human brain has a "baseline" state of metabolic activation (as reflected by oxygen uptake) reflecting "default self-monitoring."[216–218] Specific areas of brain that are active at rest (e.g., posterior cingulate cortex and ventral anterior cingulate cortex[219]) form the DMN, which deactivates during tasks that activate other areas of the brain. Data obtained from these investigators provide evidence supporting a functional role of a resting state of monitoring environmental and internal state that might be sensitive to salient events such as emotionally meaningful human speech.[219–221] Laureys and colleagues have shown that the functional integrity of connectivity within this network is correlated to the level of consciousness, demonstrating graded changes from VS (low connectivity) to patients in MCS and to healthy controls (higher connectivity).[215] Importantly, the posterior medial complex maintains the highest resting metabolic rate in the human brain.[216–218] As discussed later, a persistent abnormality of the resting EEG in posttraumatic confusional state may in part reflect a failure to restore sufficient afferent drive to maintain baseline function in this network component.[222] The suppression of DMN is also seen as a general finding in healthy volunteers undergoing general anesthesia (see later). Loss of metabolic signal measured by FDG-PET or BOLD signal in fMRI has been identified as a marker that grades correlates with level of consciousness.[215,223] Diffusion tensor imaging (DTI) tractography has also quantified correlation of the degradation of modeled fiber tracts connecting the precuneus with both cortical (temporo-parietal junction and frontal medial cortex) and subcortical (thalamus and striatum) regions with levels of recovery.

In addition to the frontoparietal network, the functional integrity of the anterior forebrain mesocircuit has shown strong relationships to outcomes following coma. Neurons within central regions of the thalamus project broadly across the frontal-striatal system[208] and have more widespread but selective anatomical connectivity across the entire forebrain.[224] A "central thalamus" is more a physiological, functional distinction[207,209,225,226] than one delineated by anatomical boundaries; these neurons have primary projection to integrative layers of the cerebral cortex, wide arborization over rostral striatum, and participate in a range of frontal executive functions such as sustained attention and working memory.[207,209,225,226] These specializations distinguishing the central thalamus (primarily the central lateral intralaminar nucleus and paralaminar regions of abutting nuclei such as the median dorsalis nucleus) provide a foundation, along with the strong input of all brainstem arousal neuronal populations, to the central thalamus's functional role in forebrain arousal regulation (see Schiff[205] for review). Consistent with this unique geometry of broad multifocal connections, pathological studies have shown strong correlation of the graded loss of central thalamic nuclei with the outcomes following severe brain injuries.[227] The "mesocircuit hypothesis" proposes that the anterior forebrain is particularly vulnerable to downregulation due to widespread cerebral deafferentation that typically occurs following multifocal brain injuries as the combined effect of loss of the arousal regulation function of the deafferented central thalamus and a contribution of additional active inhibition arising as a circuit-level consequence of impaired striatal function[213] (see Figure 9.9). A sharp decrease of central thalamic firing rates is expected as a result of the loss of corticothalamic inputs to these neurons providing an insufficient

level of background synaptic input to maintain neuronal membrane depolarization. For some components of the central thalamus, a direct inhibition arising from disinhibited globus pallidus interna neurons can also be expected. The globus pallidus interna is under tonic inhibition from the striatum in the awake healthy brain, but, following severe brain injuries, insufficient corticostriatal and thalamostriatal input to the medium spiny neurons (MSNs) of the striatum may drop below the high threshold level of incoming synaptic excitatory inputs required to keep the MSNs at their firing threshold.[228] The mesocircuit hypothesis predicts that graded downregulation of activity across the striatum, central thalamus, and frontal/prefrontal cortices will impair recovery after coma.[213]

Several studies now support the mesocircuit hypothesis and the linkage of functional activation across the anterior forebrain mesocircuit with frontoparietal network function. Figure 9.10 organizes observed changes measured in mesocircuit and frontoparietal network activity in relation to level of behavioral recovery from coma. Fridman et al.[214] compared metabolic profiles of severely brain-injured patients with DOC with healthy controls. They identified metabolic signatures associated with graded outcomes in patients with disordered consciousness, comparing those who could not follow commands (VS and MCS–) to those with behavioral evidence of following commands (MCS+, and CS, confusional state). A downregulation of central thalamic metabolism in comparison to globus pallidus metabolism showed a significant correlation with outcome in patients (Figure 9.10, left column). Additionally, a positive correlation of central thalamic metabolism with the precuneus of the dominant hemisphere in the same study supported the linkage of frontoparietal network activity to the restoration of anterior forebrain mesocircuit function; this positive correlation is consistent with patterns of innervation of the posterior medial complex by afferents from the central thalamus.[165,229] Recovery into the CS is accompanied by relative normalization of these measures, but studies of the resting EEG demonstrate a persistent abnormality of reduction of posterior parietal-occipital spectral power in the alpha

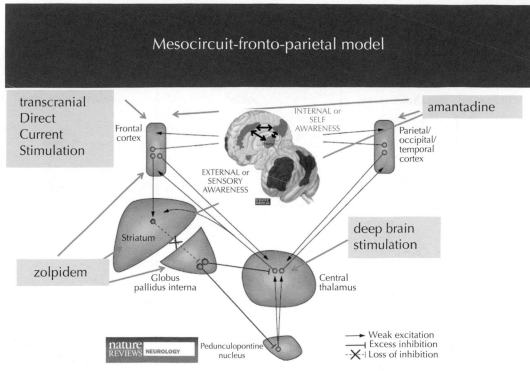

Figure 9.9 The mesocircuit-frontoparietal model. A common mechanism for downregulation of the anterior forebrain mesocircuit in severe brain injuries is illustrated (see Schiff[213] for detailed description). Reduction of thalamocortical and thalamostriatal outflow following broad cerebral deafferentation in structural brain injuries (traumatic, hypoxic, vascular, etc.) leads to loss of inputs to surviving central thalamic neurons. A resulting downregulation of activity of the central thalamic neurons withdraws important afferent drive to medial frontal cortical regions critical to arousal regulation and to the medium spiny neurons of the striatum, which may then fail to reach firing threshold because of their requirement for high levels of synaptic background activity. Loss of active inhibition from the striatum allows neurons of the globus pallidus interna to tonically fire and provide active inhibition to their synaptic targets, including relay neurons of the already strongly disfacilitated central thalamus and possibly also the projection neurons of the pedunculopontine nucleus (PPN).[230] Pallidal projections to the PPN are to glutamatergic neurons within this structure, and any interactions with the cholinergic projecting neurons from PPN that show a differentially stronger innervation of the central lateral nucleus of the human thalamus[231] are unknown. The anterior forebrain mesocircuit plays an important interactive role in supporting activity within the fronto-parietal network identified with graded outcome across disorders of consciousness.[215,232] A range of therapeutic interventions that target different components across the networks have shown efficacy in some patients with disorders of consciousness, including the medications amantadine[233] and zolpidem[24,234] and direct electrical stimulation utilizing deep brain stimulation[235] or transcranial electrical stimulation.[236]
Figure modified from Giacino et al.[166] and Thibaut and Schiff.[237]

(8–12Hz) compared to the delta (1–4Hz) frequency range that grades with depth of CS as measured by the Confusion Assessment Protocol.[222] This persistent abnormality of resting EEG activity within the posterior parietal-occipital regions likely reflects a failure to re-establish full functional activity in this region due to its high resting metabolic demands (see earlier discussion).[216] Recovery past the CS is associated with restoration of both a normal resting spectral power distribution in the EEG including these posterior parietal-occipital regions and normal resting metabolic profiles. However, consistent with the mesocircuit hypothesis, modulation of midline frontal EEG power during controlled attentional processing in patients recovered from coma to near-normal functional levels demonstrates an enduring vulnerability of the anterior forebrain mesocircuit to meet the demands of increased cognitive effort.[238]

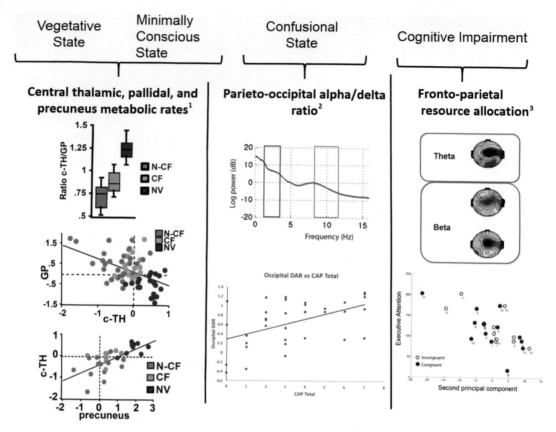

Figure 9.10 Functional correlation of linked anterior forebrain mesocircuit and fronto-parietal network activity to graded recovery from coma. Predictions of the mesocircuit hypothesis have been tested across the range of outcomes following coma from vegetative state (VS) to near full recovery in patients at the GOSE 5–7 level of independent function with persistent impairment in executive function.[214,222,238] Across several different measures, a graded relationship of increasing normalization of activity patterns within the anterior forebrain mesocircuit and frontoparietal network has been demonstrated. The first supported prediction is the existence of normalization of the ratio of metabolic activity within the central thalamus (c-TH) and globus pallidus (GP) comparing patients with disorders of consciousness arising across a wide range of etiologies and patients with and without command-following to healthy controls.[214] Top left: Normalization of the c-TH/GP ratio progressively improves from VS/minimally conscious state (MCS)– (non-command following, "N-CF") to MCS\+/confusional state (CS) (command following) to healthy controls (NV); a related measurement displayed in the bottom left panel demonstrates that central thalamic metabolism (c-TH) is linked to metabolism in the precuneus region (a critical node of the fronto-parietal network); graph shows relationship of central thalamic metabolism to left precuneus.[239] CS patients exhibit a persistent abnormality of activation in posterior parietal occipital regions, shown in middle panel. In this study, resting electroencephalogram (EEG) measures demonstrate reduction of posterior parietal-occipital spectral power in the alpha (8–12 Hz) compared to the delta (1–4 Hz) frequency range that grades with depth of CS as measured by the standard measure quantifying symptoms of confusion, the Confusion Assessment Protocol (CAP; see Shah et al.[222]). The red line indicates linear regression of occipital cortex delta-to-alpha ratio to numerical total score on CAP (beta = 2.37, p < 0.01). This persistent downregulation of the posterior parietal-occipital regions likely reflects the high metabolic demands of these regions (see Raichle et al.[216]) and failure to restore sufficient afferent input to these regions. Recovery past CS is associated with restoration of normal resting metabolic profiles measured in 18F-fluorodeoxyglucose-positron emission tomography (FDG-PET) and resting spectral power distribution in the EEG. However, persistent cognitive limitations leading to GOSE 5–7 level functional outcome after coma are associated with an incomplete restoration of a consistently observed component of the EEG activated in frontal EEG leads during performance of attentional tasks.[238] This EEG component, shown the upper right panel, shows an elevation of 2.5–7.5 Hz (theta) power during the attentional task that is associated with suppression of 12.5–22.5 Hz power and improved performance. The regression curve in the lower right panels shows the relationship between performance of an attentional task and expression of this EEG pattern; these findings demonstrate an enduring vulnerability of the anterior forebrain mesocircuit to meet demands of cognitive effort in GOSE 5–7 patients post-TBI coma (see Shah et al.[238] for details).

Collectively, the mesocircuit-frontoparietal model provides an economical explanation of the vulnerability of the anterior forebrain in patients with DOC who suffer from widespread deafferentation and neuronal cell loss and the observed patterns of graded recovery across components of these combined networks. Further supporting the joint role of these two networks are the results of neuroimaging studies of healthy volunteer subjects undergoing general anesthesia shown in Figure 9.11. Across varying types of anesthetic, suppression of both anterior forebrain mesocircuit and frontoparietal are selectively correlated with anesthetic coma.[240] Recovery of consciousness demonstrates a correlation with activation across the medial frontal and thalamic components of the anterior forebrain mesocircuit[240] and joint activation of both networks with pharmacological stimulation effective to restore command-following in an otherwise stable plane of general anesthesia.[241] Similarly, activation of the anterior forebrain mesocircuit via pharmacologic stimulation or direct electrical stimulation methods produces behavioral facilitation in some DOC patients. Paradoxically, zolpidem, a short-acting gamma-aminobutyric acid (GABA)-enhancing hypnotic, may induce marked behavioral improvements in some patients with DOC.[24,234,242–244] Chatelle et al. correlated increased brain metabolism within the dorsolateral prefrontal and mesiofrontal cortices with zolpidem-induced

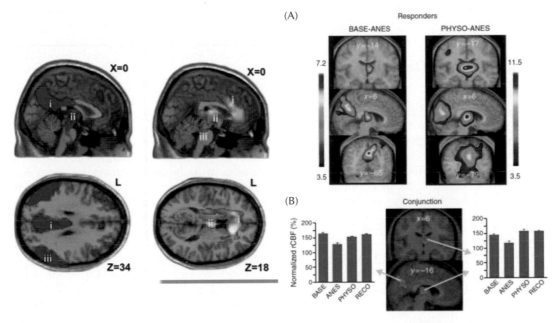

Figure 9.11 Joint modulation of anterior forebrain mesocircuit and fronto-parietal network during general anesthesia. Studies of healthy volunteers undergoing general anesthesia demonstrate similar joint relationships of the anterior forebrain mesocircuit and fronto-parietal network to the observations shown in Figure 9.10. (A) Långsjö et al.[240] examined brain regions significantly suppressed during general anesthesia and significantly activated upon return of consciousness that show a common contribution when different types of anesthesia were compared. Consistent suppression of brain activity shown in blue color occurred in posterior cingulate, inferior parietal, precuneus, thalamus, and frontal cortices during all forms of general anesthesia (left column). Regions associated with return of consciousness shown in orange-yellow (right column); increased activation observed primarily in anterior cingulate cortex, thalamus, and brainstem regions (locus ceruleus/parabrachial). (B) A study of reversal of unresponsiveness during general anesthesia employed healthy volunteers undergoing propofol general anesthesia and introduction of parental physostigmine to increase available acetylcholine and restore command-following. 15O-PET contrast images of group results from subgroup of subjects recovering command-following during anesthesia with physostigmine and those remaining in an unresponsive state during anesthesia. Co-activation of the precuneus and thalamus is seen in the group with transient recovery of command-following; this finding can be compared to the increasing central thalamic/precuneus metabolic ratio associated with recovery from disorders of consciousness shown in Figure 9.10 (also see Fridman and Schiff[239]).
Image A adapted from Långsjö et al.[240] with permission. Image B adapted from Xie et al.[241] with permission.

recovery of functional communication.[234] Zolpidem may act across several points within the anterior forebrain mesocircuit to initiate paradoxical excitation,[24] including direct excitation at the cortical level[245] and, within the striatum,[246] via inhibition of the GPi by inhibiting the $GABA_{Aa-1}$ subunit which is strongly expressed in human GPi.[247] Zolpidem may effectively restore inhibition of the GPi and increase thalamic excitation across the frontostriatal system. Direct electrical stimulation of the central thalamus has been demonstrated in single-subject study of a chronic MCS patient to restore goal-directed behavior and spoken language communication after 6 years of remaining in MCS; in this subject, cortical evoked responses generated by stimulation of individual electrode contacts were consistent with activation of the frontostriatal pathways.[235]

Cognitive Motor Dissociation

Neuroimaging and electrophysiological studies have identified an important subset of patients with severe structural brain injuries who exhibit very limited or no behavioral responses at the bedside but nonetheless retain sufficient higher level cognition to carry out motor imagery tasks to command.[165,166] As noted earlier, the term "cognitive motor dissociation" (CMD) has been proposed along with an operational definition for such patients who fulfill the behavioral criteria for coma, VS, or MCS but paradoxically demonstrate command-following capacities utilizing fMRI, EEG, or other methods of investigation.[22]

Owen and colleagues[167] first developed an fMRI imaging framework to evaluate the presence of such volitional responses in patients with DOC that addresses the ambiguities of the methods used in the Menon et al. study[188] described earlier. Applying these new methods,[167] they identified unequivocal neuroimaging evidence of a patient remaining in VS at 5 months following a severe TBI being able to follow commands to imagine various visual scenes. The commands were associated with activation of appropriate areas of the cerebral cortex (within the supplementary motor area for imagery of tennis playing and within posterior structures for spatial navigation imagery) despite lack of an external motor response. At the time of examination, the patient showed evidence of brief visual fixation, a possible transitional sign for evolution into MCS.[124] Another examination 11 months later revealed visual tracking to a mirror, another transitional sign, but no evidence of object manipulation or behavioral manifestations of command-following. Figure 9.12A shows the main result of the study. The imaging findings demonstrated preservation of cognitive function for this particular patient that the clinical bedside examination failed to reveal and indicated a cognitive level at least consistent with MCS. It is important to recognize that command-following is a cardinal feature of MCS that does not imply a capacity for communication. MCS patients may show consistent evidence of command-following with visible motor responses that cannot be used to establish communication. As a result, it is unclear from the methods used in the Owen et al. study[167] whether or not the patient's level of consciousness was consistent with MCS or a higher level of recovery.

Importantly, preservation of such capacities have been most frequently identified in patients with limited motoric function. For example, in a study of 54 patients, Monti et al.[168] found that only one subject behaviorally judged as in MCS out of 31 subjects could demonstrate neuronal activation in motor imagery tasks using fMRI responses; notably this subject's motor function was limited only to visual tracking (1.3 months) following a TBI. Conversely, in the same study, 4 out of 23 patients initially diagnosed as in VS demonstrated command-following with fMRI paradigms. Pignat et al.[248] demonstrated that more systematic search for behavioral evidence of motor response employing a measure with an expanded range of motor testing across limb, facial, ocular, and oral motricity significantly enhanced detection of consciousness and CMD. Recent studies support the inference that brain function in CMD patients is likely closer to that of healthy controls and patients in LIS than those MCS patients who can intermittently communicate or reliably show motor command-following.[142,143]

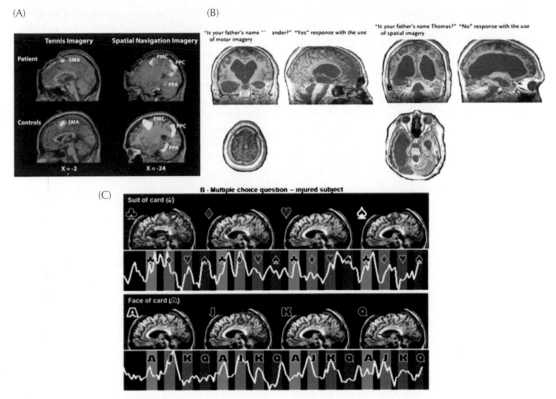

Figure 9.12 (A) Command-following in post-traumatic brain injury (TBI) vegetative state (VS) at 5 months.[167] A 23-year-old woman with clinical exam consistent with VS, with the exception of brief periods of visual fixation, following severe TBI was asked to imagine playing tennis or walking throughout her own house. The regionally selective brain activation patterns obtained from functional magnetic resonance imaging (fMRI) measurements for each condition were identical to those of normal controls. (B) A single subject judged initially as in VS demonstrated successful communication utilizing the activation methods shown in panel A (see Monti et al.[168]). (C) Demonstration of motor imagery command-following does not invariably lead to unambiguous communication with fMRI as shown by Bardin et al.[169]; the subject displayed two separate responses for the suit of a playing card shown (one correct and one incorrect), and a single incorrect response appears for the face of the card. See Bardin et al.[169] for details.
Figure elements adapted from Owen et al., Monti et al., and Bardin et al.[167–169]

However, CMD patients are distinct from those in LIS as a result of their sustaining direct injuries across the corticothalamic system in addition to severe damage to motor efferent pathways. Forgacs et al.[143] identified 4 of 44 DOC patients with limited overt behavioral responsiveness who showed fMRI evidence of command-following; all of these subjects demonstrated preserved wakeful and sleep EEG architecture and retained a preserved glucose metabolism as measured by [18]FDG-PET. Stender et al.[142] found that patients with fMRI evidence of command-following showed strong preservation of resting cerebral metabolism.

As Owen et al.[167] have originally and correctly argued, the demonstration of command following in fMRI paradigms constitutes a stringent test of forebrain function because this requires sustained neuronal activation in brain regions far from the sensory cortices supporting imagery and executive function for approximately 30 seconds at a time, in closely repeated bouts following prompts (typically for eight repetitions totaling about 4 minutes of active effort to generate a statistically significant response). Successful completion of these tasks must reflect a broad integrity of cerebral networks supporting sustained attention, working memory, and executive functions. Collectively, as noted earlier, the identification of CMD as separate category is supported by the wide range of brain structural and functional integrity measurements, including cerebral metabolism and organization of brain dynamics across the sleep–wake cycle. Although some authors have argued that no distinction should be drawn,[249] and it is certain that CMD will exist across a spectrum as well, the clustering of brain integrity measures closer to those seen in LIS identifies the urgency to evaluate and closely follow CMD patients.[250] In any CMD patient, sustained efforts should be directed toward identifying potential communication channels whether through isolated motor movements[248] or the use of augmentative technologies.[251]

Most importantly, the preservation of higher level receptive language function and cognitive systems required to perform such mental imagery tasks identifies a potential substrate for further recovery when paired with a motor output or augmentative technology to establish a communication system. Monti et al.[168] provided the first proof-of-concept of such a potential in a single-subject study (Figure 9.12B); Bardin et al.,[169] however, demonstrated that establishing command-following responses did not guarantee transfer of signaling into communication in a cohort of patients undergoing test-retest of fMRI motor imagery (Figure 9.12C). In some instances failures to communicate may arise from differences in the nature of the hemodynamic response function.[252]

Recovery of communication after severe multifocal brain injuries may be linked to a broad process of both functional and structural reorganization of intra- and interhemispheric function. Voss et al.[212] first developed evidence that slowly developing structural remodeling may be a potential source of late recovery following severe brain injury. They longitudinally characterized brain structural connectivity and resting metabolism in a 40-year-old man who recovered expressive and receptive language after remaining in MCS for 19 years after a TBI. The patient continued to improve over the next 2 years. MRI revealed extensive cerebral and subcortical atrophy particularly affecting the brainstem and frontal lobes; there

was marked volume loss throughout the brain with ventricular dilatation. However, DTI data revealed both severe diffuse axonal injury, as indicated by volume loss in the medial corpus callosum, but also large regions of increased connectivity in posterior brain white matter. Repeat imaging identified significant increases in anisotropy within the midline cerebellar white matter that correlated with significant clinical improvements in motor control over 18 months of further recovery.[212]

The findings of Voss et al.[212] suggested the possibility of structural changes within the patient's white matter playing a role in functional recovery. Similarly, Thengone et al.[170] studied the late recovery of communication prospectively in a patient with severe brainstem injuries involving both tegmental and ventral structures and the midline thalami. Local changes within the structure and function of the expressive language network within the frontal lobes and broad increases in cross-hemispheric structural and functional connections (similar to the structural changes reported by Voss et al.[212]) were associated with the patient's evolving recovery of a communication channel. Local increases in fractional anisotropy in Broca's area and occipital cortex were linked to both increased metabolism within the left frontotemporal cortices and selectively increased activation of BOLD signal within Broca's area and language-related regions in response to passive language stimuli. Increasing correlation of interhemispheric functional activation across language-responsive brain regions further correlated with the restoration of bihemispheric synchronization of sleep spindles (Figure 9.13). These results were associated with the patient's observed ability to communicate yes/no responses, albeit inconsistently, using eye movements over the course of 2.75 years. The restoration of even such limited communication resulted in a transformation of the patient's life (see Fins[253] for a detailed account).

Like the Thengone et al.[170] subject, CMD patients in chronic care facilities carry the greatest risk of ongoing recoveries of cognition going unnoticed[251,253]; thus, labeling and characterizing CMD patients as a specific group with unique physiological profiles compared to other patients with DOC after

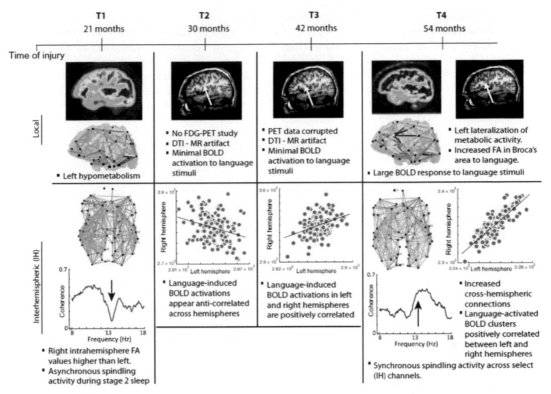

Figure 9.13 Slow structural remodeling of the adult human brain associated with emergence of a communication channel. Figure shows progressive changes in brain structural and functional measurements over a nearly three period of recovery of inconsistent communication in a patient first identified to show command-following approximately 2 years after extensive bilateral brainstem and central thalamic injuries (see Thengone et al.[170] for details). Diffusion tensor imaging revealed increasing connectivity (measured as increased fractional anisotropy) in Broca's area over time and in cross-hemispheric connections. Functional changes arising over the same time course of measurement included increases in left frontal lobe metabolic activity (measured by 18F-fluorodeoxyglucose-positron emission tomography [FDG-PET]), restoration of synchronization of sleep spindles in the sleep electroencephalogram (EEG), and increased hemispheric correlation of blood oxygen level-dependent (BOLD) response to passively presented language stimuli.
Figure from Thengone et al.[170]

severe brain injuries is a critically important step in their systematic study and in the development of effective treatment strategies. Most importantly, at least a subset of CMD patients can be expected to successfully harness bidirectional communication channels if augmentative technologies can be customized for them. However, the loss of corticothalamic connectivity in CMD patients produces impaired arousal regulation with varying contributions of specific cognitive impairments in the domains of memory, attention, and executive function. Individual patients may therefore require customization of assistive technologies even if a viable sensorimotor channel can be identified for communication. Once identified, CMD patients

need to be engaged in ongoing efforts to communicate as recovery after severe structural brain injuries may continue for years.[4,212] Recent prospective studies utilizing the resting EEG signal and network coherence measurements demonstrate a generalizability of the Thengone et al.[170] findings in a cohort of patients followed longitudinally over time; five patients who recovered communication, including the Thengone et al.[170] patient, all showed large changes in the dominant language hemisphere not present in age-matched controls.[254] Recovery in this cohort ranged across etiologies of injury to include severe TBI and diffuse hypoxic-ischemic injury; similarly recovery of communication occurred across an age range spanning the early 20s to late 50s, demonstrating a remarkable resilience of the recovery process.[254]

In this context, recent studies demonstrate that CMD patients are also misidentified in the acute intensive care setting.[141,255] A study of acutely brain injured patients in the ICU demonstrated that one out of 7 patients judged as unconscious were diagnosed as CMD using EEG methods; the CMD patients were more than 4 times more likely to recover and reach at least partial autonomy within one year.[255] These observations potentially challenge existing outcome statistics as early decisions of life-sustaining therapies are often predicated on the level of consciousness observed. Developing general screening for CMD in the acute setting is a critical near-term challenge.[144] Particular injury types may increase the risk of CMD, including basilar artery distribution infarctions, radial diffuse axonal injuries strongly impacting brainstem structures, and hypoxic-ischemic injuries impairing motor cortical and striatal function.[169,170,256]

ASSESSMENTS OF PATIENTS WITH CHRONIC DISORDERS OF CONSCIOUSNESS: AN EMPIRICAL GUIDE TO TIME-LIMITED PHARMACOLOGIC TRIALS

Given the variety of complex, nonprogressive brain injuries producing a chronic DOC, an empirical strategy for time trials of pharmacologic agents will likely remain founded on clinical experience and general principles. Data from clinical trials for each agent potentially useful in chronic DOC will never canvass the variety of mixed etiologies (e.g., trauma, hypoxic, inflammatory, postinfectious, autoimmune, and other processes), age, and specific patterns of structural brain injuries that may be present in any particular patient. Moreover, at present, there is a limited understanding of when significant residual capacity for improved function may be present. With this in mind, the following guide to assessment and time trials of pharmacologic agents is based on our own experience and the published literature reporting pharmacologic responses of severely brain-injured patients with chronic cognitive impairment. We organize our approach around the general circuit-level model for brain response to multifocal structural

brain injuries shown in Figure 9.9, which provides a framework for considering a wide range of agents for activation of the anterior forebrain.[202,213,257] The algorithm and approach suggested here reflects clinical experience but is unproven and should be seen as a guide. Several important clinical maxims should also frame the approach:

1. Patients may regress after demonstrating high-level brain function outside the period of acute injury and early convalescence without having suffered a new neurological insult. Some may have additional neurological disorders (e.g., delayed postanoxic encephalopathy or a seizure disorder). It is important that all such persons receive careful neurological re-evaluation, and they should be presumed to harbor the latent capacity to regain their previously demonstrated level of function until a compelling mechanism accounting for their decline is identified.
2. Patients with considerable preservation of brain structure who remain in coma, VS, or MCS should be aggressively evaluated for the potential for further recovery.
3. Patients with preserved corticothalamic anatomy and physiology (i.e., wake–sleep EEG architecture) along with severe brainstem injuries and motoric impairment secondary to interruption of the corticobulbar and corticospinal spinal tract pathways should always be very carefully evaluated for evidence of retained higher level brain function. Limitation of recovery of executive attention, working memory, and other high-order cognitive function may further impair the use of incomplete motor efferent systems in such patients.

It is likely that transient changes in distributed network function underlie the wide fluctuations in cognitive performance in some MCS patients and patients who immediately emerge from MCS with pharmacologic stimulation.[24,234,258] At least three different mechanisms may lead to such marked, reversible alteration of integrative brain activity following relatively focal or regionally restricted brain lesions: (1) a form of passive inhibition of broad brain regions following deafferentation of remote but strongly connected areas, (2) active inhibition resulting from altered connectivity and neuronal function following injury, and (3) persistent or paroxysmal functional activity produced by excess excitation of distributed neuronal networks and possible withdrawal of excitation from other brain regions.[259] When such local effects of injuries play a larger role in the observed behavioral state of the patient than widespread deafferentation, it reasonable to assume that a greater residual capacity exists to respond to medications.

A relatively common finding following focal ischemia or TBI is a reduction in cerebral metabolism in brain regions remote from the site of injury. This trans-synaptic (or "crossed") downregulation of distant neuronal populations (term "diaschisis" in the clinical literature) results from the loss of excitatory inputs from the damaged regions.[260] The clinical significance of these changes is unclear although electrophysiological correlates have been identified. Gold and Lauritzen[200] showed that although changes in blood flow may be modest in remote cortical regions, the trans-synaptic downregulation produces dramatic decreases in neuronal firing rates (e.g., a neuronal firing rate decreased by 80% with only a 20% reduction in regional blood flow). Thus, stable downregulation of cortical, thalamic, or basal ganglia neuronal populations through passive inhibition secondary to deafferentation is a possible source of functionally reversible alteration of cerebral network function. Intrinsic neuronal membrane properties allow nonlinear state changes on the basis of small deviations in excitation. In vivo experimental studies demonstrate that the loss of excitatory drive to neuronal populations as a result of trans-synaptic downregulation produces a powerful form of inhibition that hyperpolarizes the neuronal membrane potential.[201] In cerebral cortex[261] and basal ganglia,[262] *up* and *down* states have been identified in in vitro studies comparable to burst and tonic mode firing in the thalamus (see Chapter 1). The general circuit-level model shown in Figure 9.9 anticipates that this type of mechanism underlies the residual capacity of large connected cerebral networks, despite their remaining significantly limited in functional expression due to imbalance of neuromodulators that support a wakeful EEG and arousal pattern.[263] The most general approach underlying pharmacologic time trials is thus to attempt to broadly activate the frontal cortical and striatal system to overcome to some degree

such expected effects of broad trans-synaptic downregulation.

Other types of alteration of the balance of excitation and inhibition, particularly hypersynchronous epileptiform discharges, may play a key role in some patients with chronic DOC. Experimental studies have shown increased excitability following even modest brain trauma that may promote epileptiform activity in both cortical and subcortical regions.[264,265] Hypersynchronous activity within relatively restricted networks may underlie several different clinical phenomena following structural brain injuries. For example, a patient fluctuating from classic akinetic mutism into interactive awareness following an encephalitis had epileptiform activity measured locally within the thalamus that appeared only as surface slow waves in the EEG.[266] Such a mechanism might also explain reports of episodic akinetic mutism.[157] In one case study, a 52-year-old man remained in an akinetic mute state following the rupture of a basilar artery aneurysm with infarcts in the thalamus and basal ganglia. This behavioral state persisted without change for 17 months, at which time a spontaneous fluctuation in behavioral state occurred, described as a return to his "premorbid state, with full return of his demeanor and affect." The patient's functional recovery lasted 1 day and then relapsed.[157] One year after this event, the patient had a second "awakening" following a grand mal seizure. Electroconvulsive therapy, tried empirically, also reproduced the change. Blumenfeld and colleagues have importantly shown that focal seizures which alter consciousness may produce broad hemispheric disfacilitation similar to direct deafferentation injuries[267]; these investigators have developed evidence that thalamic inhibition underlies this linkage of paroxysmal activity and broad withdrawal of cortical excitation. Thus, the two mechanisms can be combined, as originally shown in an study by Williams and Parson-Smith.[266]

The possibility of occult underlying paroxysmal activity suggests the use of GABAergic agonists such as lorazepam or diazepam as safe diagnostic probes for initial evaluation.[157] GABAergic agents may also, however, support restoration of anterior forebrain mesocircuit function through a paradoxical excitation.[202,213,234,257] Such paradoxical effects of the drug zolpidem were first reported by

Clauss et al.[243] to underlie the late emergence from MCS in a 28-year-old man who suffered a diffuse axonal injury (presumably grade III with subcortical hemorrhages in basal ganglia, thalamus, and brainstem). Spontaneous eye opening with a GCS of 9 persisted for 3 years following injury until 10 mg of zolpidem (a $GABA_A$ positive allosteric modulator that binds to the alpha subunit) was administered. Within 15 minutes of administration, the patient began to speak and was able to respond to questions with "yes/no" answers and ultimately demonstrated intact remote and immediate memory. Temporary remission of chronic aphasia in a 52-year-old woman 3 years following administration of zolpidem has also been reported.[242] In this patient, regional cerebral blood flow measurements using single proton emission CT (SPECT) demonstrated a 35–40% increase in the medial frontal cortex bilaterally and left middle frontal and supramarginal gyri (Broca's area) 30 minutes after zolpidem ingestion. Similar mechanisms most likely underlie the well-publicized cases of Gary Dockery ("The Coma Cop") and Donald Herbert, a fireman who made international headlines in 2005 with a marked recovery of speech and cognitive function after 9 years of remaining in MCS following TBI. Electrophysiological and neuroimaging studies of small groups of zolpidem-responsive MCS patients provide evidence that bulk excitation of the anterior

forebrain mesocircuit is associated with these paradoxical behavioral improvements.[24,234]

Injury to the paramedian thalamus (intralaminar and related thalamic nuclei) and upper brainstem alone can produce widespread hemispheric trans-synaptic downregulation[268,269] as well as a variety of paroxysmal disturbances in the case of the paramedian thalamus. Most common among the types of paroxysmal alterations in brain dynamics following injury to the paramedian thalamus are generalized epileptic seizures, typically variations of the 3/s spike and wave form.[139,270] Other less well-known phenomena, such as oculogyric crises, are also associated with injuries to this region.[271] Hypersynchronous discharges restricted to the thalamostriatal system might also account for forms of catatonia[272,273] and the obsessive compulsive disorder infrequently observed after brain injuries.[274] Thus, damage to the upper brainstem and medial thalamus in combination with other cerebral injuries may lead to a variety of partially reversible mechanisms of dysfunction that could contribute to a reduced baseline activity in severely disabled patients and provide a structural basis for wide variation in functional performance.

With these general considerations in mind, Figure 9.14 shows an empirical algorithm based on our own clinical assessment of DOC patients over time. The sequence and structure

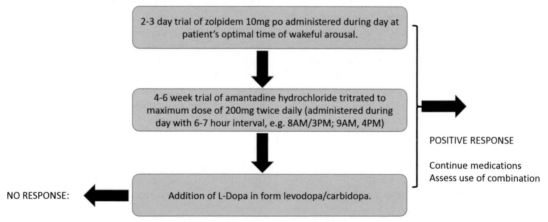

An empirical approach to pharmacologic time trials for the neurologist

2-3 day trial of zolpidem 10mg po administered during day at patient's optimal time of wakeful arousal.

4-6 week trial of amantadine hydrochloride tritrated to maximum dose of 200mg twice daily (administered during day with 6-7 hour interval, e.g. 8AM/3PM; 9AM, 4PM)

POSITIVE RESPONSE

Continue medications
Assess use of combination

NO RESPONSE: Addition of L-Dopa in form levodopa/carbidopa.

Consider use of noradrenergic, serotonergic, cholinergic agonists (see text).

If clinically suggested test with flumazenil, intravenous preparations of gabaergic agents, e.g. lorazepam, midazolam (see text)

Figure 9.14 Algorithm for time- limited pharmacologic trials.

of this algorithm derives from considerations of practicality and the general model of most common anticipated underlying mechanisms of DOC following coma reviewed earlier. As widespread cerebral deafferentation is the most typical originating cause of a chronic DOC, the initial suggested trials of pharmacologic agents are aimed at agents that will broadly activate the anterior forebrain mesocircuit. Many other possible etiologies, however, can be encountered in the patient with a chronic DOC and these less common entities also require systematic efforts to rule out.

The suggested algorithms begin with a brief time trial of zolpidem; a test dose of 10 mg given orally is suggested to be given during the day at a point of maximal alertness to support the possible elaboration of emergent behaviors. While zolpidem response is very rare, with less than 5% of patients with chronic DOC in a prospective study demonstrating a measurable effect,[244] effects are obvious when clinically meaningful. Only a few (1–3) careful evaluations should be necessary to judge the value of continued treatment with the drug. If patients are responsive, long-term use of the medication appears to have idiosyncratic effects, with some patients remaining responsive for years and others showing tolerance effects.[24,244]

Following a brief trial of zolpidem, the mainstay of pharmacologic treatment for DOC is amantadine. To date only one careful, multicenter trial has provided Class I evidence for the use of any pharmacologic agent to advance recovery after structural brain injury; Giacino et al. demonstrated that amantadine accelerated the course of recovery in posttraumatic VS and MCS within the first year following injury.[233] This observation has resulted in a treatment recommendation in the AAN/ACRM/NIDILRR Guidelines[5] which recommends that:

> Clinicians caring for patients in traumatic VS/UWS or MCS who are between 4 and 16 weeks post-injury should prescribe amantadine 100–200 mg twice daily to hasten functional recovery and reduce degree of disability after determining that there are no medical contraindications or other case-specific risks for use (Level B).[5]

While the time restriction in this recommendation originates from the limitation of

the Giacino et al.[233] study to this early intervention window during the subacute recovery process, many small studies have shown effects in patients with chronic DOC.[275] We suggest that a 4- to 6-week slowly escalating oral dose up to the AAN/ACRM/NIDILRR maximum of 200 mg twice daily be the next step in a pharmacologic time trial. Amantadine is only a weak dopamine transporter blocking agent and presynaptic dopaminergic impairment will not likely be improved with its use.[239] As a result, the addition of L-dopa (in the form of levodopa/carbidopa), or separate use if no response to amantadine is observed, should follow. In general L-dopa is well tolerated in the DOC population, and slow titration up to a 1 g/d in divided doses is safe to observe for possible response; if no benefit is evident, the drug should be slowly tapered and discontinued.

While these three steps have shown the most consistent value in our clinical judgment, other activating medications have in individual instances shown similar effects. We have observed, and the literature supports, instances of similar paradoxical responses to other sedative agents (including but not limited to midazolam, diazepam, and lorazepam). Notably, clinical experience also demonstrates that some such patients will only respond paradoxically to GABAergic agonists when delivered parentally (examples include midazolam, lorazepam, and sodium pentothal). Amantadine has strong NMDA antagonist properties and noradrenergic agonist properties.[276] Other medications with demonstrated noradrenergic agonist effects in some patients include methylphenidate (which may produce a reverse effect on frontostriatal activation in a significant fraction of the population, see Volkow et al.[277]), dextroamphetamine/amphetamine, and atomoxetine, a norepinephrine reuptake inhibitor, and perhaps in conjunction with serotoninergic reuptake inhibitors such as citalopram. Another rare underlying mechanism that produces a chronic hypersomnia that may in principle impact evaluation of DOC is the presence of an endogenous benzodiazepine-like substance which responds to treatment with flumazenil.[278] Rye and colleagues have identified a bioactive CSF component of 500–3,000 daltons present in patients with primary hypersomnia that responds to flumazenil.[279] Of note, in primary hypersomnia patients, the antibiotic clarithromycin modulates symptoms and can be considered as a potential alternative to flumazenil.[280]

REFERENCES

1. Elmer J, Torres C, Aufderheide TP, et al.; Resuscitation Outcomes Consortium. Association of early withdrawal of life-sustaining therapy for perceived neurological prognosis with mortality after cardiac arrest. *Resuscitation* 2016;102:127–135.
2. Izzy S, Compton R, Carandang R, Hall W, MuehlschlegelS. Self-fulfilling prophecies through withdrawal of care: do they exist in traumatic brain injury, too? *Neurocrit Care* 2013;19(3):347–63. doi: 10.1007/s12028-013-9925-z.
3. Turgeon AF, Lauzier F, Simard JF, et al Canadian Critical Care Trials Group. Mortality associated with withdrawal of life-sustaining therapy for patients with severe traumatic brain injury: a Canadian multicentre cohort study [published online ahead print August 29, 2011]. *CMAJ* 2011;183(14):1581–1588. doi: 10.1503/cmaj.101786.
4. Nakase-Richardson R, et al. Longitudinal outcome of patients with disordered consciousness in the NIDRR TBI Model Systems Programs. *J Neurotrauma* 2012;29:59–65.
5. Giacino JT, Katz DI, Schiff ND, et al. Comprehensive systematic review update summary: disorders of consciousness: report of the Guideline Development, Dissemination, and Implementation Subcommittee of the American Academy of Neurology; the American Congress of Rehabilitation Medicine; and the National Institute on Disability, Independent Living, and Rehabilitation Research [published online ahead of print August 8, 2018]. *Arch Phys Med Rehabil* 2018;99(9):1710–1719. doi: 10.1016/j.apmr.2018.07.002.
6. Broderick JP, Adams HP Jr, Barsan W, et al. Guidelines for the management of spontaneous intra-cerebral hemorrhage: a statement for healthcare professionals from a special writing group of the Stroke Council, American Heart Association. *Stroke* 1999;30:905–915.
7. Brain Trauma Foundation. Management and prognosis of severe traumatic brain injury. *American Association of Neurological Surgeons*, 2001.
8. Booth CM, Boone RH, Tomlinson G, et al. Is this patient dead, vegetative, or severely neurologically impaired? Assessing outcome for comatose survivors of cardiac arrest. *JAMA* 2004;291:870–879.
9. Nielsen N, Wetterslev J, Cronberg T, et al TTM Trial Investigators. Targeted temperature management at 33°C versus 36°C after cardiac arrest. *N Engl J Med* 2013;369(23):2197–2206.
10. Greer DM. Cardiac arrest and postanoxic encephalopathy. *Continuum (Minneap Minn)* 2015;21(5 Neurocritical Care):1384–1396.
11. Rossetti AO, Rabinstein AA, Oddo M. Neurological prognostication of outcome in patients in coma after cardiac arrest. *Lancet Neurol.* 2016;15(6):597–609. doi: 10.1016/S1474-4422(16)00015-6.
12. Flynn-O'Brien KT, Fawcett VJ, Nixon ZA, et al Temporal trends in surgical intervention for severe traumatic brain injury caused by extra-axial hemorrhage, 1995 to 2012. *Neurosurgery* 2015;76(4):451–460.
13. Chan PS, McNally B, Tang F, Kellermann A; CARES Surveillance Group. Recent trends in survival from out-of-hospital cardiac arrest in the United States. *Circulation.* 2014;130(21):1876–1882.
14. Nieuwkamp DJ, Setz LE, Algra A, Linn FH, de Rooij NK, Rinkel GJ. Changes in case fatality of aneurysmal subarachnoid haemorrhage over time, according to age, sex, and region: a meta-analysis. *Lancet Neurol* 2009;8(7):635–642.
15. Jennett B, Teasdale G, Braakman R, et al. Prognosis of patients with severe head injury. *Neurosurgery* 1979;4:283–289.
16. Levy DE, Bates D, Caronna JJ, et al. Prognosis in nontraumatic coma. *Ann Intern Med* 1981;94:293–301.
17. Jennett B, Bond M. Assessment of outcome after severe brain damage. *Lancet* 1975;1:480–484.
18. Wilson JT, Pettigrew LE, Teasdale GM. Structured interviews for the Glasgow Outcome Scale and the extended Glasgow Outcome Scale: guidelines for their use. *J Neurotrauma* 1998;15(8):573–585.
19. Laureys S, Celesia GG, Cohadon F, et al European Task Force on Disorders of Consciousness. Unresponsive wakefulness syndrome: a new name for the vegetative state or apallic syndrome. *BMC Med* 2010;8:68.
20. Bernat JL. Nosologic considerations in disorders of consciousness. *Ann Neurol* 2017;82(6):863–865.
21. Bruno MA, Vanhaudenhuyse A, Thibaut A, Moonen G, Laureys S. From unresponsive wakefulness to minimally conscious PLUS and functional locked-in syndromes: recent advances in our understanding of disorders of consciousness. *J Neurol* 2011;258:1373–1384.
22. Schiff ND. Cognitive motor dissociation following severe brain injuries. *JAMA Neurol* 2015;72(12):1413–1415.
23. Becker DA, Schiff ND, Becker LB, et al. A major miss in prognostication after cardiac arrest: Burst suppression and brain healing. *Epilepsy Behav Case Rep* 2016;17(7):1–5.
24. Williams ST, Conte MM, Goldfine AM, et al Common resting brain dynamics indicate a possible mechanism underlying zolpidem response in severe brain injury. *Elife.* 2013;2:e01157. doi: 10.7554/eLife.01157.
25. Consensus conference. Rehabilitation of persons with traumatic brain injury. NIH Consensus Development Panel on Rehabilitation of Persons with Traumatic Brain Injury. *JAMA* 1999;282:974–983.
26. Jennett B. Predictors of recovery in evaluation of patients in coma. *Adv Neurol* 1979;22:129–135.
27. Steyerberg EW, Mushkudiani N, Perel P, et al Predicting outcome after traumatic brain injury: development and international validation of prognostic scores based on admission characteristics. *PLoS Med.* 2008;5(8):e165; discussion e165.
28. Roozenbeek B, Chiu YL, Lingsma HF. Predicting 14-day mortality after severe traumatic brain injury: application of the IMPACT models in the brain

trauma foundation TBI-trac® New York State database. *J Neurotrauma* 2012;29(7):1306–1312.

29. Gennarelli TA, Champion HR, Copes WS, et al. Comparison of mortality, morbidity, and severity of 59,713 head injured patients with 114,447 patients with extra-cranial injuries. *J Trauma* 1994;37:962–968.

30. Narayan RK, Greenberg RP, Miller JD, et al. Improved confidence of outcome prediction in severe head injury. A comparative analysis of the clinical examination, multimodality evoked potentials, CT scanning, and intracranial pressure. *J Neurosurg* 1981;54:751–762.

31. Braakman R, Gelpke GJ, Habbema JD, et al. Systematic selection of prognostic features in patients with severe head injury. *Neurosurgery* 1980;6:362–370.

32. Choi SC, Narayan RK, Anderson RL, et al. Enhanced specificity of prognosis in severe head injury. *J Neurosurg* 1988;69:381–385.

33. Stocchetti N, Penny KI, Dearden M, et al. Intensive care management of head-injured patients in Europe: a survey from the European brain injury consortium. *Intensive Care Med* 2001;27:400–406.

34. Teasdale G, Knill-Jones R, van der SJ. Observer variability in assessing impaired consciousness and coma. *J Neurol Neurosurg Psychiatry* 1978;41:603–610.

35. Marion DW, Carlier PM. Problems with initial Glasgow Coma Scale assessment caused by prehospital treatment of patients with head injuries: results of a national survey. *J Trauma* 1994;36:89–95.

36. Jennett B, Teasdale G, Galbraith S, et al. Severe head injuries in three countries. *J Neurol Neurosurg Psychiatry* 1977;40:291–298.

37. Signorini DF, Andrews PJ, Jones PA, et al. Predicting survival using simple clinical variables: a case study in traumatic brain injury. *J Neurol Neurosurg Psychiatry* 1999;66:20–25.

38. Hukkelhoven CW, Steyerberg EW, Rampen AJ, et al. Patient age and outcome following severe traumatic brain injury: an analysis of 5600 patients. *J Neurosurg* 2003;99:666–673.

39. van Dongen KJ, Braakman R, Gelpke GJ. The prognostic value of computerized tomography in comatose head-injured patients. *J Neurosurg* 1983;59:951–957.

40. Fearnside MR, Cook RJ, McDougall P, et al. The Westmead Head Injury Project outcome in severe head injury. A comparative analysis of pre-hospital, clinical and CT variables. *Br J Neurosurg* 1993;7:267–279.

41. Carlsson CA, von Essen C, Lofgren J. Factors affecting the clinical course of patients with severe head injuries. 1. Influence of biological factors. 2. Significance of posttraumatic coma. *J Neurosurg* 1968;29:242–251.

42. Young GB. The EEG in coma. *J Clin Neurophysiol* 2000;17:473–485.

43. Young GB, Wang JT, Connolly JF. Prognostic determination in anoxic-ischemic and traumatic encephalopathies. *J Clin Neurophysiol* 2004;21:379–390.

44. Logi F, Fischer C, Murri L, et al. The prognostic value of evoked responses from primary somatosensory and auditory cortex in comatose patients. *Clin Neurophysiol* 2003;114:1615–1627.

45. Lew HL, Dikmen S, Slimp J, et al. Use of somatosensory-evoked potentials and cognitive event-related potentials in predicting outcomes of patients with severe traumatic brain injury. *Am J Phys Med Rehabil* 2003;82:53–61.

46. Schwarz S, Schwab S, Aschoff A, et al. Favorable recovery from bilateral loss of somatosensory evoked potentials. *Crit Care Med* 1999;27:182–187.

47. Robe PA, Dubuisson A, Bartsch S, et al. Favourable outcome of a brain trauma patient despite bilateral loss of cortical somatosensory evoked potential during thiopental sedation. *J Neurol Neurosurg Psychiatry* 2003;74:1157–1158.

48. Schorl M, Valerius-Kukula SJ, Kemmer TP. Median-evoked somatosensory potentials in severe brain injury: does initial loss of cortical potentials exclude recovery? *Clin Neurol Neurosurg* 2014;123:25–33.

49. Mazzini L, Zaccala M, Gareri F, et al. Long-latency auditory-evoked potentials in severe traumatic brain injury. *Arch Phys Med Rehabil* 2001;82:57–65.

50. Perrin F, Schnakers C, Schabus M, et al. Brain response to one's own name in vegetative state, minimally conscious state, and locked-in syndrome. *Arch Neurol* 2006;63:562–569.

51. Tzovara A, Rossetti AO, Spierer L, et al Progression of auditory discrimination based on neural decoding predicts awakening from coma. *Brain* 2013;136(Pt 1):81–89.

52. Pelinka LE, Kroepfl A, Leixnering M, et al. GFAP versus S100B in serum after traumatic brain injury: relationship to brain damage and outcome. *J Neurotrauma* 2004;21:1553–1561.

53. Mercier E, Boutin A, Lauzier F, et al Predictive value of S-100β protein for prognosis in patients with moderate and severe traumatic brain injury: systematic review and meta-analysis. *BMJ* 2013;346:f1757.

54. Mercier E, Boutin A, Shemilt M, et al Predictive value of neuron-specific enolase for prognosis in patients with moderate or severe traumatic brain injury: a systematic review and meta-analysis. *CMAJ Open* 2016;4(3):E371–E382.

55. Shutter L, Tong KA, Holshouser BA. Proton MRS in acute traumatic brain injury: role for glutamate/glutamine and choline for outcome prediction. *J Neurotrauma* 2004;21:1693–1705.

56. Sharma K, Stevens RD. Determinants of prognosis in neurocatastrophes. *Handb Clin Neurol* 2017;140:379–395.

57. Stevens RD1, Sutter R. Prognosis in severe brain injury. *Crit Care Med* 2013;41(4):1104–1123.

58. Perel P, Arango M, Clayton T, et al Predicting outcome after traumatic brain injury: practical prognostic models based on large cohort of international patients. *BMJ* 2008;336(7641):425–429.

59. Booth CM, Boone RH, Tomlinson G, et al. Is this patient dead, vegetative, or severely neurologically impaired? Assessing outcome for comatose survivors of cardiac arrest. *JAMA* 2004;291:870–879.

60. Rohaut B, Claassen J. Decision making in perceived devastating brain injury: a call to explore the impact of cognitive biases. *Br J of Anesthesia* 2018;120(1):5–9. PMID 29397137

61. Hamel MB, Goldman L, Teno J, et al. Identification of comatose patients at high risk for death or severe disability. SUPPORT Investigators. Understand prognoses

and preferences for outcomes and risks of treatments. *JAMA* 1995;273:1842–1848.

62. Sacco RL, VanGool R, Mohr JP, et al. Nontraumatic coma. Glasgow coma score and coma etiology as predictors of 2-week outcome. *Arch Neurol* 1990;47:1181–1184.

63. Greer DM, Yang J, Scripko PD, et al Clinical examination for outcome prediction in nontraumatic coma. *Crit Care Med* 2012;40(4):1150–1156.

64. Sasser H. *Association of Clinical Signs with Neurological Outcome After Cardiac Arrest* [dissertation]. University of Pittsburgh; 1999.

65. Geocadin RG, Wijdicks E, Armstrong MJ, et al Practice guideline summary: Reducing brain injury following cardiopulmonary resuscitation: Report of the Guideline Development, Dissemination, and Implementation Subcommittee of the American Academy of Neurology. *Neurology* 2017;88(22):2141–2149.

66. Madl C, Kramer L, Domanovits H, et al. Improved outcome prediction in unconscious cardiac arrest survivors with sensory evoked potentials compared with clinical assessment. *Crit Care Med* 2000;28:721–726.

67. Forgacs P, Devinsky O, Schiff ND. Independent functional outcomes after prolonged coma following cardiac arrest: a mechanistic hypothesis. (submitted)

68. Zandbergen EG, de Haan RJ, Stoutenbeek CP, et al. Systematic review of early prediction of poor outcome in anoxic-ischaemic coma. *Lancet* 1998;352:1808–1812.

69. Brunko E, Zegers de Beyl D. Prognostic value of early cortical somatosensory evoked potentials after resuscitation from cardiac arrest. *Electroencephalogr Clin Neurophysiol* 1987 Jan;66(1):15–24.

70. Chen R, Bolton CF, Young B. Prediction of outcome in patients with anoxic coma: a clinical and electrophysiologic study. *Crit Care Med* 1996 Apr;24(4):672–678.

71. Bender A, Howell K, Frey M, Berlis A, Naumann M, Buheitel G. Bilateral loss of cortical SSEP responses is compatible with good outcome after cardiac arrest. *J Neurol* 2012;259(11):2481–2483.

72. Karunasekara N, Salib S, MacDuff A. A good outcome after absence of bilateral N20 SSEPs post-cardiac arrest. *J Intensive Care Soc* 2016;17(2):168–170.

73. Rothstein TL, Thomas EM, Sumi SM. Predicting outcome in hypoxic-ischemic coma. A prospective clinical and electrophysiologic study. *Electroencephalogr Clin Neurophysiol* 1991;79:101–107.

74. Rothstein TL. The role of evoked potentials in anoxic-ischemic coma and severe brain trauma. *J Clin Neurophysiol* 2000;17:486–497.

75. Fischer C, Luauté J, Adeleine P, et al. Predictive value of sensory and cognitive evoked potentials for awakening from coma. *Neurology* 2004;63:669–673.

76. Mattsson N, Zetterberg H, Nielsen N, et al Serum tau and neurological outcome in cardiac arrest. *Ann Neurol* 2017;82(5):665–675.

77. Goh WC, Heath PD, Ellis SJ, et al. Neurological outcome prediction in a cardiorespiratory arrest survivor. *Br J Anaesth* 2002;88:719–722.

78. Wijdicks EF, Rabinstein AA. Absolutely no hope? Some ambiguity of futility of care in devastating acute stroke. *Crit Care Med* 2004;32:2332–2342.

79. Werhahn KJ, Brown P, Thompson PD, et al. The clinical features and prognosis of chronic posthypoxic myoclonus. *Mov Disord* 1997;12:216–220.

80. Elmer J, Rittenberger JC, Faro J, et al. Clinically distinct electroencephalographic phenotypes of early myoclonus after cardiac arrest. *Ann Neurol* 2016;80(2):175–184.

81. Reynolds AS, Holmes MG, Agarwal S, Claassen J. Phenotypes of early myoclonus do not predict outcome. *Ann Neurol* 2017;81(3):475–476.

82. Reynolds AS, Rohaut B, Holmes MG, et al Early myoclonus following anoxic brain injury. *Neurol Clin Pract* 2018;8(3):249–256.

83. Kaplan PW. The EEG in metabolic encephalopathy and coma. *J Clin Neurophysiol* 2004;21:307–318.

84. Golby A, McGuire D, Bayne L. Unexpected recovery from anoxic-ischemic coma. *Neurology* 1995;45:1629–1630.

85. Greer DM, Rosenthal ES, Wu O. Neuroprognostication of hypoxic-ischaemic coma in the therapeutic hypothermia era. *Nat Rev Neurol* 2014;10(4):190–203.

86. Wijdicks EF, Rabinstein AA. Absolutely no hope? Some ambiguity of futility of care in devastating acute stroke. *Crit Care Med* 2004;32:2332–2342.

87. Pullicino PM, Alexandrov AV, Shelton JA, et al. Mass effect and death from severe acute stroke. *Neurology* 1997;49:1090–1095.

88. Voetsch B, DeWitt LD, Pessin MS, et al. Basilar artery occlusive disease in the New England Medical Center Posterior Circulation Registry. *Arch Neurol* 2004;61:496–504.

89. Rabinstein AA, Tisch SH, McClelland RL, et al. Cause is the main predictor of outcome in patients with pontine hemorrhage. *Cerebrovasc Dis* 2004;17:66–71.

90. Hemphill JC et al. Prospective validation of the ICH Score for 12-month functional outcome. *Neurology* 2009;73:1088–1094.

91. Rost NS, et al. Prediction of functional outcome in patients with primary intracerebral hemorrhage: the FUNC score. *Stroke* 2008;39:2304–2309.

92. Report of World Federation of Neurological Surgeons Committee on a universal subarachnoid hemorrhage grading scale. *J Neurosurg* 1988;68:985–986.

93. Rosen DS, Macdonald RL. Grading of subarachnoid hemorrhage: modification of the World Federation of Neurosurgical Societies scale on the basis of data for a large series of patients. *Neurosurgery* 2004;54:566–575.

94. Schievink WI, Wijdicks EF, Piepgras DG, et al. The poor prognosis of ruptured intracranial aneurysms of the posterior circulation. *J Neurosurg* 1995;82:791–795.

95. Inamasu J, Nakae S, Ohmi T, et al The outcomes of early aneurysm repair in World Federation of Neurosurgical Societies grade V subarachnoid haemorrhage patients with emphasis on those presenting with a Glasgow Coma Scale score of 3. *J Clin Neurosci* 2016;33:142–147.

96. Suwatcharangkoon S, Meyers E, Falo C, et al. Loss of consciousness at onset of subarachnoid hemorrhage as an important marker of early brain injury. *JAMA Neurol* 2016;73(1):28–35. doi: 10.1001/jamaneurol.2015.3188. PMID: 26552033.

97. Lee VH, Ouyang B, John S, et al. Risk stratification for the in-hospital mortality in subarachnoid hemorrhage: the HAIR score. *Neurocrit Care*

2014;21(1):14–19.   doi:10.1007/s12028-013-9952-9. PMID: 24420695.

98. Witsch J, Frey HP, Patel S, et al Prognostication of long-term outcomes after subarachnoid hemorrhage: the FRESH score [published online ahead of print May 25, 2016]. *Ann Neurol* 2016;80(1):46–58. doi:10.1002/ana.24675. PMID: 27129898.

99. Lantigua H, Ortega-Gutierrez S, Schmidt JM, et al Subarachnoid hemorrhage: who dies, and why? *Crit Care* 2015;19:309. doi:10.1186/s13054-015-1036-0. PMID: 26330064.

100. Hojer C, Haupt WF. The prognostic value of AEP and SEP values in subarachnoid hemorrhage. An analysis of 64 patients [in German]. *Neurochirurgia (Stuttg)* 1993;36:110–116.

101. Ritz R, Schwerdtfeger K, Strowitzki M, et al. Prognostic value of SSEP in early aneurysm surgery after SAH in poor-grade patients. *Neurol Res* 2002;24:756–764.

102. van de Beek BD, De Gans J, Spanjaard L, et al. Clinical features and prognostic factors in adults with bacterial meningitis. *N Engl J Med* 2004;351:1849–1859.

103. Pikis A, Kavaliotis J, Tsikoulas J, et al. Long-term sequelae of pneumococcal meningitis in children. *Clin Pediatr (Phila)* 1996;35:72–78.

104. Roos KL, Tunkel AR, Scheld WM. Acute bacterial meningitis. In: Scheld WM, Whitley RJ, Marra CM, eds. *Infections of the Central Nervous System*. 3rd ed. Philadelphia: Lippincott Williams & Wilkins; 2004:347–422.

105. Muralidharan R, Mateen FJ, Rabinstein AA. Outcome of fulminant bacterial meningitis in adult patients. *Eur J Neurol* 2014;21(3):447–453.

106. Hoogman M, van de Beek D, Weisfelt M, de Gans J, Schmand B. Cognitive outcome in adults after bacterial meningitis. *J Neurol Neurosurg Psychiatry* 2007;78(10):1092–1096.

107. Xiao F, Tseng MY, Teng LJ, et al. Brain abscess: clinical experience and analysis of prognostic factors. *Surg Neurol* 2005;63:442–449.

108. Yang SY, Zhao CS. Review of 140 patients with brain abscess. *Surg Neurol* 1993;39:290–296.

109. Taira N, Kamei S, Morita A, et al Predictors of a prolonged clinical course in adult patients with herpes simplex virus encephalitis. *Intern Med* 2009;48(2):89–94.

110. Menge T, Hemmer B, Nessler S, et al Acute disseminated encephalomyelitis: an update. *Arch Neurol* 2005;62(11):1673–1680.

111. Sonneville R, Demeret S, Klein I, et al. Acute disseminated encephalomyelitis in the intensive care unit: clinical features and outcome of 20 adults. *Intensive Care Med* 2008;34(3):528–532.

112. Titulaer MJ, McCracken L, Gabilondo I, et al Treatment and prognostic factors for long-term outcome in patients with anti-NMDA receptor encephalitis: an observational cohort study [published online ahead of print January 3, 2013]. *Lancet Neurol* 2013;12(2):157–165. doi:10.1016/S1474-4422(12)70310-1. PMID: 23290630.

113. Maloney PR, Mallory GW, Atkinson JL, Wijdicks EF, Rabinstein AA, Van Gompel JJ. Intracranial pressure monitoring in acute liver failure: institutional case series. *Neurocrit Care* 2016;25(1):86–93. doi:10.1007/s12028-016-0261-y.

114. Pulver M, Plum F. Disorders of consciousness. In: Evans WR, Baskin DS, Yatsu FM, eds. *Prognosis of Neurological Disorders*. 2nd ed. New York: Oxford University Press; 2000:523–534.

115. García-Martínez R, Simón-Talero M, Córdoba J. Prognostic assessment in patients with hepatic encephalopathy. *Dis Markers* 2011;31(3):171–179.

116. Witsch J, Neugebauer H, Flechsenhar J, Jüttler E. Hypoglycemic encephalopathy: a case series and literature review on outcome determination. *J Neurol* 2012;259(10):2172–2181.

117. Ikeda T, Takahashi T, Sato A, et al Predictors of outcome in hypoglycemic encephalopathy. *Diabetes Res Clin Pract* 2013;101(2):159–163.

118. Barbara G, Mégarbane B, Argaud L, et al Functional outcome of patients with prolonged hypoglycemic encephalopathy. *Ann Intensive Care* 2017;7(1):54.

119. Farrell B, Godwin J, Richards S, et al. The United Kingdom transient ischaemic attack (UK-TIA) aspirin trial: final results. *J Neurol Neurosurg Psychiatry* 1991;54(12):1044–1054.

120. Jennett B, Plum F. Persistent vegetative state after brain damage: a syndrome in search of a name. *Lancet* 1972;1:434–437.

121. Persistent vegetative state: report of the American Neurological Association Committee on Ethical Affairs. ANA Committee on Ethical Affairs. *Ann Neurol* 1993;33(4):386–390.

122. Jennett B. *The Vegetative State: Medical Facts, Ethical and Legal Dilemmas*. Cambridge: Cambridge University Press; 2002.

123. Corazzol M, Lio G, Lefevre A, et al Restoring consciousness with vagus nerve stimulation. *Curr Biol* 2017;27(18):R994–R996.

124. Giacino JT, Ashwal S, Childs N, et al. The minimally conscious state—definition and diagnostic criteria. *Neurology* 2002;58:349–353.

125. Schiff ND, Plum F. The role of arousal and "gating" systems in the neurology of impaired consciousness. *J Clin Neurophysiol* 2000;17(5):438–452.

126. Katz DI, Alexander MP, Mandell AM. Dementia following strokes in the mesencephalon and diencephalon. *Arch Neurol* 1987;44:1127–1133.

127. The Multi-Society Task Force on PVS. Medical aspects of the persistent vegetative state (1). *N Engl J Med* 1994;330:1499–1508.

128. The Multi-Society Task Force on PVS. Medical aspects of the persistent vegetative state (2). *N Engl J Med* 1994;330:1572–1579.

129. Cairns H, Oldfield RC, Pennybacker JB, et al. Akinetic mutism with an epidermoid cyst of the 3rd ventricle. *Brain* 1941;84:272–290.

130. Otto A, Zerr I, Lantsch M, et al. Akinetic mutism as a classification criterion for the diagnosis of Creutzfeldt-Jakob disease. *J Neurol Neurosurg Psychiatry* 1998;64:524–528.

131. Nemeth G, Hegedus K, Molnar L. Akinetic mutism associated with bicingular lesions: clinicopathological and functional anatomical correlates. *Eur Arch Psychiatry Neurol Sci* 1988;237:218–222.

132. Castaigne P, Lhermitte F, Buge A, et al. Paramedian thalamic and midbrain infarct: clinical and neuropathological study. *Ann Neurol* 1981;10:127–148.

133. Segarra JM. Cerebral vascular disease and behavior. I. The syndrome of the mesencephalic

artery (basilar artery bifurcation). *Arch Neurol* 1970;22:408–418.

134. Fisher CM. Honored guest presentation: abulia minor vs. agitated behavior. *Clin Neurosurg* 1983;31:9–31.

135. Alexander GE, DeLong MR, Strick PL. Parallel organization of functionally segregated circuits linking basal ganglia and cortex. *Annu Rev Neurosci* 1986;9:357–381.

136. Mega MS, Cohenour RC. Akinetic mutism: disconnection of frontal-subcortical circuits. *Neuropsychiatry Neuropsychol Behav Neurol* 1997;10:254–259.

137. Fleet WS, Valenstein E, Watson RT, et al. Dopamine agonist therapy for neglect in humans. *Neurology* 1987;37:1765–1770.

138. Matsuda W, Matsumura A, Komatsu Y, et al. Awakenings from persistent vegetative state: report of three cases with parkinsonism and brain stem lesions on MRI. *J Neurol Neurosurg Psychiatry* 2003;74:1571–1573.

139. van Domburg PH, Ten Donkelaar HJ, Notermans SL. Akinetic mutism with bithalamic infarction. Neuro-physiological correlates. *J Neurol Sci* 1996;139:58–65.

140. Stuss DT, Guberman A, Nelson R, et al. The neuropsychology of paramedian thalamic infarction. *Brain Cogn* 1988;8:348–378.

141. Edlow BL, Chatelle C, Spencer CA, et al. Early detection of consciousness in patients with acute severe traumatic brain injury. *Brain* 2017;140(9):2399–2414.

142. Stender J, Gosseries O, Bruno MA, et al. Diagnostic precision of PET imaging and functional MRI in disorders of consciousness: a clinical validation study. *Lancet*. 2014;384(9942):514–522.

143. Forgacs PB, Conte MM, Fridman EA, Voss HU, Victor JD, Schiff ND. Preservation of electroencephalographic organization in patients with impaired consciousness and imaging-based evidence of command-following. *Ann Neurol* 2014;76(6):869–879.

144. Schiff ND. Uncovering hidden integrative cerebral function in the intensive care unit. *Brain* 2017;140(9):2259–2262.   doi:10.1093/brain/awx209.

145. Rosenberg GA, Johnson SF, Brenner RP. Recovery of cognition after prolonged vegetative state. *Ann Neurol* 1977;2:167–168.

146. Childs NL, Mercer WN. Brief report: late improvement in consciousness after post-traumatic vegetative state. *N Engl J Med* 1996;334:24–25.

147. Dyer C. PVS criteria put under spotlight. *BMJ* 1997;314(7085):919.

148. Schiff ND, Ribary U, Plum F, Llinas R. Words without mind. *J Cogn Neurosci* 1999;1(6):650–656.

149. Giacino JT, Kalmar K. The vegetative and minimally conscious states: a comparison of clinical features and functional outcome. *J Head Trauma Rehabil* 1997;12:36–51.

150. Luauté J, Maucort-Boulch D, Tell L, et al. Long-term outcomes of chronic minimally conscious and vegetative states. *Neurology* 2010;75(3):246.

151. Kotchoubey B, Lang S, Mezger G, et al. Information processing in severe disorders of consciousness: vegetative state and minimally conscious state. *Clin Neurophysiol* 2005;116(10):2441–2453.

152. Wang F, Di H, Hu X, et al. Cerebral response to subject's own name showed high prognostic value in traumatic vegetative state. *BMC Med* 2015;13:83.

153. Whyte J, Katz D, Long D, et al. Predictors of outcome in prolonged posttraumatic disorders of consciousness and assessment of medication effects: A multicenter study. *Arch Phys Med Rehabil* 2005;86:453–462.

154. Cavinato M, Freo U, Ori C, et al. Post-acute P300 predicts recovery of consciousness from traumatic vegetative state. *Brain Injury* 2009;23:973–980.

155. Bagnato S, Boccagni C, Sant'Angelo A, Prestandrea C, Mazzilli R, Galardi G. EEG predictors of outcome in patients with disorders of consciousness admitted for intensive rehabilitation. *Clin Neurophysiol.* 2015;126(5):959–966.

156. Zheng X, Chen M, Li J, Cao F. Prognosis in prolonged coma patients with diffuse axonal injury assessed by somatosensory evoked potential. *Neural Regen Res* 2013;8:948–954.

157. Burruss JW, Chacko RC. Episodically remitting akinetic mutism following subarachnoid hemorrhage. *J Neuropsychiatry Clin Neurosci* 1999;11:100–102.

158. Bernat JL. Questions remaining about the minimally conscious state. *Neurology* 2002;58:337–338.

159. Onofrj M, Thomas A, Paci C, et al. Event related potentials recorded in patients with locked-in syndrome. *J Neurol Neurosurg Psychiatry* 1997;63:759–764.

160. Leon-Carrion J, Van Eeckhout P, Dominguez-Morales MDR. Review of subject: the locked-in syndrome: a syndrome looking for a therapy. *Brain Inj* 2002;16:555–569.

161. Doble JE, Haig AJ, Anderson C, et al. Impairment, activity, participation, life satisfaction, and survival in persons with locked-in syndrome for over a decade: follow-up on a previously reported cohort. *J Head Trauma Rehabil* 2003;18:435–444.

162. Bauby J-D. *The Diving Bell and the Butterfly.* New York: Vintage International; 1997.

163. Ware JE, Snow KK, Kosinski M, et al. SF-36 Health Survey Manual and Interpretation Guide. Boston, MA: New England Medical Center, The Health Institute, 1993.

164. Laureys S, Pellas F, Van Eeckhout P, et al. The locked-in syndrome: what is it like to be conscious but paralyzed and voiceless? *Prog Brain Res* 2005;150:495–511.

165. Laureys S, Schiff ND. Coma and consciousness: paradigms (re)framed by neuroimaging. *Neuroimage* 2012;61(2):478–491.

166. Giacino JT, Fins JJ, Laureys S, Schiff ND. Disorders of consciousness after acquired brain injury: the state of the science [published online ahead of print January 28, 2014]. *Nat Rev Neurol* 2014;10(2):99–114. doi:10.1038/nrneurol.2013.279.

167. Owen AM, Coleman MR, Boly M, et al. Detecting awareness in the vegetative state. *Science* 2006;313:1402.

168. Monti MM, Vanhaudenhuyse A, Coleman et al. Willful modulation of brain activity in disorders of consciousness. *N Engl J Med* 2016;18;362(7):579–589.

169. Bardin JC, Fins JJ, Katz DI, et al. Dissociations between behavioural and functional magnetic resonance imaging-based evaluations of cognitive function after brain injury. *Brain* 2011;134(Pt 3):769–782. doi:10.1093/brain/awr005.
170. Thengone DJ, Voss HU, Fridman EA, Schiff ND. Local changes in network structure contribute to late communication recovery after severe brain injury. *Sci Transl Med* 2016;8(368):368re5.
171. Curley WH, Forgacs PB, Voss HU, Conte MM, Schiff ND. Characterization of EEG signals revealing covert cognition in the injured brain. *Brain* 2018;141(5):1404–1421.
172. Kondziella D, Friberg CK, Frokjaer VG, Fabricius M, Møller K. Preserved consciousness in vegetative and minimal conscious states: systematic review and meta-analysis. *J Neurol Neurosurg Psychiatry* 2016;87(5):485–492.
173. Levy DE, Sidtis JJ, Rottenberg DA, et al. Differences in cerebral blood flow and glucose utilization in vegetative versus locked-in patients. *Ann Neurol* 1987;22:673–682.
174. DeVolder AG, Goffinet AM, Bol A, et al. Brain glucose metabolism in postanoxic syndrome. Positron emission tomographic study. *Arch Neurol* 1990;47:197–204.
175. Tommasino C, Grana C, Lucignani G, et al. Regional cerebral metabolism of glucose in comatose and vegetative state patients. *J Neurosurg Anesthesiol* 1995;7:109–116.
176. Rudolf J, Ghaemi M, Ghaemi M, et al. Cerebral glucose metabolism in acute and persistent vegetative state. *J Neurosurg Anesthesiol* 1999;11:17–24.
177. Laureys S, Faymonville ME, Degueldre C, et al. Auditory processing in the vegetative state. *Brain* 2000;123:1589–1601.
178. Schiff ND, Ribary U, Moreno DR, et al. Residual cerebral activity and behavioural fragments can remain in the persistently vegetative brain. *Brain* 2002;125:1210–1234.
179. Blacklock JB, Oldfield EH, Di CG, et al. Effect of barbiturate coma on glucose utilization in normal brain versus gliomas. Positron emission tomography studies. *J Neurosurg* 1987;67:71–75.
180. Alkire MT, Miller J. General anesthesia and the neural correlates of consciousness. *Prog Brain Res* 2005;150:229–244.
181. Maquet P, Degueldre C, Delfiore G, et al. Functional neuroanatomy of human slow wave sleep. *J Neurosci* 1997;17:2807–2812.
182. Laureys S, Owen AM, Schiff ND. Brain function in coma, vegetative state, and related disorders. *Lancet Neurol* 22004;3:537–546.
183. Laureys S, Faymonville ME, Ferring M, et al. Differences in brain metabolism between patients in coma, vegetative state, minimally conscious state and locked in syndrome. *Eur J Neurol* 2003;10:224.
184. Laureys S, Lemaire C, Maquet P, et al. Cerebral metabolism during vegetative state and after recovery to consciousness. *J Neurol Neurosurg Psychiatry* 1999;67:121–122.
185. Laureys S, Faymonville ME, Peigneux P, et al. Cortical processing of noxious somatosensory stimuli in the persistent vegetative state. *Neuroimage* 2002;17:732–741.
186. Plum F, Schiff N, Ribary U, et al. Coordinated expression in chronically unconscious persons. *Philos Trans R Soc Lond B Biol Sci* 1998;353:1929–1933.
187. Schiff ND, Ribary U, Moreno DR, et al. Residual cerebral activity and behavioural fragments can remain in the persistently vegetative brain. *Brain* 2002;125:1210–1234.
188. Menon DK, Owen AM, Williams EJ, et al. Cortical processing in persistent vegetative state. Wolfson Brain Imaging Centre Team. *Lancet* 1998;352:1148–1149.
189. Macniven JA, Poz R, Bainbridge K, et al. Emotional adjustment following cognitive recovery from "persistent vegetative state": psychological and personal perspectives. *Brain Inj* 2003;17:525–533.
190. Schiff ND, Plum F. Cortical function in the persistent vegetative state. *Trends Cogn Sci* 1999;3:43–44.
191. Menon DK, Owen AM, Pickard JD. Response from Menon, Owen and Pickard. *Trends Cogn Sci* 1999;3:44–46.
192. Zeki S. The visual association cortex. *Curr Opin Neurobiol* 1993;3:155–159.
193. Demertzi A, Antonopoulos G, Heine L, et al. Intrinsic functional connectivity differentiates minimally conscious from unresponsive patients [published online ahead of print June 27, 2015]. *Brain.* 2015;138(Pt 9):2619–2631. doi:10.1093/brain/awv169.
194. Chennu S, Annen J, Wannez S, et al. Brain networks predict metabolism, diagnosis and prognosis at the bedside in disorders of consciousness. *Brain* 2017;140(8):2120–2132.
195. Sitt JD, King JR, El Karoui I, et al. Large scale screening of neural signatures of consciousness in patients in a vegetative or minimally conscious state. *Brain.* 137(Pt 8):2258–2270.
196. Casarotto S, Comanducci A, Rosanova M, et al. Stratification of unresponsive patients by an independently validated index of brain complexity. *Ann Neurol* 2016;80(5):718–729.
197. Casali AG, Gosseries O, Rosanova M, et al. A theoretically based index of consciousness independent of sensory processing and behavior. *Sci Transl Med* 2013;14,5(198):198ra105.
198. King JR, Sitt JD, Faugeras F, et al. Information sharing in the brain indexes consciousness in noncommunicative patients [published online ahead of print September 26, 2013]. *Curr Biol* 2013;23(19):1914–1919. doi: 10.1016/j.cub.2013.07.075.
199. Steriade M, Contreras D, Curró Dossi R, Nuñez A. The slow (< 1 Hz) oscillation in reticular thalamic and thalamocortical neurons: scenario of sleep rhythm generation in interacting thalamic and neocortical networks. *J Neurosci* 1993;13(8):3284–3299.
200. Gold L, Lauritzen M. Neuronal deactivation explains decreased cerebellar blood flow in response to focal cerebral ischemia or suppressed neocortical function. *Proc Natl Acad Sci U S A* 2002;99:7699–7704.
201. Timofeev I, Grenier F, Steriade M. Disfacilitation and active inhibition in the neocortex during the natural sleep-wake cycle: an intracellular study. *Proc Natl Acad Sci U S A* 2000;98:1924–1929.

202. Brown EN, Lydic R, Schiff ND. General anesthesia, sleep and coma. *N Engl J Med* 2010;363(27):2638–2650.

203. Krolak-Salmon P, Croisile B, Houzard C, Setiey A, Girard-Madoux P, Vighetto A. Total recovery after bilateral paramedian thalamic infarct. *Eur Neurol* 2000;44:216–218.

204. Parvizi J, Damasio AR. Neuroanatomical correlates of brainstem coma. *Brain* 2003;126:1524–1536.

205. Schiff ND. Central thalamic contributions to arousal regulation and neurological disorders of consciousness. *Ann N Y Acad Sci* 2008;1129:105–118.

206. Mair RG, Onos KD, Hembrook JR. Cognitive activation by central thalamic stimulation: the Yerkes-Dodson law revisited. *Dose Response* 2011;9(3):313–331.

207. Schiff ND Resolving the role of the paramedian thalamus in forebrain arousal mechanisms. *Annals of Neurology*. 2019;84(6):812–813.

208. Liu J, Lee HJ, Weitz AJ, et al. Frequency-selective control of cortical and subcortical networks by central thalamus. *Elife* 2015;pii: e09215. doi: 10.7554/eLife.09215.

209. Baker JL, Ryou JW, Wei XF, Butson CR, Schiff ND, Purpura KP. Robust modulation of arousal regulation, performance, and frontostriatal activity through central thalamic deep brain stimulation in healthy nonhuman primates. *J Neurophysiol* 2016;116(5):2383–2404. doi:10.1152/jn.01129.2015. PMID: 27582298.

210. Fuller PM, Sherman D, Pedersen NP, Saper CB, Lu J. Reassessment of the structural basis of the ascending arousal system. *J Comp Neurol* 2011;519(5):933–956.

211. Edlow JA, Rabinstein A, Traub SJ, Wijdicks EF. Diagnosis of reversible causes of coma. *Lancet* 2014;384(9959):2064–2076.

212. Voss HU, Ulug AM, Watts R, et al. Possible axonal regrowth in late recovery from minimally conscious state. *J Clin Invest* 2006;116:2005–2011.

213. Schiff ND. Recovery of consciousness after brain injury: a mesocircuit hypothesis. *Trends Neurosci* 2010;33(1):1–9.

214. Fridman EA, Beattie BJ, Broft A, Laureys S, Schiff ND. Regional cerebral metabolic patterns demonstrate the role of anterior forebrain mesocircuit dysfunction in the severely injured brain [published online ahead of print April 14, 2014]. *Proc Natl Acad Sci U S A* 2014;111(17):6473–6478. doi:10.1073/pnas.1320969111.

215. Vanhaudenhuyse A, Noirhomme Q, Tshibanda LJ, et al. Default network connectivity reflects the level of consciousness in non-communicative brain-damaged patients. *Brain* 2010;133:161–171.

216. Raichle ME, MacLeod AM, Snyder AZ, et al. A default mode of brain function. *Proc Natl Acad Sci U S A* 2001;98:676–682.

217. Gusnard DA, Raichle ME, Raichle ME. Searching for a baseline: functional imaging and the resting human brain. *Nat Rev Neurosci* 2001;2:685–694.

218. Gusnard DA, Akbudak E, Shulman GL, et al. Medial prefrontal cortex and self-referential mental activity: relation to a default mode of brain function. *Proc Natl Acad Sci U S A* 2001;98:4259–4264.

219. Greicius MD, Krasnow B, Reiss AL, et al. Functional connectivity in the resting brain: a network analysis of the default mode hypothesis. *Proc Natl Acad Sci U S A* 2003;100:253–258.

220. Simpson JR Jr, Snyder AZ, Gusnard DA, et al. Emotion-induced changes in human medial prefrontal cortex: I. During cognitive task performance. *Proc Natl Acad Sci U S A* 2001;98:683–687.

221. Simpson JR Jr, Drevets WC, Snyder AZ, Gusnard DA, Raichle ME. Emotion-induced changes in human medial prefrontal cortex: II. During anticipatory anxiety. *Proc Natl Acad Sci U S A* 2001;98(2):688–693.

222. Shah S, Mohamadpour M, Askin G, et al. Focal electroencephalographic changes index post-traumatic confusion and outcome [published online ahead of print June 22, 2017]. *J Neurotrauma* 2017;34(19):2691–2699. doi:10.1089/neu.2016.4911. PMID: 28462682.

223. Laureys S, Faymonville ME, Ferring M, et al. Differences in brain metabolism between patients in coma, vegetative state, minimally conscious state and locked-in syndrome. *Eur J Neurol* 2003; 10:224.

224. Van derWerf YD, Witter MP, Groenewegen HJ. The intralaminar and midline nuclei of the thalamus. Anatomical and functional evidence for participation in processes of arousal and awareness. *Brain Res Brain Res Rev* 2002;39:107–140.

225. Schiff ND, Shah SA, Hudson AE, Nauvel T, Kalik SF, Purpura KP. Gating of attentional effort through the central thalamus [published online ahead of print December 5, 2012]. *J Neurophysiol* 2013;109(4):1152–1163. doi:10.1152/jn.00317.2011.

226. Wyder MT, Massoglia DP, Stanford TR. Contextual modulation of central thalamic delay-period activity: representation of visual and saccadic goals. *J Neurophysiol* 2004;91:2628–2648.

227. Maxwell WL, MacKinnon MA, Smith DH, McIntosh TK, Graham DI. Thalamic nuclei after human blunt head injury. *J Neuropathol Exp Neurol*, 2006;65:478–488.

228. Grillner S, Hellgren J, Ménard A, Saitoh K, Wikström MA. Mechanisms for selection of basic motor programs—roles for the striatum and pallidum. *Trends Neurosci* 2005;28:364–370.

229. Schiff ND. Posterior medial corticothalamic connectivity and consciousness. *Ann Neurol* 2012;72(3):305–306.

230. Rye DB, Turner RS, Vitek JL, Bakay RAE, Crutcher MD, DeLong MR. Anatomical investigations of the pallidotegmental pathway in monkey and man. In: Ohye C, Kimura M, McKenzie JS, eds. *The Basal Ganglia V*. New York: Plenum Press; 1996: 59–75.

231. Heckers S, Geula C, Mesulam MM. Cholinergic innervation of the human thalamus: dual origin and differential nuclear distribution. *J Comp Neurol* 1992;325:68–82.

232. Laureys SL, Owen AM, Schiff ND. Brain function in coma, vegetative state and related disorders. *Lancet Neurol* 2004 3(9):537–546.

233. Giacino JT, Whyte J, Bagiella E, et al. Placebo-controlled trial of amantadine for severe traumatic brain injury. *N Engl J Med* 2012;366(9):819–826.

234. Chatelle C, Thibaut A, Gosseries O, et al. Changes in cerebral metabolism in patients with a minimally

conscious state responding to zolpidem. *Front Hum Neurosci* 2014;8:917.

235. Schiff ND, Giacino JT, Kalmar K, et al. Behavioral improvements with thalamic stimulation after severe traumatic brain injury. *Nature* 2007;448:600–603.

236. Thibaut A, Di Perri C, Chatelle C, et al. Clinical response to tDCS depends on residual brain metabolism and grey matter integrity in patients with minimally conscious state. *Brain Stimul* 2015;8(6):1116–1123.

237. Thibaut A. Schiff ND. New therapeutic options for the treatment of patients with disorders of consciousness: the field of neuromodulation. In: Schnakers C, Laureys S, eds. *Coma and Disorders of Consciousness*. Cham, Switzerland: Springer International.

238. Shah SA, Goldin Y, Conte MM, et al. Executive attention deficits after traumatic brain injury reflect impaired recruitment of resources. *Neuroimage Clin* 2017;14:233–241.   doi:10.1016/j.nicl.2017.01.010. PMID: 28180082.

239. Fridman EA, Schiff ND. Neuromodulation of the conscious state following severe brain injuries. *Curr Opin Neurobiol* 2014;29C:172–177.

240. Långsjö JW, Alkire MT, Kaskinoro K, et al. Returning from oblivion: imaging the neural core of consciousness. *J Neurosci* 2012;32(14):4935–4943.

241. Xie G, Deschamps A, Backman SB, et al. Critical involvement of the thalamus and precuneus during restoration of consciousness with physostigmine in humans during propofol anaesthesia: a positron emission tomography study. *Br J Anaesth* 2011;106(4):548–557.

242. Brefel-Courbon C, et al. Clinical and imaging evidence of zolpidem effect in hypoxic encephalopathy. *Ann Neurol* 2007;62(1):102–105.

243. Clauss RP, van der Merwe CE, Nel HW. Arousal from a semi-comatose state on zolpidem. *S Afr Med J* 2001;91:788–789.

244. Whyte J, Rajan R, Rosenbaum A, et al. Zolpidem and restoration of consciousness. *Am J Phys Med Rehabil* 2014;93(2):101–113.

245. McCarthy MM, Brown EN, Kopell N. Potential network mechanisms mediating electroencephalographic beta rhythm changes during propofol-induced paradoxical excitation. *J Neurosci* 2009;28:13488–504. doi:10.1523/JNEUROSCI.3536-08.2008.

246. McCarthy MM, Moore-Kochlacs C, Gu X, Boyden ES, Han X, Kopell N. Striatal origin of the pathologic beta oscillations in Parkinson's disease. *Proc Natl Acad Sci USA* 2011;108:11620–11625. doi: 10.1073/pnas.1107748108.

247. Waldvogel HJ, Kubota Y, Fritschy J, Mohler H, Faull RL. Regional and cellular localisation of GABA(A) receptor subunits in the human basal ganglia: an autoradiographic and immunohistochemical study. *J Comp Neurol* 1999;151:386–395.

248. Pignat JM, Mauron E, Jöhr J, et al. Outcome prediction of consciousness disorders in the acute stage based on a complementary motor behavioural tool. *PLoS One* 2016;11(6):e0156882.

249. Bayne T, Hohwy J, Owen AM. Reforming the taxonomy in disorders of consciousness. *Ann Neurol* 2017;82(6):866–872.

250. Braiman C, Fridman EA, Conte et al. Cortical response to the natural speech envelope correlates with neuroimaging evidence of cognition in severe brain injury. *Current Biology* In press;28(23):3833–3839.

251. Fins JJ, Schiff ND. In search of hidden minds. *Sci Am Mind* 2016;27:44–51.

252. Bardin JC, Schiff ND, Voss HU. Pattern classification of volitional fMRI responses in severely brain-injured subjects. *Arch Neurol* 2012;69(2):176–181.

253. Fins J. *Rights Come to Mind*. Cambridge University Press; 2015 New York, New York.

254. Nauvel TJ. *The Time Evolution of Global Brain Dynamics in the Human Electroencephalogram: Innovations in Quantitative Multi-variate Methods and Applications to Neurological Disorders* [thesis]. Weill Cornell Medicine; 2017.

255. Claassen J, Doyle K, Matory A, et al. Detection of brain activation in unresponsive patients with acute brain injury. *N Engl J Med* 2019 (in press).

256. Forgacs PB, Fridman EA, Goldfine AM, Schiff ND. Isolation syndrome after cardiac arrest and therapeutic hypothermia. *Front Neurosci* 2016;10:259. doi: 10.3389/fnins.2016.00259.

257. Schiff ND, Posner JP. Another "Awakenings." *Ann Neurol* 2007;62;5–7.

258. Schnakers C, Hustinx R, Vandewalle G. Measuring the effect of amantadine in chronic anoxic minimally conscious state. *J Neurol Neurosurg Psychiatry* 2008;79(2):225–227.

259. Schiff N.D. Modeling the minimally conscious state: measurements of brain function and therapeutic possibilities. *Prog Brain Res* 2005;150:477–497.

260. Nguyen DK, Botez MI. Diaschisis and neurobehavior. *Can J Neurol Sci* 1998;25:5–12.

261. McCormick DA, Shu Y, Hasenstaub A, et al. Persistent cortical activity: mechanisms of generation and effects on neuronal excitability. *Cereb Cortex* 2003;13:1219–1231.

262. Kasanetz F, Riquelme LA, Murer MG. Disruption of the two-state membrane potential of striatal neurones during cortical desynchronisation in anaesthetised rats. *J Physiol* 2002;543:577–589.

263. Robinson PA, Rennie CJ, Rowe DL. Dynamics of large-scale brain activity in normal arousal states and epileptic seizures. *Phys Rev E Stat Nonlin Soft Matter Phys* 2002;65:041924.

264. Santhakumar V, Ratzliff AD, Jeng J, et al. Long-term hyperexcitability in the hippocampus after experimental head trauma. *Ann Neurol* 2001;50:708–717.

265. Topolnik L, Steriade M, Timofeev I. Hyperexcitability of intact neurons underlies acute development of trauma-related electrographic seizures in cats in vivo. *Eur J Neurosci* 2003;18:486–496.

266. Williams D, Parsons-Smith G. Thalamic activity in stupor. *Brain* 1951;74:377–398.

267. Blumenfeld H, Rivera M, McNally KA, Davis K, Spencer DD, Spencer SS. Ictal neocortical slowing in temporal lobe epilepsy. *Neurology* 2004;63(6):1015–1021.

268. Szelies B, Herholz K, Pawlik G, et al. Widespread functional effects of discrete thalamic infarction. *Arch Neurol* 1991;48:178–182.

269. Caselli RJ, Graff-Radford NR, Rezai K. Thalamocortical diaschisis: single-photon emission tomographic study of cortical blood flow change after focal thalamic infarction. *Neuropsychiatry Neuropsychol Behav Neurol* 1991;4:193–214.

270. Ingvar DH. Reproduction of the 3 per second spike and wave EEG pattern by subcortical electrical stimulation in cats. *Acta Physiol Scand* 1955;33:137–150.

271. Kakigi R, Shibasaki H, Katafuchi Y, et al. The syndrome of bilateral paramedian thalamic infarction associated with an oculogyric crisis. *Rinsho Shinkeigaku* 1986;26:1100–1105.

272. Wilcox JA, Nasrallah HA. Organic factors in catatonia. *Br J Psychiatry* 1986;149:782–784.

273. Kamal AR, Schiff ND. Does the form of akinetic mutism linked to mesodiencephalic injuries bridge the double dissociation of Parkinson's disease and catatonia? *Behav Brain Sci* 2002;25:586–587.

274. Berthier ML, Kulisevsky JJ, Gironell A, et al. Obsessive compulsive disorder and traumatic brain injury: behavioral, cognitive, and neuroimaging findings. *Neuropsychiatry Neuropsychol Behav Neurol* 2001;14:23–31.

275. Zafonte R, Hammond F, Dennison A, Chew E. Pharmacotherapy to enhance arousal: what is known and what is not. *Prog Brain Res* 2009;177:293–316.

276. Sommerauer C, Rebernik P, Reither H, Nanoff C, Pifl C. The noradrenaline transporter as site of action for the anti-Parkinson drug amantadine. *Neuropharmacology* 2012;62(4):1708–1716.

277. Volkow ND, Wang GJ, Fowler JS, et al. Effects of methylphenidate on regional brain glucose metabolism in humans: relationship to dopamine D2 receptors. *Am J Psychiatry* 1997;154(1):50–55.

278. Trotti LM, Saini P, Koola C, LaBarbera V, Bliwise DL, Rye DB. Flumazenil for the Treatment of Refractory Hypersomnolence: Clinical Experience with 153 Patients. *J Clin Sleep Med* 2016;12(10):1389–1394.

279. Rye DB, Bliwise DL, Parker K, et al. Modulation of vigilance in the primary hypersomnias by endogenous enhancement of GABAA receptors. *Sci Transl Med* 2012;4(161):161ra151. doi: 10.1126/scitranslmed.3004685.

280. Trotti LM, Saini P, Bliwise DL, Freeman AA, Jenkins A, Rye DB. Clarithromycin in γ-aminobutyric acid-related hypersomnolence: A randomized, crossover trial. *Ann Neurol* 2015;78(3):454–465.

Chapter 10

Brain Death

DETERMINATION OF BRAIN DEATH

CLINICAL SIGNS OF BRAIN DEATH
Brainstem Function
Confirmatory Laboratory Tests and Diagnosis

Diagnosis of Brain Death in Profound Anesthesia
    or Coma of Undetermined Etiology
Pitfalls in the Diagnosis of Brain Death
Brain Death Versus Prolonged Coma
Management of the Brain Dead Patient

DETERMINATION OF BRAIN DEATH

Since Mollaret and Goulon[1] first examined the question in 1959, investigators have tried to establish criteria that would accurately and unequivocally determine that the brain is dead or about to die no matter what therapeutic measures one might undertake. Since that time, several committees and reviewers have sought to establish appropriate clinical and laboratory criteria for brain death based on retrospective analyses. The earliest widely known definition is that of the 1968 Ad Hoc Committee of the Harvard Medical School to examine the criteria of brain death (called, at the time, "irreversible coma"[2]) (Table 10.1). At present, in the United States the principle that brain death is equivalent to the death of the person is established under the Uniform Determination of Death Act.[3] (In fact, all death is brain death. An artificial heart can

keep a patient alive. If all the organs, save the brain, were artificial, that individual would still be alive. Conversely, when the brain is dead, sustaining the other organs by artificial means is simply preserving a dead body and not keeping the individual alive. Thus, although this chapter uses the term "brain death," the term as we use it carries the same import as death.) Detailed evidence-based guidelines and practice parameters for the clinical diagnosis of brain death are available from the American Academy of Neurology (AAN) online (http://www.aan.com). An AAN subcommittee reviewed these Guidelines in 2010 to address specific questions about possible diagnostic accuracy and aspects of the brain death assessment[4] (see the later section "Brain Death Versus Prolonged Coma").

Three medical considerations emphasize the importance of the concept of brain death: (1) transplant programs require the donation of healthy peripheral organs for

Table 10.1 Harvard Criteria for Brain Death (1968)

1. Unresponsive coma
2. Apnea
3. Absence of cephalic reflexes
4. Absence of spinal reflexes
5. Isoelectric electroencephalogram
6. Persistence of conditions for at least 24 hours
7. Absence of drug intoxication or hypothermia

From Ad Hoc Committee of the Harvard Medical School.[2]

Table 10.2 Clinical Criteria for Brain Death in Adults and Children in the United States

A. Coma of established cause
   1. No potentially anesthetizing amounts of either toxins or therapeutic drugs can be present; hypothermia below 30°C or other physiologic abnormalities must be corrected to the extent medically possible.
   2. Irreversible structural disease or a known and irreversible endogenous metabolic cause due to organ failure must be present.
B. Absence of motor responses
   1. Absence of pupillary responses to light and pupils at midposition with respect to dilation (4–6 mm)
   2. Absence of corneal reflexes
   3. Absence of caloric vestibulo-ocular responses
   4. Absence of gag reflex
   5. Absence of coughing in response to tracheal suctioning
   6. Absence of sucking and rooting reflexes
   7. Absence of respiratory drive at a $PaCO_2$ that is 60 mm Hg or 20 mm Hg above normal baseline values (apnea testing)
C. Interval between two evaluations, by patient's age
   1. Term to 2 months old, 48 hours
   2. >2 months to 1 year old, 24 hours
   3. >1 year to <18 years old, 12 hour
   4. ≥18 years old, optional
D. Confirmatory tests
   1. Term to 2 months old, two confirmatory tests
   2. >2 months to 1 year old, one confirmatory test
   3. >1 year to <18 years old, optional
   4. ≥18 years old, optional

success. The early diagnosis of brain death before the systemic circulation fails allows the salvage of such organs. However, ethical and legal considerations demand that if one is to declare the brain dead, the criteria must be clear and unassailable. (2) Even if there were no transplant programs, the ability of modern medicine to keep a body functioning for extended periods often leads to prolonged, expensive, and futile procedures accompanied by great emotional strain on family and medical staff. Conversely, the recuperative powers of the brain sometimes can seem astounding to the uninitiated, and individual patients whom uninformed physicians might give up for hopelessly brain damaged or dead sometimes make unexpectedly good recoveries (see "Pitfalls," page 445). It is even more important to know when to fight for life than to be willing to diagnose death. Extra efforts should be made to recognize and minimize the impact of cognitive biases that assume poor outcomes in patients with apparently devastating brain injury that can result in suboptimal resuscitative management approaches. This will often result in brain death as a self-fulfilling prophecy[5]. (3) Critical care facilities are limited and expensive and inevitably place a drain on other medical resources. Their best use demands that one identify and select patients who are most likely to benefit from intensive techniques so that these units are not overloaded with individuals who can never recover cerebral function.

The cornerstone of the diagnosis of brain death remains a careful and sure clinical neurologic examination (Table 10.2). In addition, a thorough evaluation of clinical history, neuroradiologic studies, and laboratory tests must be done to rule out potential confounding variables. The diagnosis of brain

death rests on two major and indispensable tenets. The first is that the cause of brain nonfunction must be inherently irreversible. This means that damage must be due to either known structural injury (e.g., cerebral hemorrhage or infarction, brain trauma, abscess) or known irreversible metabolic injury such as prolonged asphyxia. The second indispensable tenet is that the vital structures of the brain necessary to maintain consciousness and independent vegetative survival are damaged beyond all possible recovery.

The cause of brain damage must be known irreversible. This first criterion is crucial, and the diagnosis of brain death cannot be considered until it is fulfilled. The reason for stressing this point is that both in the United States and abroad often "coma of unknown origin" arising outside of a hospital is due to depressant drug poisoning. Witnesses cannot be relied upon for accurate histories under such circumstances because efforts at suicide or homicide can readily induce false testimony by companions or family. Even in patients already in the hospital for the treatment of other illnesses, drug poisoning administered by self or others sometimes occurs and at least temporarily can deceive the medical staff. Accordingly, the diagnosis of an irreversible lesion by clinical and laboratory means must be fully documented and unequivocally accurate before considering a diagnosis of brain death. The ease of being mistaken in such a diagnosis is illustrated by some of the results of a collaborative study sponsored several years ago by the National Institutes of Health.[6] The findings of toxicologic analyses revealed many more cases in which drug poisoning caused deep coma than had been suspected clinically by physicians, not all of whom had previous experiences with the ubiquity and subtlety of sedative-induced coma. The most common underlying causes of brain death are listed in Table 10.3. Documentation of structural injury explaining loss of brainstem function by computed tomography (CT) or magnetic resonance imaging (MRI) is possible in almost all patients. If scans are normal and clinical history is equivocal for the origin of cerebral demise, an examination of the cerebral spinal fluid is indicated.

A prospective study[7] evaluated 310 patients with cardiac arrest or other forms of acute medical coma who met the clinical criteria of brain death for 6 hours with no examples of recovery. Asystole occurred in all within a matter of hours or days. Jorgenson[9] systematically examined the time required for recovery of neurologic functions in 54 patients following cardiopulmonary arrest and plotted these times against eventual outcomes. For respiratory movements, pupillary light reflexes, coughing, swallowing, and ciliospinal reflexes, the longest respective times of reappearance compatible with any cerebral recovery were 15, 28, 58, and 52 minutes. In other words, if no recognizable brain function returned within an hour, the brain never recovered.

Time periods for repeated evaluations of brain death criteria may vary and are influenced by the etiology of injury. Several guidelines suggest a minimum time period of 24 hours over which human subjects must show signs of brain death following anoxic injury (or other diffuse toxic-metabolic insult; e.g. air, fat embolism, endocrine derangement) before the final diagnosis can be reached.[10] Evaluation times for identified structural injuries of the brainstem are typically shorter. Since time is so strong a safeguard, and few brain-damaged patients escape receiving at least an initial dose of a drug (alcohol or sedative outside of hospital, sedatives or anticonvulsants inside), guidelines suggest a 6-hour period of observation before making a clinical diagnosis of brain death (https://www.aan.com/Guidelines/home/ByTopic?topicId=13). This seems a reasonable time interval for cases where all circumstances of onset, diagnosis, and treatment can be fully identified.

Table 10.3 Most Common Etiologies of Brain Death

1. Traumatic brain injury
2. Aneurysmal subarachnoid hemorrhage
3. Intracerebral hemorrhage
4. Ischemic stroke with cerebral edema and herniation
5. Hypoxic-ischemic encephalopathy
6. Fulminant hepatic necrosis with cerebral edema and increased intracranial pressure

From Wijdicks,[8] with permission.

CLINICAL SIGNS OF BRAIN DEATH

All observers agree that in order to conclude that the vital functions of the brain have ceased, no behavioral or clinical reflex responses that depend on structures innervated from the supraspinal nervous system can exist. In a practical sense, because forebrain function depends on the integrity of the brainstem, the brain death examination primarily focuses on functional brainstem activity (Table 10.2). These observations may be accompanied by confirmatory tests providing evidence of absence of cerebral hemispheric and upper brainstem function, discussed later. Patients with primarily brainstem lesions pose a particular challenge and may require ancillary testing to accurately diagnose brain death.[11]

Brainstem Function

PUPILS

The pupils must be nonreactive to light. In the period immediately following brain death, the agonal release of adrenal catecholamines into the bloodstream may cause the pupils to become dilated. However, as the catecholamines are metabolized, the pupils return to a midposition. Hence, although the Harvard criteria required that the pupils be dilated as well as fixed, midposition fixed pupils are a more reliable sign of brain death, and failure of the pupils to return to midposition within several hours after brain death suggests residual sympathetic activation arising from the medulla. The pupils should be tested with a bright light and the physician should be certain that mydriatic agents, including intravenous atropine, have not been used (although conventional doses of atropine used in treating patients with cardiac arrest will not block the direct light response). Neuromuscular blocking agents, however, should not affect pupillary size as nicotinic receptors are not present in the iris. One case has been reported that described the unusual observation of persistent asynchronous light-independent pupillary activity (2.5 seconds constriction/10 seconds dilation) in an otherwise "brain dead" patient.[12]

OCULAR MOVEMENTS

Failure of brainstem function should be determined by the inability to find either oculocephalic or caloric vestibulo-ocular responses (VOR; see Chapter 2). In patients in whom a history of possible trauma has not been eliminated, cervical spine injury must be excluded before testing oculocephalic responses. Care should be taken when performing cold water caloric testing to ensure that the stimulus reaches the tympanic membrane. Up to 1 minute of observation for eye movement should follow irrigation of each side, with a 5-minute interval between each examination.

MOTOR, SENSORY, AND REFLEX ACTIVITY

The initial Harvard criteria demanded that there be an absence of all voluntary and reflex movements, including absence of corneal responses and other brainstem reflexes; no postural activity, including decerebrate rigidity; and no stretch reflexes in the extremities. Reflex responses mediated by the brainstem (e.g., corneal and jaw jerk reflexes as well as cutaneous reflexes such as snout and rooting reflexes) must be absent before making the diagnosis of brain death. The absence of a gag reflex should be tested by stimulation of the posterior pharynx but may be difficult to elicit or observe in intubated patients. Additionally, response to noxious stimulation of the supraorbital nerve or temporomandibular joints[13] should be tested during the examination. However, spinal reflex activity, in response to both noxious stimuli and tendon stretch, often can be shown to persist in experimental animals whose brains have been destroyed above the spinal level. The same reflexes can be found in the isolated spinal cord of humans following high spinal cord transection.

A variety of unusual, spinally mediated movements can appear and persist for prolonged periods during artificial life support.[14-21] Such phenomena include spontaneous movements in synchrony with the mechanical ventilator; slow body movements producing flexion at the waist, causing the body to rise to a sitting position ("Lazarus sign"); "stepping movements"; and preservation of lower body reflexes.[4] The consensus view is that in a patient in whom apneic oxygenation shows no return of breathing, such movements are generated by the spinal cord and the vital functions of the brainstem have no chance of recovery, making the diagnosis of brain death appropriate. It is important to note that spontaneous hypoxic or hypotensive events and apnea testing may precipitate these movements. Surprisingly, extensor plantar responses are not found in brain dead patients.[16] Instead, plantar responses are either flexor, absent, or consistent with undulations of toe flexion.[21]

APNEA

Spontaneous respiration must be absent. Most patients on a mechanical ventilator will have a PaO_2 above and a $PaCO_2$ below normal levels. However, the threshold for stimulation of respiratory movements by the blood gases usually is elevated in patients in deep coma, sometimes to $PaCO_2$ values as high as 50–55 mm Hg. As a result, such patients may be apneic for several minutes when removed from the ventilator, even if they have a structurally normal brainstem. To test brainstem function without concurrently inducing severe hypoxemia under such circumstances, respiratory activity should be tested by the technique of apneic oxygenation. With this technique, the patient is ventilated with 100% oxygen for a period of 10–20 minutes. The respirator is then disconnected to avoid false readings and oxygen is delivered through a catheter to the trachea at a rate of about 6 L/min. The resulting tension of oxygen in the alveoli will remain high enough to maintain the arterial blood at adequate oxygen tensions for as long as an hour or more. The $PaCO_2$ rises by about 3 mm Hg/min during apneic oxygenation in a deeply comatose or clinically brain dead patient.[22] Apneic oxygenation of 8–10 minutes thus allows the $PaCO_2$ to rise without danger of further hypoxia and ensures that one exceeds the respiratory threshold. A $PaCO_2$ that rises above 60 mm Hg without concomitant breathing efforts provides unequivocal evidence of nonfunctioning respiratory centers. The AAN guidelines for brain death (https://www.aan.com/ professionals/practice/guidelines/pda/Brain_ death_adults.pdf) accept either a $PaCO_2$ of 60 mm Hg or a value 20 mm Hg higher than baseline as the threshold for maximum stimulation of the respiratory centers of the medulla oblongata. Chronic pulmonary disease producing baseline hypercapnia may complicate the apnea testing and can be identified in initial blood gas examination by elevated serum bicarbonate concentration. In such cases, ancillary testing is recommended by current guidelines. Alternatively, hypocapnia often arises in the setting of hyperventilation to manage increased intracranial pressure (ICP). Since it is important to start the examination near a target PCO_2 of 40 mm Hg, hypocapnia should be corrected by adjusting the minute volume of ventilation through either a reduction of the tidal volume or a resetting of the respiratory rate.

During testing the patient should be observed for respiration, defined as abdominal or chest excursions.[6] If respiration occurs during apnea testing, it is usually early into the testing. After 8 minutes have elapsed, arterial blood gases should be sampled and the ventilator reconnected. The absence of respiratory movements and rise of PCO_2 past 60 mm Hg

Table 10.4 Prerequisites for Apnea Testing

1. Core temperature >36.5°C or 97°F
2. Systolic blood pressure >90 mm Hg
3. Euvolemia. *Option*: positive fluid balance in the previous 6 hours
4. Normal PCO_2. *Option*: arterial PCO_2 >40 mm Hg
5. Normal PO_2. *Option*: preoxygenation to obtain arterial PO_2 >200 mm Hg

Adapted from Wijdicks.[8]

indicates a positive apnea test. Alternatively, if respiratory movements are seen, the test is negative and retesting at a later time is indicated. Prior to initiating apnea testing, the absence of brainstem reflexes should have already been established.

Additionally, several other prerequisites for accurate determination of brain death must be established, as indicated in Table 10.4. Hypothermia must be excluded; if core temperatures obtained by rectal measurement are below 36.5°C, the patient should be warmed with a blanket. A systolic blood pressure of greater than 90 mm Hg should be maintained using dopamine infusion if required. If hypotension (systolic blood pressure less than 90 mm Hg) arises during the examination, blood samples should be promptly drawn and the ventilator immediately reconnected. Conversely, any elevation of blood pressure during testing is evidence of lower brainstem function. As diabetes insipidus is a common complication of severe brain injuries, this should be recognized if present and managed. Accordingly, efforts should ensure euvolemia or positive fluid balance for at least 6 hours prior to testing. Finally, arterial gas pressures should reflect PO_2 greater than 200 mm Hg and PCO_2 greater than or equal to 40 mm Hg prior to testing, as already discussed. Extracorporeal membrane oxygenation (ECMO) allows physicians to replace cardiac and pulmonary function but generates challenges for the diagnosis of brain death as traditional apnea testing cannot be performed and confirmatory testing is mostly not feasible. PCO_2 can be raised by decreasing the sweep gas flow and increasing the oxygen delivery via the ECMO membrane to test for breathing responses by changing the sweep on the ECMO machine[23,24].

Confirmatory Laboratory Tests and Diagnosis

When the clinical examination is unequivocal, no additional tests are required. If there is uncertainty in either establishing the clinical examination or the natural history, clinical practice guidelines suggest the potential use of confirmatory testing in the determination of brain death.[4,6] Techniques that have been used include conventional angiography, electroencephalography (EEG)/evoked potential (EP) studies, transcranial Doppler sonography (TCD), and cerebral scintigraphy; however, we recommend the use of conventional angiography or cerebral scintigraphy only. Consensus criteria for brain death determination are only available for EEG/EP studies.

STUDIES TO ESTABLISH CESSATION OF CEREBRAL BLOOD FLOW: CEREBRAL ANGIOGRAPHY, TRANSCRANIAL DOPPLER SONOGRAPHY, AND CEREBRAL SCINTIGRAPHY

Cerebral angiography is a widely accepted procedure for determination of brain death and can be used to overcome the limitation of the clinical neurologic examination due to facial trauma, baseline pulmonary disease, and other confounding factors. This procedure also has the advantage, when positive, of establishing a structural cause of brain death (i.e., absence of blood flow to the brain). In cases where the original cause of cerebral injury is not known, the absence of blood flow provides the crucial information necessary to declare brain death with certainty.

Physiologically, two events may produce failure of the cerebral circulation. First, a sudden and massive increase in ICP (e.g., during subarachnoid hemorrhage) may cause it to rise to the level of arterial perfusion pressure at which point cerebral circulation ceases. The second, and probably more common, occurrence is a progressive loss of blood flow that accompanies death of the brain. As the dead tissue becomes edematous, the local tissue pressure exceeds capillary perfusion pressure, resulting in stasis of blood flow, further edema, and further vascular stasis. If the respiratory and cardiovascular systems are kept functioning for many hours or days after brain circulation has ceased, the brain undergoes autolysis at body temperature, resulting in a soft and necrotic organ at autopsy referred to by pathologists as a "respirator brain."[25]

Demonstration of the failure of intracerebral filling at the level of entry of the carotid and vertebral arteries indicates brain death. Recently, magnetic resonance angiography (MRA) has been reported for diagnosis of brain death, but this technique is less reliable as MRA often fails to demonstrate slow flow. Additional MRI criteria for brain death include loss of the subarachnoid spaces, slow flow in the intracavernous and cervical internal carotid arteries, loss of flow void in both small and large intracranial arteries and venous sinuses, and loss of gray–white matter distinction on T1-weighted images, but "supranormal" distinction on T2-weighted images.[26] However, until additional data are available on the reliability of these indicators for determining brain death, the presence of complete cessation of brain function on examination, or complete loss of blood flow, must remain the gold standards for diagnosis. CT angiography has also been reported and used as a confirmatory test but should be advised against as technical aspects, such as contrast bolus administration and the underlying computational steps to generate the CTA images, may generate false-positive studies.[27]

Bilateral insonation of the intracranial arteries using a portable 2-MHz pulsed Doppler device (*transcranial Doppler ultrasonograph* [*TCD*]) is also variably employed as a confirmatory test for brain death.[28,29] The middle cerebral arteries are insonated on both sides through the temporal bone above the zygomatic arch (of note, up to 10% of patients may not have temporal insonation windows, limiting use of this method) and the vertebral arteries or basilar artery through a suboccipital transcranial window. Two types of abnormalities have been correlated with brain death: (1) an absence of diastolic or reverberating flow, indicating the loss of arterial contractive force; and (2) the appearance of small systolic peaks early in systole, indicative of high vascular resistance. Both abnormalities are associated with significant elevations of ICP. The technique is limited by the requirement of skill in the operation of the equipment and has a potentially high error rate for missing blood flow because of incorrect placement of the transducer. Recent studies report a sensitivity of 77% and a specificity of 100% of diagnosing brain death if both the middle cerebral arteries and the basilar artery were insonated; sensitivity improved with increasing time of evaluation following initial clinical diagnosis.[30]

Cerebral scintigraphy measures the failure of uptake of the radioisotope nuclide technetium (Tc) 99m hexametazime in brain parenchyma. This technique has shown good correlation with cerebral angiography. The test can be done at the bedside using a portable gamma camera after injection of isotope, which should be used within 30 minutes after its reconstitution. A static image of 500,000 counts obtained at several time points is recommended (taken immediately, 30–60 minutes after injection, and at 2 hours past injection time[31]). A prospective study using 99m Tc-hex-amethyl-propylamineoxime (HMPAO) single photon emission tomography (SPECT) in 50 comatose and brain dead patients to examine cerebral perfusion found the characteristic "empty skull" image indicating arrest of cerebral perfusion in 45 of 47 brain dead patients.[32] The bedside nuclide brain scan test is probably the best adjunct test to confirm the diagnosis in unclear cases. It is inexpensive, can be done without moving a patient on a ventilator, and is extremely reliable when it shows an empty skull (see Figure 10.1). This test can be considered a gold standard for use in difficult cases.

However, both SPECT scans and cerebral angiography may extremely infrequently produce a false-positive result suggesting brain death in patients with severe hypotension and use of faulty technique (i.e., errors in preparation or injection of the isotope, poor angiographic technique[33,34]). False negative results suggesting preserved cerebral blood flow in truly brain-dead patients are also very rare and mostly related to persistent blood flow in the superior sagittal sinus from extracranial sources, decompressive surgery leading to lowered ICP, and posterior fossa pathology without cerebral pathology. Interestingly, blood supply for the posterior pituitary, hypophysial stalk, and parts of the hypothalamus may be via the inferior hypophyseal artery branches off the extradural segments of the internal carotid artery, which are not subject to the elevated intracranial pressure that results cessation of intracranial blood flow[35]. This may result in the misleading finding of a central hotspot on SPECT scanning in a patient who otherwise fulfills brain death criteria and has no blood flow to the brain via the internal carotid artery.[36]

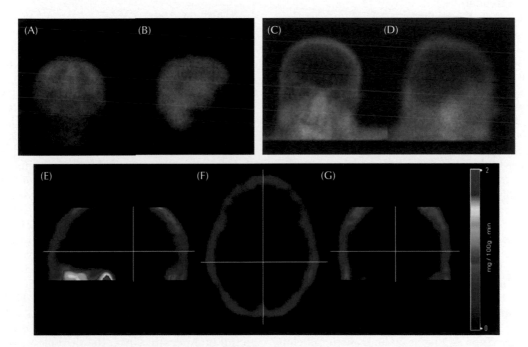

Figure 10.1 (A–D) A 50-year-old woman after cardiac arrest. Clinical exam is consistent with brain death but, due to hemodynamic instability, the team was unable to perform apnea testing. Tc-single-proton emission computed tomography (SPECT scanning demonstrates initially preserved cerebral perfusion (Panels A–B) that was absent on repeat SPECT) scanning 4 days later without any other changes in examination (Panels C–D). (E–G) Cerebral metabolism in brain death measured by 18F-fluorodeoxyglucose-positron emission tomography (FDG-PET) demonstrating the unequivocal finding of an "empty skull." (Panels E–G: Sequence of images: sagittal [left]; transverse [middle]; and coronal [right]). From Laureys et al.,[37] with permission.

ELECTROENCEPHALOGRAPHY/ EVOKED POTENTIAL MEASUREMENTS

The EEG has little place in the determination of brain death, except perhaps in those rare cases where other clinical evidence is equivocal. An isoelectric EEG, often termed *electrocerebral inactivity* by electroencephalographers, that lasts for a period of 6–12 hours in a patient who is not hypothermic and has not ingested or been given depressant drugs identifies forebrain death (because the EEG does not demonstrate brainstem activity, it can be isoelectric in patients with brainstem reflexes who are clearly not brain dead). Silverman and associates reported on a survey of 2,650 isoelectric EEGs that lasted up to 24 hours.[38] Only three patients in this group, each in coma caused by overdose of central nervous system depressant drugs, recovered cerebral function. However, Heckmann and colleagues[39] have reported a patient with an isoelectric EEG following cardiac arrest who showed residual brainstem function, including spontaneous breathing and SPECT evidence of cerebral blood flow, for 7 weeks prior to death.

Electrical interference makes artifact-free EEG or evoked potential records exceedingly difficult to obtain in the intensive care setting. Moreover, technical recording errors can simulate electrocerebral activity as well as electrocerebral inactivity, and several ostensibly isoelectric tracings must be discarded because of faulty technique. A national cooperative group has published technical requirements necessary to establish electrocerebral silence (Table 10.5) and has produced an atlas illustrating potential problems of interpretation of the EEG in coma.[40] It should be noted that the EEG is not infallible, even with anoxic-ischemic injury. Cerebral activity may be absent on the EEG for up to several hours following cardiac arrest, only to return later.[41] A prolonged vegetative state is occasionally possible in such cases despite the presence of an initially silent EEG. After depressive drug poisoning, total loss of cerebral hemispheric function and electrocerebral silence have been observed for as long as 50 hours with full clinical recovery.

Physicians have appropriately raised questions as to whether a few fragments of

Table 10.5 Electroencephalographic Recording for Diagnosing Cerebral Death

1. A minimum of eight scalp electrodes and ear reference electrodes
2. Interelectrode impedances <10,000 ohms, but >100 ohms
3. Test of integrity of recording system by deliberate creation of electrode artifact by manipulation
4. Interelectrode distances of at least 10 cm
5. No activity with a sensitivity increased to at least 2 μV/mm for 30 minutes with inclusion of appropriate calibrations
6. The use of 0.3- or 0.4-second time constants during part of the recording
7. Recording with an electrocardiogram and other monitoring devices, such as a pair of electrodes on the dorsum of the right hand, to detect extracerebral responses
8. Tests for reactivity to pain, loud noises, or light
9. Recording by a qualified technician
10. Repeat record if doubt about electrocerebral silence (ECS)
11. elephonically transmitted electroencephalograms are not appropriate for determination of ECS

From Bennett et al.[40]

cerebral electrical activity mean anything when they arise from a body that has totally lost all capacity for the brain to regulate internal and external homeostasis. Death is a process in which different organs and parts of organs lose their living properties at widely varying rates. Death of the brain occurs when the organ irreversibly loses its capacity to maintain the vital integrative functions regulated by the vegetative and consciousness-mediating centers of the brainstem. Not surprisingly, the time when the state of brain death is reached often precedes the final demise of small collections of electrically generating cells in the cerebral hemispheres, as evidenced by the observation that 20% of 56 patients meeting other clinical criteria for brain death had residual EEG activity lasting up to 168 hours.[42] Thus, EEG examinations may pick up a few patients with brainstem death who have not yet progressed to full brain death. Given the extremely poor prognosis of such individuals, using EEG as a criterion for prolonging the period of futile life support is not a service to them.

Diagnosis of Brain Death in Profound Anesthesia or Coma of Undetermined Etiology

It must be repeatedly emphasized that patients with very deep but reversible anesthesia due to sedative drug ingestion can give the clinical appearance of brain death and even can have an electrically silent EEG. Furthermore, recovery in such instances has been observed even when the EEG showed no physiologic activity for as long as 50 hours. Given such evidence, when and how is one to decide in such cases that anesthesia has slipped into death and further cardiopulmonary support is futile? Unfortunately, few empirical data provide an answer to the question, particularly if faced with the complex problem of a patient with a coma of undetermined origin. In such cases, the combination of a prolonged period of observation (more than 24 hours), loss of cerebral perfusion, and exclusion of other potential confounds is required.[43] It is important to test drug levels and follow the patient until the drug is eliminated. A general guideline proposed for known intoxications is the following: an observation period greater than four times the half-life of the pharmacologic agent should be used.[4] Of course, the presence of unmeasured metabolites, potentiation by additional medications, and impaired renal or hepatic clearance are likely to complicate individual evaluations.

Pitfalls in the Diagnosis of Brain Death

Potential pitfalls accompany the diagnosis of brain death, particularly when coma occurs in hospitalized patients or those who have been chronically ill. Almost none of these will lead to serious error in diagnosis if the examining physician is aware of them and attends to them when examining individual patients who are considered brain dead. In fact, there are no reported cases of "recovery" from correctly diagnosed brain death.

With meticulous efforts, other organs (e.g., heart, kidney, etc.) can be sustained, but usually only for hours or days.[44,45] Prolonged survival of peripheral organs is quite rare,[46,47] so

Table 10.6 Some Pitfalls in the Diagnosis of Brain Death

Findings	Possible causes
1. Pupils fixed	Anticholinergic drugs, tricyclic antidepressants
	Neuromuscular blockers
	Preexisting disease
2. No oculovestibular reflexes	Ototoxic agents
	Vestibular suppression
	Preexisting disease
	Basal skull fracture
3. No respiration	Posthyperventilation apnea
	Neuromuscular blockers
4. No motor activity	Neuromuscular blockers
	"Locked-in" state
	Sedative drugs
5. Isoelectric electroencephalogram	Sedative drugs
	Anoxia
	Hypothermia
	Encephalitis
	Trauma

Adapted from Wijdicks.[8]

much so that, in the few reported cases, one must question whether the clinical criteria were correctly met. Conversely, there are several reported cases of recovery from "cardiac" death,[48] the Lazarus phenomenon (not to be confused with Lazarus sign, a spinal reflex [see page 440]). A number of case reports describe patients with clinical and electrocardiographic cardiac arrest who, after failed attempts at resuscitation, are pronounced dead, only to be discovered to be alive later, sometimes in the mortuary.[49] Some of these pitfalls are outlined in Table 10.6.

In comatose patients, pupillary fixation does not always mean absence of brainstem function. In rare instances, the pupils may have been fixed by preexisting ocular or neurologic disease. More commonly, particularly in a patient who has suffered cardiac arrest, atropine has been injected during the resuscitation process and pupils are widely dilated; fixed pupils may result without indicating the absence of brainstem function. Neuromuscular blocking agents also can produce pupillary fixation, although in these instances the pupils are usually midposition or small rather than widely dilated.

Similarly, the absence of VORs does not necessarily indicate absence of brainstem vestibular function. Like pupillary responses, vestibulo-ocular reflexes may be absent if the end organ is either poisoned or damaged. For example, traumatic injury producing basal fractures of the petrous bone may cause unilateral loss of caloric response. Some otherwise neurologically normal patients suffer labyrinthine dysfunction from peripheral disease that predates the onset of coma. Other patients with chronic illnesses have suffered ototoxicity from a variety of drugs, including antibiotics such as gentamicin. In these patients, VORs may be absent even though other brainstem processes are still functioning. Finally, a variety of drugs, including sedatives, anticholinergics, anticonvulsants, chemotherapeutic agents, and tricyclic antidepressants, may suppress vestibular and/or oculomotor function to the point where oculo-vestibular reflexes disappear.

Pitfalls in the diagnosis of apnea in comatose patients maintained on respirators were discussed earlier.

The absence of motor activity also does not guarantee loss of brainstem function. Neuromuscular blockers are often used early in the course of artificial respiration when the patient is resisting the respirator; if suspected brain death subsequently occurs, there may still be enough circulating neuromuscular blocking agent to produce absence of motor function when the examination is carried out. One report has described the simulation of brain death by excessive sensitivity to succinylcholine[50]; in this case the presence of activity in the EEG established cerebral viability. If neuromuscular blockade has been recently withdrawn, guidelines require that a peripheral nerve stimulator be used to demonstrate transmission (e.g., a train of four stimulation pulses produces four thumb twitches).

Therapeutic overdoses of sedative drugs to treat anoxia or seizures likewise may abolish reflexes and motor responses to noxious stimuli. At least two reports document formal brain death examinations in reversible intoxications with tricyclic antidepressant and barbiturate agents.[51,52]

There are pitfalls in using the EEG as an ancillary technique in the diagnosis of cerebral death. Isoelectric EEGs with subsequent recovery have been reported with sedative drug overdoses, after anoxia, during hypothermia,

following cerebral trauma, and after encephalitis, especially in cases of diffuse acute disseminated encephalomyelitis.[5]

It is important to recognize that brain death criteria are not universal, and requirements and acceptance of confirmatory testing varies widely in different countries.[29,53] Even within the United States, the practices of who performs brain death examinations and what confirmatory testing is acceptable varies widely; additionally, religious and cultural acceptance of brain death is regionally variable (see Chapter 11). However, most mistakes in making the diagnosis of brain death are made by inexperienced practitioners, and the training and toolkits have been developed that hopefully will minimize this deficiency.[54]

Brain Death Versus Prolonged Coma

Recovery from brain death by definition can only occur in the setting of an original misdiagnosis. In the past several years controversy has surrounded a small number of cases of brain death leading to public confusion and unwarranted concern about the conceptual integrity of the entity[55–57]. Patients approximating the features of brain death but not fulfilling the full criteria are in a prolonged coma. Deviations from the complete fulfillment of the clinical criteria for brain death thus create an unknown but finite risk that other abnormalities on the clinical exam may not reflect irreversible damage. In 2010, the AAN updated the 1995 Brain Death Guidelines and addressed five specific questions surrounding possible pitfalls in the assessment of brain death.[4] This evidence-based review found: (1) no evidence of verified examples in which patients who fulfilled clinical criteria for brain death recovered brain function; (2) insufficient evidence to establish a minimally acceptable observation period to ensure that neurologic functions have ceased irreversibly; (3) examples of complex, non–brain mediated movements in some patients diagnosed as brain dead that can falsely suggest retained brain function, including, ventilator autocycling which may on occasion be misinterpreted as well as falsely suggesting patient-initiated breathing; (4) the safety of apneic oxygenation diffusion to determine apnea without sufficient evidence to determine the comparative safety of other techniques to assess apnea; and (5) insufficient evidence to determine value for ancillary tests. The 2010 update also concluded that alternatives to apnea testing be evaluated and that protocols and examiners be subject to auditing procedures to improve the universality of implementation of brain death assessments. Ultimately, expert reviewers have concluded that accurate application of the clinical brain death examination techniques have not resulted in late recovery in any verified instance (see Fins Chapter 11 for additional discussion).

Management of the Brain Dead Patient

Major physiologic changes occur as patients transition to brain death, and these require aggressive critical care measures for those patients who are potential organ donors (Society of Critical Care Medicine/American College of Chest Physicians/Association of Organ Procurement Organizations Consensus Statement, 2015). While neuroendocrine function may be preserved in some brain dead patients, supplementation of pituitary axes hormones is frequently practiced.[58] This includes administration of levothyroxine, Solu-Medrol, and vasopressin, which often stabilizes the patients hemodynamically. Adequate end organ perfusion frequently requires fluid administration and vasopressors support. Additional medications such as antibiotics are frequently given to optimize organ conditions prior to transplantation. Diagnostic tests such as cultures, bronchoscopy, cardiac catheterization, liver biopsy, and other tests may be required to risk-stratify organs for transplantation.

REFERENCES

1. Mollaret P, Goulon M. [The depassed coma (preliminary memoir)]. *Rev Neurol (Paris)* 1959;101:3–15.
2. A definition of irreversible coma. Report of the Ad Hoc Committee of the Harvard Medical School to Examine the Definition of Brain Death. *JAMA* 1968;205:337–340.
3. Uniform Determination of Death Act 320. In: *Uniform Laws Annotated.* St. Paul, MN: West Group;1990.
4. Wijdicks EF, Varelas PN, Gronseth GS, Greer DM; American Academy of Neurology. Evidence-based guideline update: determining brain death in adults: report of the Quality Standards Subcommittee of the American Academy of Neurology.

Neurology 2010;74(23):1911–1918. doi: 10.1212/WNL.0b013e3181e242a8.
5. Rohaut B, Claassen J. Decision making in perceived devastating brain injury: a call to explore theimpact of cognitive biases. *Br J Anaesth* 2018 Jan;120(1):5–9.
6. An appraisal of the criteria of cerebral death. A summary statement. A collaborative study. *JAMA* 1977;237:982–986.
7. Bates D, Caronna JJ, Cartlidge NE, et al. A prospective study of nontraumatic coma: methods and results in 310 patients. *Ann Neurol* 1977;2:211–220.
8. Wijdicks EF. The diagnosis of brain death. *N Engl J Med* 2001;344:1215–1221.
9. Jorgensen EO. Spinal man after brain death. The unilateral extension-pronation reflex of the upper limb as an indication of brain death. *Acta Neurochir (Wien)* 1973;28:259–273.
10. President's Commission for the Study of Ethical Problems in Medicine and Biomedical Behavioral Research. *Defining death: medical, legal and ethical issues in the determination of death.* Washington, DC: Author;1981.
11. Walter U, Fernández-Torre JL, Kirschstein T, Laureys S. When is "brainstem death" brain death? The case for ancillary testing in primary infratentorial brain lesion. *Clin Neurophysiol* 2018. pii: S1388-2457(18)31195-7.
12. Shlugman D, Parulekar M, Elston JS, et al. Abnormal pupillary activity in a brainstem-dead patient. *Br J Anaesth* 2001;86:717–720.
13. Wijdicks EFM. Temporomandibular joint compression in coma. *Neurology* 1996;46:1774.
14. Christie JM, O'Lenic TD, Cane RD. Head turning in brain death. *J Clin Anesth* 1996;8:141–143.
15. Hanna JP, Frank JI. Automatic stepping in the pontomedullary stage of central herniation. *Neurology* 1995;45:985–986.
16. de Freitas GR, Andre C. Absence of the Babinski sign in brain death: a prospective study of 144 cases. *J Neurol* 2005;252:106–107.
17. Martí-Fàbregas J, López-Navidad A, Caballero F, et al. Decerebrate-like posturing with mechanical ventilation in brain death. *Neurology* 2000;51:224–227.
18. Ropper AH. Unusual spontaneous movements in brain-dead patients. *Neurology* 1984;34:1089–1092.
19. Saposnik G, Bucri JA, Mauriño J, et al. Spontaneous and reflex movements in brain death. *Neurology* 2000;54:221–223.
20. Saposnik G, Maurino J, Saizar R, et al. Spontaneous and reflex movements in 107 patients with brain death. *Am J Med* 2005;118(3):311–314.
21. McNair NL, Meador KJ. The undulating toe flexion sign in brain death. *Mov Disord* 1992;7:345–347.
22. Schafer JA, Caronna JJ. Duration of apnea needed to confirm brain death. *Neurology* 1978;28:661–666.
23. Smilevitch P, Lonjaret L, Fourcade O, Geeraerts T. Apnea test for brain death determination in a patient on extracorporeal membrane oxygenation. *Neurocrit Care* 2013;19(2):215–217. doi: 10.1007/s12028-013-9845-y.
24. Saucha W, Solek-Pastuszka J, Bohatyrewicz R, Knapik P. Apnea test in the determination of brain death in patients treated with extracorporeal membrane oxygenation (ECMO). *Anaesthesiol Intensive Ther* 2015;47(4):368–371.
25. Walker AE, Diamond EL, Moseley J. The neuropathological findings in irreversible coma. A critique

of the "respirator brain." *J Neuropathol Exp Neurol* 1975;34(4):295–323.

26. Lee DH, Nathanson JA, Fox AJ, et al. Magnetic resonance imaging of brain death. *Can Assoc Radiol J* 1995;46:174–178.

27. Greer DM, Strozyk D, Schwamm LH. False positive CT angiography in brain death. *Neurocrit Care* 2009;11(2):272–275. doi: 10.1007/s12028-009-9220-1.

28. Sloan MA, Alexandrov AV, Tegeler CH, et al. Assessment: transcranial Doppler ultrasonography: report ofthe Therapeutics and Technology Assessment Subcommittee of the American Academy of Neurology. *Neurology* 2004;62:1468–1481.

29. Greer DM, Wang HH, Robinson JD, Varelas PN, Henderson GV, Wijdicks EF. Variability of brain death policies in the United States. *JAMA Neurol* 2016;73(2):213–218. doi: 10.1001/jamaneurol.2015.3943.

30. Kuo JR, Chen CF, Chio CC, et al. Time dependent validity in the diagnosis of brain death using transcranial Doppler sonography. *J Neurol Neurosurg Psychiatry* 2006;77:646–649.

31. Bonetti MG, Ciritella P, Valle G, et al. 99mTc HM-PAO brain perfusion SPECT in brain death. *Neuro-radiology* 1995;37:365–369.

32. Facco E, Zucchetta P, Munari M, et al. 99mTc-HMPAO SPECT in the diagnosis of brain death. *Intensive Care Med* 1998;24:911–917.

33. Young GB, Lee D. A critique of ancillary tests for brain death. *Neurocrit Care* 2004;1(4):499–508.

34. Zuckier LS, Kolano J. Radionuclide studies in the determination of brain death: criteria, concepts, and controversies. *Semin Nucl Med* 2008;38(4):262–273. doi: 10.1053/j.semnuclmed.2008.03.003.

35. Leclercq TA, Grisoli F. Arterial blood supply of the normal human pituitary gland. An anatomical study. *J Neurosurg* 1983;58(5):678–681.

36. Busl KM, Greer DM. Pitfalls in the diagnosis of brain death. *Neurocrit Care*. 2009;11(2):276–287.

37. Laureys S, Owen AM, Schiff ND. Brain function in coma,vegetative state, and related disorders. *Lancet Neurol* 2004;3:537–546.

38. Silverman D, Masland RL, Saunders MG, et al. Irreversible coma associated with electrocerebral silence. *Neurology* 1970;20:525–533.

39. Heckmann JG, Lang CJ, Pfau M, et al. Electrocerebral silence with preserved but reduced cortical brain perfusion. *Eur J Emerg Med* 2003;10:241–243.

40. Bennett DR, Hughes JR, Korein J. *Atlas of Electroencephalography in Coma and Cerebral Death. EEG at the Bedside or in the Intensive Care Unit*. San Diego: Raven Press; 1976.

41. Jorgensen EO. Clinical note. EEG without detectable cortical activity and cranial nerve areflexia as parameters of brain death. *Electroencephalogr Clin Neurophysiol* 1974;36:70–75.

42. Grigg MM, Kelly MA, Celesia GG, et al. Electroencephalographic activity after brain death. *Arch Neurol* 1987;44:948–954.

43. The Quality Standards Subcommittee of the American Academy of Neurology. Practice parameters for determining brain death in adults (summary statement). *Neurology* 1995;45:1012–1014.

44. Yoshioka T, Sugimoto H, Uenishi M, et al. Prolonged hemodynamic maintenance by the combined administration of vasopressin and epinephrine in brain death: a clinical study. *Neurosurgery* 1986;18:565–567.

45. Hung TP, Chen ST. Prognosis of deeply comatose patients on ventilators. *J Neurol Neurosurg Psychiatry* 1995;58:75–80.

46. Shewmon DA. Chronic "brain death": meta-analysis and conceptual consequences. *Neurology* 1998;51:1538–1545.

47. Repertinger S, Fitzgibbons WP, Omojola MF, et al. Long survival following bacterial meningitis-associated brain destruction. *J Child Neurol* 2006;21:591–595.

48. Maleck WH, Piper SN, Triem J, et al. Unexpected return of spontaneous circulation after cessation of resuscitation (Lazarus phenomenon). *Resuscitation* 1998;39:125–128.

49. Mullie A, Miranda D. A premature referral to the mortuary. Cerebral recovery with barbiturate therapy. *Acta Anaesthesiol Belg* 1979;30:145–148.

50. Tyson RN. Simulation of cerebral death by succinylcholine sensitivity. *Arch Neurol* 1974;30:409–411.

51. Grattan-Smith PJ, Butt W. Suppression of brainstem reflexes in barbiturate coma. *Arch Dis Child* 1993;69:151–152.

52. Yang KL, Dantzker DR. Reversible brain death. A manifestation of amitriptyline overdose. *Chest* 1991;99:1037–1038.

53. S, Wijdicks EF, Patel PV, Greer DM, Hemphill JC 3rd, Carone M, Mateen FJ. Brain death declaration: practices and perceptions worldwide. *Neurology* 2015;84(18):1870–9. doi: 10.1212/WNL.0000000000001540.

54. MacDougall BJ, Robinson JD, Kappus L, Sudikoff SN, Greer DM. Simulation-based training in brain death determination. *Neurocrit Care* 2014 Dec;21(3):383–391.

55. Aviv R. The death debate. *The New Yorker* February 5, 2018:30–41.

56. Lewis A, Greer D. Current controversies in brain death determination. *Nat Rev Neurol* 2017;13(8):505–509.

57. Truog RD. Defining death-making sense of the case of Jahi McMath. *JAMA* 2018 Apr 9. doi: 10.1001/jama.2018.3441.

58. Nair-Collins M, Northrup J, Olcese J. Hypothalamic-pituitary function in brain death: a review. *J Intensive Care Med* 2016;31(1):41–50. doi: 10.1177/0885066614527410.

Chapter 11

Disorders of Consciousness in Clinical Practice

Ethical, Legal and Policy Considerations

Joseph J. Fins

PROFESSIONAL OBLIGATIONS AND CLINICAL DISCERNMENT

It is the professional obligation of the physician caring for individuals with a disorder of consciousness to bring evolving scientific knowledge to the bedside and use it to inform the decision-making process with surrogates. It especially critical that surrogates understand that the probability of the recovery of consciousness is dynamic and depends upon anatomic locale, etiology, and duration.[1]

To this end, physicians should use their knowledge of the evolution of brain states to strategically orchestrate discussions at key clinical milestones that have prognostic significance, recognizing that these categorizations still remain crude and mostly descriptive compared to other domains in medicine. Because of the rudimentary nature of this emerging nosology, it is inevitable that patients with variable injuries and outcomes will be included in diagnostic categories that are too broad and heterogeneous. This can make prognostication difficult and complicate efforts to achieve greater diagnostic clarity.[1,2]

Despite the injunction to categorically avoid a nihilistic stance, the prognosis for many who become comatose is grim (as reviewed in Chapter 9). It is especially critical that surrogate decision-makers have accurate information about potential outcomes informed by the clinician's knowledge of the etiology of the insult, its location in the brain, and our evolving understanding about the natural history of disorders of consciousness over time.[3,4]

The ethical obligations of clinicians caring for patients with disorders of consciousness are complex. When speaking with surrogates, a delicate balance needs to be achieved between too quickly foreclosing any prospect of recovery and the offering of false hope. Yet even "favorable" outcomes marked by survival and recovery often force difficult quality of life choices for those whose existence has been irrevocably altered by a disorder of consciousness and an alteration of one's very self.

To mitigate these challenges clinicians must assume a fiduciary obligation on behalf of patients entrusted to their care. The physician must ensure that the patient has received the appropriate evaluation and requisite amount of clinical care—diagnostic,

therapeutic, and rehabilitative—that would allow for informed decisions by surrogates about treatment decisions. At times this will mean respecting decisions to forgo life-sustaining therapies when surrogates believe that ongoing treatment would be burdensome and result in an existence that would have been unacceptable to the patient or inconsistent with his or her prior wishes.

In sum, clinicians have a bifurcated set of responsibilities. They must be stalwart advocates for patient care. And even as they help patients work toward recovery, they must accept that this pursuit may entail disproportionate burdens. This creates a complex ethos of care which must at once must affirm a right to care and yet preserve a right to die.[5] In this chapter, we will provide strategies to help clinicians navigate their responsibilities to better meet the needs of patients with disorders of consciousness and their families.

AN EMERGING NOSOLOGY AND ETHIC OF CARE

One of the ethical challenges at this juncture in the history of our evolving knowledge of disorders of consciousness is that, as we learn more about brain states, there is more uncertainty about the choices that need to be made. Just a couple of decades ago, before the advent of more sophisticated imaging data, clinicians would make determinations based on bedside assessment. Opinions were often expressed categorically with value-laden statements like there "was no hope for meaningful recovery."[6] Acculturated to the futility of these brain states, these presumptions were not questioned and left to silently direct care and sustain a nihilistic bias toward this patient population whose care was viewed as hopeless.

A decade ago, Wijdicks and Rabinstein advised practitioners to lower their expectations for patients in the comatose state. They counseled, "The attending physician of a patient with a devastating neurologic illness will have to come to terms with the futility of care . . . Those families who are unconvinced should be explicitly told they should have markedly diminished expectations for what intensive care can accomplish and that withdrawal of life support or abstaining from performing complex interventions is more commensurate with the neurologic status."[7]

More recent studies have shown the persistence of these views, with 70.2% of the 31.7% in-hospital mortality for disorders of consciousness patients stemming from a decision to withdraw life-sustaining therapy.[8] But even amid a culture of therapeutic nihilism, with practitioners taking false comfort in our biases and relative ignorance of the underlying biology of recovery and resilience, some early experts were more prudential in their stance. As early as the late 1970s, Fred Plum warned against being overly nihilistic. Where others saw only futility, Dr. Plum also saw the utility of ongoing care and assessment. In an unpublished manuscript in his papers, he wrote:

> We have studied over a 100 patients . . . can identify within 24 hrs by their neurological signs alone who will not recover above a vegetative level . . . who will do well . . . This leaves a middle group for whom more information is needed but where presenting every effort at treatment must be made to know their maximal potential and how to judge their early signs.[9]

While others were asserting the relationship of a right to die to severe brain injury, Dr. Plum was also thinking about a right to care. This was a point made explicitly in earlier volumes of this text.[10]

Implicit in Plum's analysis was the recognition that there was a fluidity to these brain states.[11] Although we think of these categories as if they were diagnoses, they are not fixed and immutable but rather *syndromic* and based on clinical features, as James L. Bernat has importantly noted.[12] Historically, this classification has been based on phenotypes and less on underlying pathophysiology, leading to variable outcomes and making prognostication difficult. Dr. Plum's wisdom has become even more apparent, as the dynamic nature of these brain states and how they can evolve (as reviewed in Chapter 9) makes clear. This makes clinical assessment more complicated with clinical and ethical consequences for prognosis, communication with families, and the patient's ability to perceive pain and experience suffering.

The dynamic quality of these brain states is further complicated by the fact that the clinical neurology of disorders of consciousness is undergoing a profound transition from behavioral assessment, done classically at the bedside, to a more mechanistic and circuit-based approach utilizing neuroimaging and electrophysiological data. The challenge is that, in some circumstances, there may be a discordance between what is observed in the bedside exam and what may be occurring within the brain when assessed by other measures.

While diagnostic criteria have traditionally been governed by observable clinical data, this approach is becoming increasingly less tenable, creating uncertainty as to whether to rely on historical clinical methods or to utilize neuroimaging or electrophysiologic metrics, which remain investigational.

At the core of the ethical challenges posed by this new neuroscience is covert consciousness and the challenge of cognitive motor dissociation (CMD).[13] With the advent of neuroimaging, patients who appear at the bedside as unconscious may in fact demonstrate evidence of responsiveness to their environment via neuroimaging.[14] Covert consciousness may also be implied by variations in electroencephalographic (EEG) signals in some patients.[15] This creates a discordance between observed behaviors and the underlying ability of patients to perceive their environment. This disconnect has profound normative implications.[16]

Historically, as we will see, the first brain state where there was evidence of a discordance between what was thought to be observed at the bedside and the patient's actual brain state was the minimally conscious state (MCS). In the early part of this century much of the clinical and ethics literature centered on the distinction between the vegetative state and the MCS. This remains a critical distinction because patients who are minimally conscious are conscious, whereas vegetative state patients, with whom they are confused and classically conflated, are not. But it would be a mistake to think that cognitive motor dissociation only applies to the difference between the vegetative state and the MCS.

Our concerns began with that distinction but do not end there. In many respects they were our canary in the coal mine, alerting us to the possibility that patients who appeared to be unconscious may have been conscious, albeit liminally so. We now appreciate that the possibility of covert consciousness and CMD is a far broader—and thus worrisome—category which applies to those in the MCS to those in the locked-in state who have normal consciousness but no motor output, save for the cranial nerves. There are profound ethical consequences for patient care and well-being when any of these patients are misdiagnosed due to either episodic or a paucity of behavioral or motor signs.

Of course, we cannot always know when and if a patient has covert consciousness because their behaviors may be intermittent and our methods remain imprecise. But knowledge of the possibility of covert consciousness and CMD brings doubt to the standard bedside assessment, even though use of the behavioral neuropsychologic test, Coma Recovery Scale-Revised (CRS-R), remains the most accurate means to assess patients with disorders of consciousness.[17] At this stage of our knowledge, the clinician is advised to engage in nested judgments in which no test alone is viewed as dispositive and efforts are made to obtain mutually reinforcing data to confirm one diagnostic assessment.

In the aggregate, these factors place diagnostic assessment into a liminal state similar to what Thomas Insel, former head of the National Institute of Mental Health (NIMH), has proposed for psychiatry. While psychiatry has emphasized descriptive and epidemiological classifications found in the *Diagnostic and Statistical Manual of Nervous Disorders*, Insel maintains that it needs to evolve to a more circuit-based approach to describe psychiatric conditions,[18] as exemplified by emerging neuroimaging data describing the phenomenology of depression and its subtypes.[19,20] In fact, this classic problem of dissociation of cognitive function and overt behavior originally drove Hans Berger to develop the EEG (see Chapter 1).

While this transition will cause confusion in the short term, a more precise understanding of these brain states will inevitably lead to more accurate assessment and improved therapeutics. As the great physician William Osler observed in *Aequanimitas*, "The determination of structure with a view to the discovery of function has been the foundation of progress."[21] More than a century after he authored these words, his admonition pertains

to our growing knowledge of disorders of consciousness as we move from a purely descriptive characterization of these brain states to one that is more scientifically informed.[22]

BRAIN STATES

Let us now turn to major brain states constituting disorders of consciousness and consider how developments in the neuroscience of brain injury have begun to alter this nosology and reframe our normative considerations.

Coma

Coma is an eyes-closed state of unresponsiveness. It is typically self-limited and either progresses to full recovery (as after anesthesia-induced coma), death (as progressing to brain death), or to the vegetative state (the isolated survival of brainstem function) or the MCS (which also includes some pockets of preserved but integrated cerebral function). While coma is often erroneously conflated with the brain states that follow in common parlance—and sometimes in careless medical practice—it is important to communicate with surrogates that coma is self-limited and is pluripotential in its outcome, depending on its etiology. This range of prognostic outcomes is important to convey as surrogates may assume that this initial loss of consciousness is permanent and make precipitate judgments in light of this misinformation.

Brain Death

Brain death is defined as irreversible cessation of function of the whole brain including brainstem and higher brain functions. Patients who have sustained prolonged cerebral anoxia or ischemia or have sustained severe traumatic injury or cerebral edema are at risk of brain death, as reviewed in Chapter 10. While brain death remains a viable clinical construct (see Chapter 10), methods for identifying it at the bedside remain controversial.

Brain death, as a clinical entity, was first proposed in 1968 by an Ad Hoc Committee at the Harvard Medical School. Their deliberations followed the first cardiac transplant by Dr. Christian Barnard in South Africa in 1967.[23] This redefining of death has been instrumental in permitting retrieval of viable organs for transplantation that would have otherwise have been lost. Viewing brain death as the ultimate in medical futility, Committee Chair Henry K. Beecher advanced the radical proposition that organs be retrieved from the "hopelessly comatose" patient.[24] Adopting a utilitarian stance, Beecher argued that to not harvest organs from these patients would result in a

> . . . desperately radical result: the curable, the salvageable, can thus be sacrificed to the hopelessly damaged and unconscious who consume the time and space and money better devoted to those who could be helped. To pretend otherwise is nonsense: what one gets the other is deprived of.[24]

Beecher moderated his position limiting organ retrieval to brain death, but the cultural linkage between disorders of consciousness and hopelessness had been established.[25]

Since 1968, brain death has been widely accepted and seen as integral to organ retrieval and transplantation. That definition advanced the notion that death can be legally defined as the irreversible cessation of whole brain function independent of either a cardiac arrest or cessation of pulmonary function.[26] Following that effort, the construct of brain death was endorsed by a presidential commission charged with the study of ethical issues in medicine,[27] incorporated into the Uniform Determination of Death Act,[28] adopted into state laws, and has become part of routine clinical practice as the legal standard for the declaration of death in 48 states.

However, the achievement of this utilitarian greater good at the expense of individual beliefs has not been without some contention. Although generally accepted in professional circles,[29] the concept of brain death is not well understood among lay people when consent for organ donation is sought.[30] To lay observers, patients appear alive, well perfused, with a heart beat on the cardiac monitor, even as neuroimaging studies like radionucleotide imaging demonstrate a lack of perfusion. It is hard to grasp that a body that seems viable has

a brain that is not. In brain death, the patient looks better than the scan.[31]

Even clinicians can find the presentation of brain death paradoxical, as was the case of an intensivist who had just completed a positive apnea test with a lack of spontaneous respiration following a 20 mm Hg increase in pco_2. After "proclaiming" the patient dead, the patient demonstrated a classic spinally mediated response, or what has been described as a *Lazarus reflex,* in which the arms rise and the hands come together at the midline as if to pray.[32] Shaken by this observation and despite his own calculations of the blood gases which informed the brain death determination, this intensivist reached for his stethoscope to check for respirations. The experience, despite his grounding in science was counterintuitive and emotionally disturbing.

A more challenging issue is that some segments of our society reject this definition of death, most notably members of some orthodox religious groups[33] and others with cultural roots in Asia, most notably Japan, which has only recently legalized brain death determinations.[34] In response, New York State requires *reasonable accommodation* for religious or moral objections but does not preclude a medical determination of death based on criteria of cessation of all brain functions.[35] More categorically, New Jersey requires a declaration of cardiac death if there is a family objection because brain death would violate religious beliefs.[36]

Working with surrogates who reject brain death standards requires cultural sensitivity and the use of cultural intermediaries to enhance communication.[37] In our experience working with Orthodox Jewish patients, it is helpful to not insist on the cogency of the scientific construct, or secular law, but rather to reframe the clinical dilemma in terms of their religious tradition. First, it is critical to determine if an objection to brain death is an idiosyncratic grief reaction or truly founded on a theological objection. Even within the Orthodox Jewish tradition, there are subsects that accept brain death and others that do not. Second, if a tradition rejects brain death, it is helpful to cast care decisions within religious law. For example, in Orthodox Judaism there is a mandate to preserve life as well as not prolong the dying process once the patient has been deemed a *Goses* or one who is imminently dying. The argument is that it is God alone who determines who lives or dies, and either accelerating the process or delaying the call from the divine is an act of human hubris. This tension can be helpfully discussed with families as they consider right courses of action consistent with their beliefs. These discussions can be guided with an appeal to rabbinic authorities who can often provide assistance and comfort families.

These conversations have become more complicated given high-profile cases, such as that of Jahi McMath, in which a brain death diagnosis has been disputed.[38] While it is beyond the scope of this text to discuss the details of a case which as yet has not been fully disclosed in the peer review medical literature, there are ways in which the diagnosis could be made in error. Absence of brainstem reflexes may be due to inadequate exclusion of historical confounders like sedative agents or hypothermia. Practically there could be inadequate adherence to established guidelines set out by the American Academy of Neurology[39,40] at either the institutional policy level[41] (although data indicate improving uniformity)[42] or through the practices of individual practitioners who either fail to conform to national guidelines or their local hospital policies.[43] In addition, the literature suggests variance in practice based on field of specialty tasked to do these tests within institutions,[41] with it being delegated to neurologists, neurosurgeons, or neurocritical care physicians as compared to more generalist practitioners.[44] In the aggregate, these shortcomings can result in procedural errors which undermine the perceived cogency of brain death as a diagnostic construct.

Ancillary testing may help validate or confirm diagnostic assessment (see Chapter 10) in the setting of religious or moral objections to brain death, but this approach is not without the risk of false-negative data. To increase support for brain death in Israel among Orthodox Jews who might be opposed, the Israeli Brain Death Act was modified in 2009 to include mandatory use of ancillary tests in addition to bedside evaluation, which included apnea testing. Initially these tests included one of the following: transcranial Doppler (TCD), computed tomographic angiography (CTA), or auditory brainstem-evoked potentials. Radionucleotide angiography using HM-PAO single-photon emission CT (SPECT) was added as an alternative in 2011. CTA may show persistent blood flow in the face

of clinical evidence of brain death.[45] Other investigators have found SPECT to be a more reliable mode of assessment.[46] As the Israeli example illustrates, ancillary testing, if improperly chosen, may provide unreliable information that can create more uncertainty and complicate discussions with families who object to brain death testing.

At the interface of law and medicine, Troug and Miller have contested the view of the President's Commission that brain death can be equated with death because these patients have lost integrative biological function, retaining the ability to maintain many other critical functions like circulation, digestion, wound healing, temperature control, and even the ability to bring a pregnancy to term with ongoing ventilatory support and hormonal replacement. While these scholars admit that there might be *public policy* reasons to view these patients as legally dead, they are in fact "biologically alive but psychologically dead."[47] This is a distinction that has been made elsewhere in the bioethics literature, with scholars debating whether death of the person and personhood was equivalent to a definition of biological death which hinged on biological functioning of the organism and which was not grounded in a psychological formulation.[48] A major confound in these arguments is that the preservation of endocrine and autonomic functions implies survival of the hypothalamus, which means that the patient has not had "cessation of all functions of the brain." However, the standard brain death exam, as used clinically, does not contain tests of hypothalamic functions, and so, in the absence of an ancillary study that proves lack of blood flow to the brain, there may be areas of tissue preservation in the hypothalamus and perhaps elsewhere in the forebrain.

Many commentators viewing brain death biologically point to the necessity of an integrative homeostatic function for life and the lack of this function in brain death versus the vegetative state. In brain death, the minimal autonomic control provided by the brainstem seen in the vegetative state is absent even as higher cortical integrative function is absent in the vegetative state.[49] An additional distinction following the syndromic argument laid out by Bernat is that while brain death is a condition from which patients cannot evolve, if properly diagnosed, patients can evolve to higher levels of recovery from the vegetative state,[50] even when it has become chronic.[51]

Returning to the McMath case, Troug points to these two perspectives on brain death and the differing functions of biology and the law. He argues that the law requires bright line distinctions (e.g., when to declare death), whereas "biology tends to be continuous." In his formulation, these opposing needs cause confusion in her case. While he does not believe that cases like McMath "present a fundamental challenge to the diagnosis of death by neurological criteria," he does urge additional clarification about how the bright line distinctions of the law can incorporate the continuity of biological processes.[52] Elsewhere, Troug and Miller suggest that the dead-donor rule be abandoned with respect to organ donation to address this quandary.[53] It is an argument that is reminiscent of Beecher's argument to retrieve organs from those he described as "hopelessly comatose" before he settled on the narrower category of brain death.[24]

Vegetative State

The vegetative state is a paradoxical condition. As Jennett and Plum classically described it, patients are in a state of wakeful unresponsiveness in which the eyes are open but there is no awareness of self, others, or environment. If eyes are the metaphorical window to the soul, it can be disheartening for families to learn that the opening of the eyes of a loved one in the vegetative state as they emerge from coma are unseeing and unknowing. In her autobiography, Mrs. Quinlan spoke of the tragic moment when she realized that her daughter, Karen, was unaware even as her brainstem recovered and her eyes opened. After the initial excitement that "she had come back," the stark reality of the vegetative state sunk in when she wasn't tracking or focusing:

 . . . that was the most disheartening development of all, watching her eyes look into space, or move all around the room, as though she was looking and looking for something—and
finally forcing ourselves to realize she couldn't see.[54]

Surrogates need to appreciate that the behaviors that are seen in the vegetative state—sleep–wake cycles, blinking, eye movements, and even the startle reflex—are not purposeful and do not indicate consciousness or awareness of self, others, or the environment.[55] This is a hard concept for lay people to get their arms around. They need to appreciate that these are autonomic behaviors, much like breathing and the maintenance of a heartbeat, controlled by brainstem activity. Explicating this distinction is important when the patient first enters the vegetative state, lest these behaviors be understood as evidence of awareness or consciousness.

Discussions about prognosis will be further complicated by the fact that, following coma, the vegetative state may be transient or more prolonged depending on the inciting event, with traumatic brain injury (TBI) having a more favorable prognosis for recovery of consciousness than anoxia. This is a point even lost on clinicians who may erroneously believe, or may have been taught, that the persistent vegetative state is invariably permanent.[6] Indeed, in cases of TBI, a patient who remains in a persistent vegetative state 6 months after initial injury has up to a 20% chance of regaining consciousness.[50]

This variable outcome should be explained once the surrogate appreciates that the patient has become vegetative. The sequence of recovery that may occur—and its probabilistic likelihood depending on known etiology—should be shared with surrogates. This can be tremendously helpful to them because it prepares them for what the future might hold and milestones that require due attention. Insight into these markers is especially empowering to surrogates once the patient has left the acute care setting and the standards of assessment are more variable.[56]

Having said this, it is especially important to appreciate that discussions about the vegetative state and its prognosis occur in a societal context. This is a critical backdrop for discussions at the bedside, and it is important for clinicians to understand that the vegetative state has an outsized place in the history of bioethics and the evolution of the right to die.

Since the late 1960s, bioethics has been predicated on the evolution of self-determination and autonomy. One central area where this has evolved has been in the negative right to be left alone. The right to die was established in American jurisprudence through cases involving patients in the vegetative state.[57] This right was established in the landmark case of Karen Ann Quinlan, a young woman left in a vegetative state from a presumptive drug overdose.[58] Her parents appealed to the New Jersey Supreme Court to allow for the removal of her ventilator, and this request was granted based on the futility of continued care and the irreversible loss of a cognitive, sapient state.[59,60]

Fred Plum, co-originator of the term "persistent vegetative state" with the Scottish neurosurgeon Bryan Jennett in a landmark 1972 *Lancet* article, was asked to testify by Chief Judge Richard Hughes. Plum confirmed the diagnosis, and Judge Hughes cites Plum's findings in his opinion:

> It was indicated by Dr. Plum that the brain works in essentially two ways, the vegetative and the sapient . . . We have no hesitancy in deciding . . . that no external compelling interest of the State should compel Karen to endure the unendurable, only to vegetate a few more measurable months with no realistic possibility of returning to any semblance of cognitive or sapient life.[58]

In this historical frame, the vegetative state was identified with medical futility and, as such, as a case in which surrogates would be granted the discretion to withdraw life-sustaining therapy.[61]

In the ensuing decades, physicians became acculturated to a right to die, and the vegetative state became the ultimate in medical futility. Nothing could or should be done because once the permanent vegetative state was reached it was immutable. This logic and public endorsement of an autonomy ethic held in two other cases involving individuals in the vegetative state: Nancy Beth Cruzan[62] and Terri Schiavo.[63]

In 1990, the US Supreme Court heard an appeal to remove Ms. Cruzan's feeding tube. The Court ruled that patients have a right to refuse life-sustaining therapy, including the right to refuse artificial nutrition and hydration. The Court did not create an expansive federal right but said it was up to the States to determine what kind of evidentiary knowledge would allow surrogates to makes decisions on an incapacitated patient's behalf. Ms. Cruzan's

feeding tube was removed when her case was again heard in her native Missouri.

The increasing recognition of the importance of advance care planning—or the use of living wills or healthcare proxies—was also a byproduct of *Cruzan*. As a part of her ruling in *Cruzan*,[64] Justice Sandra Day O'Connor suggested a greater role for advance care planning, a mechanism for patients to express their wishes before decisional incapacity.[65] Through the use of a living will or durable power of attorney, patients could make their wishes known.

The lack of such an advance directive became part of the conflict in the case of Terri Schiavo. Ms. Schiavo fell into a permanent vegetative state following a cardiac arrest and anoxic brain injury in 1990.[66] Her case gained national prominence in 2003 and again in 2005, when family members disputed the ethical propriety of the removal of her feeding tube. Multiple courts ruled that her prior wishes were known and that her husband, who advocated the removal of her percutaneous gastrostomy tube, was the appropriate surrogate decision-maker under state law.

In the aggregate, these three cases helped shape attitudes toward the vegetative state and tightly linked the condition with the evolution of the right to die and with a negative prognostic bias toward patients who were vegetative or appeared so.

Since Jennett and Plum's original formulation of the persistent vegetative state—as one of wakeful unresponsiveness in which there is no awareness of self, other, or the environment—the classification of this brain state has evolved. In 1994, the Multi-Society Task Force (MSTF) determined that the vegetative state became *persistent* once it has persisted for 1 month and that it became *permanent* 3 months following *anoxic* injury and 12 months after TBI.[50] These milestones assumed that patients were properly assessed at these endpoints for possible migration into the MCS (see later discussion).

Presciently, the authors of the MSTF hedged on the question of permanence once these milestones were crossed, noting that "the persistent vegetative state is a diagnosis and that the permanent vegetative state is a prognosis."[50] This was prompted by the rare outlier cases who seemed to recover beyond the aforementioned temporal milestones. More recent Guidelines on Disorders of Consciousness developed jointly by the American Academy of Neurology (AAN), the American College of Rehabilitation Medicine (ACRM), and National Institute on Disability, Independent Living, and Rehabilitation Research (NIDILRR) now estimate that upward of 20% of patients who were thought to be in the permanent vegetative state may actually recover consciousness.[51] This estimate comes from a reanalysis of the data used by the MSTF, new epidemiological data, and evidence from neuroimaging that points to covert consciousness. For this reason, the AAN/ACRM/NIDILRR guideline recommend that the permanent vegetative state be reclassified as the *chronic* vegetative state.[51]

This represents a sea change in nosology, broader medico-legal norms, and cultural expectations about this condition, the futility of which served as the predicate of the right to die movement since the *Quinlan* decision. While patients no longer need to be in the vegetative state to withdraw life-sustaining therapy, this right to die did begin in this population.[67] At a national level, questioning the immutability of this condition could rekindle the debate over the well-established right to die. And, at the bedside, one could well imagine families confronted with the vegetative diagnosis asking why their loved one might not be among the 20% who might recover consciousness.

Ethically, the possibility that 1 in 5 patients might make an additional recovery will present a challenge for families and clinicians. To avoid too broad an overgeneralization of this possibility, it is useful to consider which patients might fall into this 20% category and distinguish among them.[68] The first group are patients who were misdiagnosed and appeared vegetative but were in fact in the MCS. Schnakers et al. have found that 41% of patients in chronic care thought to be in the vegetative state following TBI were in fact in MCS.[69] This finding has been observed by other investigators. Patients constituting a second group would be those who appeared vegetative but had the potential to undergo a state change when stimulated by a drug or neuroprosthetic device like deep brain stimulation (DBS), transcranial magnetic stimulation (TCMS), or vagus nerve stimulation (VNS). In contrast to true vegetative patients who do not have the intact neural networks necessary to sustain consciousness, these patients had intact but unactivated neural networks, as would be found in MCS. Without stimulation,

these patients would behaviorally appear to be vegetative. A third category of patients would be those who were in CMD, where there was a discordance between volitional responsiveness seen on neuroimaging and behavioral manifestations at the bedside. Patients in CMD could constitute a large functional span from MCS to the locked-in state. A fourth category of patients includes those who undergo structural changes establishing new neural networks *after* the prior milestone for permanence had passed, a phenomena described longitudinally in MCS.[70] Patients who sustained late structural changes could either manifest overt behaviors consistent with consciousness or have covert consciousness with CMD.

Redesignating the permanent vegetative state as the chronic vegetative state also raises the question of how long families should wait and the distributive justice issues that follow when the costs of continued care are considered. It is fair to ask how long is too long, and how the needs of patients and the preferences of their families can be balanced against inevitable questions about limited resources. While individual physicians should be fiduciaries for their patients, we also need to address these broader policy questions at a societal level.

One way to mitigate these concerns is to risk-stratify the potential for the late recovery of consciousness. Given the uncertainty now associated with the chronic vegetative state, prudence would dictate—and the AAN/ACRM/NIDILRR guideline call for—comprehensive assessment of these patients when continued treatment would be consistent with the patient's prior wishes and the family's preferences.[51] This evaluation should center on mitigating errors in mistaking MCS patients as vegetative; identifying covert consciousness with use of volitional neuroimaging; attempting to induce a state change to activate latent networks; and identifying structural changes, such as axonal sprouting, that might undergird neural networks necessary to sustain consciousness. These assessments can help frame probabilities of additional recovery, identify subsets of patients within the putative 20% who might recover, and inform family choices.[51] Ultimately, data collected from these assessments will bring greater prognostic clarity and provide guidance about which patients are likely to recover and those who will in fact remain permanently unconscious. But to obtain this information, diagnostic registries will be necessary to make generalizable recommendations which are not possible at this time.[71,72]

While this approach may help with risk stratification, it will not immediately answer all questions about prognosis and whether a patient will end up in the vegetative state or regain additional functional status. This will lead to uncertainty for family members who will need to be given the requisite information about what is known and what remains unclear. If we take informed consent and informed refusal as an ethical norm, the task is to disclose and inform and accommodate the uncertainty, not act as if it were not there. That is disingenuous and undermines trust.

Unresponsive Wakefulness Syndrome

Some scholars have proposed the use of the *unresponsive wakefulness syndrome* (UWS) as a pseudonym for the vegetative state.[73] Some have objected to the term "vegetative state" because it connotes a disrespect for persons in that brain state, implying that these individuals were akin to "vegetables." This would be a simplistic and uninformed reading of a complex etymology related to Jennett and Plum's nomenclature for this brain state. In 1998, Plum et al. addressed this criticism noting:

> How did the vegetative state get its name? Not as the reader might think. Patients' families sometimes challenge us, implying that we have re-graded the sufferer as a vegetable. Not so! The conception of a vegetative nervous system goes a long way back.[74]

Recently, Zoe Adams and I have written how Plum traced the lineage of the vegetative state to the French physician Xavier Bichat (1771–1802) and the American neurologist and endocrinologist Walter Timme (1874–1956), each of whom invoke *De Anima*, Aristotle's treatise on the soul.[75] In that mid–fourth-century BCE work, Aristotle writes of a "vegetative faculty" of the soul.[76]

Beyond the provenance of the phrase's intellectual history, the vegetative state is ensconced in current American jurisprudence related to end-of-life care and the right to die.[57,77] The alternate formulation of UWS is not cited in current law, and this could create problems in some jurisdictions about decisions to withhold or withdraw life-sustaining therapies.

Beyond the historical and potential legal challenges of redesignating the vegetative state as the UWS, there are conceptual ones as well that should be considered. While the UWS echoes the language of Jennett and Plum's original *Lancet* paper, where they described the patient in the persistent vegetative state as "it seems wakefulness without awareness."[55] Given this, it is regressive to adopt a *phenotypic* description of this condition because neuroimaging data suggest that patients who appear unresponsive and wakeful may actually have covert consciousness.[68,78] This term, more commonly applied to the vegetative state outside of the United States, focuses on the observable bedside characteristics of the patient and not the underlying pathophysiology associated with consciousness. This approach can conflate the truly vegetative patient with one who appears to be so at the bedside but who displays evidence of covert consciousness when undergoing volitional tasking on neuroimaging. If we return to Jennett and Plum's original description, we note their careful addition of the word "seems" to the observation of "wakefulness without awareness,"[55] a caution which now accommodates the possibility of the discordance observed in patients with CMD.

The Minimally Conscious State

The MCS was codified in a 2002 consensus statement.[79] This liminal state of consciousness is distinct from the vegetative state in that patients are aware of self, others, and their environment. They may say their name, track objects and persons in their environment, and perform simple tasks. The challenge is that these behaviors are episodic and intermittent and not reliably reproduced. The episodic nature of these behaviors, coupled with the chronic care setting to which many of these patients are placed, results in a staggering rate of misdiagnosis. Families who report observed behaviors to clinicians who are then unable to elicit them are viewed as unreliable historians even though this lack of reproducibility is consistent with the biology of the condition. This discounting of family observations is further entrenched when clinicians view disorders of consciousness through the prism of a rigid diagnostic frame and fail to appreciate that a patient admitted to chronic care in the vegetative state could evolve to MCS. In the aggregate, these factors have led to 41% of patients with TBI in the vegetative state being identified as in MCS when carefully evaluated.[69]

MCS is also the plateau from which patients may regain consistent evidence of consciousness; an awareness of self, others, and their environment; and, most critically, the ability to engage in functional communication. Emergence from MCS is a major milestone for several key reasons. First, when patients arrive at this functional level, they are able to consistently engage others. This will make the question of whether or not the patient is conscious or not less disputable and less open to charges of familial emotionality or denial. Unlike the MCS, during which patients will demonstrate episodic evidence of consciousness, emerged patients do this consistently and reliably. Second, at this more evolved state of consciousness, patients more fully recapture personhood lost as the result of their injury. As the philosopher William Winslade observed in an early exploration of ethical issues following TBI, "Being persons requires having a personality, being aware of ourselves and our surroundings, and possessing human capacities, such as memory, emotions, and the ability to communicate and interact with other people."[80]

An additional point about emergence from MCS is that the potential for recovery is open-ended and unpredictable. Functional capability beyond mere emergence is an active area of study in rehabilitation, with novel concepts like the level of early impaired self-awareness being considered as a marker for predicting complex functional activities later in the course of recovery from TBI.[81] This suggests the need for ongoing assessment of capabilities and aggressive physical and occupational therapy for patients who have managed to recover to this state.

A final note on *diagnostics* is in order. Families may want confirmatory studies to convince them of the solidity of the clinical diagnosis, trusting the "objectivity" of a scan over the analysis of the clinician. Expectations are raised by the advent of "neuroethics" articles in the popular culture asserting the potential of neuroimaging technologies to read minds and refine marketing techniques.[82,83] Because of these trends, surrogates will invest imaging technologies with more diagnostic reliability than they currently possess and seek clear-cut answers through this visual medium. It is important to be clear that although progress is being made with neuroimaging, especially in the identification of covert consciousness (see later discussion), the assessment of patients with disorders of consciousness is a clinical task best accomplished by a competent history and neurological exam using the CRS-R.[51]

Although families may request them, these technologies are best applied in research settings and at best can be ancillary to clinical evaluation. They must be interpreted in light of the history and neurological and neurobehavioral examination. It is important to be transparent when discussing the capabilities of current technology to assess brain states, indicate that this is an active area of research, and caution that many of the *experimental* protocols portrayed in the media are being utilized in patients who have already been diagnostically assessed.[84]

NEUROETHICS OF COVERT CONSCIOUSNESS

The advent of neuroimaging and its ability to reconfigure our understanding of the injured brain and our normative obligations to patients and their families is reminiscent of what the American philosopher John Dewey wrote about the power of technology to change our obligations and ends. In *Common Sense and Scientific Inquiry* Dewey wrote, "inventions of new agencies and instruments create new ends; they create new consequences which stir men to form new purposes."[85] What was true when Dewey wrote those words in 1938 is true today as we are prompted to increasingly appreciate that CMD, made apparent by neuroimaging, is in fact an ethical issue that should stir the profession "to form new purposes."

Normative Significance of Covert Consciousness

The presence of covert consciousness has profound normative significance for patients and families. If patients are conscious, their consciousness deserves to be recognized. A failure to recognize consciousness, when it can be identified, is a disrespect of personhood. Practically, a failure to recognize that a patient is conscious deprives him or her of the possibility of engagement with family, friends, and others. As social creatures, to inflict isolation on a conscious being is to deprive some of the most vulnerable among us of human companionship. This also deprives their family from knowing that they are there. And, even more fundamentally, if a patient is conscious and has intact neural networks capable of supporting consciousness, then the patient is also likely to experience pain. If a patient is mistakenly thought to be vegetative, a class of patients who do not activate distributed pain networks when exposed to painful stimuli in experimental conditions,[86] then conscious patients will be treated as if they are unconscious and possibly deprived of appropriate pain and symptom management. This is an inhumane omission compounded by the fact that many MCS and CMD patients may be unable to express the distress they might experience because they do not have access to functional communication.

The realization that some patients may appear unconscious but not be so raises the question of what the clinical community is to do with data about MCS and CMD that are gleaned from experimental protocols that have not yet been validated as clinical methods. That is, as we move beyond behavioral criteria, can neuroimaging be used to assess covert consciousness while it is still experimental and not yet a vetted clinical tool? And, if it is used, how should results, both "positive" and "negative" be understood and conveyed to families?

Ancillary Care Obligations

One of the challenges investigators and clinicians will face is how to utilize emerging methods to detect covert consciousness using means that are still investigational. What are the putative benefits and risks of these methods and associated risks? And how might that they be mitigated through procedural safeguards and prudential interpretation of data? To address these questions, we need to address whether these methods are research or therapy, and, if they are the latter, whether they have a role in clinical practice.

Historically, there has been a rather bright-line distinction between research and clinical practice because of historical abuse of research subjects, often in the name of clinical care.[87–89] The Tuskegee syphilis study comes to mind as an example where more than 400 African Americans were told they were being treated in an observational "study" while antibiotics were withheld.[87] Tuskegee, and an awareness of research ethics abuses during the Holocaust and in contemporary American practice,[90] led Congress to pass the National Research Act of 1974,[91] which recognized the vulnerability of research subjects, articulated governing principles to promote their protection, and established the modern Institutional Review Board (IRB) regulatory framework.

These are critical protections, but, more recently, the stark research–practice dichotomy of that earlier era is being questioned. Susan Wolf, a leading bioethicist and law professor, has noted that there is "an emerging view that researchers bear some clinical responsibility toward research subjects."[92] The use of research data in the context of clinical care can be appropriate based on whether there is actionable information that might emerge from the data. Her criteria for this assessment include its potential health or reproductive significance, the validity of the test, the risks and benefits of disclosure, and the utility of the information.

It is our view that the identification of covert consciousness has high utility. As I have written elsewhere, "Nothing is more important than knowing that a patient may be conscious, especially when there is a paucity of motor output and the possibility that neuroimaging data, obtained through research or not, might suggest that an individual thought to be vegetative might actually be aware."[25] Interactions with family change, isolation can be mitigated, and the presence of pain addressed. Moreover, when a patient is appreciated as conscious, neuroprosthetics and pharmacologic interventions can be utilized to try to establish a channel for functional communication.

For the aforementioned reasons, investigators have what the philosopher Henry S. Richardson has described as "ancillary care obligations"[93] to those conscious subjects with disorders of consciousness who might otherwise be mistaken as unconscious.[94] If research data must be shared with their families, it must be done in conjunction with the patient's doctors responsible for providing clinical care. This obligation is heightened by the vulnerability of this population and the high risk they face of misdiagnosis and incomplete assessment.

Translating Research to Practice

Even if covert consciousness should be pursued using emerging methods of assessment, there remain unresolved methodological questions about sensitivity and specificity and the important distinction between a positive and negative result. How do we know if a patient is conscious?

This is a question that is complex in its simplicity and applies to all with whom we interact. It has been argued that the only consciousness we truly know is our own. We can only infer the consciousness of another through their response to an outward expression of our own sentience. We say something to another, we see a raised eyebrow, a smile, or hear a comment that suggests agreement or dissent with what we have said. These responses suggest the presence of a conscious entity from which the response originates. While this threshold does not conclusively suggest consciousness if we consider the responses we can glean from our cell phones, it does suggest that some degree of processing of information and output is necessary if not sufficient to infer consciousness.

Taking this threshold to the experimental evidence regarding covert consciousness, or CMD, is the methodological and thereby ethical distinction between the utility of passive versus volitional activation. The response of MCS patients to family narratives played forward versus backward (and thus with the same frequency spectrum) reported by Schiff et al. was highly suggestive of language processing[95] and thus potentially ethically significant in suggesting sentience in these patients.[96] Nonetheless, such passive responses are *less* convincing than a positive activation in a volitional paradigm where a subject is asked to imagine doing a task with expected activations of regions of interest.[97] In these examples, the paradigm requires the subject to both receive and process the information and willingly imagine doing the task.

For this reason, a positive test, for example volitional response on neuroimaging, would be highly suggestive of consciousness. These data would be actionable, leading to triage toward early rehabilitation and greater sensitivity to the patient's need for human engagement and proper pain management and neuropalliative care (see later discussion). In contrast, a negative result in isolation cannot be taken as dispositive because it might constitute a type II error that fails to identify consciousness when it is present. As has been noted in Chapter 9, a percentage of healthy controls do not demonstrate activation in regions of interest with motor imagery tests. This makes "negative" studies highly problematic and of dubious utility.

Another area for concern is timing and the risk of stigmatization. A patient who has a negative test for consciousness may be labeled as unconscious and later evolve out of the vegetative state to MCS or beyond and be saddled with this "objective" assessment.[98] Given the fluidity of syndromic brain states,[11] there is a risk of premature moral closure when imaging studies fail to demonstrate consciousness, if this were to curtail further surveillance for its reemergence.

This temporal concern is of heightened importance given emerging data that suggest that there is an ongoing regenerative recovery process in the severely injured brain. Thengone et al. demonstrated the longitudinal strengthening of bilateral functional and structural white matter connections across the hemispheres and Broca's area in a patient in MCS over a 54 month period.[70] These data, coupled with the AAN/ACRM/NIDILRR guideline on disorders of consciousness, which has renamed the permanent vegetative state as "chronic,"[51] (see earlier discussion) and thus open to evolution, suggest that any labels attached to the recovering brain through early functional imaging need to be interpreted as a provisional finding when covert consciousness is *not* identified. To do otherwise is to prematurely discount the potentiality of further recovery. Given the recency of our ability to test cognitive function with neuroimaging, it will require repeated longitudinal evaluation, from the earliest stages of coma, in a large cohort of patients before we can say with any degree of confidence at what point the capacity for recovery to a conscious state has been exhausted.

Over the lifetime of this book, hypotheses will evolve, diagnostic and therapeutic methods will be refined, and investigational methods will mature into established clinical practice and an established standard of care.[99] Until that time, investigators should engage in prospective discussions with surrogates about the nature and scope of potential disclosure of research data, focusing on information that is both credible and actionable, and collaborate with the patient's *treating* physician when sharing results. A critical ethical dilemma emerges when the treating clinician is also an investigator. To avoid conflicts of interest, it is essential that the physician seek the input of the governing institutional review board and/or hospital ethics committee to advise on role sequestration.

CAPACITY, COMPETENCE, AND SURROGATE DECISION-MAKING

By its nature, care decisions for patients with severe disorders of consciousness generally involve surrogates. Patients so impaired have lost their decision-making capacity and the ability to direct their own care. Surrogates—family members, friends, other intimates, or court-appointed guardians—must step in and make decisions about ongoing care or its withdrawal. In this section, we will consider the special challenges faced by surrogate decision-makers entrusted with the care of a patient with a disorder of consciousness and delineate what practitioners might do to ease their burden by improving the process of communication and deliberation.

Decision-Making Capacity

A surrogate decision-maker is a person, other than the patient, who directs care when the patient is decisionally incapacitated and unable to provide informed consent or informed refusal for a medical intervention. A patient is

considered to lack decision-making capacity when he or she is unable to understand the risks, benefits, and alternatives to a diagnostic or therapeutic procedure. Patients who have the capacity to consent or refuse a medical intervention need to evidence sufficient understanding of their choice to demonstrate that they have brought a rational standard of decision-making to the process.

This standard of assessment is important because the ability to communicate is necessary to evidence understanding. For example, a patient who has CMD may understand the risks, benefits, and alternatives posed by a treatment choice but not be able to express that choice. And, without that expression, we cannot know whether the patient truly understands the choice that is under consideration. Absent that expression of understanding, a patient will necessarily be found to lack capacity, presenting an ethically troubling scenario in which a patient who might understand a choice at hand cannot tell us his or her preferences.

Because this is an ethically fraught situation, every effort must be made to provide such patients with assistive devices that might allow them to express their preferences lest they be treated over their objections, with such interventions potentially disrespecting "personhood." Devices like word boards and eye-tracking devices have been used productively in these situations, as has the consultation of skilled physical and speech therapists who can help patients express themselves.

Having said this, patients suspected of having CMD, who are thought to understand what is being asked of them but for whom a communication channel cannot be established, are nonetheless considered to lack decision-making capacity and thus deemed incompetent to legally consent or refuse a medical intervention because they can neither demonstrate their thinking nor be in a position to defend their interests. In addition, many patients may be unable to ask questions about treatment choices because they cannot communicate or because they don't have the ability to initiate the kind of queries that decisionally capacitated patients might ask. This puts these patients at a disadvantage and ultimately deprives them of the ability to make decisions because they cannot fully express their self-determination or defend their autonomy because of their inability to communicate.

While depriving patients thought to have capacity of the right to make choices may seem an abridgement of their self-determination, competence as a legal right needs to be binary and follow a bright-line distinction, even if decision-making capacities exist on an ethical continuum.

Surrogate Decision-Making

When a patient lacks capacity, we need to turn to surrogate decision-makers for guidance. Under prevailing legal and ethical norms, surrogates should make decisions based on a decision-making hierarchy that prizes the patient's expressed choices while able to do so (e.g., an advance directive).[100] Thus, surrogates should follow known *expressed wishes* of the patient when they are known and invoke *substituted judgment*—what is believed or inferred about patient choices—when actual preferences are unknown. In the absence of any evidence of prior wishes or known patient values, surrogates should invoke a *best interests standard*. This is a generic standard intended to represent what an average person would do when confronted by prevailing circumstances.

When working with surrogate decision-makers, it is important to know who among many family members has standing and priority.[101] A surrogate designated by the patient while still decisionally capacitated through advance care planning has precedence over other potential decision-makers because he or she was expressly chosen by the patient. This exercise of patient self-determination can take place through an advance directive, variably called a *durable power attorney for healthcare, healthcare agent,* or *healthcare proxy.*[102,103]

Alternately, a patient without a designated surrogate can express substantive preferences in an advance directive document called a *living will*. A living will details patient wishes but does not authorize a designated spokesperson. If there is no designated surrogate, family members and close friends can be turned to in order of their relationship to the patient.

Reemergent Agency

Clinically, the distinction between capacity and competence is a critical one. While a patient may be found to be incompetent, leaving his

surrogate (a family member for example) or a court-appointed guardian to make decisions on his behalf, it remains ethically important to engage the patient in decisions as much as is possible. This is important for three reasons. First, it enhances patient adherence and compliance if he or she is part of the decision. Second, many clinicians will find it objectionable to treat a patient over his or her objection. Third, patients—even those with diminished capacity—retain rights of self-dominion over decisions of great personal importance. While they may not be entrusted to make decisions unilaterally, their views still matter both operationally (for adherence and cooperation) and normatively.

For patients with disorders of consciousness, especially those who are minimally conscious or who have CMD, two categories of decision-making (assent and dissent) are particularly relevant. A patient who assents agrees with a treatment or diagnostic recommendation even if he or she does not fully understand the choice at hand. Conversely, the dissent of the patient signifies an unwillingness to agree to an intervention even if the individual does not fully grasp the consequences of the refusal. While neither assent nor dissent rise to the level of consent or refusal as seen in competent patients, each has moral valence because it provides some evidence of patient preferences and thus should be cultivated.

This can be accomplished through assisted decision-making in which surrogates and professionals aid the patient with decisions both conceptually and with assisted devices that help create a communication channel. This can be achieved with neuroprosthetic devices and drugs which improve the patient's ability to communicate. As a first step, clinicians can ask the patient to participate in simpler decisions for which he or she may have the ability to participate. This engages the patient in the care plan and also is consistent with the ethical and legal view that capacity is specific to the task at hand and not a more global assessment. Ethically, this narrower frame allows for patient participation in some decisions, thus maximizing their self-determination as appropriate.

Mosaic Decision-Making

Involving the patient with reemergent agency, the ability to represent his or her interests to some extent in decisions about his or her care presents both philosophical and practical challenges beyond the traditional framework of the patient or a surrogate making decisions. Here, instead of a traditional doctor–patient or doctor–surrogate dyad, there is a triad with the addition of a patient whose decision-making abilities are incomplete and potentially evolving. The challenge is to involve such patients as much as possible without asking them to make decisions for which they are unprepared.

In our experience, when patients are legally incompetent, clinicians generally turn to surrogates and discount the possibility that the patient might be able to contribute at some level to decisions about their care and well-being. Turning exclusively to the surrogate is simpler, but it is ethically problematic. The patient has a stake in decisions about his or her care and should be included.

Sadly, historically, people with disabilities have been excluded from the conversation to the point that a slogan in the disabilities rights community is "nothing about us without us."[104] So the clinical challenge is to engage patients in a proportionate way and not discount their voices while remaining cognizant of their limited ability to fully participate in the decision-making process.

In many ways, the situation is reminiscent of the developmental process in which an individuating child or adolescent gains an ability to make and be responsible for decisions.[105] The difference for adult patients with disorders of consciousness is that, before their injuries, they had decision-making capacity and prior preferences and values, unlike children who had yet to form their values and preferences.

Making decisions which involve a patient who had past preferences and is regaining decision-making capacity includes calculating the valence given to prior wishes as opposed to current claims and desires. There is no easy calculus to know how to incorporate a patient's reemerging voice into decisions, but a process of *mosaic decision-making* may be useful.[106] Mosaic decision-making incorporates the patient's prior preferences and current choices with views of the surrogate decision-maker, the patient's physician, and a patient advocate in a deliberative process that seeks to pull these differing perspectives together into a discernible pattern, much as shards coalesce to create

a mosaic, to invoke a useful metaphor.[107] In this way, the current voice of the patient, his past, and the reemergent self are brought into constructive conversation with his surrogate and physician, as well as with an advocate who will seek to ensure that he is heard and acknowledged.

COMMUNICATION STRATEGIES

Beyond process questions and the professional obligation to exchange information with surrogates, it is also important to appreciate that probabilities about survival and functional status do not easily translate into value choices.[108] Sharing prognostic probabilities is not, in itself, sufficient to improve the deliberative process or to effect outcome decisions.

Given the complexity of the decision-making process, this is not wholly unexpected. The quality of how information is conveyed is difficult to assess and may be as critical as what has been conveyed. Families may be distrustful of clinicians and systems of care that are not designed for longitudinal chronic care.[2] They may have been the recipients of misinformation about the patient's brain state and be wary of family meetings that they worry might try to engineer a decision to withhold or withdraw care.[109] They are also generally unaware of the brain states that comprise disorders of consciousness and have a knowledge deficit amid a time of great stress.[25] Because clinicians have superior knowledge, they have a superior obligation to explain these brain states patiently and carefully to families who are facing unanticipated decisions for which most will be wholly unprepared.

Communication with surrogates would present formidable challenges even if there were continuity of care and ongoing doctor–patient/family relationships. In the setting of shifting venues of care from the acute hospital setting to rehabilitation and long-term care facilities, the challenge of building trust is formidable. To help build such relationships, it is critical to be empathic and supportive and try to imagine what has eloquently been described as "the loneliness of the long-term care-giver"[110] faced with social isolation and family members whose injury has altered them and their relationships with those who hold them dear.

These longitudinal stresses, the dependency of loved ones, coupled with the prognostic uncertainties, suggest the need for compassion when working with families touched by a disorder of consciousness.

Time-Delimited Communication

To ensure that these decisions are indeed informed, it is essential that there is proper information flow between clinical staff and surrogates at key junctures of care when clinical findings warrant discussion or when a prognostic milestone is reached. How much information is conveyed to achieve this objective and how determinative it can be will depend on clinical circumstances.

For example, it may be justified to provide an early and definitive prognosis of permanent unconsciousness or death while a patient is comatose following an out-of-hospital cardiac arrest if there are clear negative prognostic predictors, as reviewed in Chapters 4 and 8, including loss of pupillary function, corneal reflexes, and bilateral absence of somatosensory evoked responses.

In contrast, it would seem inappropriate, and premature, to offer a conclusive prognosis in the comatose TBI patient who demonstrates brainstem function and appears to be moving quickly into the vegetative state. The rate of recovery of such patients might warrant a cautiously optimistic approach[111] delineated by a *prognostic time trial* in which the clinician gives a *time-delimited prognosis*.[112]

A useful metaphor to guide communication with families is drawn from storm prediction during the hurricane season. As a tropical storm leaves the west coast of Africa and travels across the Atlantic toward the Eastern Seaboard of North America, it is impossible to predict how strong it will be and where it will land. But, as the storm makes its crossing and gains directionality, predicting its strength and landfall becomes possible. Meteorologists depict this improving confidence interval with a cone of uncertainty that narrows over time. A similar process can guide family communication with patients with disorders of consciousness.

It is equally unwise for clinicians to be categorical about a patient's prognosis prematurely, except in the most dire or hopeful of

circumstances, as discussed in Chapter 9. In intermediate cases, which comprise most clinical scenarios, they need to guard against a negative prognostic bias and help families accept the inherent uncertainty of the situation, explaining that the passage of time often, but not always, provides increasing clarity.

To that end, it is helpful to engage in *time-delimited communication* in which patient progress is explained to anxious families in tandem with the patient's trajectory. Discussions are tracked and contextualized against certain temporal milestones, such as the patient's passage from one brain state to the next. While progression to a conscious state would be preferable to evolution into the vegetative state, it is important to explain that the early cessation of coma with rapid movement into the vegetative state can be a favorable prognostic sign.[112]

Several factors have prognostic significance and should be communicated with families. The first is the degree of structural injury in the brain. Second is the rapidity with which the patient moves out of coma. All of these factors require a balanced presentation to families because the road to recovery or chronic unconsciousness is indeterminate, and a combination of time courses and brain states may follow the cessation of the comatose phase. This indeterminacy of evolution to brain states from coma to full recovery needs to be stressed. This is often not appreciated by surrogates who may be unduly pessimistic or optimistic. At this juncture, it may be prudent to caution surrogates to avoid making a potentially premature decision and waiting until prognostication can be informed by *how* and *when* the patient evolves from coma.

Clearly if the patient regains consciousness quickly, this is prognostically favorable, but so, too, is rapid evolution into a vegetative state, even though surrogates may perceive this as invariably negative. While recovery of consciousness is optimal, surrogates need to appreciate that the vegetative state is not an immutable condition and that patients can progress beyond it, especially when the patient quickly evolves to the vegetative state out of a coma. This can be explained as the recovery of brainstem function in the absence of, as yet, higher cortical activity. In contrast, late emergence from coma to the vegetative state may be prognostically more worrisome.

Having said this, it is also important to explain that prognosis degrades the longer the patient is in the vegetative state. Under earlier nomenclature, at the 1-month interval following onset of the vegetative state, it was said that the vegetative state became persistent, and permanent 3 months after anoxic injury and 1 year after traumatic injury. As noted earlier, permanence is no longer an operative category following upon the new AAN/ACRM/NIDILRR guideline, thus injecting more uncertainty into family deliberations[51,68] and suggesting that there may be limited mobility into the MCS even after these previously delineated milestones.

Despite this ambiguity, it is helpful to structure conversations with families and give them a timeline when you will provide regular updates.[25,68] We recommend revisiting any assessment a month after cessation of coma and after the vegetative state has persisted for a month. Since 80% of anoxic and traumatic persistent vegetative states (i.e., no recovery at 1 month) will become "permanent," discursive discussions at this stage and after 3 months (for anoxic coma) and 12 months (for TBI) respectively, are also warranted. At these junctures, the task is a complicated one: explaining that the data suggest that more than 75% of patients in vegetative state at 1 month will *not* recover. The goal at this milestone is to explain what will be done to clarify the patient's brain state and track any changes longitudinally while not overly heightening expectations.

This is uncharted territory. It is important to try to minimize uncertainty by seeking to exclude covert consciousness and an unidentified MCS because MCS patients have a more open-ended prognosis and additional responsiveness to therapeutic engagement.

Unfortunately, at this point, the depiction of recovery is no longer linear as the time course to emergence from MCS is highly variable and examples of recovery to a level of severe disability with preserved personality and ability to communicate arising years or even decades following entry into MCS have been documented (as reviewed in Chapter 9).[113] Nonetheless, the movement into MCS is significant because it signals the presence of some degree of consciousness and potentially heralds the regaining of functional communication and consistent evidence of consciousness.

Goals of Care

While time can be helpful in clarifying outcomes, this is not always the case because of the *syndromic* uncertainty of these conditions. An alternative approach to attempting to formulate *goals of care* can be especially valuable in two circumstances: when the patient's brain state is unclear, and when the potential for additional functional recovery cannot be precisely predicted. In these circumstances, it is helpful to pivot from the question of brain state to thinking more broadly about the patient's likely functional status and whether this degree of recovery would be consistent with the patient's goals of care as known by their surrogates. Contextualizing care decisions against goals of care discussions can be very helpful.

Surrogates will articulate a broad range of preferences, depending on the patient's values and their own sense of what constitutes proportionate care: from the rejection of brain death to the decision to remove artificial nutrition and hydration in a patient who is in a MCS. In most cases, however, surrogates will struggle with the more nuanced question of the *degree* of loss of self that would make a life worth living.

This is a highly personal question. Families may benefit by your asking them to consider the ability to relate to others in the context of a broader consideration about the goals of care.[114] As for achieving a degree of functional communication, this level of relationality is not reached until the patient has recovered to the upper end of MCS or emerged from that state. Although all may not agree with the centrality of functional communication, this may be a helpful goal of care when speaking with family members. Narrative and empirical data both suggest that restoring the ability to communicate is a priority for families.[25,115]

Consider a patient who is on the cusp of the vegetative and minimally conscious states, a quandary that cannot be resolved in the immediate or intermediate future. In this scenario, it is helpful to pivot from the question of brain states and consider whether the functional status they will likely reach will allow them to achieve their goals of care. What did the patient hope to achieve? What would make life tolerable or intolerable? Could this goal of care drive treatment decisions? And would their likely brain state allow them to pursue these goals? This process places prognosis into the context of the patient's narrative and can provide useful guidance to families. While they may still have the burden of prognostic uncertainty, they may know enough—even with a large confidence interval—to be able to make choices about care.

We recall the case of a woman with a history of substance abuse who was admitted with a hypoglycemic coma that later progressed to the vegetative state. Whether she had progressed to the MCS was unclear, and this uncertainty prompted an ethics consultation. Instead of seeking to resolve this imponderable, the consultant asked about the patient's life and goals. After overcoming her addiction, she returned to school, came to love books, and either wanted to become a librarian or work in a book store. While it was unclear whether she was in the MCS or would evolve there, it was clear that she would never be able to have a bibliophilic existence, her life goal. This provided the family with clarity and informed their decision regarding life-sustaining therapy. Invoking a helpful aphorism, they let the goals drive the therapies, not the therapies drive the goals.[114]Fundamentally, the ethical analysis of these cases on the margins hinge less on the diagnosis than on articulating and then seeking to achieve goals of care important to the patient and family.

Finally, it is also important to disaggregate neurological prognostication from the impact of distinct medical comorbidities that can affect the course of intensive care. For example, sepsis, hypoxia, and metabolic disturbances can cloud assessment of the patient's underlying disorder of consciousness. When these conditions are remediable, it is best to defer neurologic assessment. When they are not, the intractability of the comorbidity can help clarify goals of care as the issue is not a patient's potential brain state but rather whether a trilobar pneumonia and bacteremia with resistant organisms is survivable.

Another prognostic concern that needs to be considered are the underlying conditions that precipitated the neurologic event. This is less critical when the etiology is trauma and more important in anoxic events. For example, if a cardiac arrest from a massive myocardial infarction led to anoxic brain injury, discussions with families should consider the patient's cardiac status, ejection fraction, and need for revascularization. When significant comorbid or precipitating conditions are present, they may more clearly drive prognostic thinking than the patient's brain state. Although neurologists will be focused on the patient's state of consciousness, it is critical to view prognosis within a global frame and not discount other variables. In addition, comorbidities like delirium from electrolyte disturbances or sepsis may cloud prognostication and should be normalized before making neurological assessments.

In all of these conversations, it may be helpful to reach out to the hospital's ethics committee, which will have additional expertise to help surrogates interpret technical information such patient as diagnosis and prognosis in light of the patient's prior wishes, preferences, and values.[116]

INSTITUTIONAL CONTEXT OF CARE

The provision of care can often be influenced by where it is provided and prevailing cultural norms that govern behaviors and attitudes of practitioners in that practice space. These venues can create biases and engender expectations about "right behaviors" that can lead to distortions of care. To engage in inquiry about decisions prompted under these circumstances, the clinician needs to become aware of these problematic situations and make them explicit so that they can be addressed. Here we focus on three key phases of patient care: the intensive care unit, hospital discharge planning, and rehabilitation.

Intensive Care

Outcomes for patients with severe brain injury who require intensive care differ depending on concomitant trauma, medical comorbidities, and where treatment is received. Neurocritical care is associated with lower mortality and a greater likelihood of recovery as compared to less specialized units.[117] For patients with concomitant trauma, trauma and neuro ICUs have similar mortality, with trauma units having better mortality data when the patient has multiple injuries. For patients with multiple injuries, mixed medical-surgical units have the highest mortality risk.[118] Delirium and depressed sensorium following brain injury are more likely seen in older ICU patient with medical comorbidities and dementia.[119]

In addition to the distinct expertise and epidemiology of differing ICUs, each venue has its own culture of care with complex interpersonal relationships influencing how ethical choices are made.[120] Families of patients with TBI, for example, experience stress differently than other families with loved ones in intensive care.[121]

Families shortly after the onset of a devastating injury associated with unconsciousness are fragile and search for guidance from healthcare providers. This is problematic if the healthcare provider is unable to dissociate his or her assessments of prognosis from prevalent, but mostly unfounded, biases about prognosis. Healthcare professionals, unfortunately, out of fear of coming across as not knowledgeable, often simplify the complex medical issue of prognostication and misguide families. Biases in providing guidance are prevalent, and, if honest guidance is the goal, they need to be recognized and actively addressed.[122]

Clinicians need to be cognizant of these practice variables in order not to fall prey to routines of care that may distort decision-making. For example, in the medical context (e.g., the treatment of progressive and life-threatening illnesses), the loss of decision-making capacity is often taken as a major prompt to withhold life-sustaining therapy. Most do not resuscitate (DNR) orders are authorized by surrogates who perceive the loss of capacity, which is often associated with stupor or coma, as the end of a debilitating process and the harbinger of an impending death.[123] (See the section "Withholding and Withdrawing Life-Sustaining Therapy.")

This experience drawn from the general medical context presents a paradox for those entrusted with the care of patients with a disorder of consciousness. In these cases, the loss of consciousness is quite different. It could result in death *or be the start of a recovery process.* Because perceptions of outcome hinge so strongly on the question of the recovery of consciousness,[25] it is important that practitioners and surrogate decision-makers do not draw a false analogy to the loss of decision-making capacity in most medical contexts and consider

its distinct significance in the setting of severe brain injury. The recognition of this problematic situation[124] is especially critical given the aforementioned data that 70% of in-patient hospital mortality for patients with disorders of consciousness is accounted for by decisions to withdraw life-sustaining therapy.[8]

Appreciating that the loss of consciousness following brain injury is distinct from that which emanates from advanced life-threatening medical illness is especially important given recent research conducted by Edlow et al. who detected covert consciousness in vegetative and MCS ICU patients 9–10 days following admission by assessing volitional command following using functional magnetic resonance imaging (fMRI) and EEG.[125] CMD was not identified in comatose patients. These research findings, coupled with the rush to judgment about the prognostic implications regarding the loss of consciousness in the ICU, have profound implications for end-of-life decision-making in critical care settings. During the life span of this edition of *Stupor and Coma*, it is likely that these methods will mature and that investigational efforts to identify CMD patients in the ICU will evolve and become the standard of care.

Discharge Planning

Hospital discharge can be a precarious time for patients and their families. Data from family narratives indicate that discharges are often precipitous and sudden, with little prospective planning.[109] Families report that discharge planning is often an after-thought and that they are presented few options for placement. They are often directed to "custodial care" care facilities that are ill-suited to patients' ongoing medical needs and which do not provide rehabilitation.[25,126]

It is important that clinicians view discharge placement as a critical juncture in the patient's care trajectory that can determine long-term outcomes. A patient who is sent to a nursing home versus rehabilitation is less likely to regain function or undergo proper longitudinal evaluation as his or her brain states progress.[25,126] For these critical reasons the acute care physicians who were instrumental in saving a patient's life have an ongoing ethical obligation and a forward-looking responsibility to ensure a safe discharge plan that maximizes the patient's potential for additional recovery. To think that one's fiduciary responsibility to patient care ends at the ambulance bay undermines all the brilliant neurosurgical and neurointensive care that made hospital discharge possible. To turn away and feel no responsibility for the course of post-hospital care could be said to violate the ethical prohibition against non-abandonment.

There is tremendous vulnerability at this care milestone, and patients who are sent to chronic care in lieu of rehabilitation are likely never to leave the chronic care sector, have their brain states properly reevaluated, or receive the physical therapy, assistive devices, and/or pharmacologic agents that might prompt additional progress. The mission statement of the Spanish Federation for Brain Injury captures the importance of ensuring that acute care is followed by rehabilitative interventions that can maximize recovery: *una vida salvada merce ser vivida*—a life that is saved deserves to be lived.[127]

Rehabilitation and Long-Term Care

Access to rehabilitation is an integral aspect of the care of patients with disorders of consciousness. While a comprehensive treatment of the means and modes of rehabilitation available for this population is beyond the scope of this chapter, it is within our purview to assert that clinicians have an ethical obligation to ensure that patients received rehabilitation and ongoing assessment following acute hospitalization.[72] This responsibility is consistent with recent the AAN/ACRM/NIDILRR guideline that views rehabilitation as the standard of care for this population.[51]

This is a worthy aspirational statement that will face barriers to implementation in practice. One challenge that patients encounter is what has been described as the "improvement standard"—a requirement that rehabilitation will only be provided if the patient demonstrates improvement. While this was never federal Medicare policy, it became something of an urban myth, distorting practice patterns and access. This often deprived patients with severe brain injury rehabilitation because their potential for improvement was felt to be improbable.[25]

In 2011, the improvement standard was challenged in federal court in *Jimmo et al. v. Sebelius.* Plaintiffs with chronic conditions requiring rehabilitation sued then Secretary of Health and Human Services Kathleen Sebelius, alleging the misapplication of Medicare policies.[128] When Chief Judge Christina C. Reiss of the Federal District Court in Vermont found the evidence plausible and set a trial date, the plaintiffs and the Center for Medicaid and Medicare Services (CMS) reached an agreement to extensively modify the Medicare Policy Manual.[129] These revisions asserted that there was no improvement standard and that restoration of function was *not* required to provide skilled services which could serve to preserve capabilities or prevent deterioration. As importantly, assessments of patient eligibility could not be based on "rule of thumb" or generic assessments, which were viewed as often prejudicial. While this was a major victory for patients in need of chronic rehabilitative services, local practices do not always comport with Federal Medicare guidelines, with challenges coming from local care determinations (LCDs).[130] Clinicians can serve as advocates for their patients by working with social work colleagues and legal representatives of families to help ensure that patients receive access to the rehabilitation to which they are legally entitled.

Families with private insurance also face significant challenges securing rehabilitation. Many policies have caps which limit the amount and quality of rehabilitation, making families pay for services out of pocket. Many are unable to do so. Those who can often do so at great sacrifice. Many families touched by severe brain injury enter into bankruptcy because of the uncovered cost of care. The rate of bankruptcy is higher among families of patients with TBI and spinal cord injury versus randomly selected petitioners.[131]

To further complicate matters, some insurance benefit managers have restrictive policies which disallow discharge to rehabilitation until the patient can participate in "active" rehabilitation. While it is a reasonable premise to await the return of consciousness so as to allow participation in rehabilitation, members of the American College of Rehabilitation Medicine have challenged these restrictive policies. They counter that the pervasive failure to properly identify patients with covert consciousness in the chronic care sector means patients who might evolve into MCS or CMD will neither be properly identified nor given access to rehabilitation. These advocates argue for screening assessments of patients by trained neuropsychologists and neurorehabilitation so that those who might be able to engage in rehabilitation can be given that opportunity.[25,132] Surveillance of this sort, made necessary by the syndromic nature of these conditions, is also consistent with the policy recommendations of the AAN/ACRM/NIDILRR guideline.[51]

Forward-looking surveillance of patients is also consistent with the emerging epidemiology and dynamic biology of these brain states. As noted earlier, some 20% of patients once thought to be in the permanent (now chronic) vegetative state will regain some degree of consciousness.[51] And, as notably, patients in MCS have been shown to engage in axonal sprouting and pruning, a neurodevelopmental mechanism, in the service of brain repair. If normal brain development takes decades to occur, bolstered by years of primary and secondary education, is it not reasonable to expect that brain recovery after injury—which invokes a similar mechanism—will take longer than the brief time generally allotted to rehabilitation?[25] Given this homology, I suggested a paradigm shift in which clinicians and policymakers view rehabilitation after injury as more akin to childhood education, expanding both its scope and duration.[133,134]

NEUROPALLIATIVE CARE

Patients with disorders of consciousness are vulnerable to the undertreatment of pain and often receive inadequate symptom management because they are often misdiagnosed as vegetative and thought insensate when they are in fact conscious and thus able to perceive pain and distress. This creates a moral imperative for neuropalliative care to attend to their pain and symptom management.[135]

This process begins with properly assessing patients for the presence of covert consciousness and being attentive to mischaracterization of patients as vegetative who are in MCS or have CMD.[136] In contrast to vegetative patients who do not activate the pain network and only the primary sensory area, MCS and CMD patients may have the capacity to experience pain.[136] This suggests a role for neuropalliation for these patients in order to address and mitigate distress.[137]

Pain and Suffering

While many traditionally think of palliative care as being synonymous with the care of the dying, increasingly there is a trend to move palliation upstream to respond to life-altering illness or injury,[114] and thus patients with disorders of consciousness are worthy recipients of this focused care. Patients with disorders of consciousness are especially in need of pain and symptom relief because they can experience pain, perhaps suffer, and may be unable to voice their distress. Families are equally stressed and could be said to experience a prolonged period of anticipatory grief and prolonged bereavement. Having said this, disorders of consciousness pose clinical challenges because clinicians cannot always determine if a patient is in pain and because patients may not be able to convey their distress.[138]

While unexplained autonomic signs may signal untreated pain, it is difficult to assess the patient's quality of life without seeking the input of family members.[139-141] The CRS-R does evaluate a patient for the ability to localize to noxious stimuli. While a positive response would indicate that a patient was able to perceive pain,[79] a nonresponse would not preclude it, for example, in a patient with CMD. Some behavioral responses evinced independent of painful stimuli may not indicate the presence of pain, causing the potential for the misinterpretation of these signs in some patients.[142] Recent work has shown a high correlation of the Nociception Coma Scale-Revised (NCS-R) with level of consciousness as determined by the CRS-R, suggesting an important relationship between levels of consciousness and the ability to perceive pain.[143] This instrument might also play a role in independently assessing pain management in patients with disorders of consciousness.

The recent AAN/ACRM/NIDILRR guideline acknowledges the challenge of pain assessment in this population and urges that "clinicians should be cautious in making definitive conclusions about pain and suffering in individuals with DoC."[51] While this admonition could be viewed as urging clinicians to neither overlook pain when it is present nor overestimate it when it is not, we believe that errors of omission are more egregious in this especially vulnerable population than mistakenly thinking a patient incapable of perceiving pain is in distress. For this reason, we urge the invocation of the *precautionary principle* and the use of "universal pain precautions" as a clinical and normative approach to pain management for this patient population.[68]

Withholding and Withdrawing Life-Sustaining Therapy

Clinicians must work with families to affirm the right to care and also accept—and preserve—the right to die.[5] This is a complicated balance given the aforementioned history of the vegetative state and the right to die in the history of medical ethics and the law.[25] It is even more challenging at the familial level.

Decisions to withhold or withdraw life-sustaining therapy can be among the most difficult that families confront. After surviving the illness or injury which led to the disorder of consciousness, families may reach the point where care may seem disproportionate, conferring more burdens than benefits. At this juncture, surrogates have a right to withhold or withdraw life-sustaining therapy by consenting to a DNR order or agreeing to the removal of mechanical ventilation or artificial nutrition and hydration. These decisions should be based on the decision-making hierarchy delineated earlier and be consistent with the patient's prior wishes if they are known or as more formally conveyed in an advance directive. Short of that information, families may make a judgment as surrogates based on their perception of what is in the best interests of the patient. In this context, decisions are assessed based on the proportionality of ongoing care and the relative relationship of burdens and benefits. Because evidentiary criteria for surrogate decision-making varies by local jurisdiction, clinicians would be advised to seek the guidance of their hospital ethics committee.

We believe that raising the question of withholding or withdrawing life-sustaining therapy with families is a delicate one. Many families will not fully appreciate that end-of-life choices can be made. Because of this, clinicians should speak about care options and have goals of care discussions (see earlier discussion) with families. When introducing the possibility of withholding or withdrawing life-sustaining care, it is important not to engineer an outcome or to be paternalistic. It is better to approach the topic with questions about what the family knows and understands, processing and clarifying their response, and suggesting a path forward. If that means broaching an end-of-life decision, it is helpful to offer information versus providing an outright recommendation which might come across as overly directive.[144] Instead of being determinative, we suggest language that says, "some families in this situation, might think about a decision to withhold certain kinds of treatments. . . . " This allows for a more open-ended response and does not predetermine or paternalistically dictate a family's decision.

Short of medical complications like multisystem organ failure, where ongoing medical treatment is likely to be futile, decisions to withhold or withdraw care in these patients are generally not about an inability to maintain life. Instead, the decision reflects the realization that care has become disproportionate and burdensome. Clinicians should support family decisions and help ensure that that the decision is an informed refusal, consistent with the doctrine of informed consent and informed refusal.

Whether these discussions occur in the acute phase of illness or injury or during rehabilitation or convalescence, the realization that therapeutic goals and aspirations will not be achieved can be devastating. During the acute hospitalization, the unforeseen circumstances encountered by families can make the accommodation of new information difficult. It is prudent to provide families with time to make choices and be patient as they accommodate themselves to realities wholly unexpected days earlier.

Later in the course of care, it is important to acknowledge the family's investment in their loved one's care and be supportive of their decision. It is helpful to suggest that fiduciary obligations can take on a different shape over time.[114] While the pursuit of recovery might have been appropriate at the outset, ongoing treatments can be understood as burdensome late in the course of care. Families who make choices to limit care often do so charitably, forsaking erstwhile hopes for recovery and time together. This can be heart-breaking for families and the clinicians who have stood faithfully by their side.

Finally, it is important to appreciate that different families will make distinct choices given the same clinical circumstances. Some will continue life-sustaining therapy while others will make decisions to discontinue it given the same diagnostic and, more importantly, prognostic data. This variance should not prompt the clinician's disapprobation but rather an appreciation that each family unit will bring their values to bear upon these difficult circumstances. The clinician's responsibility is to ensure that these are informed decisions and to be supportive. It is inappropriate to impose one's own moral views on surrogates when they act in good faith and in accordance with prevailing ethical norms and the law. Such actions may lead to complicated and iatrogenic bereavement.

Family Burden and Bereavement

It is said in palliative medicine that the "family is the unit of care," and this is certainly the case when one considers the burdens that family assume when caring for a loved one with a disorder of consciousness.[145] They operate under tremendous stress, grapple with uncertainty and guilt over decisions made, or not made. Family units and hierarchies are profoundly disrupted with parents caring for adult children. Relationships are frozen in time, sometimes haunted by unresolved conflicts that will never be resolved, leaving survivors guilt-ridden,[25] with surrogate expectations in part driven by the nature of their preexisting relationship with the patient.[146] The cumulative strain takes its toll on families;[147] causes financial stress,[131] decreased well-being, and illness[148]; and leads to social isolation.[149] A recent study showed increased inflammatory cytokines in female spouses of veterans with TBI.[150] In the aggregate, experiencing both the presence and absence of a loved one with severe brain injury constitutes what has been described as "ambiguous loss" for informal caregivers.[151] The needs of families of patients with disorders of consciousness should thus form part of a broader constellation of care.

RIGHTS COME TO MIND

The British polymath Sir C. P. Snow once observed that "scientists, by the very nature of their subject, have the future in their bones."[152] With an eye toward that future, it is not premature to imagine how the neuroscience of consciousness will evolve over the coming decade and how this progress will reshape clinical ethics and the law.

In the decades since the publication of the first edition of *Stupor and Coma* in 1966, we have witnessed nosological advance. When first published, neither the vegetative nor the minimally conscious state had been identified. Over the subsequent decades, we can fully expect further diagnostic refinement, as exemplified by the chronic vegetative state advanced by the AAN/ACRM/NIDILRR guideline.[51] Just as this categorization was prompted by reanalysis of epidemiological and trial data,[153] future refinements will likely be informed by a deeper understanding of underlying circuits and mechanisms of recovery.[154,155] Collectively, these data will improve diagnosis and prognosis and catalyze therapeutic trials to restore and augment disordered consciousness.

At the center of these efforts will be the quest to restore functional communication to patients who are currently sequestered from family, friends, and the broader human community due to their inability to communicate. Here, the restoration of functional communication helps rebuild community and places patients back into the mainstream, less isolated in the chronic care sector where many linger far from rehabilitation and the recoveries that may yet be achieved.

Progress has already been made with the advent of deep brain stimulation[156] and its derivative approaches using transcranial magnetic stimulation[157] and directed ultrasound;[158] the use of volitional neuroimaging;[159,160] and pharmaceuticals that have accelerated[161] or prompted state changes[162] resulting in the recovery of consciousness. The results are still in the proof of principle stage, but the trend is promising and clear.

Integrating patients back into their communities is consistent with a disability rights paradigm which is well-suited to understanding our obligations to this population.[25] Both the United Nations Declaration on the

Rights of Persons with Disabilities[163] as well as the United States' Americans with Disabilities Act[164] call for the maximal integration of people with disabilities. In earlier phases of a march to equality for people with disabilities, the focus was on physical access—the cut in the sidewalk so individuals could make their way to work and more fully engage in communal life.[133] In our context, the restoration of communication becomes a means to overcome the segregation that is imposed by their injuries and too often compounded by societal neglect.

Viewing the needs of patients with disorders of consciousness through the prism of civil and disability rights properly broadens the question of what is owed those in liminal states of consciousness from an access to care question to one about fundamental human rights.[25,165] We hope that this approach will lead to more humane care that is guided by the best science and the best intentions. Only so informed can clinicians hope to achieve the delicate balance of restoration, palliation, and compassion that patients with disorders of consciousness require.

REFERENCES

1. Hauber RP, Testani-Dufour L. Living in limbo: the low-level brain-injured patient and the patient's family. *J Neurosci Nurs* 2000;32(1):22–26.
2. Fins JJ. Clinical pragmatism and the care of brain damaged patients: toward a palliative neuroethics for disorders of consciousness. *Prog Brain Res* 2005;150:565–582.
3. Fins JJ. The ethics of measuring and modulating consciousness: the imperative of minding time. *Prog Brain Res* 2009;177C:371–382.
4. Taylor CM, Aird VH, Tate RL, Lammi MH. Sequence of recovery during the course of emergence from the minimally conscious state. *Arch Phys Med Rehabil* 2007;88(4):521–525.
5. Fins JJ. Affirming the right to care, preserving the right to die: disorders of consciousness and neuroethics after Schiavo. *Support Palliat Care* 2006;4(2):169–178.
6. Fins JJ. Rethinking disorders of consciousness: new research and its implications. *Hastings Center Rep* 2005;35(2):22–24.
7. Wijdicks EFM, Rabinstein AA. The family conference: end-of-life guidelines at work for comatose patients. *Neurology* 2007;68:1092–1094.
8. Turgeon AF, Lauzier F, Simard JF, et al. Mortality associated with withdrawal of life-sustaining therapy for patients with severe traumatic brain injury: a Canadian multicentre cohort study. *CMAJ* 2011;183:1581–1588.
9. Fred Plum Archives. New York Presbyterian Weill Cornell Medicine Archives: FP Archives, Box 2, undated ms, circa late 1970s.
10. Plum F, Posner JB. *The Diagnosis of Stupor and Coma*, 3rd edn. New York: Oxford University Press, 1982.
11. Fins JJ, Schiff ND. Differences that make a difference in disorders of consciousness. *Am J Bioethics-Neuroethics* 2017;8(3):131–134.
12. Bernat JL. Nosologic considerations in disorders of consciousness. *Ann Neurol* 2017;82:863–865.
13. Schiff ND. Cognitive motor dissociation following severe brain injury. *JAMA Neurology* 2015;72(12):1413–1415.
14. Giacino JT, Fins JJ, Laureys S, Schiff ND. Disorders of consciousness after acquired brain injury: the state of the science. *Nat Rev Neurol* 2014;10(2):99–114.
15. Curley WH, Forgacs PB, Voss HU, Conte MM, Schiff ND. Characterization of EEG signals revealing covert cognition in the injured brain. *Brain* 2018;141(5):1404–1421.
16. Fins JJ, Schiff ND. Shades of gray: new insights from the vegetative state. *Hastings Center Rep* 2006;36(6):8.
17. Giacino JT, Kalmar K, Whyte J. The JFK Coma Recovery Scale-Revised: measurement characteristics and diagnostic utility. *Arch Phys Med Rehabil* 2004;85(12):2020–2029.
18. Insel TR, Quirion R. Psychiatry as a clinical neuroscience discipline. *JAMA* 2005;294(1):2221–2224.
19. Mayberg HS, Lozano AM, Voon V, et al. Deep brain stimulation for treatment-resistant depression. *Neuron* 2005;45(5):651–660.
20. Drysdale AT, Grosenick L, Downar J, et al. Resting-state connectivity biomarkers define neurophysiological subtypes of depression. *Nat Med* 2017;23(1):28–38.
21. Osler WO. The leaven of science. In *Aequanimitas*. London: 1904.
22. Insel TR, Cuthbert BN. Brain disorders? Precisely. *Science* 2015;348(6234):499–500.
23. Barnard C. *One Life*. New York: Macmillan, 1969.
24. Beecher HK. Ethical problems created by the hopelessly unconscious patient. *N Engl J Med* 1968;278:1425–1430.
25. Fins JJ. *Rights Come to Mind: Brain Injury, Ethics and the Struggle for Consciousness*. New York: Cambridge University Press, 2015.
26. Ad Hoc Committee of the Harvard Medical School to Examine the Definition of Brain Death. A definition of irreversible coma. *JAMA* 1968;205:337–340.
27. President's Commission for the Study of Ethical Problems in Medicine and Biomedical and Behavioral Research. *Defining Death: Medical, Legal and Ethical Issues in the Determination of Death*. Washington, DC: Government Printing Office, 1981.
28. Uniform Determination of Death Act. 12 Uniform Laws Annotated 320 (1990 Supp.).
29. Bernat JL. Whither brain death? *Am J Bioethics* 2014;14(8):3–8.
30. Siminoff LA, Mercer MB, Arnold R. Families' understanding of brain death. *Prog Transplant* 2003;13(3):218–224.
31. Fins JJ. Neuroethics, neuroimaging & disorders of consciousness: promise or peril? *Trans Am Clin Climatol Assoc* 2010;122:336–346.

32. Fins JJ. When brain death pulls at the heart strings. In *Caring for the Dying, Identification and Promotion of Physician Competency: New Additions to Personal Narratives*. Philadelphia: American Board of Internal Medicine, 1999.
33. The New York State Task Force on Life and the Law. *The Determination of Death*. Minority report by Rabbi J. David Bleich, 2nd edn. New York: New York State Department of Health, 1989.
34. Kimura R. Japan's dilemma with the definition of death. *Kennedy Inst Ethics J* 1991;1(2):123–131.
35. New York State Department of Health. Determination of Death. Adopted Regulation 10 N.Y.C.R.R. 400.16.
36. The New Jersey Declaration of Death Act. P.L. 1991, Chapter 90 (To be codified as Chapter 6A of Title 26 of the Revised Statutes.) Section 5: Exemption to Accommodate Personal Religious Beliefs. *Kennedy Institute of Ethics Journal* 1991;1(4):289–292.
37. Fins JJ. Across the divide: religious objections to brain death. *J Religion Health* 1995;34(1):33–39.
38. Aviv R. What does it mean to die? *The New Yorker.* February 5, 2018. https://www.newyorker.com/magazine/2018/02/05/what-does-it-mean-to-die. Accessed May 7, 2018.
39. The Quality Standards Subcommittee of the American Academy of Neurology. Practice parameters for determining brain death in adults (summary statement). *Neurology* 1995;45(5):1012–1014.
40. Wijdicks EF, Varelas PN, Gronseth GS, Greer DM; American Academy of Neurology. Evidence-based guideline update: determining brain death in adults: report of the Quality Standards Subcommittee of the American Academy of Neurology. *Neurology* 2010;74(23):1911–1918.
41. Greer DM, Wang HH, Robinson JD, Varelas PN, Henderson GV, Wijdicks EF. Variability of Brain Death Policies in the United States. *JAMA Neurol* 2016;73(2):213–218.
42. Wang HH, Varelas PN, Henderson GV, Wijdicks EF, Greer DM. Improving uniformity in brain death determination policies over time. *Neurology* 2017;88(6):562–568.
43. Schappell CN, Frank JL, Husari K, Sanchez M, Goldenberg F, Ardelt A. Practice variability in brain death determination: a call to action. *Neurology* 2013;81:2009–2014.
44. Pandey A, Sahota P, Nattanmai P, Newey CR. Variability in diagnosing brain death at an academic medical center. *Neurosci J* 2017;6017958.
45. Cohen J, Askenazi T, Katvan E, Singer P. Brain death determination in Israel: the first two years experience following changes to the brain death law—opportunities and challenges. *Am J Transplantation* 2012;12:2514–2518.
46. Munari M, Zucchetta P, Carollo C, et al. Confirmatory tests in the diagnosis of brain death: comparison between SPECT and contrast angiography. *Crit Care Med* 2005;33(9):2068–2073.
47. Troug RD, Miller FG. The meaning of brain death: a different view. *JAMA Intern Med* 2014;174:1215–1216.
48. Belkin GS. *Death and Dying: History, Medicine, and Brain Death*. New York: Oxford University Press, 2014.
49. Schiff ND, Fins JJ. Brain death and disorders of consciousness. *Curr Biol* 2016;26:R543–R576.
50. Multi-Society Task Force on PVS. Medical aspects of the persistent vegetative state. Parts I and II. *N Engl J Med* 1994;330:1499–1508, 1572–1579.
51. Giacino JT, Katz DI, Schiff ND, et al. Practice guideline: disorders of consciousness. *Neurology* 2018;91(10):450–460. Simultaneously published in *Arch Phys Med Rehabil* 2018;99(9):1710–1719.
52. Troug RD. Defining death—making sense of the case of Jahi McMath. *JAMA* 2018;319(18):1859–1860.
53. Troug RD, Miller FG, Halpern SD. The dead-donor rule and the future of organ donation. *N Engl J Med* 2013;369(14):1287–1289.
54. Quinlan J, Quinlan JD. *Karen Ann: The Quinlans Tell Their Story*. Garden City, NY: Doubleday & Co., 1977.
55. Jennett B, Plum F. Persistent vegetative state after brain damage: a syndrome in search of a name. *Lancet* 1972;1(7753):734–737.
56. Fins JJ. Letter to the Editor in response to Joan Didion piece on Terri Schiavo. *The New York Review of Books*. August 11, 2005. Volume LII, Number 13, page 63.
57. Fins JJ. Constructing an ethical stereotaxy for severe brain injury: balancing risks, benefits and access. *Nature Rev Neurosci* 2003;4:323–327.
58. *Matter of Karen Quinlan*, 70 N.J. 10, 335 A.2d 677 (1976).
59. Cantor NL. Twenty-five years after Quinlan: a review of the jurisprudence of death and dying. *J Law Med Ethics* 2001 Summer;29 (2):182–196.
60. Annas GJ. The "right to die" in America: sloganeering from Quinlan and Cruzan to Quill and Kevorkian. *Duquesne Law Rev* 1996;34(4):875–897.
61. Cranford RE. Medical futility: transforming a clinical concept into legal and social policies. *J Am Ger Soc* 1994;42:894–898.
62. Wolf SM. Nancy Beth Cruzan: in no voice at all. *Hastings Center Rep* 1990;20(1):38–41.
63. Blendon RJ, Benson JM, Hermann MJ. The American public and the Terri Schiavo case. *Arch Int Med* 2005;165(22):2580–2584.
64. *Cruzan v Director*, Missouri Department of Health, 110 S. Ct. 2841 (1990).
65. McCloskey EL. The Patient-Self Determination Act. *Kennedy Inst Ethics J* 1991;1(2):163–169.
66. Annas GJ. "Culture of life" politics at the bedside: the case of Terri Schiavo. *N Engl J Med* 2005;352(16):1710–1715.
67. Fins JJ, Plum F. Neurological diagnosis is more than a state of mind: diagnostic clarity and impaired consciousness. *Arch Neurol* 2004;61(9):1354–1355.
68. Fins JJ, Bernat JL. Ethical, palliative, and policy considerations in disorders of consciousness. *Neurology* 2018;91:471–475. Simultaneously published in *Arch Phys Med Rehabil* 2018;99(9):1927–1931.
69. Schnakers C, Vanhaudenhuyse A, Giacino J, et al. Diagnostic accuracy of the vegetative and minimally conscious state: clinical consensus versus standardized neurobehavioral assessment. *BMC Neurol* 2009;9:35.
70. Thengone DJ, Voss HU, Fridman EA, Schiff ND. Local changes in network structure contribute to late communication recovery in severe brain injury. *Sci Trans Med* 2016;8(368):368re5.

71. Fins JJ, Master MG, Gerber LM, Giacino JT. The minimally conscious state: a diagnosis in search of an epidemiology. *Arch Neurol* 2007;64(10):1400–1405.

72. Fins JJ, Schiff ND, Foley KM. Late recovery from the minimally conscious state: ethical and policy implications. *Neurology* 2007;68:304–307.

73. Laureys S, Celesia GG, Cohadon F, et al.; European Task Force on Disorders of Consciousness. Unresponsive wakefulness syndrome: a new name for the vegetative state or apallic syndrome. *BMC Med* 2010;8:68.

74. Plum F, Schiff N, Ribary U, Llinas R. Coordinated expression in chronically unconscious persons. *Philosoph Trans Biol Sci* 1998;353:1929–1933.

75. Adams ZM, Fins JJ. The historical origins of the vegetative state: received wisdom and the utility of the text. *J History Neurosci* 2017;26(2):140–153.

76. Aristotle. *On The Soul (De Anima)*. Hett Q, trans., Greek text, translation, and notes. Cambridge, MA: Harvard University Press, 1957.

77. Fins JJ. *A Palliative Ethic of Care: Clinical Wisdom at Life's End*. Sudbury, MA: Jones and Bartlett, 2006.

78. Fins JJ. Border zones of consciousness: another immigration debate? *Am J Bioethics-Neuroethics* 2007;7(1):51–54.

79. Giacino JT, Ashwal S, Childs N, et al. The minimally conscious state: definition and diagnostic criteria. *Neurology* 2002;58(3):349–353.

80. Winslade W. *Confronting Traumatic Brain Injury: Devastation, Hope and Healing*. New Haven: Yale University Press, 1998.

81. Sherer M, Hart T, Nick TG, Whyte J, Thompson RN, Yablon SA. Early impaired self-awareness after traumatic brain injury. *Arch Phys Med Rehabil* 2003;84(2):168–176.

82. *The Economist*. Inside the mind of the consumer. June 10, 2004 Accessed at https://www.economist.com/technology-quarterly/2004/06/10/inside-the-mind-of-the-consumer. Access date 31 March 2019.

83. Farah MJ, Wolpe PR. Monitoring and manipulating brain function, new neuroscience technologies and their ethical implications. *Hastings Center Rep* 2004;34(3):35–45.

84. Fins JJ. The Orwellian threat to emerging neurodiagnostic technologies. *Am J Bioethics* 2005; 5(2):56–58.

85. Dewey J. Common sense and scientific inquiry. In: Boydston JA, ed. *Logic. The Theory of Inquiry*. Collected in *John Dewey, The Later Works, 1925–1953. Volume 12:1938*. Carbondale and Edwardsville, IL: Southern Illinois University Press; 1991:66–85.

86. Laureys S, Faymonville ME, Peigneux P, et al. Cortical processing of noxious somatosensory stimuli in the persistent vegetative state. *Neuroimage* 2002;17(2):732–741.

87. National Commission for the Protection of Human Subjects of Biomedical and Behavioral Research. *The Belmont Report: Ethical Principles and Guidelines for the Protection of Human Subjects of Research*. Washington, DC: Government Printing Office, 1979.

88. Beauchamp TL, Saghai Y. The historical foundations of the research-practice distinction in bioethics. *Theor Med Bioethics* 2012;33:45–46.

89. Fins JJ. In reply: commentary: deep brain stimulation as clinical innovation: an ethical and organizational framework to sustain deliberations about psychiatric deep brain stimulation *Neurosurgery* 2017;80(6): E271–272.

90. Jonsen AR. *The Birth of Bioethics*. New York: Oxford University Press, 1998.

91. National Research Service Award Act of 1974. (Pub. L. 93-348).

92. Wolf SM, Lawrenz FP, Nelson CA, et al. Managing incidental findings in human subjects research: analysis and recommendations. *J Law Med Ethics* 2008;36(2):219–248, 211.

93. Richardson HS. *Moral Entanglements: The Ancillary-Care Obligations of Medical Researchers*. New York: Oxford University Press, 2012.

94. Fins JJ. A Review of *Moral Entanglements: The Ancillary-Care Obligations of Medical Researchers* by Henry S. Richardson. New York: Oxford University Press, 2012. *Notre Dame Philosophical Reviews*. May 19, 2013. http://ndpr.nd.edu/news/40053-moral-entanglements/

95. Schiff ND, Rodriguez-Moreno D, Kamal A, Kim K, Giacino J, Plum F, Hirsch J. fMRI reveals large scale network activation in minimally conscious patients. *Neurology* 2005;64:514–523.

96. Carey B. New signs of awareness in some brain-injured patients. *The New York Times*. February 8, 2005. A-1.

97. Owen AM, Coleman MR, Boly M, et al. Willful modulation of brain activity in disorders of consciousness. Detecting awareness in the vegetative state. *Science* 2006;313(5792):1402.

98. Weijer C, Bruni T, Gofton T, Young GB, Norton L, Peterson A, Owen AM. Ethical considerations in functional magnetic resonance imaging in acutely comatose patients. *Brain* 2016;139 (Pt1):292–299.

99. Fins JJ. Deep Brain Stimulation. In: Jennings B, ed., *Encyclopedia of Bioethics*, 4th edn. Farmington Hills, MI: MacMillan Reference USA; 2014: vol. II, 817–823.

100. Sachs GA, Siegler M. Guidelines for decision-making when the patient is incompetent. *J Crit Illness* 1991;6:348–359.

101. Terry PB, Vettese M, Song J, et al. End-of-life decision-making: when patients and surrogates disagree. *J Clin Ethics* 1999;10(4):286–293.

102. The New York State Task Force on Life and the Law. *When Others Must Choose: Deciding for Patients Without Capacity*. The New York State Task Force on Life and the Law. New York, 1992:47–69.

103. Brock DW. Trumping advance directives. Special Supplement. *Hastings Center Rep* 1991;21: S5–6.

104. Charlton JI. *Nothing About Us Without Us: Disability Oppression and Empowerment*. Berkeley: University of California Press, 2000.

105. Wright MS, Kraft C, Ulrich MR, Fins JJ. Capacity, competence, and the minimally conscious state: lessons from a developmental model. *Am J Bioethics-Neurosci* 2018;9:56–64.

106. Fins JJ. Mosaic decision-making and reemergent agency following severe brain injury. *Cambridge Q Healthc Ethics* 2018;27(1):163–174.

107. Fins JJ. Mosaic decisionmaking and severe brain injury: adding another piece to the argument. *Cambridge Q Healthc Ethics*. In Press.

108. Fins JJ. Beyond good and evil: doing concrete ethics in the clinic. *J Religion Health*. 2019;58:368–371.

109. Fins JJ, Hersh J. Solitary advocates: the severely brain injured and their surrogates. In: Hoffman B, Tomes N, Schlessinger M, Grob R, eds., *Transforming Healthcare from Below: Patients as Actors in U.S. Health Policy*. New Brunswick, NJ: Rutgers University Press; 2011:21–42.

110. Levine C. The loneliness of the long-term care giver. *N Engl J Med* 1999;340(20):1587–1590.

111. Whyte J, Katz D, Long D, et al. Predictors of outcome in posttraumatic disorders of consciousness and assessment of medication effects: a multicenter study. *Arch Phys Med Rehabil* 2005;86(3):453–462.

112. Fins JJ. Ethics of clinical decision-making and communication with surrogates. In: Posner J, Saper C, Schiff ND, Plum F, eds., *Plum and Posner's Diagnosis of Stupor and Coma*, 4th edn. New York: Oxford University Press; 2007.

113. Lammi MH, Smith VH, Tate RL, Taylor CM. The minimally conscious state and recovery potential: a follow-up study 2 to 5 years after traumatic brain injury. *Arch Phys Med Rehabil* 2005;86(4):746–754.

114. Fins JJ. *A Palliative Ethic of Care: Clinical Wisdom at Life's End*. Boston: Jones and Bartlett, 2006.

115. Jox RJ, Kuehlmeyer K, Klein AM, et al. Diagnosis and decision-making for patients with disorders of consciousness: a survey among family members. *Arch Phys Med Rehabil* 2015;96(2):323–330.

116. Agrawal SK, Fins JJ. Ethics committees and case consultation in the hospital setting. In: Siegler E, Mirafzali S, Foust JB, eds. *A Guide to Hospitals and Inpatient Care*. New York: Springer; 2003: 256–267.

117. Kramer AH, Zygun DA. Neurocritical care: why does it make a difference? *Curr Opin Crit Care* 2014;20(2):174–181.

118. Lombardo S, Scalea T, Sperry J, et al. Neurotrauma, or med/surg intensive care unit: does it matter where multiple injuries patients with traumatic brain injury are admitted? Secondary analysis of the American Association for the Surgery of Trauma Multi-Institutional Trials Committee decompressive craniectomy study. *J Trauma Acute Care Surg* 2017;82(3):489–496.

119. Singh TD, O'Horo JC, Gajic O, et al. Risk factors and outcomes of critically ill patients with acute brain failure: a novel end point. *J Crit Care* 2018;43:42–47.

120. Sur MD, Angelos PS. Ethical issues in surgical critical care: the complexity of interpersonal relationships in the surgical intensive care unit. *J Intensive Care Med* 2016;31(7):442–450.

121. Warren AM, Rainey EE, Weddle RJ, Bennett M, Roden-Foreman K, Foreman ML. The intensive care unit experience: psychological impact on family members of patients with and without traumatic brain injury. *Rehabil Psychol* 2016;61(2):179–185.

122. Rohaut B, Claassen J. Decision-making in perceived devastating brain injury: a call to explore the impact of cognitive biases. *Br J Anaesthesia* 2018;120:5–9.

123. Fins JJ, Miller FG, Acres CA, Bacchetta MD, Huzzard LL, Rapkin BD. End-of-life decision-making in the hospital: current practices and future prospects. *J Pain Sympt Manag* 1999;17(1):6–15.

124. Fins JJ, Bacchetta MD, Miller FG. Clinical pragmatism: a method of moral problem solving. *Kennedy Institute Ethics J* 1997;7(2):129–145.

125. Edlow BL, Chatelle C, Spencer CA, et al. Early detection of consciousness in patients with severe traumatic brain injury. *Brain* 2017;140(9):2399–2414.

126. Fins JJ. Disorders of consciousness and disordered care: families, caregivers and narratives of necessity. *Arch Phys Med Rehabil* 2013;94(10):1934–1939.

127. Fins JJ. *Trastornos de Conciencia y Los Derechos Humanos: Una Nueva Frontera Ética y Científica*. Solemne Sesión de Toma de Posesión como Académico de Honor del Dr. Joseph J. Fins. Con Laudatio del Excmo. Sr. D. Diego Gracia Guillén. Madrid: Instituto de Espana, Real Academia Nacional de Medicina, Año 2014—Tomo CXXXI. Cuaderno Sgundo, 631–667.

128. Glenda Jimmo, KR by her guardian Kenneth Roberts, et al., Plaintiffs, v. Kathleen Sebelius, in her official capacity as Secretary of Health and Human Services, Defendant. Case No. 5:11-cv-17. United States District Court, D. Vermont. October 25, 2011.

129. Fins JJ, Wright MS, Kraft C, Rogers A, Romani MB, Goodwin S, Ulrich MR. Whither the "improvement standard"? coverage for severe brain injury after *Jimmo v. Sebelius*. *J Law Medicine Ethics* 2016;44(1):182–193.

130. Gladieux JE, Basile M. *Jimmo* and the improvement standard: implementing medicare coverage through regulations, policy manuals and other guidance. *Am J Law and Medicine* 2014;40(1):7–25.

131. Relyea-Chew A, Hollingworth W, Chan L, Comstock BA, Overstreet KA, Jarvik JG. Personal bankruptcy after traumatic brain or spinal cord injury: the role of medical debt. *Arch Phys Med Rehabil* 2009;90(3):413–419.

132. Whyte J. Personal communication with: Joseph Fins. 28 May 2013. Accompanying email to the author detailing the history of the Disorders of Consciousness Special Interest Group of the NIDDR Traumatic Brain Injury Model Systems communications with McKesson concerning their admission criteria for acute rehabilitation.

133. Fins JJ. Brain injury and the civil right we don't think about. *The New York Times*. August 24, 2017. https://www.nytimes.com/2017/08/24/opinion/minimally-conscious-brain-civil-rights.html?_r=0. Accessed 31 March 2019.

134. Wright MS, Fins JJ. Rehabilitation, education, and the integration of individuals with severe brain injury into civil society: towards an expanded rights agenda in response to new insights from translational neuroethics and neuroscience. *Yale J Health Policy, Law, Ethics* 2016;16(2):233–288.

135. Fins JJ. Neuroethics and disorders of consciousness: a pragmatic approach to neuro-palliative care. In: Laureys S, Tononi G, eds., *The Neurology of Consciousness, Cognitive Neuroscience and Neuropathology*. New York: Academic Press-Elsevier; 2008:234–244.

136. Schnakers C, Chatelle C, Majerus S, Gosseries O, De Val M, Laureys S. Assessment and detection of pain in noncommunicative severely brain-injured patients. *Expert Rev Neurother* 2010;10(11):1725–1731.

137. Fins JJ, Pohl BR. Neuro-palliative care and disorders of consciousness. In: Hanks G, Cherny NI, Christakis NA, Fallon M, Kassa S, Portenoy RK, eds., *Oxford Textbook of Palliative Medicine*, 5th edn. Oxford: Oxford University Press; 2015:285–291.

138. Laureys S, Boly M. What is it like to be vegetative or minimally conscious?. *Curr Opin Neurol* 2007;20:609–613.

139. Bullinger M, et al. Quality of life in patients with traumatic brain injury—basic issues, assessments and recommendations. *Restor Neurol Neurosci* 2002;20:111–124.

140. Phipps E, Whyte J. Medical decision-making with persons who are minimally conscious. *Am J Phys Med Rehabil* 1999;78:77–82.

141. Phipps E, Di Pasquale M, Blitz CL, White J. Interpreting responsiveness in persons with severe traumatic brain injury: beliefs in families and quantitative evaluations. *J Head Trauma Rehabil* 1997;12:52–69.

142. Bernat JL. Chronic consciousness disorders. *Annu Rev Med* 2009;60:381–392.

143. Chatelle C, Hauger SL, Martial C, et al. Assessment of nociception and pain in participants with unresponsive or minimally conscious state after acquired brain injury: the relationship between the Coma Recovery Scale-Revised and the Nociception Coma Scale-Revised. *Arch Phys Med Rehabil* 2018;99(9):1755–1762.

144. Buckman R. *How to Break Bad News.* Baltimore: Johns Hopkins University Press, 1992.

145. Leonardi M, Giovannetti AM, Pagani M, Raggi A, Sattin D; National Consortium Functioning and Disability in Vegetative and in Minimal Conscious State Patients. Burden and needs of 487 caregivers of patients in vegetative state and in minimally conscious state: results from a national study. *Brain Inj* 2012;26(10):1201–1210.

146. Suppes A, Fins JJ. Surrogate expectations in severe brain injury. *Brain Inj* 2013;27(10):1141–1147.

147. Fins JJ, Master MG. Disorders of consciousness and neuro-palliative care: towards an expanded scope of practice for the field. In: Youngner SJ, Arnold R, eds., *Oxford Handbook of Ethics at the End of Life.* New York: Oxford University Press; 2017:154–169.

148. Brickell TA, French LM, Lippa SM, Lange RT. Characteristics and health outcomes of post-9/11 caregivers of US service members and veterans following traumatic brain injury. *J Head Trauma Rehabil* 2018;33(2):133–145.

149. Manskow US, Friborg O, Røe C, Braine M, Damsgard E, Anke A. Patterns of change and stability in caregiver burden and life satisfaction from 1 to 2 years after severe traumatic brain injury: a Norwegian longitudinal study. *NeuroRehabilitation* 2017;40(2):211–222.

150. Saban KL, Mathews HL, Collins EG, et al. The man I once knew: grief and inflammation in female partners of veterans with traumatic brain injury. *Biol Res Nurs* 2016;18(1):50–59.

151. Giovannetti AM, Černiauskaitė M, Leonardi M, Sattin D, Covelli V. Informal caregivers of patients with disorders of consciousness: experience of ambiguous loss. *Brain Inj* 2015;29(4):473–480.

152. The many-sided life of Sir Charles Snow. *Life Magazine.* April 7, 1961; 134–136.

153. Giacino JT, Katz DI, Schiff ND, et al. Comprehensive systematic review update summary: disorders of consciousness: report of the Guideline Development, Dissemination, and Implementation Subcommittee of the American Academy of Neurology; the American Congress of Rehabilitation Medicine; and the National Institute on Disability, Independent Living, and Rehabilitation Research. *Neurology* 2018;91(10):461–470. Published simultaneously in *Arch Phys Med Rehabil* 2018;99(9):1710–1719.

154. Fins JJ. Deep brain stimulation as a probative biology: scientific inquiry & the mosaic device. *AJOB-NeuroScience* 2012;3(1):4–8.

155. Bodien YG, Chatelle C, Edlow BL. Functional networks in disorders of consciousness. *Semin Neurol* 2017;37(5):485–502.

156. Schiff ND, Giacino JT, Kalmar K, et al. Behavioral improvements with thalamic stimulation after severe traumatic brain injury. *Nature* 2007;448(7153):600–603.

157. Ragazzoni A, Cincotta M, Giovannelli F, Cruse D, Young GB, Miniussi C, Rossi S. Clinical neurophysiology of prolonged disorders of consciousness: from diagnostic stimulation to therapeutic neuromodulation. *Clin Neurophysiol* 2017;128(9):1629–1646.

158. Monti MM, Schnakers C, Korb AS, Bystritsky A, Vespa PM. Non-invasive ultrasonic thalamic stimulation in disorders of consciousness after severe brain injury: a first-in-man report. *Brain Stimul* 2016;9(6):940–941.

159. Monti MM, Vanhaudenhuyse A, Coleman MR, et al. Willful modulation of brain activity in disorders of consciousness. *N Engl J Med* 2010;362(7):579–589.

160. Bardin JC, Fins JJ, Katz DI, et al. Dissociations between behavioural and functional magnetic resonance imaging-based evaluations of cognitive function. *Brain* 2011;134(3):769–782.

161. Giacino JT, Whyte J, Bagiella E, et al. Placebo-controlled trial of amantadine for severe traumatic brain injury. *N Engl J Med* 2012;366(9):819–826.

162. Brefel-Courbon C, Payoux P, Ory F, et al. Clinical and imaging evidence of zolpidem effect in hypoxic encephalopathy. *Ann Neurol* 2007;62(1):102–105.

163. United Nations. 2007. *Convention on the Rights of Persons with Disabilities.* http://www.un.org/disabilities/convention/conventionfull.shtml. Accessed November 4, 2016.

164. *Americans with Disabilities Act,* 42 U.S.C. 12101 (1990).

165. Fins JJ, Wright MS. Rights language and disorders of consciousness: a call for advocacy. *Brain Inj* 2018;32(5):670–674.

Index

Note: Page numbers followed by *f, t,* or *b* denote figures, tables, or boxes respectively.